PROGRESS IN BRAIN RESEARCH

VOLUME 134

VISION: FROM NEURONS TO COGNITION

Other volumes in PROGRESS IN BRAIN RESEARCH

Volume 106: Current Neurochemical and Pharmacological Aspects of Biogenic Amines, by P.M. Yu, K.F. Tipton and A.A. Boulton (Eds.) – 1995, ISBN 0-444-81938-X.
Volume 107: The Emotional Motor System, by G. Holstege, R. Bandler and C.B. Saper (Eds.) – 1996, ISBN 0-444-81962-2.
Volume 108: Neural Development and Plasticity, by R.R. Mize and R.S. Erzurumlu (Eds.) – 1996, ISBN 0-444-82433-2.
Volume 109: Cholinergic Mechanisms: From Molecular Biology to Clinical Significance, by J. Klein and K. Löffelholz (Eds.) – 1996, ISBN 0-444-82166-X.
Volume 110: Towards the Neurobiology of Chronic Pain, by G. Carli and M. Zimmermann (Eds.) – 1996, ISBN 0-444-82149-X.
Volume 111: Hypothalamic Integration of Circadian Rhythms, by R.M. Buijs, A. Kalsbeek, H.J. Romijn, C.M.A. Pennartz and M. Mirmiran (Eds.) – 1996, ISBN 0-444-82443-X.
Volume 112: Extrageniculostriate Mechanisms Underlying Visually-Guided Orientation Behavior, by M. Norita, T. Bando and B.E. Stein (Eds.) – 1996, ISBN 0-444-82347-6.
Volume 113: The Polymodal Receptor: A Gateway to Pathological Pain, by T. Kumazawa, L. Kruger and K. Mizumura (Eds.) – 1996, ISBN 0-444-82473-1.
Volume 114: The Cerebellum: From Structure to Control, by C.I. de Zeeuw, P. Strata and J. Voogd (Eds.) – 1997, ISBN 0-444-82313-1.
Volume 115: Brain Function in Hot Environment, by H.S. Sharma and J. Westman (Eds.) – 1998, ISBN 0-444-82377-8.
Volume 116: The Glutamate Synapse as a Therapeutical Target: Molecular Organization and Pathology of the Glutamate Synapse, by O.P. Ottersen, I.A. Langmoen and L. Gjerstad (Eds.) – 1998, ISBN 0-444-82754-4.
Volume 117: Neuronal Degeneration and Regeneration: From Basic Mechanisms to Prospects for Therapy, by F.W. van Leeuwen, A. Salehi, R.J. Giger, A.J.G.D. Holtmaat and J. Verhaagen (Eds.) – 1998, ISBN 0-444-82817-6.
Volume 118: Nitric Oxide in Brain Development, Plasticity and Disease, by R.R. Mize, T.M. Dawson, V.L. Dawson and M.J. Friedlander (Eds.) – 1998, ISBN 0-444-82885-0.
Volume 119: Advances in Brain Vasopressin, by I.J.A. Urban, J.P.H. Burbach and D. De Wied (Eds.) – 1999, ISBN 0-444-50080-4.
Volume 120: Nucleotides and their Receptors in the Nervous System, by P. Illes and H. Zimmermann (Eds.) – 1999, ISBN 0-444-50082-0.
Volume 121: Disorders of Brain, Behavior and Cognition: The Neurocomputational Perspective, by J.A. Reggia, E. Ruppin and D. Glanzman (Eds.) – 1999, ISBN 0-444-50175-4.
Volume 122: The Biological Basis for Mind Body Interactions, by E.A. Mayer and C.B. Saper (Eds.) – 1999, ISBN 0-444-50049-9.
Volume 123: Peripheral and Spinal Mechanisms in the Neural Control of Movement, by M.D. Binder (Ed.) – 1999, ISBN 0-444-50288-2.
Volume 124: Cerebellar Modules: Molecules, Morphology and Function, by N.M. Gerrits, T.J.H. Ruigrok and C.E. De Zeeuw (Eds.) – 2000, ISBN 0-444-50108-8.
Volume 125: Volume Transmission Revisited, by L.F. Agnati, K. Fuxe, C. Nicholson and E. Syková (Eds.) – 2000, ISBN 0-444-50314-5.
Volume 126: Cognition, Emotion and Autonomic Responses: The Integrative Role of the Prefrontal Cortex and Limbic Structures, by H.B.M. Uylings, C.G. Van Eden, J.P.C. De Bruin, M.G.P. Feenstra and C.M.A. Pennartz (Eds.) – 2000, ISBN 0-444-50332-3.
Volume 127: Neural Transplantation II. Novel Cell Therapies for CNS Disorders, by S.B. Dunnett and A. Björklund (Eds.) – 2000, ISBN 0-444-50109-6.
Volume 128: Neural Plasticity and Regeneration, by F.J. Seil (Ed.) – 2000, ISBN 0-444-50209-2.
Volume 129: Nervous System Plasticity and Chronic Pain, by J. Sandkühler, B. Bromm and G.F. Gebhart (Eds.) – 2000, ISBN 0-444-50509-1.
Volume 130: Advances in Neural Population Coding, by M.A.L. Nicolelis (Ed.) – 2001, ISBN 0-444-50110-X.
Volume 131: Concepts and Challenges in Retinal Biology, by H. Kolb, H. Ripps, and S. Wu (Eds.), – 2001, ISBN 0-444-506772.
Volume 132: Glial Cell Function, by B. Castellano López and M. Nieto-Sampedro (Eds.) – 2001, ISBN 0-444-50508-3.
Volume 133: The Maternal Brain. Neurobiological and neuroendocrine adaptation and disorders in pregnancy and post partum, by J.A. Russell, A.J. Douglas, R.J. Windle and C.D. Ingram (Eds.) – 2001, ISBN 0-444-50548-2.

PROGRESS IN BRAIN RESEARCH

VOLUME 134

VISION: FROM NEURONS TO COGNITION

EDITED BY

CHRISTIAN CASANOVA

MAURICE PTITO

École d'Optométrie et Centre de Recherche en Sciences Neurologiques, Université de Montréal, Montreal, PQ H3C 3J7 Canada

ELSEVIER

AMSTERDAM – LONDON – NEW YORK – OXFORD – PARIS – SHANNON – TOKYO

2001

ELSEVIER SCIENCE B.V.
Sara Burgerhartstraat 25
P.O. Box 211, 1000 AE Amsterdam, The Netherlands

First edition 2001

Library of Congress Cataloging in Publication Data
Vision : from neurons to cognition / edited by Christian Casanova, Maurice Ptito.
p. cm. – (Progress in brain research; v. 134)
Includes bibliographical references and index
ISBN 0-444-50586-5 (hardcover) – ISBN 0-444-80104-9 (series)
1. Vision–Congresses. 2. Visual perception–Congresses. 3. Visual cortex–Congresses.
I. Casanova, Christian. II. Ptito, Maurice. III. Series

QP376 .P7 vol. 134
[QP474]
612.8 s–dc21
[612.8'4]

2001040569

British Library Cataloguing in Publication Data
Vision : from neurons to cognition. – (Progress in brain research ; v. 134)
1. Vision
I. Casanova, Christian II. Ptito, Maurice
612.8'4
ISBN 0444505865

ISBN: 0-444-50586-5 (volume)
ISBN: 0-444-80104-9 (series)

∞ The paper used in this publication meets the requirements of ANSI/NISO Z39.48-1992 (Permanence of Paper).
Printed in The Netherlands.

List of Contributors

C.L. Baker, Jr., Department of Ophthalmology, McGill University, 687 Pine Avenue, WH4-14, Montreal, PQ H3A 1A1, Canada

M.T. Banich, Department of Psychology, University of Colorado at Boulder, E213 E Muenzinger Hall, 345 UCB, Boulder, CO 80309-0202, USA

L.L. Barnes, Rush Alzheimer's Disease Center, 1645 W. Jackson, Chicago, IL 60612, USA

E. Benardete, NYU School of Medicine, New York, NY 10016, USA

A. Bergeron, Department of Neurology and Neurosurgery, Montreal Neurological Institute, McGill University, Montreal, PQ H3A2B4, Canada

D. Boire, School of Optometry, University of Montreal, 3744 rue Jean-Brillant, CP 6128, Succ. Centre-Ville, Montreal PQ H3C 3J7, Canada

J. Bullier, Centre de Recherche Cerveau et Cognition, CNRS-UPS UMR 5549, Université Paul Sabatier, 133 Route de Narbonne, 31062 Toulouse Cedex, France

W. Burke, Department of Physiology, Institute for Biomedical Research, The University of Sydney, NSW 2006, Australia

M.B. Calford, Discipline of Human Physiology, School of Biomedical Sciences, Faculty of Medicine and Health Sciences, University of Newcastle, Callaghan, NSW 2308, Australia

C. Casanova, École d'Optométrie, Laboratoire des Neurosciences de la Vision, Centre de Recherche en Sciences Neurologiques, Université de Montréal, CP 6128, Succ. Centre-Ville, Montreal, PQ H3C 3J7, Canada

L.M. Chalupa, Section of Neurobiology, Physiology, and Behavior, University of California, Davis, CA 95616, USA

N.J. Cohen, The Beckman Institute, University of Illinois at Urbana-Champaign, Urbana, IL 61801, USA

A. Cowey, University of Oxford, Department of Experimental Psychology, South Parks Road, Oxford OX1 3UD, UK

B.G. Cumming, University Laboratory of Physiology, Parks Road, Oxford OX1 3PT, UK

A. Desautels, École d'Optométrie, Laboratoire des Neurosciences de la Vision, Centre de Recherche en Sciences Neurologiques, Université de Montréal, CP 6128, Succ. Centre-Ville, Montreal, PQ H3C 3J7, Canada

V. Diaconu, School of Optometry, University of Montreal, 3744 rue Jean-Brillant, Montreal PQ H3T 1P1, Canada

B. Dreher, Department of Anatomy and Histology, Institute for Biomedical Research (F13), The University of Sydney, NSW 2006, Australia

J. Faubert, School of Optometry, University of Montreal, 3744 rue Jean-Brillant, Montreal PQ H3T 1P1, Canada

R. Fendrich, Center for Cognitive Neuroscience, Dartmouth College, Hanover, NH 03755-3547, USA

A. Fortin, Montreal Neurological Institute and Hospital, McGill University, 3801 University Street, Montreal PQ H3A 2B4, Canada and School of Optometry, University of Montréal, 3744 Jean-Brillant Street, Montreal, PQ H3C 3J7, Canada

G.A. Fowler, Department of Biological Structure, Box 35-7420, University of Washington, Seattle, WA 98195, USA
R.D. Freeman, Group in Vision Science, School of Optometry, University of California, Berkeley, CA 94720-2020, USA
D.O. Frost, Department of Pharmacology and Experimental Therapeutics, University of Maryland, School of Medicine, 655 West Baltimore Street, Baltimore, MD 21201, USA
M.S. Gazzaniga, Center for Cognitive Neuroscience, Dartmouth College, Hanover, NH 03755-3547, USA
J.-F. Giguère, Département de Psychologie, Université de Montréal, CP 6128, Montreal, PQ H3C 3J7, Canada
P. Girard, Centre de Recherche Cerveau et Cognition, CNRS-UPS UMR 5549, Université Paul Sabatier, 31062 Toulouse Cedex, France
M.A. Goodale, Departments of Psychology and Physiology, University of Western Ontario, London, ON N6A 5C2, Canada
D. Guitton, Department of Neurology and Neurosurgery, Montreal Neurological Institute, McGill University, Montreal, PQ H3A2B4, Canada
R. Hamilton, Department of Neurology, Beth Israel Deaconess Medical Center, Harvard Medical School, Brookline Avenue, Boston, MA 02215, USA
K.P. Hoffmann, LS Allgemeine Zoologie und Neurobiologie, Ruhr-Universität Bochum, Universitatsstr. 150, 44780 Bochum, Germany
J. Hupé, Center for Neural Science, New York University, New York, NY 10003, USA
M. Iordanova, Department of Psychology, Concordia University, 7141 Sherbrooke Street West, Montreal, PQ H4B 1R6, Canada
B.L. Jacobson, Department of Psychology, University of Colorado at Boulder, E213 E Muenzinger Hall, 345 UCB, Boulder, CO 80309-0202, USA
A.C. James, Centre de Recherche Cerveau et Cognition, CNRS-UPS UMR 5549, Université Paul Sabatier, 31062 Toulouse Cedex, France
W. Jiang, Department of Neurobiology and Anatomy, Wake Forest University, School of Medicine, Winston-Salem, NC 27157-1010, USA
J.H. Kaas, Department of Psychology, 301 Wilson Hall, Vanderbilt University, 111 21st Avenue South, Nashville, TN 37203, USA
E. Kaplan, The Mount Sinai/NYU School of Medicine, One Gustave Levy Place, New York, NY 10029, USA
R. Kleiser, LS Allgemeine Zoologie und Neurobiologie, Ruhr-Universität Bochum, Universitatsstr. 150, 44780 Bochum, Germany
A.F. Kramer, The Beckman Institute, University of Illinois at Urbana-Champaign, Urbana, IL 61801, USA
L.C. Liets, Section of Neurobiology, Physiology, and Behavior, University of California, Davis, CA 95616, USA
S.G. Lomber, Cerebral Systems Laboratory, School of Human Development, University of Texas at Dallas, Richardson, TX 75083-0688, USA
L. Lunenburger, LS Allgemeine Zoologie und Neurobiologie, Ruhr-Universität Bochum, Universitatsstr. 150, 44780 Bochum, Germany
D.C. Lyon, Department of Psychology, 301 Wilson Hall, Vanderbilt University, 111 21st Avenue South, Nashville, TN 37240, USA
I. Mareschal, Center for Neural Science, Room 809, New York University, New York NY 10003, USA

L. Merabet, École d'Optométrie, Laboratoire des Neurosciences de la Vision, Centre de Recherche en Sciences Neurologiques, Université de Montréal, CP 6128, Succ. Centre-Ville, Montreal, PQ H3C 3J7, Canada

M.P. Milham, The Beckman Institute, University of Illinois at Urbana-Champaign, Urbana, IL 61801, USA

L.E. Miller, Department of Physiology, Northwestern University Medical School, Chicago, IL 60611, USA

K. Minville, École d'Optométrie, Laboratoire des Neurosciences de la Vision, Centre de Recherche en Sciences Neurologiques, Université de Montréal, CP 6128, Succ. Centre-Ville, Montreal, PQ H3C 3J7, Canada

J.K. Nelson, Department of Psychology, University of Michigan, Ann Arbor, MI 48109-1109, USA

I. Ohzawa, Department of Biophysical Engineering, Osaka University, Osaka 560-8531, Japan

A.J. Parker, University Laboratory of Physiology, Parks Road, Oxford OX1 3PT, UK

A. Pascual-Leone, Department of Neurology, Beth Israel Deaconess Medical Center, Harvard Medical School, Brookline Avenue, Boston, MA 02215, USA

A. Ptito, Montreal Neurological Institute and Hospital, McGill University, 3801 University Street, Montreal, PQ H3A 2B4, Canada

M. Ptito, Montreal Neurological Institute and Hospital, McGill University, 3801 University Street, Montreal, PQ H3A 2B4, Canada *and* School of Optometry, 3744 Jean-Brillant Street, University of Montreal, Montreal, PQ H3C 3J7, Canada

P.A. Reuter-Lorenz, Department of Psychology, University of Michigan, Ann Arbor, MI, 48109-1109, USA

P.H. Schiller, Department of Brain and Cognitive Sciences, Massachusetts Institute of Technology, Cambridge, MA 02139, USA

H. Sherk, Department of Biological Structure, Box 35-7420, University of Washington, Seattle, WA 98195, USA

S.M. Sherman, Department of Neurobiology, State University of New York, Stony Brook, NY 11794-5230, USA

T.R. Stanford, Department of Neurobiology and Anatomy, Wake Forest University, School of Medicine, Winston-Salem, NC 27157-1010, USA

B.E. Stein, Department of Neurobiology and Anatomy, Wake Forest University, School of Medicine, Winston-Salem, NC 27157-1010, USA

V. Stuphorn, LS Allgemeine Zoologie und Neurobiologie, Ruhr-Universität Bochum, Universitatsstr. 150, 44780 Bochum, Germany

E.J. Tehovnik, Department of Brain and Cognitive Sciences, Massachusetts Institute of Technology, Cambridge, MA 02139, USA

H. Théoret, Laboratory for Magnetic Brain Stimulation, Behavioral Neurology Unit, Beth Israel Deaconess Medical Center, Harvard Medical School, 330 Brookline Avenue KS-454, Boston, MA 02215, USA

T.R. Vidyasagar, Psychobiology Laboratory and Center for Visual Sciences, School of Psychology, Australian National University, Canberra, ACT 0200, Australia

M.W. von Grünau, Department of Psychology, Concordia University, 7141 Sherbrooke Street West, Montreal, PQ H4B 1R6, Canada

M.T. Wallace, Department of Neurobiology and Anatomy, Wake Forest University, School of Medicine, Winston-Salem, NC 27157-1010, USA

G. Walker, Guidant Corporation, 1525 O'Brien Dr., Menlo Park, CA 94025, USA

V. Walsh, University of Oxford, Department of Experimental Psychology, South Parks Road, Oxford OX1 3UD, UK

A. Webb, The Beckman Institute, University of Illinois at Urbana-Champaign, Urbana, IL 61801, USA

M. Wessinger, Center for Cognitive Neuroscience, Dartmouth College, Hanover, NH 03755-3547, USA

T. Wszalek, The Beckman Institute, University of Illinois at Urbana-Champaign, Urbana, IL 61801, USA

Preface

The visual system has emerged as the model *par excellence* for the experimental investigation of brain sensory functions and is consequently the domain in which we have the greatest knowledge. This interest in the visual system is surely related to the fact that most of our knowledge of the external world comes from vision, that the activity of approximately one-third of our cortex is related to this function, and that the partial or total loss of vision seriously reduces the ability of a subject to interact with its environment. In addition, the stimuli used to activate visual neurons in the brain can be generally controlled with more accuracy and ease than those used to stimulate other systems.

Historically, the extraordinary progress in understanding visual functions occurred within the fields of experimental psychology and neuropsychology. In the former, there were attempts to identify how different visual stimuli led to different subjective experiences. With the advent of the objective methodology of psychophysics, there was a quantitative appreciation of the elements of visual stimuli such as color, brightness, and motion, and ideas on how they might be represented in the brain started to take form. Neuropsychology on the other hand, through the study of brain lesioned subjects (animals and humans), helped to identify brain regions that subserved visual functions. It was found then that the occipital lobe of the cerebral cortex played an essential role in the processing of visual information. We have come a long way since then and the marriage between experimental psychology and neuropsychology has significantly increased our knowledge on how the human brain processes visual information.

The technical advance of single-unit physiology has also largely contributed to understanding the neuronal processing of visual information. One can recall the pioneering work of Hartline in the early 1930s who recorded from single cells in the eye of the horseshoe crab and later from axons in the frog's optic nerve. Two major important discoveries were then made: the notion of receptive fields and the importance of contrast. The tradition of single neuron studies continued through the 1940s and the 1950s with an emphasis on mammals and has provided us with notions that became a part of our daily vocabulary. The subsequent studies by S. Kuffler on the retina and D.H. Hubel and T.N. Wiesel beyond the retina (e.g., the lateral geniculate nucleus and the primary visual cortex or V1) have provided us with a hierarchical model of visual processing, later followed by the notion of parallel streams. These two models are not mutually exclusive: incoming information of different types, having reached the primary visual cortex is then channelled through different streams, such that the output of each stream serves a unique function. It is now widely accepted that beyond area V1, the ventral stream is involved in the definition of the attributes of the visual stimulus (*what*) whereas the dorsal one is concerned with the spatial localization of that stimulus (*where*). It now also believed that those pathways can be distinguished on the basis of perceptual representation and visuomotor control (perception *versus* action).

Visual processing does not, of course, terminate in area V1 and much attention has been given in the second part of the past century to the extrastriate visual cortex. A large number of electrophysiological and anatomical studies were performed and have led to the current knowledge that the cortex can be subdivided into more than thirty distinct modules. Little is yet known of the specific role 'assigned' to the vast majority of these modules and one of the challenges of the coming years is to determine the specialization of each subdivision, and to discover how they interact to yield an unified perception of the external world.

Another tenet of modern neuroscience is that stages of brain development correspond to specific stages in the development of perceptual abilities. These stages, known as critical periods, are characterized by an extraordinary degree of neuronal plasticity. This plastic process is such that it is possible, for example, to manipulate the anatomical organization of the visual pathways and induce novel visual projections to non-visual structures. Other promising avenues concern the use of growth factors to protect neurons from injury and induce sprouting of their axons.

Thanks to the development of new powerful techniques (e.g., neuroimaging, transcranial magnetic stimulation) and to the progressive contribution of researchers from other disciplines (e.g., physics, bio-genetics), there has been in recent years, a tremendous increase in our knowledge of the mechanisms underlying vision. Recent symposiums and books have been devoted to very specific topics such as progress in retinal, extrageniculate, or cortical network research. Such symposia and ensuing books have not provided an overall view of how retinal, sub-cortical, and cortical systems interact and work together to permit the perception of an image and subsequent appropriate behavior. For all these reasons, we considered that it was an opportune time to organize a general meeting on visual processing. This meeting, titled "Vision: From Neurons to Cognition" was the XXII international meeting of the *centre de recherche en sciences neurologiques* of the *Université de Montréal*, and was held in May 2000 in the beautiful city of Montreal. Montreal was indeed the perfect place to organize this symposium not only because it has a tradition of excellence in neurosciences but also because it has one of the most active visual neuroscience communities in Quebec and Canada. Another reason may be its francophone characteristics, fine cuisine, and lively nightlife . . .

During two and a half days, internationally renowned researchers from Australia, Canada, England, France, Germany, and the United States got together and discussed how the various parts of the brain process and integrate visual signals. We are grateful to our colleagues (lecturers and invited contributors) for having made the symposium a success and for providing thirty chapters in which the reader will find up to date original findings, reviews, and theoretical proposals. We are also indebted to David Hubel, a former citizen of Montreal, for having given the symposium's closing lecture.

This book will not only address the basic mechanisms of visual perception but also issues such as neuronal plasticity, functional reorganization and recovery, residual vision, and sensory substitution. Knowledge of the basic mechanisms by which our brain can analyze, reconstruct, and interpret images in the external world is of fundamental importance for our capacity to understand the nature and causes of visual deficits, such as those resulting from ischemia, abnormal development, neuro-degenerative disorders, and normal aging. It is also essential for our goal of developing better therapeutic strategies, such as early diagnosis, visual training, behavioral rehabilitation of visual functions, and visual implants.

We are grateful to Le Ministère de la Recherche, de la Science et de la Technologie du Québec, le centre de recherche en sciences neurologiques de l'Université de Montréal, la Fondation Savoy (Épilepsie/Epilepsy), the Canadian Institutes of Health Research, le Fonds de la recherche en santé du Québec (FRSQ), l'École d'optométrie de l'Université de Montréal, l'Université de Montréal, le Fonds pour la Formation de Chercheurs et l'Aide à la Recherche (FCAR), le Réseau FRSQ en santé de la vision du Québec, le groupe de recherche en neuropsychologie expérimentale de l'Université de Montréal, Frederick Haer and Co., Bausch and Lomb, Cambridge Electronic Design Ltd., CIBA Vision, and Instruments ophtalmiques Innova Inc, for their financial contribution that made the symposium which resulted in this volume. We are also grateful to Mr. Daniel Cyr, Mrs. Karine Minville, and Mrs. Chantal Nault for their precious help and excellent work. Finally, many thanks to Tom Merriweather for believing in this project from the beginning and for helping us in the making of this *Progress in Brain Research* volume.

Christian Casanova
Maurice Ptito

Contents

C. Casanova and M. Ptito (Eds.)
Progress in Brain Research, Vol. 134

CHAPTER 1

Glutamate-mediated responses in developing retinal ganglion cells

L.C. Liets * and L.M. Chalupa

Section of Neurobiology, Physiology, and Behavior, University of California, Davis, CA 95616, USA

Abstract: Glutamate has been suggested to regulate the development of retinal ganglion cells, but little is known about the functional properties of glutamate receptors during ontogeny of these neurons. Using whole-cell and outside-out patch-clamp recordings, we have characterized the pharmacological, rectification, and kinetic properties of ionotropic glutamate receptors in ganglion cells isolated from fetal and postnatal cat retinas. The fetal cells were studied at embryonic day 33 (E33) to E38, before significant outgrowth of their dendritic processes and prior to the formation of synaptic contacts in the inner plexiform layer. In several respects, the functional properties of early fetal ganglion cells were found to be remarkably similar to those of postnatal cells. In both age groups, glutamate and AMPA produced fast desensitizing currents, kainate yielded large steady-state currents, while applications of NMDA resulted in multiple channel openings. The shapes and amplitudes of these glutamate-gated currents were also similar and the current–voltage relations were nearly linear, with reversal potentials near 0 mV. Moreover, the dose–response curves (to kainate) were virtually identical in the fetal and postnatal neurons. The proportion of neurons responsive to NMDA and non-NMDA agonists was nearly the same in both age groups. This early functional expression of glutamate receptors cannot be involved in the transmission of electrical information in the developing retina because at this stage few ganglion cells are capable of generating action potentials (Skaliora et al., 1993). It is suggested that the early activation of NMDA and non-NMDA receptors in fetal ganglion cells may regulate the outgrowth and stabilization of dendritic processes in these neurons. Our data also revealed some differences in the responses of fetal and postnatal cells to glutamate and its agonists. Thus, the unitary NMDA conductance was found to decrease with age, while the rate of glutamate receptor desensitization increased with age. Also, while virtually all postnatal cells responded to glutamate, the proportion of fetal cells that manifested glutamate-mediated responses was lower. These maturational changes presumably allow retinal ganglion cells to integrate synaptic inputs for the transmission of electrical signals to the visual centers of the brain.

Introduction

In the developing nervous system, neurotransmitters have been implicated in a variety of ontogenetic events independent of their mature synaptic functions (Ben-Ari et al., 1997; Cameron et al., 1998; Vallano, 1998; Fox et al., 1999). For instance, glutamate, the primary excitatory neurotransmitter in the adult brain, has been reported to regulate neuronal migration (Komuro and Rakic, 1993, 1996; Behar et al., 1999), cell differentiation (Gleason and Spitzer, 1998; Morrison and Mason, 1998; Yuan et al., 1998), growth and elaboration of dendritic processes (Metzger et al., 1998; Rajan and Cline, 1998; Cuppini et al., 1999; Rajan et al., 1999), as well as refinement of early axonal projections (Simon et al., 1992; Schlaggar et al., 1993; Li et al., 1994; Fox et al., 1996). Patch-clamp recording studies in several systems have also shown that neurons can express glutamate receptors at very early stages of development, even before synaptogenesis (Dupont et al., 1987; LoTurco et al., 1991; Blanton and Kriegstein, 1992).

* Corresponding author: L.C. Liets, Section of Neurobiology, Physiology, and Behavior, University of California, Davis, CA 95616, USA. Tel.: +1-530-752-3897; Fax: +1-530-752-3451; E-mail: lcliets@ucdavis.edu.

Several lines of evidence suggest that glutamate also plays diverse roles in the development of retinal ganglion cells. Thus, high levels of extracellular glutamate have been documented at early stages of retinal development, even before traditional synapses are formed (Haberecht and Redburn, 1996). During synaptogenesis activation of NMDA and non-NMDA receptors has been found to affect the rate and extent of movements manifested by dendritic processes of retinal ganglion cells (Wong and Wong, 2000). Moreover, glutamate-mediated activity regulates the stratification of ganglion cell dendrites into On and Off sublaminae of the inner plexiform layer (Bodnarenko and Chalupa, 1993; Bodnarenko et al., 1995; Bisti et al., 1998). Glutamate activation of developing retinal ganglion cells has also been found essential for the generation of 'spontaneous' waves of retinal activity during the period when retinogeniculate On and Off pathways are being formed (Wong, 1999; Wong et al., 2000).

In view of the evidence implicating glutamate in the development of retinal ganglion cells and their patterns of projections, surprisingly little is known about the functional properties of glutamate receptors in immature ganglion cells. It has been reported that retinal ganglion cells are responsive to applications of glutamate and NMDA in the embryonic mouse (Rörig and Grantyn, 1994). Imaging studies of the developing rabbit retina have also revealed that non-NMDA receptors can mediate internal calcium fluctuations earlier than NMDA receptors (Wong, 1995). While these studies provide evidence of functional NMDA and non-NMDA receptors in developing ganglion cells, they did not attempt to characterize the functional properties of glutamate responses in such neurons.

In the present study, we compared NMDA and non-NMDA responses of early fetal ganglion cells with those of postnatal cells harvested from cat retinas. The fetal cells were harvested at a very early stage of development, between embryonic ages 33 (E33) and E38. (Gestation in the cat is about 65 days.) By E38, all ganglion cells have been generated (Rapaport et al., 1985), but dendritic processes are still sparse and synapses are lacking (Maslim and Stone, 1986). Moreover, few retinal ganglion cells are capable of generating action potentials prior to E38, reflecting their low density of sodium voltage-gated channels (Skaliora et al., 1993). Thus, any glutamate responses manifested by retinal ganglion cells at this fetal age cannot be involved in the transmission of electrical signals. Rather, the functional attributes of glutamate receptors would more likely be associated with dendritic outgrowth in these neurons, a process that is just beginning at this stage of development. (Maslim et al., 1986; Ramoa et al., 1988).

Methodological considerations

All procedures were carried out in compliance with National Institute of Health guidelines, and in accordance with protocols approved by the campus animal use committee.

Recordings were made from a total of 243 ganglion cells isolated from the retinas of fetal and postnatal cats between embryonic days E33 and E38 and 1 and 2 weeks of age, respectively. Previous studies have shown that the intrinsic membrane properties as well as spiking properties of these neurons are adult-like by 2 weeks of age (Skaliora et al., 1993, 1995).

Retrograde labeling and preparation of retinal ganglion cells

To unequivocally distinguish ganglion cells from other retinal cells, these neurons were retrogradely labeled by injections of rhodamine latex microspheres using a modification of procedures described previously (Skaliora et al., 1993, 1995). For fetal experiments, timed-pregnant animals were anesthetized with halothane and nitrous oxide and cesarian sections were performed to expose the cranium. Postnatal animals were anesthetized with an intramuscular injection of Telozol (15 mg/kg). Following anesthesia, the primary retinorecipient nuclei (lateral geniculate nucleus and superior colliculus) and optic tract were injected with rhodamine fluorescent beads. Heart rate and respiration were monitored throughout these procedures.

After a survival period of 24–36 h, the animals were administered a lethal dose of sodium pentobarbital and enucleated binocularly. The retinas were dissected free of the choroid and sclera and enzymatically digested using the procedure described by Karschin and Wässle (1990). Following the enzymatic treatment, the cells were triturated and plated onto glass coverslips treated with Cel-Tak® or poly-D-lysine and laminin, and maintained in an incubator at 5% CO_2 and 37°C. They were fed every 2–3 days by replacing half the media in each well.

To avoid space clamp problems, recordings in the whole-cell configuration were made within the first 36 h in culture, before the occurrence of significant process outgrowth. Outside-out patch recordings were made from fetal cells between the day of plating (0 days in vitro, DIV0) and DIV2 and from postnatal cells by DIV5, with a few postnatal cells recorded as late as DIV7. No differences were seen in the glutamate-mediated responses as a function of time in culture (see Discussion and Fig. 7).

Electrophysiology

Voltage-clamp recordings were performed at room temperature from cells in the whole-cell and outside-out configurations of the patch-clamp technique using an Axopatch-1D amplifier (Hamill et al., 1981; Edwards et al., 1989). Due to the sustained nature of currents elicited by applications of kainate, these currents could be measured in the whole-cell configuration. Responses to glutamate and AMPA were characterized by fast transient currents so drugs could be applied sufficiently fast to elicit these currents only in the outside-out configuration. Single-channel currents in response to application of NMDA were also recorded in the outside-out configuration. Cells were visualized on an inverted epifluorescence microscope and only fluorescently labeled cells with a healthy, non-granular appearance were selected for recordings.

During whole-cell recordings, the series resistance was measured (10–30 MΩ) and reduced by >50% with electronic compensation. Capacitive transients were compensated using the calibrated adjustment on the amplifier and typically had values of 6–25 pF.

Data were digitized at intervals ranging between 65 µs and 1 ms and the signals were low-pass filtered at 500 Hz to 5 kHz with a 4-pole Bessel filter. Reported current recordings are averages of 10–20 individual traces. Dose–response data and decay phases of current records were fit using the least squares method. The time course of current decay was fit with a single (Eq. 1) and double (Eq. 2) exponential function of the forms:

$$I = A\mathrm{e}^{-(t-K/\tau)} + C \tag{1}$$

$$I = A_1\mathrm{e}^{-(t-K_1/\tau_2)} + A_2\mathrm{e}^{-(t-K_1/\tau_2)} + C \tag{2}$$

where I is the current (pA), A is the amplitude (pA), t is the time (ms), K is the time (ms) of the peak current, τ is the decay time constant, and C is the steady-state constant. To determine whether a single exponential provided an adequate fit, the steady-state current was subtracted from the trace and the data were plotted on a log scale along with the single and double exponential fit. A double exponential fit was utilized when the data deviated from the linear single exponential fit. The dose–response data were normalized for each cell and the average responses were plotted versus the log of the agonist concentration. The mean data were fit with the Hill equation of the form:

$$I = I_{\mathrm{max}}/1 + (\mathrm{EC}_{50}/C)^h \tag{3}$$

where I is the current (pA), I_{max} is the maximum current (pA), C is the ligand concentration (M), h is the Hill coefficient, and EC_{50} is the concentration at the half maximal response (M). Events-list and all-points single-channel histograms are displayed with bin widths of 0.2 pA and were fit with Gaussian distributions. The mean amplitude levels were obtained from these fits and used to calculate unitary conductance by the formula $\gamma = i/(V_{\mathrm{cmd}} - V_{\mathrm{rev}})$, where i is the observed single-channel current, V_{cmd} is the holding potential and V_{rev} is the reversal potential. Numerical values are given as means ± SEM, and error bars reflect the standard error about the mean. Differences between groups were tested with a randomized Student's t-test and were considered significant at $P < 0.05$.

Recording and test solutions

Electrodes were filled with a solution containing 140 mM CsCl, 10 mM NaCl, 1 mM $CaCl_2$, 1 mM $MgCl_2$, 1.1 mM EGTA, 10 mM HEPES and 3 mM ATP. Cesium was included to block voltage-gated potassium currents. The recording chamber was continuously perfused with an extracellular solution containing

140 mM NaCl, 5 mM KCl, 2 mM $CaCl_2$, 1 mM $MgCl_2$, 10 mM HEPES, and 15–30 mM glucose. In most whole-cell recordings, 2.5 mM $CoCl_2$ and 300 nM tetrodotoxin (TTX) were included to block voltage-gated calcium and sodium channels, respectively. No differences in glutamate-gated responses were noted in these experiments. Recordings were obtained with 1 mM $MgCl_2$ and 2 μM glycine in the extracellular solution unless otherwise noted. Glucose concentration was adjusted to bring the solution to 300 mOsm.

For whole-cell recordings, drugs were applied using a modification of the microperfusion system described by Krishtal and Pidoplichko (1980). This perfusion system yielded an average onset rate of 10.62 ± 3.00 ms. For recordings from isolated patches, rapid solution changes were achieved using a piezo-activated θ-pipette. Solutions could be applied to (τ_{on} = 425 ± 147 μs) and removed (τ_{off} = 459 ± 177 μs) from the patch reliably in <500 μs.

Results

NMDA and non-NMDA receptor-mediated currents

Whole-cell and outside-out patch recordings were made from 99 fetal and 144 postnatal cat retinal ganglion cells. Isolated cells were identified by the presence of rhodamine microspheres, and some neurons were filled with Lucifer Yellow as shown in Fig. 1. In some cases, extensive processes could be visualized that extended for more than 100 μm from the soma. The extent of dendritic growth and the complexity of the secondary and tertiary branches was greater in postnatal neurons than in fetal cells (compare Fig. 1A and C), but there was no indication that the glutamate responses correlated with the extent of process outgrowth in either the fetal or postnatal cells.

Representative responses recorded from fetal cells (Fig. 2A) and postnatal cells (Fig. 2B) are shown in Fig. 2. In both instances, focal application of 300 μM kainate to whole cells elicited a sustained inward current when the cell was held near the resting potential (V_h = −60 mV). The inward current continued for up to 2 s (not shown) after withdrawal of the agonist reflecting the long interval for agonist removal when recording in the whole-cell configuration. To facilitate acquisition of fast peak currents, recordings were also made using the outside-out patch-clamp configuration and a fast ligand application system. As may be seen in Fig. 2, focal application of 1 mM AMPA and 1 mM glutamate elicited inward currents at −60 mV that displayed a fast rising phase followed by a rapid decay to near baseline levels. Application of kainate to outside-out patches yielded non-desensitizing inward currents similar to those seen in the whole-cell configuration (data not shown).

Stimulation with 1 mM NMDA, in the presence of 2 μM glycine and the absence of extracellular magnesium, elicited multiple single-channel events (Fig. 2, bottom traces). In addition, single NMDA channel activity could sometimes be resolved in individual glutamate-induced current recordings following the decay of the fast initial non-NMDA receptor-mediated inward current (see Fig. 5A).

Peak current amplitudes in response to application of 1 mM glutamate ranged between 3 and 58 pA (mean: 28.8 ± 24.15, n = 11) in fetal cells and between 9 and 68 pA (mean: 34.97 ± 22.7, n = 7) for postnatal cells. Peak currents elicited by applications of 1 mM AMPA ranged from 7 to 53 pA (mean: 27.05 ± 19.6, n = 6) for fetal cells and from 4 to 29 pA (mean: 17.67 ± 10.9, n = 6) for postnatal cells. There were no significant differences in the glutamate- and in the AMPA-induced peak currents recorded from fetal and postnatal cells. The variability in these recordings was considerable, however, most likely reflecting variations in patch size as well as regional differences in channel density.

Activation of KA channels (300 μM KA) in fetal cells yielded current amplitudes between 14 and 311 pA (mean: 118.47 ± 98.05, n = 7). Currents recorded from postnatal cells ranged between 47 and 411 pA (mean: 267.8 ± 171.9, n = 6). When current amplitudes were normalized for cell size, responses from fetal and postnatal cells did not differ significantly (current density: fetal, 16.8 ± 11.9 pA/pF, n = 7; postnatal, 35.2 ± 24.4 pA/pF, n = 6). It may also be seen in Fig. 2 that the general shape and time-course of glutamate-, KA-, and AMPA-activated currents are similar in early fetal and postnatal cells.

The bottom traces in Fig. 2 (A and B) depict representative examples of single-channel activity

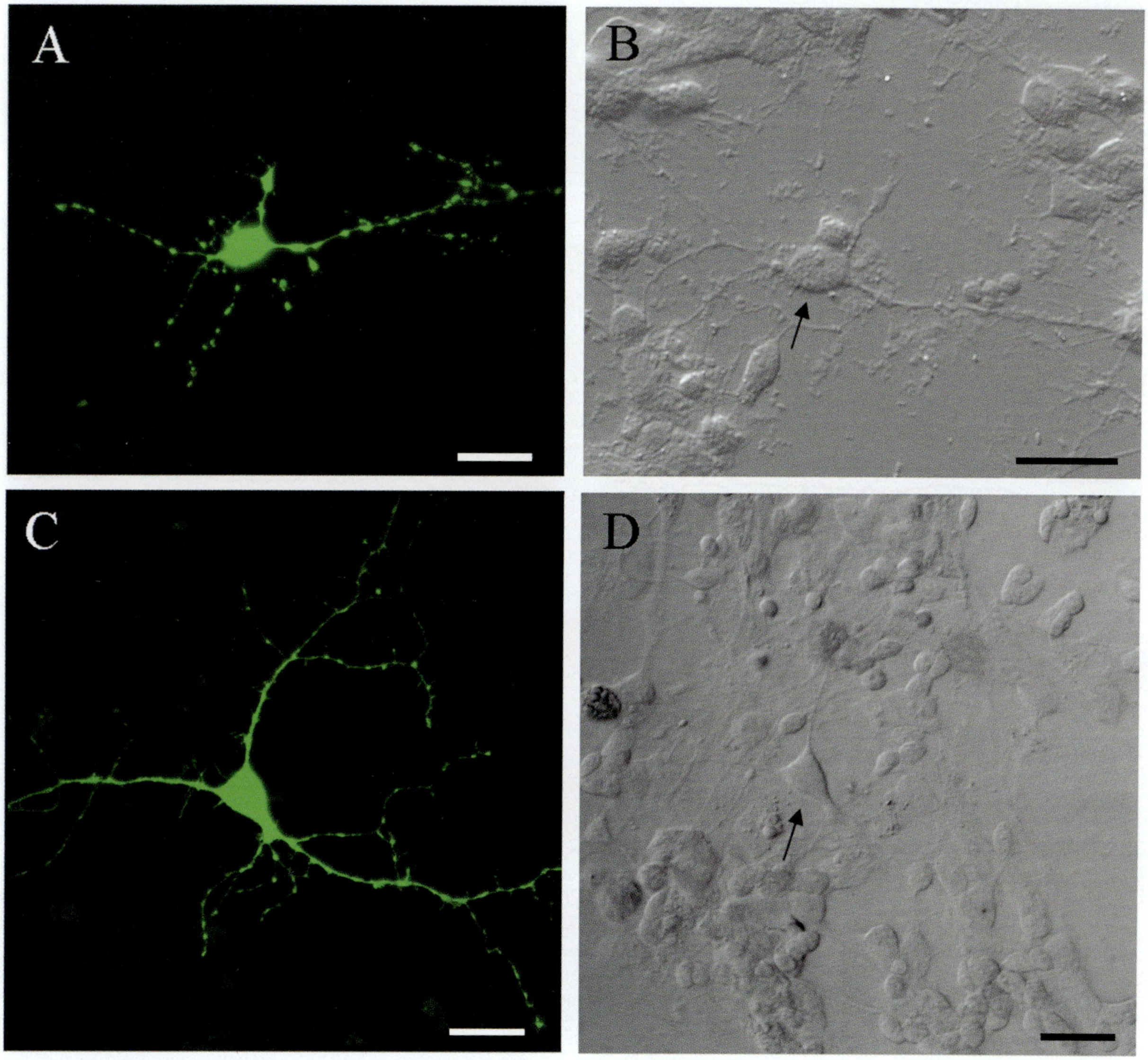

Fig. 1. Cell prepared for patch clamp recordings. (A) Ganglion cell from an E35 retina. The cell was filled with Lucifer Yellow and has been in culture for 2 days. (B) Same cell as in A (indicated by black arrow) shown in bright field to demonstrate culture preparation. (C) Retinal ganglion cell from a P10 retina filled with Lucifer Yellow. This cell has been in culture 3 days. (D) Same cell as in C (indicated by black arrow) shown in bright field. Cells were fixed overnight in 4% paraformaldehyde. Scale bars: 30 μm.

initiated by applications of NMDA to outside-out patches. All patches from fetal cells and most from postnatal cells expressed relatively few active NMDA channels since even high concentrations of NMDA (1 mM in Fig. 2) elicited few overlapping channel openings. Some patches from postnatal cells, however, contained several active channels (see Fig. 5D).

The proportions of postnatal and fetal cells (ranging in age between E35 and E38) expressing functional glutamate receptors are indicated in Table 1. Recordings to NMDA and glutamate application were also made at earlier ages (E33 and E34) from a smaller sample of cells. In this younger group, the incidence of responsive neurons was lower with 43% glutamate sensitive ($n = 14$ at E34)

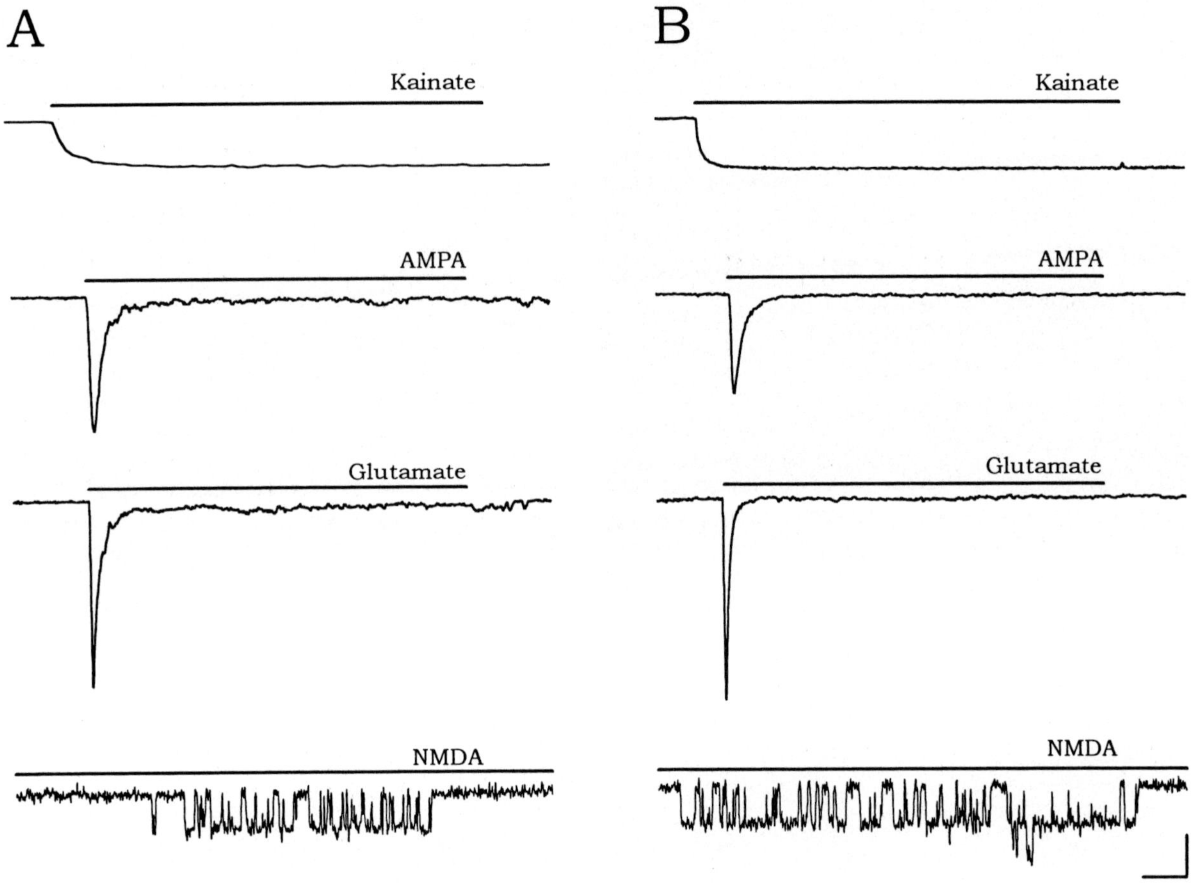

Fig. 2. Representative examples of responses to glutamate and its major agonists. (A) Responses to 300 μM kainate, 1 mM AMPA, 1 mM glutamate, and 1 mM NMDA recorded from tissue obtained from fetal animals. (B) Responses (same concentrations of agonists as in A) recorded from tissue obtained from postnatal animals. Kainate responses were recorded in the whole-cell configuration of the patch-clamp technique and drugs were applied using the U-tube application system. AMPA, glutamate and NMDA responses were recorded in outside-out patches and drugs were applied using the fast-application system. Magnesium was omitted from the extracellular solution during recordings of NMDA responses. Bars indicate duration of ligand application. Cells and patches were held at −60 mV. Scale bar: 75 ms/250 pA (kainate), 20 ms/12 pA (AMPA), 20 ms/20 pA (glutamate), 25 ms/4 pA (NMDA).

TABLE 1

Fetal and postnatal cell responsiveness

	E35–E38	P6–P14
Glutamate	77% ($n = 18$)	96% ($n = 51$)
AMPA	75% ($n = 20$)	98% ($n = 51$)
Kainate	80% ($n = 15$)	100% ($n = 25$)
NMDA	100% ($n = 10$)	100% ($n = 22$)

Percentage of cells responsive to each agonist at a given age.

and 39% responding to NMDA application ($n = 22$ at E33/E34).

Rectification properties and dose–response characteristics

Current–voltage (I/V) relations for glutamate, AMPA and kainate are shown in Fig. 3. Filled circles represent recordings from fetal cells while responses from postnatal cells are indicated by the open circles. Each I/V relation is composed of the normalized average responses recorded at holding potentials

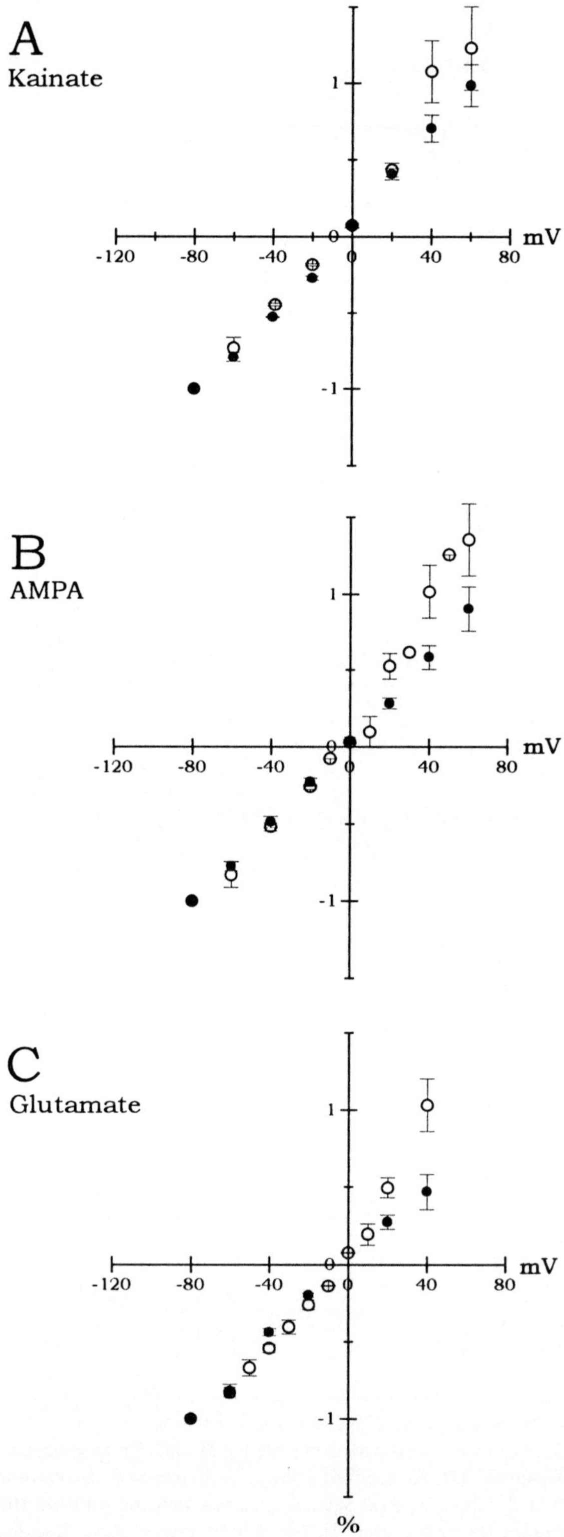

ranging from −80 to +60 mV from 4 to 7 cells. All agonists yielded nearly linear I/V relations with reversal potentials near 0 mV (KA: postnatal, $V_{rev} = -4.94 \pm 3.75$ mV, $n = 4$; fetal, $V_{rev} = -4.94 \pm 5.34$ mV, $n = 5$; AMPA: postnatal, $V_{rev} = -5.59 \pm 6.18$ mV, $n = 6$; fetal, $V_{rev} = -2.62 \pm 4.30$ mV, $n = 7$; glutamate: postnatal, $V_{rev} = -6.93 \pm 3.85$ mV, $n = 7$; fetal, $V_{rev} = -2.60 \pm 7.92$ mV, $n = 6$). Current–voltage relations generated from responses to all three agonists were only slightly more outwardly rectifying in the postnatal cells, as evidenced by a larger average g_{+40}/g_{-40} chord conductance ratio (KA: postnatal (open circles), 1.85; fetal (closed circles), 1.04; AMPA: postnatal (open circles), 1.48; fetal (closed circles), 1.05; glutamate: postnatal (open circles), 1.33; fetal (closed circles), 0.93; calculated from V_{rev} and the current values at −40 mV and +40 mV).

Responses from representative postnatal cells to different concentrations of KA, AMPA and glutamate, recorded with the membrane held at −60 mV, are shown in Fig. 4A, B, and C, respectively. Current amplitudes varied as a function of agonist concentration. The mean normalized steady-state responses for KA or peak responses for AMPA and glutamate were plotted on a logarithmic scale (Fig. 4D) and fit with the Hill function. The lowest concentration of agonists yielding measurable responses ranged between 3 and 10 μM, while concentrations yielding responses near I_{max} (calculated from the Hill equation, see methods) were in the mM range. Postnatal cells were most sensitive to KA (Fig. 4D, squares) which had an average half maximal (EC_{50}) steady-state concentration of 220 μM with a Hill coefficient

Fig. 3. Current–voltage relations in fetal and postnatal cells. Current responses for each cell were normalized to the response obtained while holding the membrane potential at −80 mV with responses obtained at other holding potentials expressed as a percentage of the response at −80 mV. The normalized average current–voltage relations were plotted in response to applications of 300 μM kainate (A), 1 mM AMPA (B), and 1 mM glutamate (C). Recordings were made in the whole-cell configuration for KA and in outside-out patches for AMPA and glutamate. Records obtained from fetal cells are indicated by the closed circles, while those obtained from postnatal cells are indicated by the open circles. Data points represent the average (±SEM) of recordings from 5 to 8 cells.

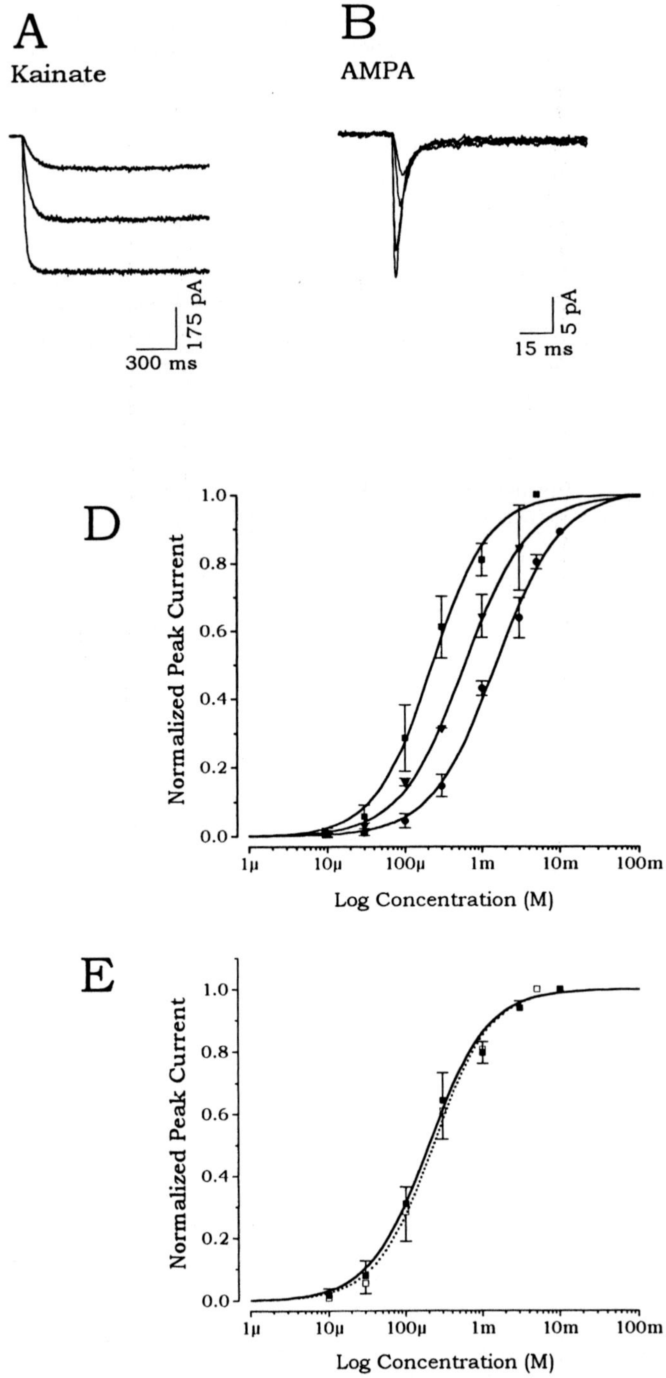

Fig. 4. Glutamate receptor sensitivity in fetal and postnatal cells. (A) Responses obtained in the whole-cell configuration to applications of 100 μM, 300 μM and 5 mM kainate. (B) Responses obtained from an outside-out patch to applications of 100 μM, 300 μM, 1 mM, and 3 mM AMPA. (C) Responses obtained from an outside-out patch to applications of 100 μM, 300 μM, 1 mM, and 5 mM glutamate. The cell and patches used in A, B, and C were obtained from postnatal animals. (D) Normalized average dose–response curves from postnatal tissue for glutamate (closed circles), AMPA (closed triangles), and kainate (closed squares). Curves were fit with the Hill equation using the least squares method. Data from 4 to 7 cells were averaged for each ligand. (E) Normalized average dose–response curves obtained from fetal (open circles) and postnatal (closed circles; same as shown in D) cells in response to applications of kainate. Data from 5 to 6 cells were averaged at each age. All cells and patches were held at −60 mV.

of 1.18 ($n = 5$). Peak currents elicited by applications of AMPA and glutamate yielded higher EC_{50} values (590 μM, $h = 1.05$, $n = 9$, triangles; 1.5 mM, $h = 1.04$, $n = 5$, circles, respectively), suggesting a lower affinity for these agonists.

We also compared the dose–response curves of fetal and postnatal cells to kainate application. (Such comparisons were not made for the other agonists because it was problematic to make the lengthy recordings required to obtain such functions.) Fig. 4E illustrates postnatal (closed squares) and fetal (open squares) dose response curves for kainate. Note that the two populations displayed nearly identical Hill functions (EC_{50} values: postnatal, 220 μM; fetal, 230 μM and Hill coefficients: postnatal, 1.18; fetal, 1.14).

NMDA channel properties during development

The responses to glutamate were composed of two components: a fast initial peak current followed by a small steady-state current. In normal physiological solution, NMDA channels are blocked at resting potential by the extracellular Mg^{2+} and the steady-state component of the glutamate response is very small (see glutamate trace in Fig. 2B). When NMDA channel activity was not blocked at negative holding potentials by the presence of extracellular Mg^{2+}, individual NMDA channel openings could often be resolved in the steady-state region of individual glutamate-induced current traces (Fig. 5A). These traces combined to yield an average glutamate trace with a larger steady-state current in the absence of extracellular Mg^{2+} (Fig. 5B).

Fig. 5C and D depict amplitude histograms for representative fetal and postnatal patches, respectively. The amplitude histogram shown for the fetal cell was fit with a single Gaussian distribution and yielded a unitary main-state conductance of 49 pS. Fig. 5D shows a patch excised from a postnatal cell which contained several active channels. The amplitude histogram constructed from these data was fit with the sum of five Gaussian distributions. The largest peak reflects the majority of data points at the baseline current, while the other 4 peaks are separated by approximately equal current values (−2.68, −5.26, −7.93, and −10.62 pA) yielding a unitary conductance of 45 pS. In patches excised from both fetal and postnatal cells, NMDA channel openings to smaller conductance states were observed. These conductance levels were not systematically analyzed because they occurred very infrequently and were difficult to resolve above the baseline noise. To determine the average unitary main-state conductance for the two age groups unitary currents were elicited at holding potentials ranging from −80 to +60 mV and the average slope conductance was calculated by the fit of a linear regression. Six fetal cells (Fig. 5E) yielded an average slope conductance of 51.68 ± 2.28 pS and an average reversal potential of -3.88 ± 2.12 mV. Records from five postnatal patches (Fig. 5F) yielded a smaller average slope conductance of 44.86 ± 1.11 pS ($P < 0.01$) with a reversal potential of -3.71 ± 2.32 mV. This suggests that NMDA channels in fetal ganglion cells could allow slightly more current to pass than in postnatal cells.

Development of glutamate receptor kinetics

Desensitization kinetics of glutamate-mediated currents were also analyzed. Fig. 6A shows an example of currents elicited by different concentrations of glutamate in the absence of extracellular magnesium recorded from a patch excised from a postnatal cell. Higher concentrations yielded higher peak amplitudes and faster decay kinetics. The desensitization time constant decreased from 12 ms at 100 μM glutamate to 5 ms at 5 mM glutamate ($n = 5$; Fig. 6B). The kinetics of current responses to applications of 1 mM glutamate in normal physiological solution were compared for fetal and postnatal cells (Fig. 6C). The average fetal and postnatal responses are plotted together and normalized to peak currents to facilitate comparison. Note that the glutamate-mediated current desensitization is slower for the fetal patches. Postnatal responses decay (τ) in 2.58 ± 1.09 ms ($n = 9$), while fetal responses decay in 4.65 ± 0.68 ms ($n = 11$, $P < 0.01$).

Discussion

In this study, we compared the functional properties of ionotropic glutamate receptors in early fetal and postnatal ganglion cells of the cat retina. Before discussing our findings and their implications we will consider some of the limitations of this study. One

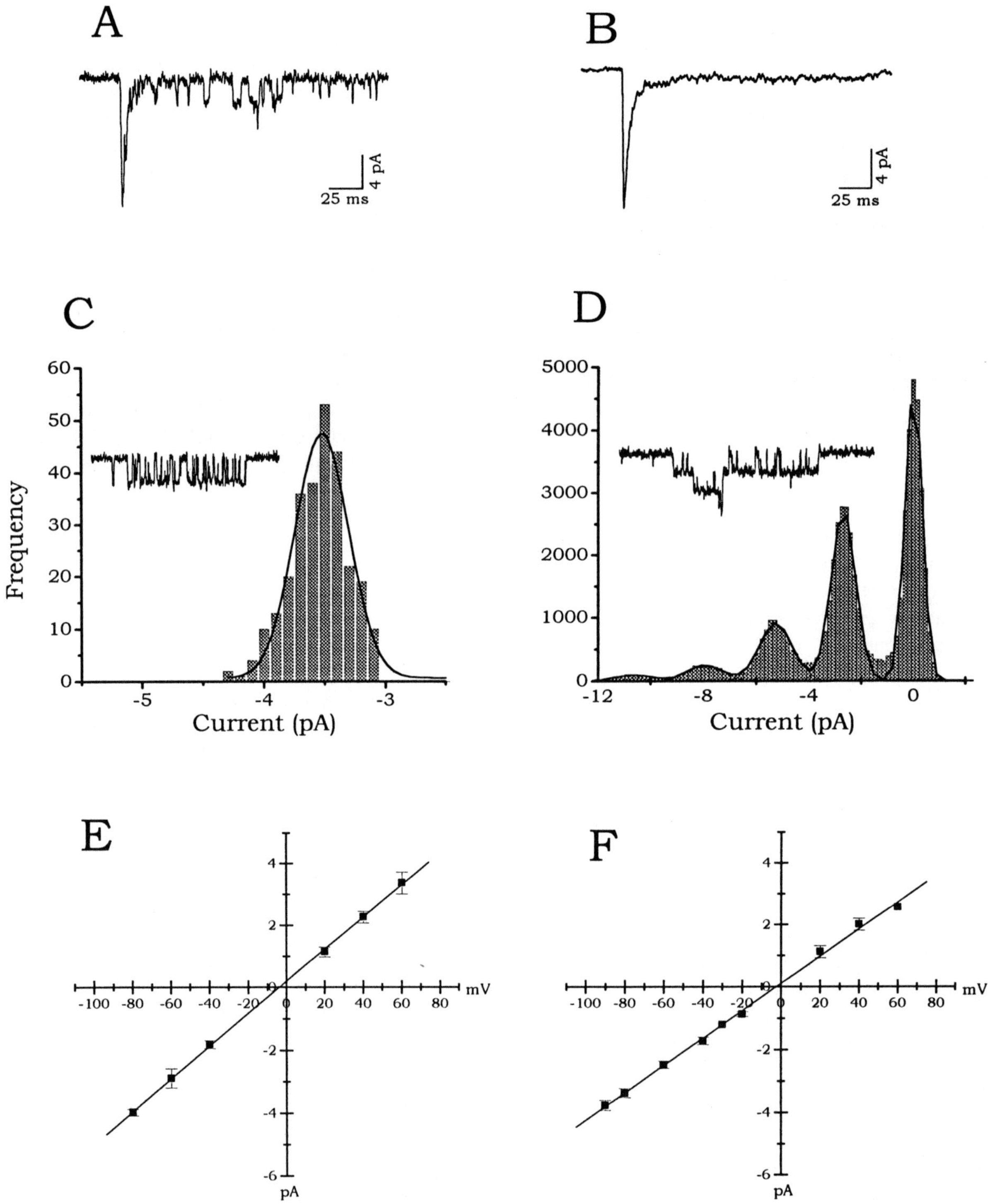
A
4 pA
25 ms
B
4 pA
25 ms
C
Frequency
Current (pA)
D
Current (pA)
E
mV
pA
F
mV
pA

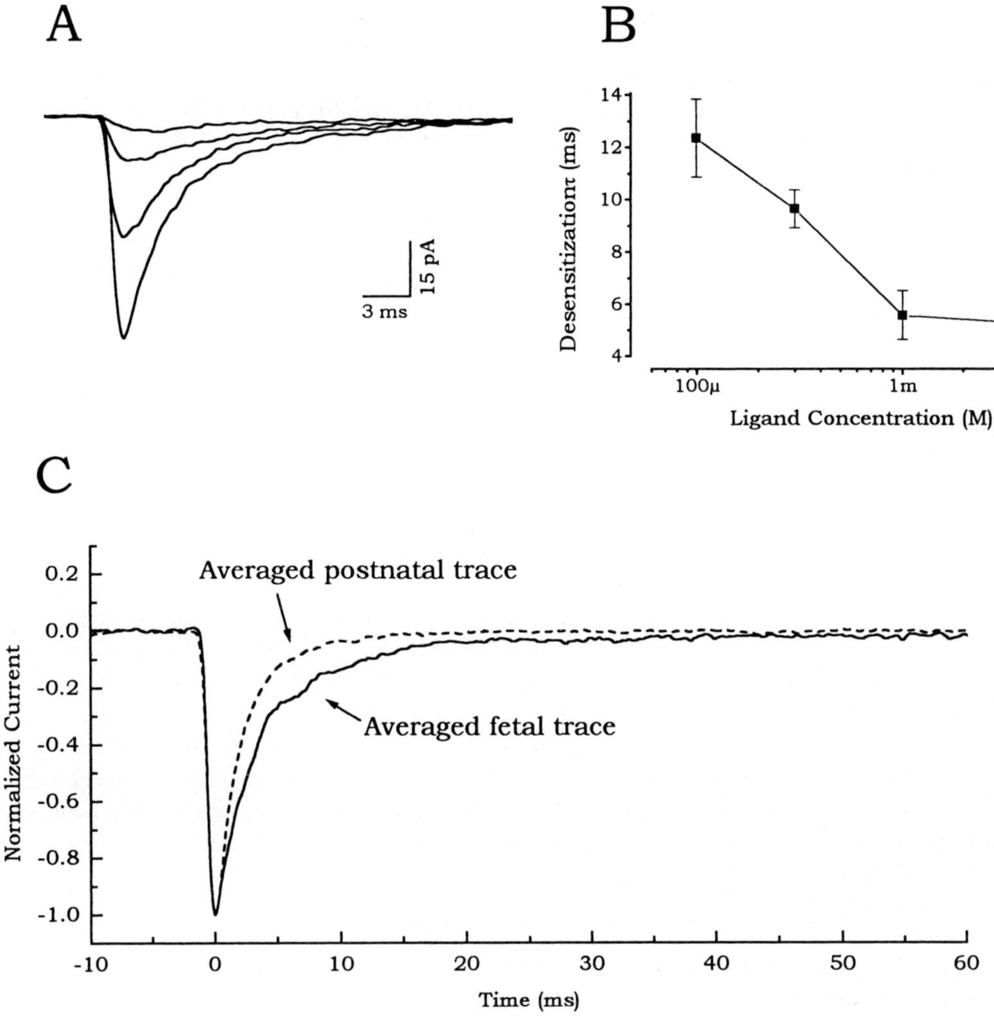

Fig. 6. Glutamate receptor desensitization. (A) Responses in an outside-out patch from a postnatal animal to applications of 100 μM, 300 μM, 1 mM, and 5 mM glutamate. (B) Average desensitization time constant (τ) plotted against glutamate concentration. Data points represent averages of 5 patches including that shown in A recorded in magnesium-free extracellular solution. (C) Average glutamate receptor desensitization in response to applications of 1 mM glutamate in fetal (solid line) and postnatal (dashed line) patches recorded in normal physiological solution, including magnesium and 2 μM glycine. Traces were normalized to peak current and overplotted to facilitate comparison. Patches were held at −60 mV and desensitization time constants were derived from the least squares fit of an exponential equation.

Fig. 5. NMDA responses in fetal and postnatal cells. (A) Individual trace obtained from a postnatal patch in response to application of 1 mM glutamate in the presence of 2 μM glycine and absence of extracellular magnesium. Individual channel openings can be observed in the latter portion of the trace. (B) Average of 15 individual responses to applications of 1 mM glutamate including the one shown in A. (C) Cumulative amplitude histogram fit with a single Gaussian distribution. (D) All-points histogram fit with the sum of five Gaussian distributions. Peaks are separated by approximately equal intervals indicating the existence of several active channels within the patch. Portions of the records from which the histograms in C and D were generated are shown in the insets. Fits were conducted using the least squares method. (E) Average current–voltage relation for NMDA channel activity recorded in six fetal patches including that shown in C. The solid line is a linear regression through the data yielding a slope conductance of 51.7 pS and a reversal potential of −3.88 mV. (F) Average current–voltage relation for NMDA channel activity recorded in five postnatal patches including that shown in D. The solid line is a linear regression through the data yielding a slope conductance of 44.9 pS and a reversal potential of −3.71 mV. Data shown in A–F were generated from records obtained in the presence of 2 μM glycine and the absence of extracellular magnesium.

potential problem is that we employed dissociated ganglion cells rather than retinal slices or wholemounts. The use of dissociated cells provides certain technical advantages as well as disadvantages. Drugs can be delivered directly to the cell from which recordings are being made and this decreases the possibility of response contamination by other neurons in the circuit. A potential drawback of this approach, however, is that dendritic processes are lost or severely truncated by the dissociation procedure so the responses primarily represent receptors expressed on the soma. This is not a factor when considering recordings from the fetal cells since in vitro these neurons have yet to show significant outgrowth of dendrites (Maslim et al., 1986; Ramoa et al., 1988). It is also the case that studies of ganglion cells dissociated from the mature rat (Aizenman et al., 1988) and goldfish (Yazejian and Fain, 1992) retinas have shown that functional NMDA and non-NMDA glutamate receptors are expressed on somal membranes.

Another potential limitation is that recordings were made from cultured cells to allow for an extended recording period. Typically, we recorded from fetal cells no more than 2 days in culture and postnatal cells within 4 days, with some recordings of postnatal cells lasting up to 7 days. Conceivably, the glutamate-mediated responses could have been affected by the time in culture, but the available evidence indicates that this was not the case. As may be seen in Fig. 7A, the percentage of cells responsive to the different glutamate agonists remained constant even when maintained 7 days in culture. A comparison of glutamate and NMDA activated currents also showed that these did not vary appreciably with time in culture (Fig. 7B). Furthermore, responses to all agonists were seen in freshly dissociated cells which argues against the possibility that the mature-like currents recorded in the fetal cells were ‘induced’ by formation of synapses in culture.

Since our objective was to compare and contrast the overall NMDA and non-NMDA responses in fetal and postnatal ganglion cells, we did not attempt to differentiate between the AMPA preferring and kainate preferring receptors, nor did we seek to identify the subunits contributing to the glutamate responses. Such finer grain assessments of developing glutamate receptors remain for future studies.

Functional properties of fetal and postnatal glutamate receptors

Based on their pharmacology, kinetics and rectification properties we found remarkable similarities as well as clear-cut differences between the glutamate receptors of early fetal and postnatal retinal ganglion cells (RGCs). With respect to the similarities, four points appear noteworthy. First, application of glutamate and AMPA yielded fast desensitizing currents and KA yielded large steady-state current, while application of NMDA initiated multiple single-channel openings in fetal as well as in postnatal cells. Second, the shape and amplitude of glutamate-gated currents were not appreciably different in fetal and postnatal cells. Third, the I/V relations of the responses from fetal and postnatal cells were nearly linear with reversal potentials near 0 mV. Fourth, the dose–response curves (obtained for kainate) were virtually identical in both age groups, indicating that the pharmacological sensitivity of glutamate receptors is equivalent in fetal and postnatal cells.

Our results also reveal some differences in the responses to glutamate of fetal and postnatal cells. Thus, the unitary main-state NMDA channel conductance was found to decrease with development, suggesting that a given stimulus would lead to a larger response in ganglion cells of younger animals. At the same time, the time-course of glutamate receptor desensitization increased with age, so that activation of these channels in younger animals would tend to lead to longer responses. Finally, while virtually all postnatal cells responded to application of glutamate or its agonist, a substantial proportion of the fetal cells could not be activated in this manner. Most likely, this reflects a true maturational difference rather than some methodological factor (e.g. the viability of the cell during the recording) because in all cases the voltage-gated currents of the unresponsive neurons appeared normal.

There was no indication from our recordings that the functional properties of NMDA receptors mature earlier than non-NMDA receptors. This relates to the concept of silent synapses, where AMPA receptors are inserted at synapses that initially contain only NMDA receptors. Such a mechanism has been proposed to account for the maintenance of LTP (Isaac et al., 1995; Liao et al., 1995) as well as for the

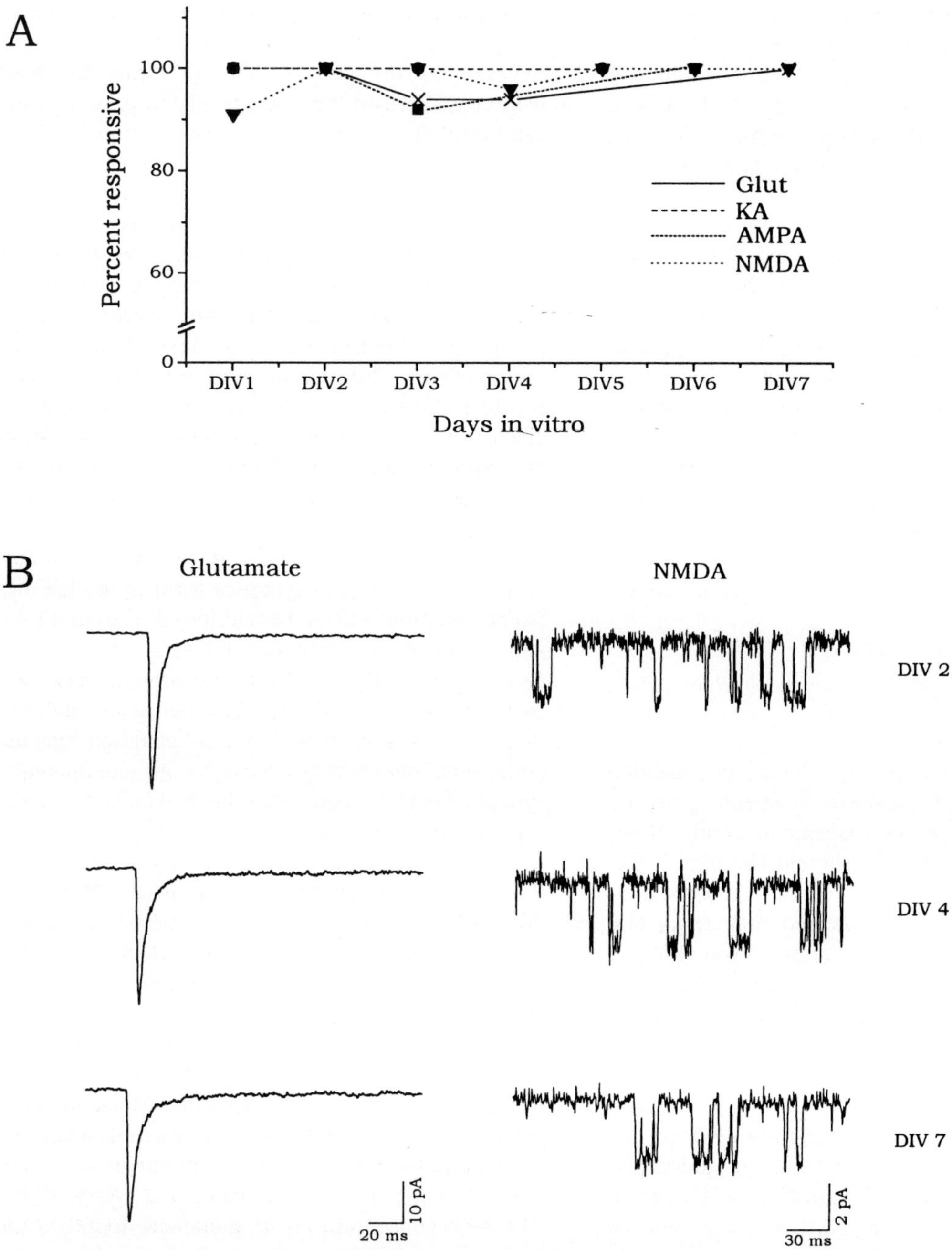

Fig. 7. Glutamate receptor-mediated responses during period in culture. (A) Percentage of postnatal cells responsive to glutamate (5), kainate (λ), AMPA (υ), and NMDA (τ) between DIV1 and DIV7. B. comparison of responses at different times in culture to applications of 500 μM glutamate and 500 μM NMDA. Example responses from six different cells are shown at DIV2, DIV4, and DIV7 for glutamate and NMDA.

stabilization of connections in the developing nervous system (Durand et al., 1996; Wu et al., 1996; Isaac et al., 1997; Li and Zhuo, 1998; Rumpel et al., 1998; Liao et al., 1999; Petralia et al., 1999). In particular, Cline and colleagues have shown that NMDA receptors are functionally expressed prior to AMPA receptors in the *Xenopus* retinotectal pathway, and that NMDA activation is required for elongation of tectal dendrites (Rajan and Cline, 1998; Rajan et al., 1999). Recently, it has been reported that this involves a pathway that decreases RhoA GTPase activity (Li et al., 2000). In the present study, recordings from fetal and postnatal ganglion cells revealed few overlapping channel openings, suggesting a low density of NMDA channels. Moreover, the glutamate I/V curves for peak responses recorded in normal magnesium were nearly linear for both fetal and postnatal cells. This implies that NMDA receptors may not contribute significantly to glutamate-mediated peak responses at either developmental stage.

Comparison with glutamate receptors in RGCs of other species

A number of investigators have documented ionotropic glutamate responses in mature ganglion cells of different species (Aizenman et al., 1988; Yazejian and Fain, 1992; Rörig and Grantyn, 1993; Cohen et al., 1994). Using a retinal slice preparation, Cohen et al. (1994) showed that alpha and beta cells in the mature cat retina respond in an equivalent manner to application of glutamate and its agonists. The current–voltage relations reported in this study were similar to those we obtained in dissociated cells. While the dose response characteristics of glutamate-activated currents have not been studied previously in retinal ganglion cells of any species, our EC_{50} (220 μM) value for kainate is within the range reported for goldfish RGCs (Yazejian and Fain, 1992). The NMDA component of the glutamate-gated response in the present study was also similar to that reported previously in retinal ganglion cells (Yazejian and Fain, 1992). Thus, the available evidence indicates that retinal ganglion cells in several different species express NMDA and non-NMDA receptors with similar functional properties.

Early functional expression of glutamate receptors

Because the ontogeny of the cat retina has been well characterized the findings of the present study can be related to several key features of retinal development. Our recordings were made shortly after ganglion cells have completed their final cell division and have migrated to the ganglion cell layer (Rapaport and Stone, 1982; Walsh et al., 1983). At this early stage (E33–E38), ganglion cell axons have already innervated their central target structures (Shatz, 1983; Williams and Chalupa, 1982), but the outgrowth and differentiation of dendritic processes is still rudimentary so that different morphological classes of cells cannot be distinguished (Maslim et al., 1986; Ramoa et al., 1988). Furthermore, the period of programmed ganglion cell death has yet to begin, so at this stage there are 5–6 times as many ganglion cells as will survive to maturity (Williams et al., 1986). The first synapses form in the IPL between ganglion cells and amacrine cells around E45, and glutamatergic synapses between bipolar cells and ganglion cells are established about a week later (Maslim and Stone, 1986). Thus, our results indicate that glutamate receptors in fetal cat ganglion cells become functional several weeks before glutamatergic synaptic contacts become established and prior to the time when these neurons are capable of generating spiking activity (Skaliora et al., 1993). This means that the early functional expression of NMDA and non-NMDA receptors in retinal ganglion cells is not associated with the transmission of electrical signals in the developing retina. More likely, the early responses to glutamate described here may presage the forthcoming rapid outgrowth of dendritic processes (Ramoa et al., 1988). This suggestion is in line with the recent finding that activation of NMDA and non-NMDA glutamate receptors induces movement and extension of dendritic processes in ganglion cells of the embryonic chick retina (Wong and Wong, 2000). The high concentrations of glutamate found in the neonatal retina (Haberecht and Redburn, 1996) also signify that glutamate receptors can be activated in vitro in these early fetal cells.

At later stages of development, ionotropic glutamate receptors complete their functional maturation. As shown here, this involves a decrease in the unitary main-state NMDA channel conductance, an increase in the time-course of the glutamate receptor desensitization, and an increase in the proportion of cells responsive to glutamate and its agonists. Presumably, these maturational changes in glutamate ionotropic receptors allow ganglion cells to integrate synaptic events prior to transmission of information to the retinorecipient structures of the brain.

Acknowledgements

Supported by grants from the National Eye Institute of the NIH and the National Science Foundation. We thank our colleagues Drs. Andrew Ishida and Martin Wilson for their comments on an earlier draft of this paper.

References

Aizenman, E., Frosch, M.P. and Lipton, S.A. (1988) Responses mediated by excitatory amino acid receptors in solitary retinal ganglion cells from rat. *J. Physiol.*, 396: 75–91.

Behar, T.N., Scott, C.A., Greene, C.L., Wen, X., Smith, S.V., Maric, D., Liu, Q.Y., Colton, C.A. and Barker, J.L. (1999) Glutamate acting at NMDA receptors stimulates embryonic cortical neuronal migration. *J. Neurosci.*, 19: 4449–4461.

Ben-Ari, Y., Khazipov, R., Leinekugel, X., Caillard, O. and Gaiarsa, J.L. (1997) GABAA, NMDA and AMPA receptors: a developmentally regulated 'ménage à trois'. *Trends Neurosci.*, 20: 523–529.

Bisti, S., Gargini, C. and Chalupa, L.M. (1998) Blockade of glutamate-mediated activity in the developing retina perturbs the functional segregation of ON and OFF pathways. *J. Neurosci.*, 18(13): 5019–5025.

Bodnarenko, S.R. and Chalupa, L.M. (1993) Stratification of ON and OFF ganglion cell dendrites depends on glutamate-mediated afferent activity in the developing retina. *Nature*, 364(6433): 144–146.

Bodnarenko, S.R., Jeyarasasingam, G. and Chalupa, L.M. (1995) Development and regulation of dendritic stratification in retinal ganglion cells by glutamate-mediated afferent activity. *J. Neurosci.*, 15: 7037–7045.

Blanton, M.G. and Kriegstein, A.R. (1992) Properties of amino acid neurotransmitter receptors of embryonic cortical neurons when activated by exogenous and endogenous agonists. *J. Neurophysiol.*, 67: 1185–1200.

Cameron, H.A., Hazel, T.G. and McKay, R.D. (1998) Regulation of neurogenesis by growth factors and neurotransmitters. *J. Neurobiol.*, 36: 287–306.

Cohen, E.D., Zhou, Z.J. and Fain, G.L. (1994) Ligand-gated currents of alpha and beta ganglion cells in the cat retinal slice. *J. Neurophysiol.*, 72(3): 1260–1269.

Cuppini, R., Sartini, S., Ambrogini, P., Falcieri, E., Maltarello, M.C. and Gallo, G. (1999) Control of neuron outgrowth by NMDA receptors. *J. Submicrosc. Cytol. Pathol.*, 31(1): 31–40.

Dupont, J.L., Gardette, R. and Crepel, F. (1987) Postnatal development of the chemosensitivity of rat cerebellar Purkinje cells to excitatory amino acids. An in vitro study. *Brain Res.*, 431: 59–68.

Durand, G.M., Kovalchuk, Y. and Konnerth, A. (1996) Long-term potentiation and functional synapse induction in developing hippocampus. *Nature*, 381(6577): 71–75.

Edwards, F.A., Konnerth, A., Sakmann, B. and Takahashi, T. (1989) A thin slice preparation for patch clamp recordings from neurones of the mammalian central nervous system. *Pflugers Arch. Eur. J. Physiol.*, 414: 600–612.

Fox, K., Schlaggar, B.L., Glazewski, S. and O'Leary, D.D. (1996) Glutamate receptor blockade at cortical synapses disrupts development of thalamocortical and columnar organization in somatosensory cortex. *Proc. Natl. Acad. Sci. USA*, 93(11): 5584–5589.

Fox, K., Henley, J. and Isaac, J. (1999) Experience-dependent development of NMDA receptor transmission. *Nat. Neurosci.*, 2: 297–299.

Gleason, E.L. and Spitzer, N.C. (1998) AMPA and NMDA receptors expressed by differentiating *Xenopus* spinal neurons. *J. Neurophysiol.*, 79(6): 2986–2998.

Haberecht, M.F. and Redburn, D.A. (1996) High levels of extracellular glutamate are present in retina during neonatal development. *Neurochem. Res.*, 21(2): 285–291.

Hamill, O.P., Marty, A., Neher, E., Sakmann, B. and Sigworth, F.J. (1981) Improved patch-clamp techniques for high-resolution current recording from cells and cell-free membrane patches. *Pflugers Arch. Eur. J. Physiol.*, 391: 85–100.

Isaac, J.T., Nicoll, R.A. and Malenka, R.C. (1995) Evidence for silent synapses: implications for the expression of LTP. *Neuron*, 15: 427–434.

Isaac, J.T., Crair, M.C., Nicoll, R.A. and Malenka, R.C. (1997) Silent synapses during development of thalamocortical inputs. *Neuron*, 18(2): 269–280.

Karschin, A. and Wässle, H. (1990) Voltage- and transmitter-gated currents in isolated rod bipolar cells of rat retina. *J. Neurophysiol.*, 63: 860–876.

Komuro, H. and Rakic, P. (1993) Modulation of neuronal migration by NMDA receptors. *Science*, 260: 95–97.

Komuro, H. and Rakic, P. (1996) Intracellular Ca2+ fluctuations modulate the rate of neuronal migration. *Neuron*, 17: 275–285.

Krishtal, O.A. and Pidoplichko, V.I. (1980) A receptor for protons in the nerve cell membrane. *Neuroscience*, 5: 2325–2327.

Li, P. and Zhuo, M. (1998) Silent glutamatergic synapses and nociception in mammalian spinal cord. *Nature*, 393(6686): 695–698.

Li, Y., Erzurumlu, R.S., Chen, C., Jhaveri, S. and Tonegawa, S. (1994) Whisker-related neuronal patterns fail to develop in the trigeminal brainstem nuclei of NMDAR1 knockout mice. *Cell*, 76: 427–437.

Li, Z., Aelst, L.V. and Cline, H.T. (2000) Rho GTPases regulate distinct aspects of dendritic arbor growth in *Xenopus* central neurons in vivo. *Nat. Neurosci.*, 3(3): 217–225.

Liao, D., Hessler, N.A. and Malinow, R. (1995) Activation of postsynaptically silent synapses during pairing-induced LTP in CA1 region of hippocampal slice. *Nature*, 75(6530): 400–404.

Liao, D., Zhang, X., O'Brien, R., Ehlers, M.D. and Huganir, R.L. (1999) Regulation of morphological postsynaptic silent synapses in developing hippocampal neurons. *Nat. Neurosci.*, 2(1): 37–43.

LoTurco, J.J., Blanton, M.G. and Kriegstein, A.R. (1991) Initial expression and endogenous activation of NMDA channels in early neocortical development. *J. Neurosci.*, 11: 792–799.

Maslim, J. and Stone, J. (1986) Synaptogenesis in the retina of the cat. *Brain Res.*, 373: 35–48.

Maslim, J., Webster, M. and Stone, J. (1986) Stages in the structural differentiation of retinal ganglion cells. *J. Comp. Neurol.*, 254(3): 382–402.

Meister, M., Wong, R.O., Baylor, D.A. and Shatz, C.J. (1991) Synchronous bursts of action potentials in ganglion cells of the developing mammalian retina. *Science*, 252: 939–943.

Metzger, F., Wiese, S. and Sendtner, M. (1998) Effect of glutamate on dendritic growth in embryonic rat motoneurons. *J. Neurosci.*, 18(5): 1735–1742.

Morrison, M.E. and Mason, C.A. (1998) Granule neuron regulation of Purkinje cell development: striking a balance between neurotrophin and glutamate signaling. *J. Neurosci.*, 18(10): 3563–3573.

Petralia, R.S., Esteban, J.A., Wang, Y.X., Partridge, J.G., Zhao, H.M., Wenthold, R.J. and Malinow, R. (1999) Selective acquisition of AMPA receptors over postnatal development suggests a molecular basis for silent synapses. *Nat. Neurosci.*, 2: 31–36.

Rajan, I. and Cline, H.T. (1998) Glutamate receptor activity is required for normal development of tectal cell dendrites in vivo. *J. Neurosci.*, 18: 7836–7846.

Rajan, I., Witte, S. and Cline, H.T. (1999) NMDA receptor activity stabilizes presynaptic retinotectal axons and postsynaptic optic tectal cell dendrites in vivo. *J. Neurobiol.*, 38: 357–368.

Ramoa, A.S., Campbell, G. and Shatz, C.J. (1988) Dendritic growth and remodeling of cat retinal ganglion cells during fetal and postnatal development. *J. Neurosci.*, 8(11): 4239–4261.

Rapaport, D.H. and Stone, J. (1982) The site of commencement of maturation in mammalian retina: observations in the cat. *Brain Res.*, 281: 273–279.

Rapaport, D.H., Robinson, S.R. and Stone, J. (1985) Cytogenesis in the developing retina of the cat. *Aust. New Zealand J. Ophthalmol.*, 13: 113–124.

Rörig, B. and Grantyn, R. (1993) Glutamatergic and GABAergic synaptic currents in ganglion cells from isolated retinae of pigmented rats during postnatal development. *Dev. Brain Res.*, 74(1): 98–110.

Rörig, B. and Grantyn, R. (1994) Ligand- and voltage-gated ion channels are expressed by embryonic mouse retinal neurones. *NeuroReport*, 5: 1197–1200.

Rumpel, S., Hatt, H. and Gottmann, K. (1998) Silent synapses in the developing rat visual cortex: evidence for postsynaptic expression of synaptic plasticity. *J. Neurosci.*, 18(21): 8863–8874.

Schlaggar, B.L., Fox, K. and O'Leary, D.D. (1993) Postsynaptic control of plasticity in developing somatosensory cortex. *Nature*, 364: 623–626.

Shatz, C.J. (1983) The prenatal development of the cat's retinogeniculate pathway. *J. Neurosci.*, 3: 482–499.

Skaliora, I., Scobey, R.P. and Chalupa, L.M. (1993) Prenatal development of excitability in cat retinal ganglion cells: action potentials and sodium currents. *J. Neurosci.*, 13: 313–323.

Skaliora, I., Robinson, D.W., Scobey, R.P. and Chalupa, L.M. (1995) Properties of K+ conductances in cat retinal ganglion cells during the period of activity-mediated refinements in retinofugal pathways. *Eur. J. Neurosci.*, 7: 1558–1568.

Simon, D.K., Prusky, G.T., O'Leary, D.D. and Constantine-Paton, M. (1992) N-Methyl-D-aspartate receptor antagonists disrupt the formation of a mammalian neural map. *Proc. Natl. Acad. Sci. USA*, 89: 10593–10597.

Vallano, M.L. (1998) Developmental aspects of NMDA receptor function. *Crit. Rev. Neurobiol.*, 12: 177–204.

Walsh, C., Polley, E.H., Hickey, T.L. and Guillery, R.W. (1983) Generation of cat retinal ganglion cells in relation to central pathways. *Nature*, 302: 611–614.

Williams, R.W. and Chalupa, L.M. (1982) Prenatal development of retinocollicular projections in the cat: an anterograde tracer transport study. *J. Neurosci.*, 2: 604–622.

Williams, R.W., Bastiani, M.J., Lia, B. and Chalupa, L.M. (1986) Growth cones, dying axons, and developmental fluctuations in the fiber population of the cat's optic nerve. *J. Comp. Neurol.*, 246: 32–69.

Wong, R.O. (1995) Effects of glutamate and its analogs on intracellular calcium levels in the developing retina. *Vis. Neurosci.*, 12: 907–917.

Wong, R.O. (1999) Retinal waves: stirring up a storm. *Neuron*, 24(3): 493–495.

Wong, W.T. and Wong, R.O.L. (2000) Rapid dendritic movements during synapse formation and rearrangement. *Curr. Opin. Neurobiol.*, 10: 118–124.

Wong, R.O., Meister, M. and Shatz, C.J. (1993) Transient period of correlated bursting activity during development of the mammalian retina. *Neuron*, 11(5): 923–938.

Wong, W.T., Myhr, K.L., Miller, E.D. and Wong, R.O.L. (2000) Developmental changes in the neurotransmitter regulation of correlated spontaneous retinal activity. *J. Neurosci.*, 20(1): 351–360.

Wu, G., Malinow, R. and Cline, H.T. (1996) Maturation of a central glutamatergic synapse. *Science*, 274: 972–976.

Yazejian, B. and Fain, G.L. (1992) Excitatory amino acid receptors on isolated retinal ganglion cells from the goldfish. *J. Neurophysiol.*, 67: 94–107.

Yuan, X., Eisen, A.M., McBain, C.J. and Gallo, V. (1998) A role for glutamate and its receptors in the regulation of oligodendrocyte development in cerebellar tissue slices. *Development*, 125(15): 2901–2914.

C. Casanova and M. Ptito (Eds.)
Progress in Brain Research, Vol. 134

CHAPTER 2

The dynamics of primate retinal ganglion cells

Ehud Kaplan [1,*] and Ethan Benardete [2]

[1] *Departments of Ophthalmology/Biophysics, The Mount Sinai School of Medicine, One Gustave Levy Place, New York, NY 10016, USA*
[2] *NYU School of Medicine, New York, NY 10029, USA*

Abstract: A knowledge of the dynamics (temporal properties) of neuronal populations is essential for an understanding of their function, and is also crucial when one attempts to develop computational or mathematical models of the neurons. Here we review the temporal properties of the receptive fields (RFs) of the two best-studied types of ganglion cells in the primate retina, those that project to the parvocellular (P) and magnocellular (M) layers of the dorsal lateral geniculate nucleus. The center and surround mechanisms of the P RFs are approximately linear, and their impulse responses are very similar, although the surround lags the center by a few milliseconds. The center and surround are chromatically opponent. With the appropriate stimulus, one can find significant nonlinearities in their responses, and also in the interaction between the center and surround. The phase lag between the responses of the center and surround depends on the temporal frequency, so that at high temporal frequency the antagonism between them is reduced or abolished. The temporal responses of M cells are nonlinear, and with increasing contrast they show the effects of a contrast gain control. The different dynamical properties of the two populations suggest that M cells participate in motion analysis, while P cells are used for the analysis of form, texture, and perhaps color.

Introduction

In this section, we shall review briefly the properties and anatomical organization of the neuronal populations that we shall consider, and provide the motivation for a discussion of the dynamical aspects of their function.

Parallel pathways from retina to cortex

The vertebrate retina is a complex structure, with well over 100 million neural elements, which include approximately 80 different cell types (Dacey, 2000), arranged in five major layers. The retina converts the visual image that impinges on its photoreceptors into a spatiotemporal pattern of neural signals, and after significant processing, which lasts for an astonishing 15–35 ms (see, for example, Maunsell et al., 1999), the results are delivered to the rest of the brain via axons of the retinal ganglion cells (RGCs), which together make up the optic nerve. In the primate, each optic nerve contains approximately one million axons, 90% of which project to the lateral geniculate nucleus (LGN).

It is now well established that — at least in the primate retina — the ganglion cells include several classes, with distinct anatomical and physiological properties (for a review, see Rodieck, 1988; Kaplan et al., 1990). The two best-studied classes of RGCs are the M and P cell classes, which project, respectively, to the magnocellular and parvocellular layers of the LGN. They correspond to the anatomically identified parasol and midget retinal ganglion cells, described by Polyak (1941). These two cell types are sometimes referred to as P_α and P_β (Perry and Cowey, 1981): the P is for Primate, and the α and β subscripts are a reference to the α and β ganglion cell

* Corresponding author: E. Kaplan, Departments of Ophthalmology/Biophysics, The Mount Sinai School of Medicine, One Gustave Levy Place, New York, NY 10029, USA. Tel.: +1-212-241-9607; Fax: +1-212-289-5984; E-mail: kaplane@rockvax.rockefeller.edu

types of the cat retina (Boycott and Wässle, 1974). In the LGN, a third type, usually referred to as K (koniocellular), has been added more recently. It represents the intercalated cells, which account for approximately 9% of the cells in the LGN (Casagrande, 1994; Hendry and Yoshioka, 1994). The identity of the retinal cells that project to it is still under active investigation, and they will not be discussed here.

The first report of a functional difference between the M and the P neuronal types focused on their dynamical (and chromatic) properties: Gouras (1968) reported that some primate ganglion cells were *phasic* (and chromatically broad-band), while others were *tonic* (and chromatically antagonistic) in their responses to steps of light increments. These have later become known as M (transient) and P (sustained) cells. These two types were later shown to differ in their size and projection patterns: the tonic cells project to the upper 4 layers of the monkey LGN, which contain small cells (parvocellular), while the phasic cells project to the lower two layers, those that contain large cells (magnocellular) (Perry et al., 1984).

The three neural streams (M, P and K) project from the LGN to distinct layers and compartments of the primary visual cortex. The magnocellular axons terminate in layers $4C_\alpha$ and 4B, while the parvocellular axons project to $4C_\beta$. The axons of the K group project to layers 2–3 and terminate in the cytochrome oxidase blobs (Carroll and Wong-Riley, 1984; Casagrande, 1994; Hendry and Yoshioka, 1994; Livingstone and Hubel, 1984). There is some evidence that the segregation persists beyond V1 as well (Wong-Riley and Carroll, 1984), although functionally there is evidence for mixing of the signals that are conveyed by the M and P streams (Merigan and Maunsell, 1993). Our knowledge of the third group is much more limited at the present.

In addition to the difference in their temporal response patterns, the M and P streams have been shown to differ in several other important ways (for a review, see Kaplan et al., 1990). The M cells (and their magnocellular LGN targets) have larger receptive fields and cell bodies, have higher sensitivity to luminance contrast (Kaplan and Shapley, 1986), and, as noted earlier, show little or no chromatic antagonism (but see Derrington et al., 1984 and Smith et al., 1992). The P cells (and their parvocellular LGN targets) have smaller receptive fields and somas, their luminance contrast sensitivity is lower, and most of them show clear chromatic opponency (Wiesel and Hubel, 1966; De Monasterio and Gouras, 1975; Derrington et al., 1984). It is this constellation of different properties, together with the distinct projection patterns of the two streams, that has led to the notion that the two are engaged in parallel processing of different aspects of the visual scene (Livingstone and Hubel, 1988; Zeki and Shipp, 1988).

Why neuronal dynamics is worth studying

We use the term *dynamics* to describe processes that evolve in time. Much of what is interesting about the *function* of various systems in the body, including the nervous system, is dynamical. The dynamical properties of a neuron (such as the time course of its response, the latency, the temporal spectrum of its sensitivity or of its response) serve at least two important functions: (1) they suggest a possible function for the neuron or neuronal stream; and (2) they inform us about the possible cellular (or network) mechanisms that are involved in shaping the dynamical properties. For example, the short latency and transient response of the Y ganglion cells in the cat retina suggest that they might be involved in temporal analysis or in an alerting response, while the more sustained response of X cells makes them more suitable for the (spatial) analysis of form. In addition, dynamical analysis of the responses of Y ganglion cells from the cat retina has suggested the existence of rectifying ‘nonlinear subunits’ that are responsible for some of the features of the responses from these cells (Enroth-Cugell and Robson, 1966; Hochstein and Shapley, 1976a,b). Such insights are useful in directing further exploration of the anatomical circuitry and biophysical properties of neurons.

The rich anatomical diversity of retinal ganglion cells is bewildering (see, for example, Watanabe and Rodieck, 1989; Rodieck and Watanabe, 1993; Dacey, 1999a, 2000). One possible reason for it is that each of the various cell types carves out a temporal niche for itself, and together they cover the entire dynamical spectrum that the animal requires. For example, cells that report diurnal changes in light level do not need a high temporal resolution, but cells that track possible predators do. In addition, it is possible that some of the morphological diversity has to do with chromatic selectivity, or some other kind of selectivity. After all, the number of aspects of the visual environment that the visual system must analyze is unknown, but it is probably not small.

Knowledge of the dynamical properties of the neuronal streams that we consider is useful in another context. Quantitative modeling of (any part of) the visual system requires a reasonably detailed understanding of their temporal capabilities. In addition, such knowledge can be used in the interpretation of experimental data. For instance, when one examines recordings that reflect the responses of many cells, such as the electroretinogram (ERG), electroencephalogram (EEG), or data obtained with various imaging methods (magnetoencephalogram, MEG, or functional magnetic resonance imaging, fMRI), one might be able to discern in the records the typical dynamical signature of one cell type or another (for example, Baseler and Sutter, 1997; Klistorner et al., 1997; Valberg and Rudvin, 1997; Rudvin et al., 2000).

Finally, certain aspects of the dynamics have some theoretical importance. For example, some hypotheses about the function of some of the types of primate ganglion cells hold only if they are linear (for example, Ingling and Martinez-Uriegas, 1983). It is important, therefore, to study the neuronal dynamics with the appropriate experimental and analytical tools in order to establish the limits of linearity.

In the following sections, we shall review the dynamics of the major classes of retinal ganglion cells in the primate retina. In each subsection we shall consider first linear responses, followed by a discussion of the nonlinear behavior.

Dynamics of the magnocellular pathway

Linear responses

The M class of primate RGCs projects to the two most ventral layers of the LGN (Perry and Cowey, 1981). A number of investigators have recognized the unique properties of this type of RGC. In particular, four aspects were emphasized: the transient response to flashes, the larger size of the receptive field, the lack of clear chromatic opponency and the relatively high sensitivity to luminance contrast (Gouras, 1968; Kaplan and Shapley, 1986; Kaplan et al., 1990; Croner and Kaplan, 1995).

Benardete and Kaplan (1999b) wished to characterize in more detail the temporal properties of M cells, and used a temporally broadband stimulus, composed of a sum of several frequencies. They found that at low luminance contrast (<2%), M cells have a temporal frequency response that peaks at approximately 10 Hz, similar to what was found for P cells (Benardete and Kaplan, 1997a; Fig. 1). However, even at low contrast, the response of M cells shows less phase lag than that of P cells, indicating that it peaks earlier than the response of P cells.

Early experiments indicated that the temporal frequency responses of both On and Off M cells depended on stimulus contrast (Benardete et al., 1992; Lee et al., 1994). For a typical M cell, as contrast increased from 1 to 12%, the peak of the temporal frequency response shifted from 8 to 16 Hz. To see the effect more clearly, we calculate the contrast gain, which is the response divided by the stimulus contrast, a quantity that has units of impulses/s-% contrast. As contrast increases, the contrast gain at low temporal frequencies decreases (Fig. 2). In addition, the phase of the sinusoidal response advances (Fig. 1). If the frequency response of an M cell is transformed into the time domain, it is evident that with increased contrast the response of an M cell to a pulse of unit contrast becomes smaller and less delayed (Fig. 3).

In the cat retina, it was observed previously that both X and Y RGCs show a selective attenuation of contrast gain at low temporal frequency and phase advance with increasing contrast. Shapley and Victor (1978, 1979) termed the nonlinear mechanism that regulates this change in gain 'the contrast gain control.' While the same phenomenon is observed in M cells, it is not observed in P cells, suggesting a possible homology between the M cell population and some of the RGCs of lower mammals (Benardete et al., 1992).

Teleologically, the contrast gain control mechanism allows the M cell to function as a selective filter. As contrast in the visual scene (and with it, the signal-to-noise ratio) increases, the low temporal frequencies that dominate the visual environment can be relatively attenuated, to allow the finer temporal detail (the higher frequencies) to stand out. A similar theory has been used to explain the spatial selectivity

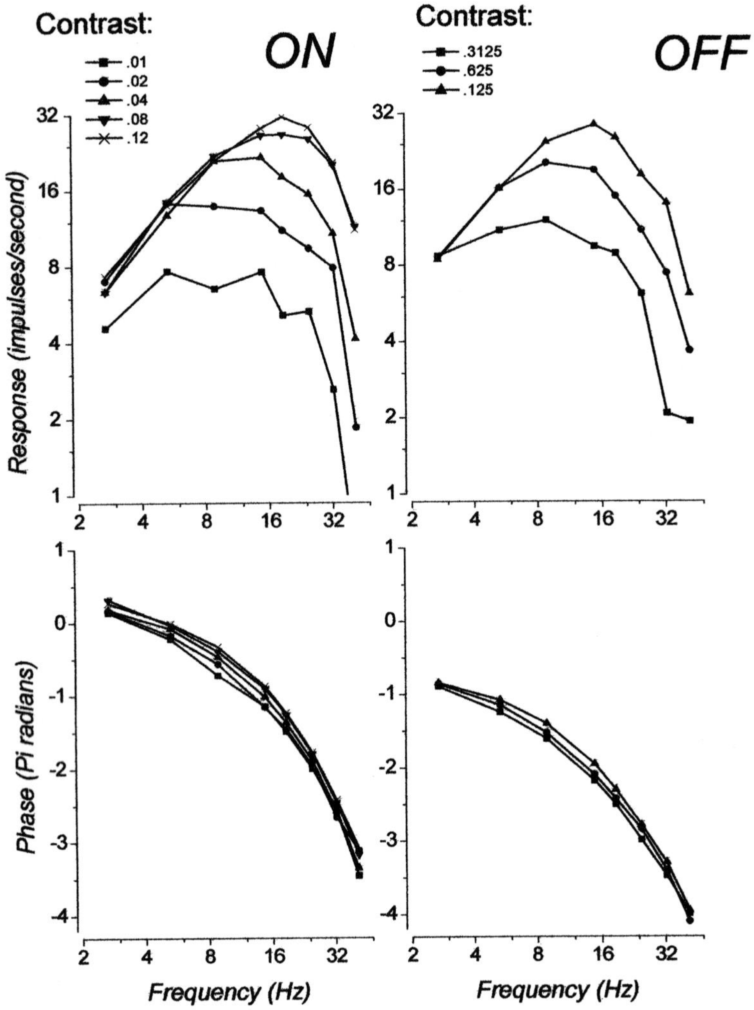

Fig. 1. The temporal frequency response of two representative M cells: an On cell (left) and an Off cell (right) at several contrasts. The upper row shows the amplitude of the response and the bottom row shows the phase. The contrasts used in each case are listed in the upper left of each column. The stimulus was an achromatic grating modulated by a sum-of-sinusoids. Note that amplitude of the response increases more at high temporal frequency as contrast increases; the phase of the response also advances (from Benardete and Kaplan, 1999b).

of RGCs (Atick and Redlich, 1992). Experimentally, this has been demonstrated by observing that the response of M cells to steps of contrast becomes more transient as contrast in the step increases (Benardete and Kaplan, 1999b).

Nonlinear responses

Because of the contrast gain control mechanism, the temporal frequency responses of M cells are nonlinear, except at very low contrast (<1%). In other words, the response does not scale linearly with contrast. As in the cat (Shapley and Victor, 1979), most of the contrast signal that controls the contrast gain originates in the surround of the M cell receptive field, and is spatial-phase insensitive (Benardete and Kaplan, 1999b).

Another manifestation of the nonlinearity of M cells is the X/Y classification adapted from the experiments of Enroth-Cugell and Robson (1966) and of Hochstein and Shapley (1976b) on the cat retina. Kaplan and Shapley (1982) have reported that a mi-

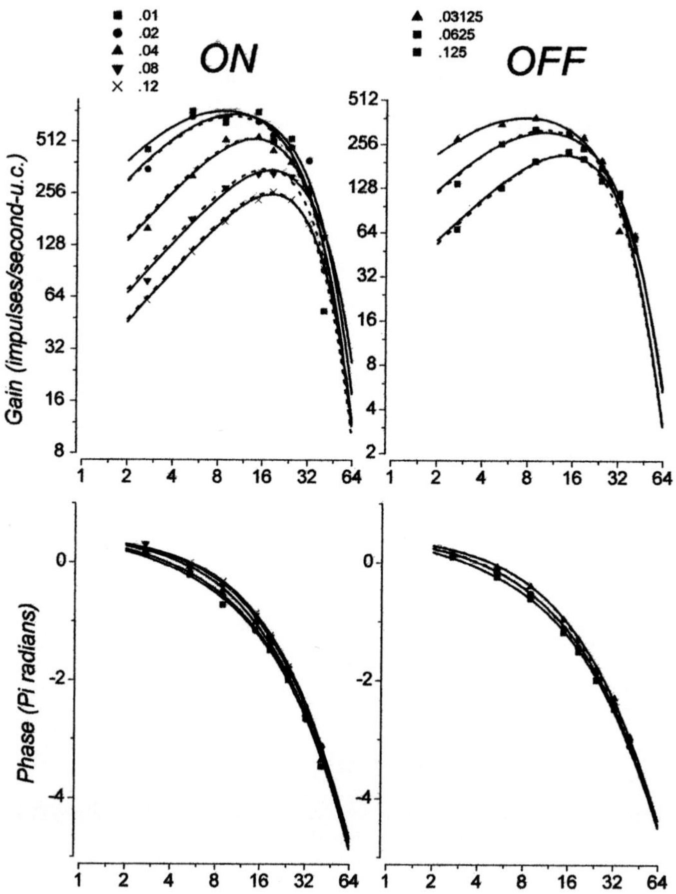

Fig. 2. The contrast gain (response/contrast) of M cells depends on both temporal frequency and contrast. The experimental data from Fig. 1 has been fitted with a model (Victor, 1987) that consists of a series of low-pass filters and a high-pass filter. Note that as contrast increases, the contrast gain at low temporal frequencies decreases for both On and Off cells (from Benardete and Kaplan, 1999b).

nority of M cells in the primate retina are Y-type when classified according to the linearity of spatial summation within their receptive fields, as Enroth-Cugell and Robson did originally for cat RGCs. These cells have spatial-phase insensitive responses that are mostly at *twice* the frequency of the stimulus. This nonlinearity was thoroughly investigated in cat Y RGCs by Shapley and Victor (1979), and there it was found to depend on input from a collection of small, nonlinear receptive field subunits. However, the Y-type M RGCs seem to be much less numerous than the X-type (Kaplan and Shapley, 1982; Derrington et al., 1984; Benardete and Kaplan, 1999b). Although both types of M cells demonstrate the contrast gain control mechanism, only M cells of the Y-type show strong frequency doubled responses. Lee et al. (1989b) have shown that, as was found in the cat, the M cells' frequency doubled response reflects the activity of a spatially extended mechanism, since small spots centered on the middle of the receptive field failed to elicit such responses.

Dynamics of the parvocellular pathway

Linear responses

P cells make up the majority of the RGCs in the primate retina. The temporal responses of these cells have been usually characterized as being predominately linear (for example, Smith et al., 1992). In general, however, these studies employed stimuli of low contrast. In order to verify and expand upon

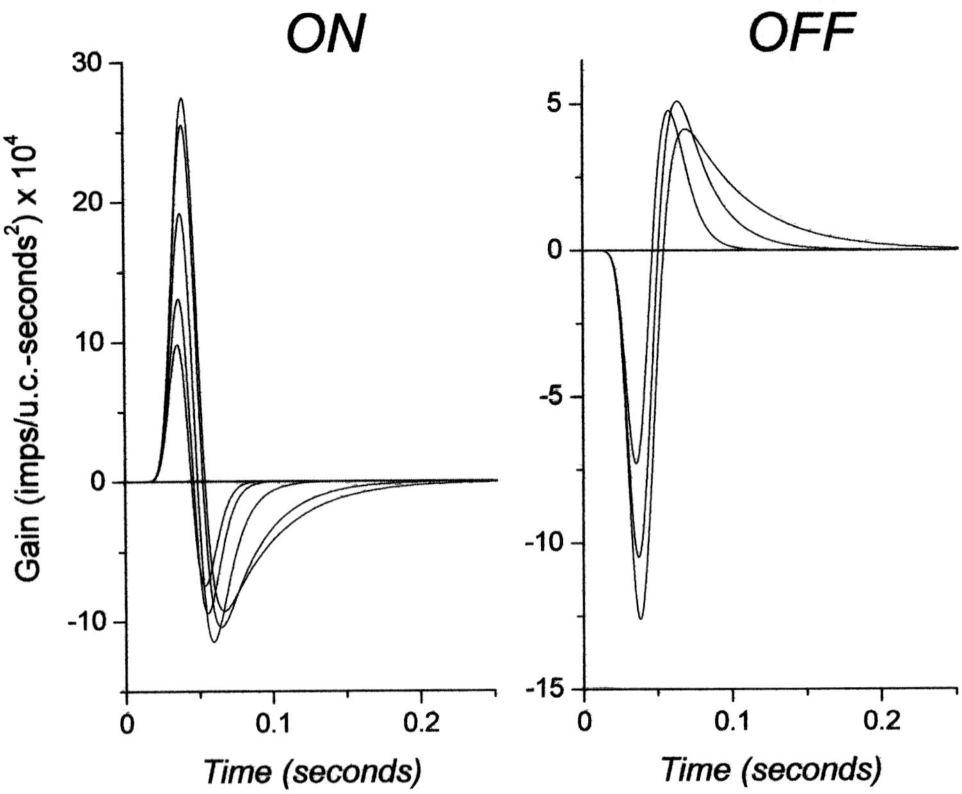

Fig. 3. The impulse response of M cells changes with increasing contrast. Data from two typical cells are illustrated: On cell (left) and Off cell (right). The impulse responses were calculated as the inverse Fourier transforms of the data shown in Fig. 2. Note that as contrast increases, the size of the impulse response decreases and the peak of the impulse response becomes less delayed (from Benardete and Kaplan, 1999b).

these results, Benardete and Kaplan used sinusoidal gratings as well as spots and annuli modulated by a pseudorandom sequence ('m-sequences', Sutter, 1987) of contrast pulses to determine the temporal response of P cells to chromatic and achromatic modulations over a wide range of contrasts (Benardete and Kaplan, 1997a,b). The center and surround of the receptive field of P cells were stimulated with spots and annuli, respectively. The responses of both center and surround regions were found to scale linearly with contrast (Fig. 4). The center response peaks around 40–50 ms when measured in the LGN as a synaptic (S) potential, a measurement that includes the conduction time from the retina to the LGN and the synaptic delay within the LGN (see Kaplan and Shapley, 1984). The surround response, measured with a large annulus, is delayed, on average, an additional 5–10 ms. This value is similar to the 3–8-ms delay reported by Smith et al. (1992). The response of the P cell to a large spot is predicted reasonably well by the linear addition of the center and surround responses. The linear prediction failed only at high luminance contrast and with low spatial frequency stimulation.

To investigate further the dynamics of the cone input to the center and surround mechanisms of the receptive field, Benardete and Kaplan employed an extension of the m-sequence technique (Benardete and Victor, 1994). They modulated *simultaneously* but *independently* two chromatic sinusoidal gratings in the receptive field of an individual P cell. The chromaticity of each grating was adjusted to stimulate only a *single* cone class (so-called 'cone-isolating gratings', see Estévez and Spekreijse, 1982). The results confirmed what has been observed in the previous experiments that used spots and annuli:

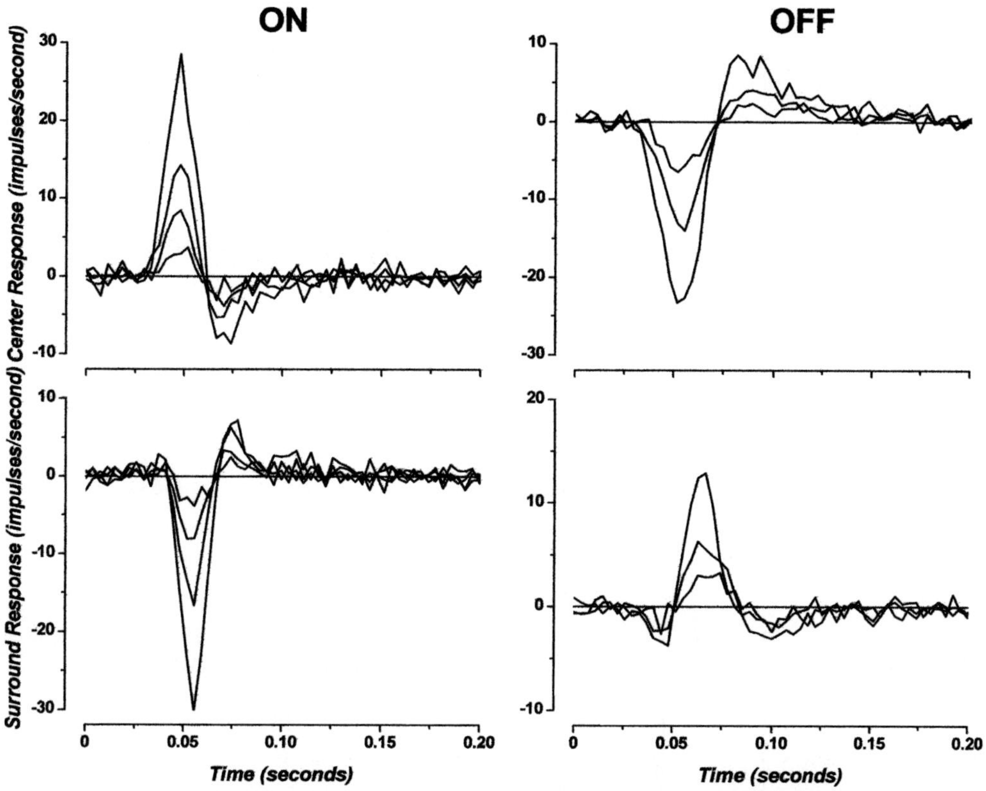

Fig. 4. The first-order responses of a P cell center and surround. The response of the center (upper row) was determined with a small spot modulated with an m-sequence. The response of the surround (lower row) was determined with an annulus modulated with another m-sequence. The various lines show responses to various contrasts. For the On cell (left) the contrasts were: 0.0625, 0.125, 0.25 and 0.5. For the Off cell (right) the contrasts were: 0.125, 0.25 and 0.5. Note that the first order responses of both center and surround mechanisms scale approximately linearly with contrast (from Benardete and Kaplan, 1997a).

the center and surround of the P cell receptive field are chromatically opponent, with each mechanism dominated by a single cone class, e.g. M (middle wavelength) or L (long wavelength) cones in the center and L (or M) cones in the surround (Fig. 5). This similarity of the temporal behavior of the center and the surround of P cells is consistent with earlier results obtained by Gielen et al. (1982), who used white noise stimulation to measure the temporal properties of monkey LGN cells, and with the results of Smith et al. (1992).

The chromatic opponency of P cells and their parvocellular LGN targets is well known (Wiesel and Hubel, 1966; De Monasterio and Gouras, 1975; Derrington et al., 1984). Furthermore, the center and surround again behaved linearly with increasing cone contrast, and their responses summed in a linear way. The peak of the center response occurs at approximately 40–50 ms, similar to the results obtained with small spots. The surround response is delayed by an additional 3–5 ms under conditions of chromatic isolation (Fig. 5). The optimal temporal frequency for both the center and surround responses is approximately 8 Hz. The phase of the surround response typically lags that of the center response (Fig. 6). Once again, the overall linearity of the P cell response seems to be violated only at high luminance contrasts and low spatial frequencies.

Spatiotemporal coupling and center-surround phase lag

When the response of a system (in our case, a receptive field of a RGC) can be described as the product

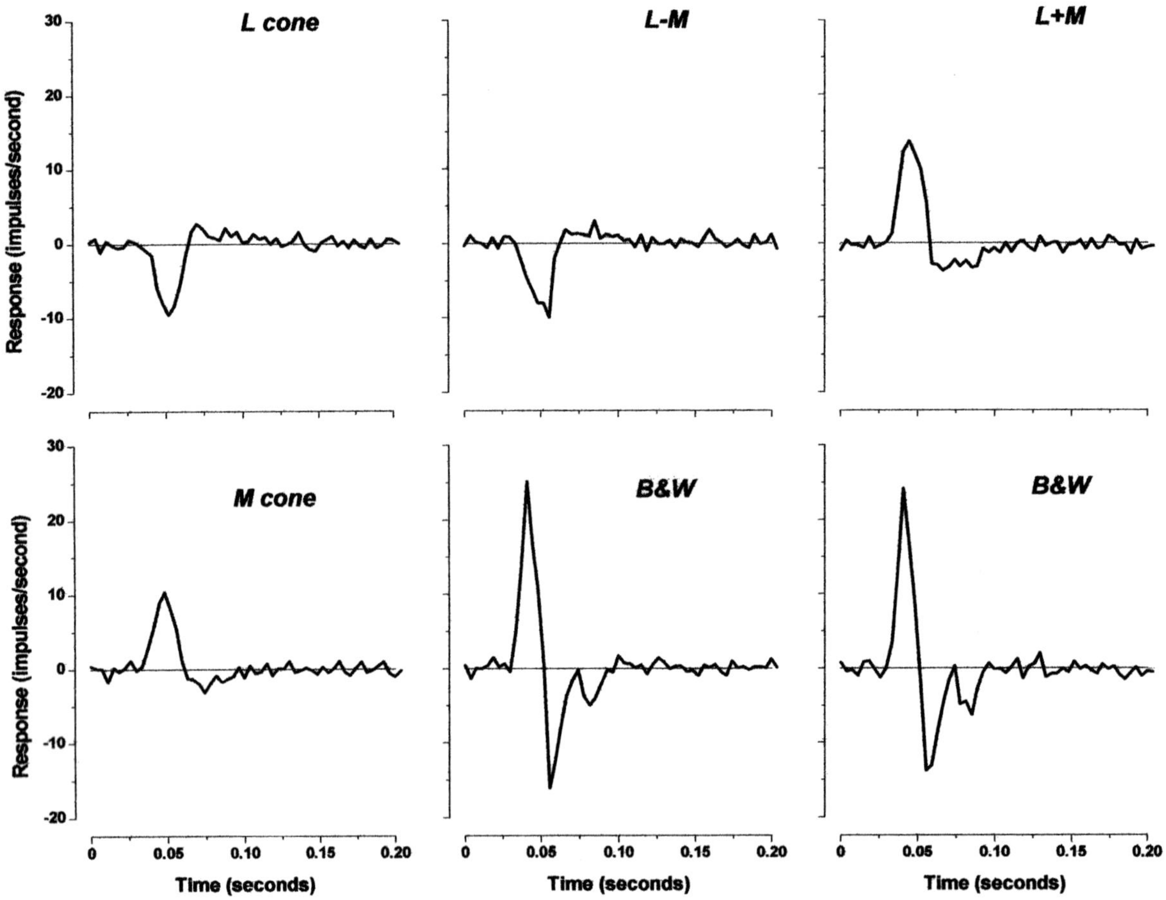

Fig. 5. The first order responses of a P On cell to two coarse gratings (spatial frequency: 0.145 c/deg) presented simultaneously, each modulated by its own m-sequence. Each row represents the response of the cell as calculated from the data recorded during the simultaneous stimulation. Left column: the center and surround of this cell responded to M and L cone isolating gratings, respectively. Middle column: the response of the same cell to a simultaneously modulated isoluminant red–green and black–white grating. Right column: the response of the same cell to a simultaneously modulated L+M grating (stimulating a mixture of L and M cones) and a black–white grating (from Benardete and Kaplan, 1999a).

of two functions, one dependent on space and the other dependent on time, the system is said to be *spatiotemporally separable*. In that case, the spatial properties of the receptive field do not depend on the temporal frequency at which they are measured, and the temporal properties are independent of the spatial parameters of the stimulus used to measure them. RGCs in the primate retina, however, are not spatiotemporally separable, as is shown in a typical example from a P Off cell in Fig. 7. Similar results for the cat RGCs were reported by Dawis et al. (1984) and by Frishman et al. (1987). As Fig. 7 shows, at high temporal frequency the receptive field becomes less selective for size: the attenuation at low spatial frequencies is reduced, compared to what is seen at low temporal frequencies. This reduction in spatial antagonism could, in principle, be due to the surround being slower than the center, or to a change in the phase relationships between the center and surround as temporal frequency increases. Fig. 6 shows that the high frequency cutoff of the surround mechanism is similar to that of the center, and that the phase difference between the responses of these two mechanisms *increases* as temporal frequency increases. This results in the loss of spatial antagonism that is depicted in Fig. 7.

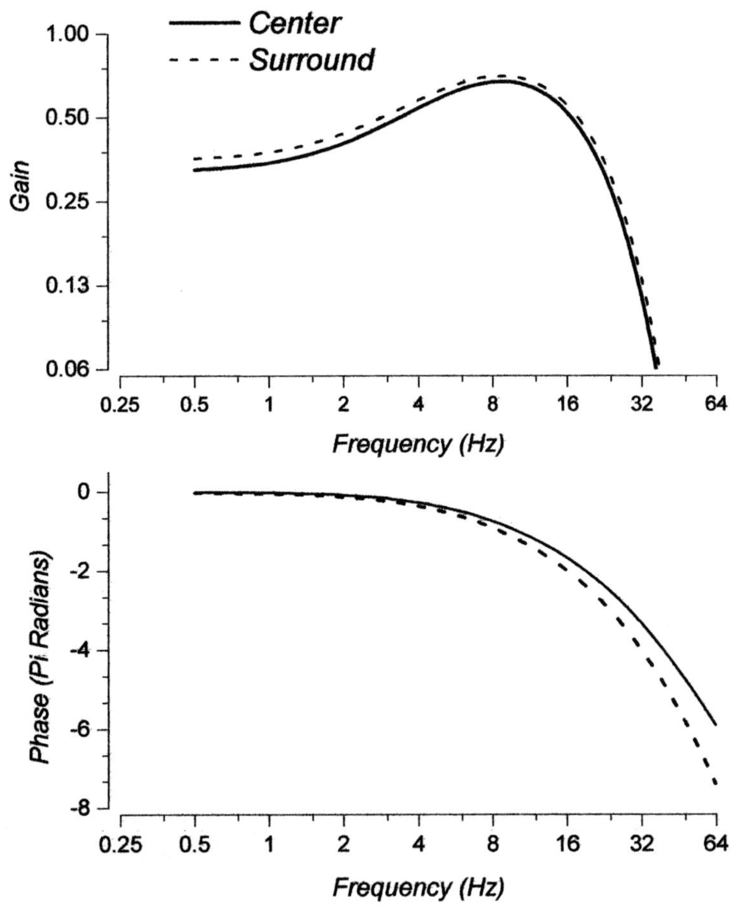

Fig. 6. The temporal frequency responses of the P cell center and surround mechanisms, derived from the population average of the model fits. Note that the center and surround amplitude response are rather similar, but the phase of the surround lags that of the center (from Benardete and Kaplan, 1999a).

The dependence of the center-surround phase lag on temporal frequency also abolishes the chromatic antagonism that is observed in parvocellular neurons (Wiesel and Hubel, 1966; De Monasterio and Gouras, 1975; Gouras and Zrenner, 1979; Benardete et al., 1992; Smith et al., 1992). A similar loss of spatial antagonism at higher temporal frequencies had been reported for the celebrated lateral eye of the horseshoe crab, *Limulus* (Ratliff et al., 1969, 1970) and in the receptive fields of cells in the cat LGN (Kaplan et al., 1979).

The results just cited tell us that the classical view of the center and surround receptive fields as mutually *antagonistic* mechanisms (Kuffler, 1953) holds *only* at those (low) temporal frequencies where the phases of the responses elicited from them are approximately opposite. At other frequencies, the center and surrounds responses add constructively, and their summed response is *larger* than the response of either the center or the surround mechanism alone.

Nonlinear responses

When one is investigating the linearity of a system, it is best to use specialized methods that are appropriate for the task. For that reason, and to further investigate the nonlinearity of P cells at high luminance contrast, Benardete and Kaplan (1997b) used the extended m-sequence method again to modulate simultaneously a spot and an annulus in the receptive

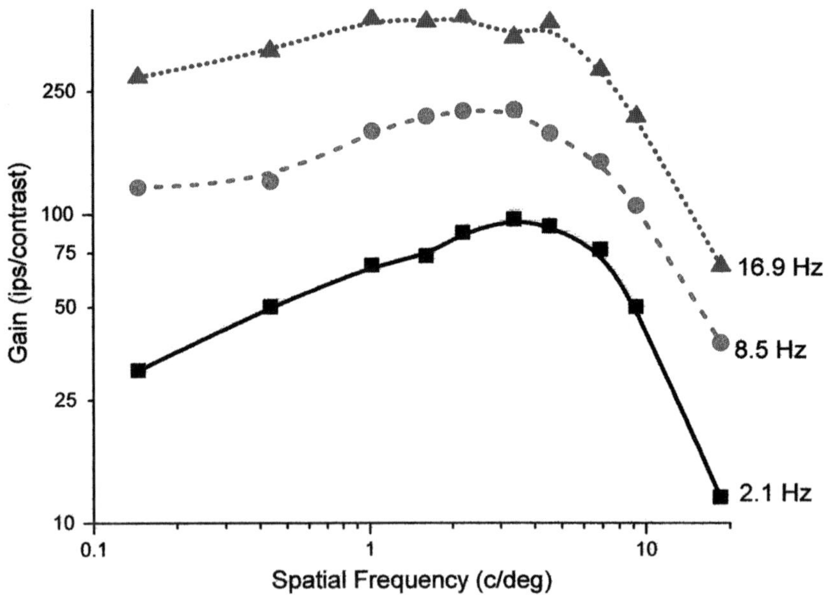

Fig. 7. The spatial frequency response of a P Off RGC measured with a drifting black–white grating at three temporal frequencies, indicated on the right. Note that as temporal frequency increases, the attenuation at low spatial frequency decreases.

field of a P cell. Significant second-order responses were detected in both On and Off P cells, and these responses originated from the center, from the surround, and also from the interaction of the two. The nonlinear response of the center mechanism is illustrated in Fig. 8. These second-order responses were consistent with a nonlinear mechanism acting in the P cell pathway. This mechanism can be mathematically modeled by a linear-nonlinear-linear (LNL) filter 'sandwich', suggesting that this second-order response does not represent a trivial nonlinearity like saturation or spike truncation.

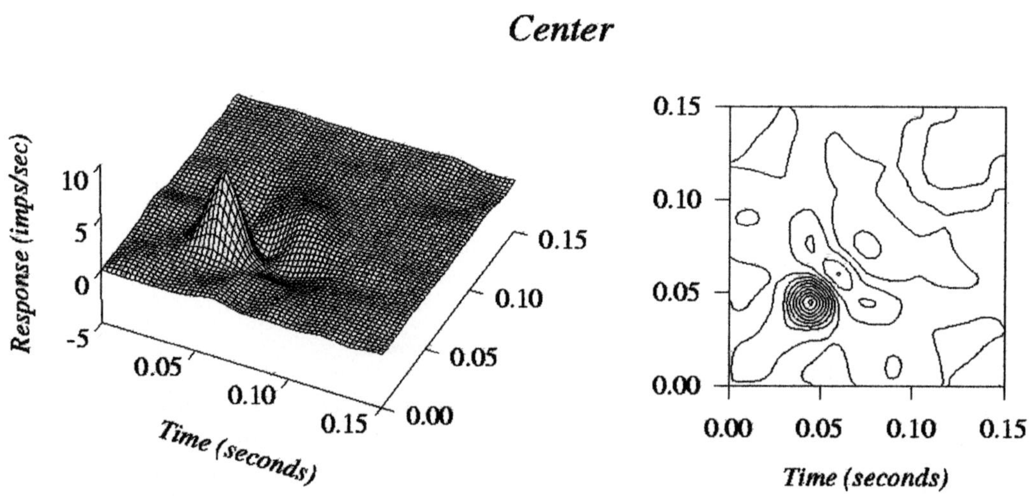

Fig. 8. The second-order response of the center of a P On cell, shown in a wire mesh plot (left) and in a contour plot (right). The stimulus was a 0.25° spot, centered on the receptive field and modulated by a sum of two independent m-sequences. Although we illustrate here only the center's non-linear response, the surround mechanism shows such behavior as well, and so does the center–surround interaction (from Benardete and Kaplan, 1997b).

A clue to the possible function of this nonlinearity was found by Kaplan and Shapley (1989), who found that steady illumination of the surround of P cells' receptive fields modulates the gain of the center. This phenomenon represents a true nonlinear interaction between the center and surround mechanisms, since summation of the two responses no longer explains the responses. As the luminance of the P On cell surround increases, the response of the center becomes less delayed and has a *lower* amplitude (Fig. 9). For P Off cells, as surround illumination increases, the center response becomes less delayed but *increases* in amplitude. Thus, the nonlinear interaction between center and surround of the P cell receptive field represents a fast adaptation mechanism that adjusts the gain of the P cell center according to the ambient illumination over a large region of the retina. Perhaps P cells take advantage of the higher signal-to-noise ratio that is available at high illumination by increasing the speed of their response.

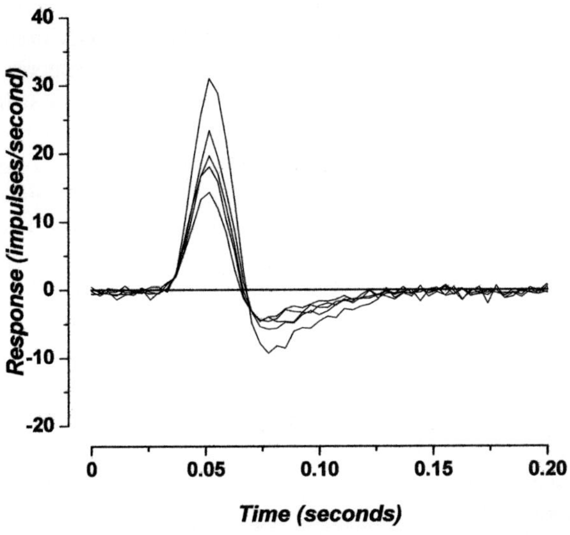

Fig. 9. The responses of the P On cell center at 4 levels of illumination of the receptive field surround provided by a steady annulus. As surround illumination increases, the response of the P cell center becomes smaller. The largest response was obtained when the surround illumination was the dimmest. Note that the steady surround illumination is capable of reducing the response to (modulated) center stimulation by a factor of ~3 (Benardete and Kaplan, 1997b).

Discussion

Comparison with other species

Cat

Linear and nonlinear subunits. The cat retina has been studied intensively in the past, and therefore we have a rather detailed description of the dynamics of the RGCs of this nocturnal mammal. The discovery of the X and Y types of RGC (Enroth-Cugell and Robson, 1966), which differ in the linearity of spatial summation within their receptive fields, focused attention on further distinctions between these two types. It was evident early on that Y cells are more transient than X cells, and several groups (for example, Cleland et al., 1971) based the dichotomous classification of cat RGCs on the time course of their responses to steps of light, or on their responses to moving targets. Hochstein and Shapley (1976a,b) applied Fourier analysis to the averaged responses of cat RGCs, and showed that the receptive fields of Y cells had nonlinear subunits, which rectified the time-varying input to produce a 'frequency doubling' response. They also showed that these subunits, which were smaller than the center mechanism of the Y cell's receptive field, extended across the entire receptive field.

Contrast gain control. Shapley and Victor (1978, 1979) pursued the matter further, and demonstrated that the nonlinear subunits endowed the Y cells with a *contrast gain control*, a spatially extended mechanism that regulated the gain of the cell according to the ambient contrast. This gain control acts just like light adaptation: it reduces the cell's response to a stimulus. However, here the adapting influence is due not to the ambient light, but to the ambient contrast. Like light adaptation, the contrast gain control affects not only the *gain* of the cell, but also its *dynamics*: responses to low temporal frequencies are attenuated more than the responses to high temporal frequencies. The result is that the cell is now more transient, and can follow flickering light up to higher frequencies (see De Lange, 1958a,b and Dodge et al., 1968 for similar effects due to light adaptation). The contrast gain control mechanism has one additional interesting effect on the response. As contrast increases, the response *phase* is advanced. This is seen clearly in M cells, but not in P cells (Smith et al., 1992; Benardete and Kaplan, 1999b).

Models of receptive field dynamics. The dynamics of the receptive fields of X and Y cells was further investigated by Victor (1987, 1988). He has developed a comprehensive mathematical model, which accounts rather well for the temporal properties measured experimentally. Victor (1987) has shown that the nonlinear behavior observed in the ganglion cell response is not due to the nonlinear nature of the biophysical process of converting the (analog) membrane potential into a spike train. It must, therefore, represent a *network* property.

Homology. Initially, it had appeared that there was a natural parallel or homology between the two pairs of functional streams, the M/P of the primate and the Y/X of the cat. The similarities were appealing: the M/Y streams are both transient, fast conducting, with large receptive fields, axons and dendritic trees. The P/X streams are both tonic, with slower conduction velocities, and smaller axons, dendritic trees and receptive fields. However, the usefulness of this homology in understanding the function or the circuitry of the two species is not established. Note that the diurnal old world primates, with their trichromatic, high resolution retina, must have optimized the circuitries of their retinas and subsequent visual stages for tasks that the nocturnal cat faces only rarely outside the laboratory.

A more appealing alternative is the view that the old world primate has added the P stream, or at least part of it, to address the needs for high spatial resolution, which produced, as a bonus, the gift of well developed color vision (Boycott and Wässle, 1999).

The 'multiplex' hypothesis

The phase lag between center and surround and its dependence on temporal frequency had been used to explain the loss of chromatic opponency seen in parvocellular neurons at high temporal frequencies (Gouras and Zrenner, 1979). Another approach was taken by Ingling and Martinez-Uriegas (1983), who pointed out that r-g parvocellular LGN cells will report the difference between their center and surround responses at *low* spatial frequencies, to which both center and surround are responsive, and the sum of the activation of center and surround at *high* spatial frequencies, to which only the (smaller) center can respond (see also Mullen and Kingdom, 1991). They thus viewed the r-g parvocellular cells as multiplexing luminance information (at high spatial frequencies) and chromatic information (at low spatial frequencies) information. This view requires a strict linearity of the receptive field dynamics of these cells, and, as we have shown above, this hypothesis needs to be re-examined in view of the various nonlinear interactions reported by Benardete and Kaplan (1997b). Nevertheless, at low contrast, below 10%, the parvocellular cells are reasonably linear (Derrington et al., 1984; Smith et al., 1992; Lee et al., 1994), and the multiplex hypothesis appears reasonable for those cells under these conditions.

Cone input to the surround of P cells

The analysis of Ingling and Martinez-Uriegas (1983) also relies on the separation of cone signals to the center and surround of the parvocellular r-g cells, following the early description of Type I LGN cells (Wiesel and Hubel, 1966). The issue of the selectivity of cone input to the surround of these cells is still a controversial one. Anatomical evidence does not support a surround mechanism with selective cone input of the type required by the results of Wiesel and Hubel (1966) or Reid and Shapley (1992), because both horizontal cells and amacrine cells make promiscuous connections with the various cones they happen to find within the reach of their dendritic trees (Boycott et al., 1987; Calkins and Sterling, 1999). We note, however, that a mixed cone input to the surround probably makes little difference to the response of the cells, or to color vision as a whole (see Paulus and Kröger-Paulus, 1983; Lennie et al., 1991).

Effects of light adaptation

As we mentioned above, light adaptation has a profound effect on the dynamics of the visual system, and that effect starts with the photoreceptors: the response to a brief flash (the 'impulse response') is monophasic in the dark-adapted state, and biphasic in the light-adapted state. In the frequency domain, that change translates to a temporal transfer function that is *low pass* when the eye is dark adapted, and *band pass* when the eye is light adapted (Dodge et al., 1968; De Lange, 1958a,b). The effect of light adaptation is propagated to the ganglion cells. Enroth-Cugell and Shapley (1973) have shown that in the cat retina there is a simple relationship between the summing area of a receptive field center of a ganglion cell and its state of adaptation: at any given light level, cells with larger receptive fields are more light adapted than cells with smaller receptive fields, simply because they capture more photons. The receptive fields of M cells are significantly larger than those of P cells at any retinal eccentricity (Croner and Kaplan, 1995), and, therefore, they should be more light adapted — and more transient — than P cells.

The effect of retinal illumination on the dynamics of monkey RGCs was investigated by Purpura et al. (1990). They found that increasing the retinal illumination affected the dynamics in much the same way that it affects photoreceptors (Dodge et al., 1968), turtle horizontal cells (Tranchina et al., 1984) and the human observer when studied psychophysically (De Lange, 1958a,b). Light-adapted transfer functions were band pass and dark-adapted ones were low pass. A linear model with a negative feedback, similar to the one that accounted for the response of turtle horizontal cells (Tranchina and Peskin, 1988), accounted well for the changes in the RGCs dynamics. It thus seems that the psychophysical effects of light adaptation on the temporal performance of the visual system can all be accounted for by retinal processing.

How important are the nonlinearities?

In this review, we have summarized recent data that show that, under appropriate conditions, significant nonlinearities can be detected in the responses of P cells (Figs. 8 and 9). These cells have been traditionally described as linear, and their linearity has been used (for instance, Ingling and Martinez-Uriegas, 1983) as a guide to their possible function in vision, as discussed above. Smith et al. (1992) have used an elegant experimental approach to dissect the various components that contribute to the response of primate RGCs. They varied the temporal phase between red and green light emitting diodes that were modulated sinusoidally, and measured the effect of this phase relationship on the cells' responses at several temporal frequencies. They were able to account for the results from most cells with a model that included only linear interactions among the cone contributions. Similarly, Lee et al. (1989a,b, 1989c, 1994) concluded that significant nonlinearities could be found only in M cells, and only when a spatially extended stimulus (or a high contrast one) was used.

This raises the possibility that there are subpopulations of RGCs with varying degrees of temporal nonlinearity, or that the stimuli used in some studies failed to elicit significant nonlinear interactions. It should be pointed out that the nonlinearities observed in the responses of P cells are not trivial: although the linear component of the response is larger than the second-order response shown in Fig. 8, it is still substantial, and, as Fig. 9 shows, the nonlinear interaction between center and surround is capable of reducing the center response by a factor of $\sim$3. Such nonlinearities point to significant interactions in the dynamical retinal circuit, and these interactions should prompt a search for their underlying physiological, biophysical and anatomical substrates.

The underlying retinal circuitry

Functionally, the receptive field of most ganglion cells (except, perhaps, for the blue On, yellow Off ganglion cell; see Dacey, 1999b, 1999a and below) appears to include (at least) 3 distinct components:

(1) A narrow (linear) center, which could be excited by either increments or decrements of light (On or Off).
(2) A broader (linear) antagonistic surround, which produces a response whose phase is opposite (at low temporal frequencies) to that of the center's response.
(3) A nonlinear (rectifying) mechanism, which extends far beyond the boundaries of the receptive field surround or the dendritic tree of the cell.

The first two mechanisms are simply the ones described half a century ago by Kuffler (1953). The third, nonlinear mechanism, is associated with the nonlinear subunits of Hochstein and Shapley

(1976a), and with the contrast gain control of Shapley and Victor (1979), and is probably the same mechanism that is responsible for the 'McIlwain effect' and the 'shift effect', as well as other spatially extended nonlinear effects (McIlwain, 1966; Krüger and Fischer, 1973; Enroth-Cugell and Jakiela, 1980).

Currently, it is thought that the center mechanism is produced (primarily) by the responses of bipolar cells. The surround antagonism is thought to be due to a negative feedback from horizontal cells onto cones, and the nonlinear responses are often attributed to the activity of amacrine cells, which contribute a significant synaptic input to the ganglion cells (Werblin and Dowling, 1969; Hochstein and Shapley, 1976b; Wässle and Boycott, 1991; Sterling, 1998; Calkins and Sterling, 1999; Demb et al., 1999). Note that this suggested correspondence between anatomical cell types and functional components of the receptive field is not the only possible one. It is possible, for instance, that the H1 and H2 types of horizontal cells, each of which tiles the retina (Wässle et al., 2000), contribute differently to the linear and nonlinear components of the receptive field. However, the overall wiring scheme of the retina suggests that the two layers that are arranged for lateral transmission of information, the outer and inner plexiform layers, will *both* contribute to the spatially extended computation that involves the surround mechanism.

The precise combination of cone inputs to the center, surround and the nonlinear mechanisms is still controversial, and it is likely that with time, additional mechanisms will be added to this hypothetical scheme. The great diversity of cell types and neurotransmitters in the inner plexiform layer (see, for example, McNeil and Masland, 1998) makes such an expansion highly probable.

Our current understanding of the structure of the receptive field can thus be summarized by the scheme shown in Fig. 10.

The blue On, yellow Off ganglion cell appears to differ from this general scheme, since its antagonistic center and surround regions appear to be coextensive (Dacey, 1999b). However, the notion that both plexiform layers contribute their individual part to the surround mechanism probably holds for these cells as well.

This general scheme of a surround with (at least) two components is consistent with several recent reports. Thus, for instance, Smith et al. (1992) reported evidence for an additional chromatically opponent mechanism in the surround of M cells. In addition, Calkins and Sterling (1999) reported anatomical evidence of synaptic input from amacrine cells to both M and P RGCs. These could provide the nonlinear elements of the surround mechanism.

Functional implications

The distinct dynamical properties of the M and P populations, taken together with the ensemble of their other differences, suggest strongly that each is dedicated to a different set of visual tasks. The high temporal resolution, high contrast sensitivity, and coarse mosaic of the M cells (Kaplan and Shapley, 1986; Kaplan et al., 1990; Croner and Kaplan, 1995) point to their role in motion analysis. The small receptive field, dense mosaic, chromatic organization, and tonic responses of the P cells suggest that they are used for spatial tasks, such as the analysis of shape, texture and color. A deeper understanding of their roles in perception must await more information about the fate of their signals once they reach the visual cortex.

Conclusions

We conclude with a brief summary of the facts as we currently know them, and a list of the things that are yet to be determined.

What is known

(1) The center and surround of P cells are approximately linear at low contrasts.
(2) Significant nonlinearities emerge in the P cell responses as contrast increases.
(3) The interaction between the center and surround of P cells includes a nonlinear component.
(4) The center and surround of P cells are chromatically opponent.
(5) The phase lag between center and surround of P cells depends on temporal frequency, so that at high frequencies the center and surround are no longer antagonistic.
(6) The M cell responses are nonlinear.

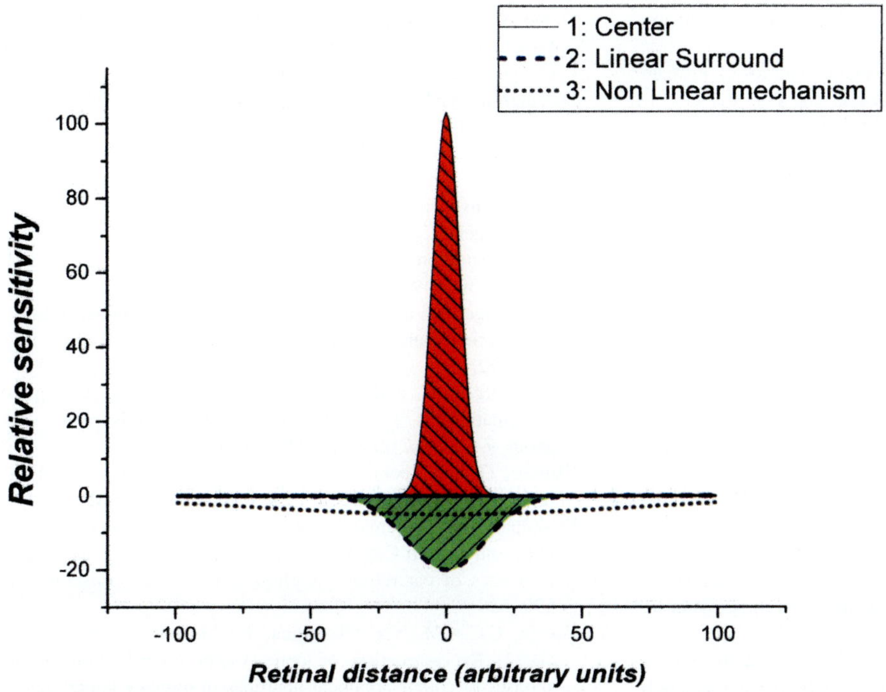

Fig. 10. The sensitivity profile of the three components that make up the receptive field of ganglion cells. The abscissa is drawn intentionally with arbitrary units, to allow cells of various sizes, including both M and P cells. The numbers in the legend correspond to the numbered list above.

(7) With increasing contrast, M cells show the effects of a contrast gain control, similar to the one found in cat Y ganglion cells.
(8) Most M cells show linear spatial summation (X like), with a minority showing nonlinear spatial summation (Y like).

What is still missing

(1) Are there different dynamical subtypes within the major 3 streams (M, P, K)?
(2) If so, are they related to other aspects (morphology, connectivity, neurochemistry, biophysics)?
(3) To what extent are the dynamical properties of the various types due to the *network* in which the neurons are embedded?
(4) What are the dynamical properties of the Koniocellular neurons?
(5) What are the contributions of the various anatomical cell types in the retina to the various functional components of the receptive field of the ganglion cell?

Acknowledgements

This work was supported by NIH Grants: EY 11276, MH50166, EY01867, and Research to Prevent Blindness. E.K. is the Jules and Doris Stein Research to Prevent Blindness Professor at the Departments of Ophthalmology, Physiology and Biophysics at the Mount Sinai/NYU School of Medicine, New York.

References

Atick, J.J. and Redlich, A.N. (1992) What does the retina know about natural scenes? *Neural Comput.*, 4: 196–210.

Baseler, H.A. and Sutter, E.E. (1997) M and P components of the VEP and their visual field distribution. *Vision Res.*, 37: 675–690.

Benardete, E. and Kaplan, E. (1997a) The receptive field of the primate P retinal ganglion cell. I: Linear dynamics. *Vis. Neurosci.*, 14: 169–185.

Benardete, E. and Kaplan, E. (1997b) The receptive field of the primate P retinal ganglion cell. II: Nonlinear dynamics. *Vis. Neurosci.*, 14: 187–205.

Benardete, E.A. and Kaplan, E. (1999a) Dynamics of primate P retinal ganglion cells: responses to chromatic and achromatic stimuli. *J. Physiol.*, 519: 775–790.

Benardete, E. and Kaplan, E. (1999b) The Dynamics of Primate M Retinal Ganglion Cells. *Vis. Neurosci.*, 16: 355–368.

Benardete, E.A. and Victor, J.D. (1994) An extension of the m-sequence technique for the analysis of multiple-input nonlinear systems. In: V.Z. Marmarelis (Ed.), *Advanced Methods of Physiological Systems Modeling. Vol. 3*. Plenum Press, New York, pp. 87–110.

Benardete, E.A., Kaplan, E. and Knight, B.W. (1992) Contrast gain control in the primate retina: P cells are not X-like, some M cells are. *Vis. Neurosci.*, 8: 483–486.

Boycott, B.B. and Wässle, H. (1974) The morphological types of ganglion cells of the domestic cat's retina. *J. Physiol. (Lond.)*, 240: 397–419.

Boycott, B. and Wässle, H. (1999) Parallel processing in the mammalian retina: the Proctor Lecture.. *Invest. Ophthalmol. Vis. Sci.*, 40: 1313–1327.

Boycott, B.B., Hopkins, J.M. and Sperling, H.G. (1987) Cone connections of the horizontal cells of the rhesus monkey's retina. *Proc. R. Soc. Lond. Ser. B.*, 229: 345–379.

Calkins, D.J. and Sterling, P. (1999) Evidence that circuits for spatial and color vision segregate at the first retinal synapse. *Neuron*, 24: 313–321.

Carroll, E.W. and Wong-Riley, M.T.T. (1984) Quantitative light and electron microscopic analysis of cytochrome oxidase-rich zones in the striate cortex of the squirrel monkey. *J. Comp. Neurol.*, 222: 1–17.

Casagrande, V.A. (1994) A third visual pathway to primate area V1. *Trends Neurosci.*, 17: 305–310.

Cleland, B.G., Dubin, M.W. and Levick, W.R. (1971) Sustained and transient neurones in the cat's retina and lateral geniculate nucleus. *J. Physiol. (Lond.)*, 217: 473–496.

Croner, L.J. and Kaplan, E. (1995) Receptive fields of P and M ganglion cells across the primate retina. *Vision Res.*, 35: 7–24.

Dacey, D.M. (1999a) Primate retina: cell types, circuits and color opponency. *Prog. Retinal Eye Res.*, 18: 737–763.

Dacey, D. (1999b) Origin of spectral opponency in primate retina. In: J.-I. Toyoda, M.M. Murakami, A. Kaneko and T. Saito (Eds.), *The Retinal Basis of Vision*. Elsevier, Amsterdam, pp. 215–230.

Dacey, D.M. (2000) Parallel pathways for spectral coding in primate retina. *Annu. Rev. Neurosci.*, 23: 743–775.

Dawis, S., Shapley, R., Kaplan, E. and Tranchina, D. (1984) The receptive field organization of X-cells in the cat: spatiotemporal coupling and asymmetry. *Vision Res.*, 24: 549–564.

De Lange, H. (1958a) Research into the dynamic nature of the human fovea-cortex systems with intermittent and modulated light: I. Attenuation characteristics with white and colored light. *J. Opt. Soc. Am.*, 48: 777–784.

De Lange, H. (1958b) Research into the dynamic nature of the human fovea-cortex systems with intermittent and modulated light. II. Phase shift in brightness and delay in color perception. *J. Opt. Soc. Am.*, 48: 784–789.

De Monasterio, F.M. and Gouras, P. (1975) Functional properties of ganglion cells of the rhesus monkey retina. *J. Physiol. (Lond.)*, 251: 167–195.

Demb, J.B., Haarsma, L., Freed, M.A. and Sterling, P. (1999) Functional circuitry of the retinal ganglion cell's nonlinear receptive field. *J. Neurosci.*, 19: 9756–9767.

Derrington, A.M., Krauskopf, J. and Lennie, P. (1984) Chromatic mechanisms in lateral geniculate nucleus of macaque. *J. Physiol. (Lond.)*, 357: 241–265.

Dodge, F.A., Knight, B.W. and Toyoda, J. (1968) Voltage noise in *Limulus* visual cells. *Science*, 160: 88–90.

Enroth-Cugell, C. and Jakiela, H.G. (1980) Suppression of cat retinal ganglion cell responses by moving patterns. *J. Physiol. (Lond.)*, 302: 49–72.

Enroth-Cugell, C. and Robson, J.G. (1966) The contrast sensitivity of retinal ganglion cells of the cat. *J. Physiol. (Lond.)*, 187: 517–552.

Enroth-Cugell, C. and Shapley, R.M. (1973) Flux, not retinal illumination, is what cat retinal ganglion cells really care about. *J. Physiol. (Lond.)*, 233: 311–326.

Estévez, O. and Spekreijse, H. (1982) The 'silent substitution' method in visual research. *Vision Res.*, 22: 681–691.

Frishman, L.J., Freeman, A.W., Troy, J.B., Schweitzer-Tong, D.E. and Enroth-Cugell, C. (1987) Spatiotemporal frequency responses of cat retinal ganglion cells. *J. Gen. Physiol.*, 89: 599–628.

Gielen, C.C.A.M., van Gisbergen, J.A.M. and Vendrik, A.J.H. (1982) Reconstruction of cone-system contributions to responses of colour-opponent neurones in monkey lateral geniculate. *Biol. Cybern.*, 44: 211–221.

Gouras, P. (1968) Identification of cone mechanisms in monkey ganglion cells. *J. Physiol. (Lond.)*, 199: 533–547.

Gouras, P. and Zrenner, E. (1979) Enhancement of luminance flicker by color-opponent mechanisms. *Science*, 205: 587–589.

Hendry, S.H.C. and Yoshioka, T. (1994) A neurochemically distinct third channel in the macaque dorsal lateral geniculate nucleus. *Science*, 264: 575–577.

Hochstein, S. and Shapley, R.M. (1976a) Quantitative analysis of retinal ganglion cell classifications. *J. Physiol. (Lond.)*, 262: 237–264.

Hochstein, S. and Shapley, R.M. (1976b) Linear and nonlinear spatial subunits in Y cat retinal ganglion cells. *J. Physiol. (Lond.)*, 262: 265–284.

Ingling, C.R. and Martinez-Uriegas, E. (1983) The relationship between spectral sensitivity and spatial sensitivity for the primate r-g X channel. *Vision Res.*, 23: 1495–1500.

Kaplan, E. and Shapley, R.M. (1982) X and Y cells in the lateral geniculate nucleus of macaque monkeys. *J. Physiol. (Lond.)*, 330: 125–143.

Kaplan, E. and Shapley, R. (1984) The origin of the S (slow) potential in the mammalian lateral geniculate nucleus. *Exp. Brain Res.*, 55: 111–116.

Kaplan, E. and Shapley, R.M. (1986) The primate retina contains two types of ganglion cells, with high and low contrast sensitivity Proc. *Proc. Natl. Acad. Sci. USA*, 83: 2755–2757.

Kaplan, E. and Shapley, R.M. (1989) Illumination of the receptive field surround controls the contrast gain of macaque P retinal ganglion cells. *Soc. Neurosci. Abstr.*, 15(1): 174 (#75.1).

Kaplan, E., Marcus, S. and So, Y.T. (1979) Effects of dark adaptation on spatial and temporal properties of receptive fields in cat lateral geniculate nucleus. *J. Physiol. (Lond.)*, 294: 561–580.

Kaplan, E., Lee, B.B. and Shapley, R.M. (1990) New views of primate retinal function. In: N.N. Osborne and G.J. Chader (Eds.), *Progress in Retinal Research*, Vol. 9. Pergamon Press, New York, pp. 273–336.

Klistorner, A., Crewther, D.P. and Crewther, S.G. (1997) Separate magnocellular and parvocellular contributions from temporal analysis of the multifocal VEP. *Vision Res.*, 37: 2161–2169.

Krüger, J. and Fischer, B. (1973) Strong periphery effect in cat retinal ganglion cells. Excitatory responses in ON- and OFF-center neurones to single grid displacements. *Exp. Brain Res.*, 18(3): 316–318.

Kuffler, S.W. (1953) Discharge patterns and functional organization of mammalian retina. *J. Neurophysiol.*, 16: 37–68.

Lee, B.B., Martin, P.R. and Valberg, A. (1989a) Amplitude and phase of responses of macaque retinal ganglion cells to flickering stimuli. *J. Physiol. (Lond.).*, 414: 245–263.

Lee, B.B., Martin, P.R. and Valberg, A. (1989b) Nonlinear summation of M- and L-cone inputs to phasic retinal ganglion cells of the macaque. *J. Neurosci.*, 9: 1433–1442.

Lee, B.B., Martin, P.R. and Valberg, A. (1989c) Sensitivity of macaque retinal ganglion cells to chromatic and luminance flicker. *J. Physiol. (Lond.)*, 414: 223–243.

Lee, B.B., Pokorny, J., Smith, V.C. and Kremers, J. (1994) Responses to pulses and sinusoids in macaque ganglion cells. *Vision Res.*, 34: 3081–3096.

Lennie, P., Haake, P.W. and Williams, D.R. (1991) The design of chromatically opponent receptive fields. In: M.S. Landy and J.A. Movshon (Eds.), *Computational Models of Visual Processing*. MIT Press, Cambridge, MA, pp. 71–82.

Livingstone, M.S. and Hubel, D.H. (1984) Specificity of intrinsic connections in primate primary visual cortex. *J. Neurosci.*, 4: 2830–2835.

Livingstone, M. and Hubel, D. (1988) Segregation of form, color, movement, and depth: anatomy, physiology, and perception. *Science*, 240: 740–749.

Maunsell, J.H.R., Ghose, G.M., Assad, J.A., McAdams, C.J., Christen, E. and Noerager, B.D. (1999) Visual response latencies of magnocellular and parvocellular LGN neurons in macaque monkeys. *Vis. Neurosci.*, 16: 1–14.

McIlwain, J.T. (1966) Some evidence concerning the physiological basis of the periphery effect in the cat's retina. *Exp. Brain Res.*, 1: 265–271.

McNeil, M.A. and Masland, R.H. (1998) Extreme diversity among amacrine cells: implications for function. *Neuron*, 20: 971–982.

Merigan, W.H. and Maunsell, J.H.R. (1993) How parallel are the primate visual pathways? *Annu. Rev. Neurosci.*, 16: 369–402.

Mullen, K.T. and Kingdom, F.A.A. (1991) Colour contrast in form perception. In: P. Gouras (Ed.), *Vision and Visual Dysfunction (The Perception of Colour)*, Vol. 6. pp. 198–217, Macmillan Press, New York.

Paulus, W. and Kröger-Paulus, A. (1983) A new concept of retinal colour coding. *Vision Res.*, 23: 529–540.

Perry, V.H. and Cowey, A. (1981) The morphological correlates of X- and Y-like retinal ganglion cells in the retina of monkeys. *Exp. Brain Res.*, 43: 226–228.

Perry, V.H., Oehler, R. and Cowey, A. (1984) Retinal ganglion cells that project to the dorsal lateral geniculate nucleus in the macaque monkey. *Neuroscience*, 12: 1101–1123.

Polyak, S.L. (1941) *The Retina*, The University of Chicago Press, Chicago.

Purpura, K., Tranchina, D., Kaplan, E. and Shapley, R.M. (1990) Light adaptation in the primate retina: analysis of changes in gain and dynamics of monkey retinal ganglion cells. *Vis. Neurosci.*, 4: 75–93.

Ratliff, F., Knight, B.W. and Graham, N. (1969) On tuning and amplification by lateral inhibition. *Proc. Natl. Acad. Sci. USA*, 62: 733–740.

Ratliff, F., Knight, B.W. and Milkman, N. (1970) Superposition of excitatory and inhibitory influences in the retina of *Limulus*: effect of delayed inhibition. *Proc. Natl. Acad. Sci. USA*, 67: 1558–1564.

Reid, R.C. and Shapley, R.M. (1992) Spatial structure of cone inputs to receptive fields in primate lateral geniculate nucleus. *Nature*, 356: 716–718.

Rodieck, R.W. (1988) The primate retina. In: *Comparative Primate Biology, Vol. 4. Neurosciences*, Alan R. Liss, New York, pp. 203–278.

Rodieck, R.W. and Watanabe, M. (1993) Survey of the morphology of macaque retinal ganglion cells that project to the pretectum, superior colliculus, and parvicellular laminae of the lateral geniculate nucleus. *J. Comp. Neurol.*, 338: 289–303.

Rudvin, I., Valberg, A. and Kilavik, B.E. (2000) Visual evoked potentials and magnocellular and parvocellular segregation. *Vis. Neurosci.*, 17: 579–590.

Shapley, R.M. and Victor, J.D. (1978) The effect of contrast on the transfer properties of cat retinal ganglion cells. *J. Physiol. (Lond.)*, 285: 275–298.

Shapley, R.M. and Victor, J.D. (1979) Nonlinear spatial summation and the contrast gain control of cat retinal ganglion cells. *J. Physiol. (Lond.)*, 290: 141–161.

Smith, V.C., Lee, B.B., Pokorny, J., Martin, P.R. and Valberg, A. (1992) Responses of macaque ganglion cells to the relative phase of heterochromatically modulated lights. *J. Physiol. (Lond.)*, 458: 191–221.

Sterling, P. (1998) Retina. In: G.M. Shepherd (Ed.), *The Synaptic Organization of the Brain*. Oxford University Press, New York, pp. 205–213.

Sutter, E.E. (1987) A practical nonstochastic approach to nonlinear time-domain analysis. In: V.Z. Marmarelis (Ed.), *Advanced Methods of Physiological Systems Modeling*, Vol. 1. University of Southern California, Los Angeles.

Tranchina, D. and Peskin, C.S. (1988) Light adaptation in the turtle retina: embedding a parametric family of linear models in a single nonlinear model. *Vis. Neurosci.*, 1: 339–348.

Tranchina, D., Gordon, J. and Shapley, R.M. (1984) Retinal light adaptation-evidence for a feedback mechanism. *Nature*, 310: 314–316.

Valberg, A. and Rudvin, I. (1997) Possible contributions of magnocellular and parvocellular-pathway cells to transient VEPs. *Vis. Neurosci.*, 14: 1–11.

Victor, J.D. (1987) The dynamics of the cat retinal X cell centre. *J. Physiol. (Lond.)*, 386: 219–246.

Victor, J.D. (1988) The dynamics of the cat retinal Y cell subunit. *J. Physiol. (Lond.)*, 405: 289–320.

Wässle, H. and Boycott, B.B. (1991) Functional architecture of the mammalian retina. *Physiol. Rev.*, 71: 447–480.

Wässle, H., Dacey, D.M., Haun, T., Haverkamp, S., Grünert, U. and Boycott, B.B. (2000) The mosaic of horizontal cells in the macaque monkey retina: With a comment on the biplexiform ganglion cells. *Vis. Neurosci.*, 17: 591–608.

Watanabe, M. and Rodieck, R.W. (1989) Parasol and midget ganglion cells of the primate retina. *J. Comp. Neurol.*, 289: 434–454.

Werblin, F.S. and Dowling, J.E. (1969) Organization of the retina of the mudpuppy, *Necturus maculosus*. II. Intracellular recording. *J. Neurophysiol.*, 32: 339–355.

Wiesel, T.N. and Hubel, D.H. (1966) Spatial and chromatic interactions in the lateral geniculate body of the rhesus monkey. *J. Neurophysiol.*, 29: 1115–1156.

Wong-Riley, M.T.T. and Carroll, E.W. (1984) Quantitative light and electron microscopic analysis of cytochrome oxidase-rich zones in V II prestriate cortex of the squirrel monkey. *J. Comp. Neurol.*, 222: 18–37.

Zeki, S. and Shipp, S. (1988) The functional logic of cortical connections. *Nature*, 335: 311–317.

C. Casanova and M. Ptito (Eds.)
Progress in Brain Research, Vol. 134

CHAPTER 3

BDNF/trkB signaling in the developmental sculpting of visual connections

Douglas O. Frost *

Department of Pharmacology and Experimental Therapeutics, Department of Anesthesiology and Neuroscience Program, University of Maryland School of Medicine, Baltimore, MD 21201, USA

Abstract: Neurotrophins are a family of secreted molecules that have multiple, profound actions on the structure and function of both developing and mature neurons. Neurotrophins exert their influences by signaling through the trk family of receptor tyrosine kinases and the p75 low affinity neurotrophin receptor. Here we review the contributions of neurotrophins to the development of neural circuitry in the mammalian visual system. We emphasize: (1) the role of neurotrophins as components of the cellular mechanisms by which neuroelectric activity sculpts pattern of brain connectivity; and (2) the results of recent experiments suggesting that the trafficking of neurotrophin proteins may be activity dependent.

Introduction

A recurrent theme in developmental neurobiology is that the assembly of neural circuits is both a constructive and a destructive process: neurons and the connections among them are overproduced and subsequently, they are selectively reduced by activity-dependent and activity-independent processes. Consequently, sensory experience, by modulating neuronal activity, can exert a powerful influence on the sculpting of neural circuits in the developing brain. Here we review experiments that investigate the role of brain-derived neurotrophic factor (BDNF), signaling through the trkB receptor, in the mechanisms by which visually evoked activity modulates the development of the mammalian visual system. The phenomenological relationships among visual experience, electrical activity, BDNF/trkB signaling and neural circuitry are schematized in Fig. 1.

* Corresponding author: D.O. Frost, Department of Pharmacology and Experimental Therapeutics, University of Maryland School of Medicine, 655 West Baltimore St., Baltimore, MD 21201, USA. Tel.: +1-410-706-0413; Fax: +1-410-706-0032; E-mail: dfrost@umaryland.edu

Activity-dependent regulation of BDNF mRNA and protein and its consequences in the developing visual cortex

Neurotrophins modulate the survival, differentiation and connectivity of developing neurons

BDNF and other neurotrophins, when bound to the pan-neurotrophin receptor, p75, or members of the trk family, have pleiotropic effects on developing and mature neurons and glia (reviews: Korsching, 1993; Davies, 1994; Thoenen, 1995; Snider and Lichtman, 1996; Shatz, 1997). The role of trk receptors with full-length catalytic domains in mediating these functions is well-established; trk receptors with truncated catalytic domains appear to act as negative regulators of the full-length trks, in part by sequestering ligand (Palko et al., 1999). Early studies emphasized the survival-promoting effects of neurotrophins on immature peripheral sensory and sympathetic neurons (reviews: Cowan et al., 1984; Oppenheim, 1991; Lewin and Barde, 1996). The survival-promoting effects of neurotrophins on developing central nervous system (CNS) neurons in vivo are controversial (review: Ma et al., 1998), although evidence for such effects is accumulating (see below; also Cui and Harvey, 1994; Von Bartheld et al., 1994; Primi and

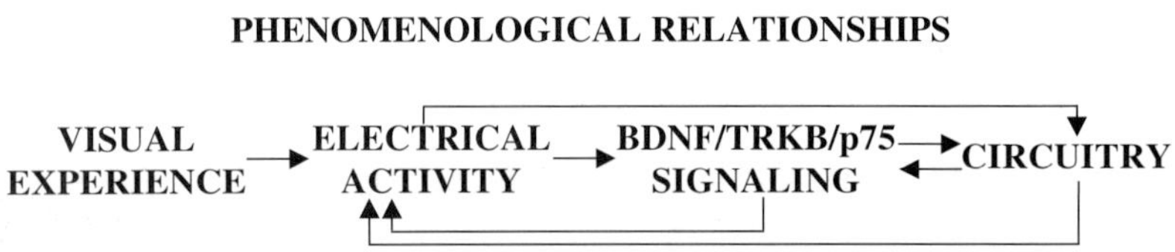

Fig. 1. Schematic diagram of the phenomenological relationships among visual experience, electrical activity, BDNF signaling through its receptors and neural circuitry.

Clarke, 1996; Alcántara et al., 1997; Frade et al., 1997; Johnson et al., 1997; Schwartz et al., 1997; Ma et al., 1998; Frost et al., 1998; Alonso-Vanegas et al., 1999; Pollock et al., 2000, 2001b). Neurotrophins, signaling through the p75 receptor, can also promote the death of immature neurons (Frade et al., 1996; Majdan et al., 1997; Bamji et al., 1998; Frade and Barde, 1998, 1999; Kohn et al., 1999). Modulation of the stabilization/elimination of developing neurons is only one means by which neurotrophins can influence patterns of neuronal circuitry: Neurotrophins, including BDNF, can also affect neuronal maturation (phenotype) (Wright et al., 1992), modulate the elaboration and stabilization of dendritic (McAllister et al., 1995, 1997, 1999; Schwartz et al., 1997; Xu et al., 2000) and axonal (Johnson et al., 1986; Hoyle et al., 1993; Cabelli et al., 1995, 1997; Cohen-Cory and Fraser, 1995; Cohen-Cory, 1999; Isenmann et al., 1999; Lein et al., 1999) arbors and regulate synaptic density (Causing et al., 1997; Cellerino et al., 1998; Vicario-Abejón et al., 1998). These actions can be mediated by the p75 receptor, in addition to the trk family (Kohn et al., 1999; Kaplan and Miller, 2000). BDNF may also contribute to the activity-dependent modification of neural circuitry by its actions as a classical neurotransmitter (Kafitz et al., 1999).

BDNF contributes to the developmental segregation of eye-specific thalamocortical axon arbors within ocular dominance columns. Infusion of V1 with BDNF or NT4 (another high-affinity ligand of trkB) blocks the developmental segregation of LGN axons (Cabelli et al., 1995). Cortical infusion with trkB-Fc receptor bodies that deplete endogenous trkB ligands has a similar effect (Cabelli et al., 1997).

Multiple signaling pathways mediate the effects of the neurotrophins

At least for peripheral neurons, the survival signal induced by nerve growth factor (NGF) involves activation and/or retrograde trafficking of trk receptors (review: Kaplan and Miller, 2000; also Zhang et al., 2000) and subsequent activation of the Ras/PI3-kinase (PI3K)/Akt pathway (review: Kaplan and Miller, 2000). Local signals requiring trkA regulate growth at peripheral axon tips (Fagan et al., 1996; Patel et al., 2000). TrkB signaling initiated by binding of BDNF or NT4 is more complex. TrkB activation can induce gene expression by activation of the CREB transcription factor through the Ras/MEK/MAP kinase- or CAMIV kinase pathways (Finkbeiner et al., 1997; Wu et al., 2001). In mammalian primary sympathetic neurons, BDNF promotes both cell survival and axonal growth by activation of at least two pathways (Fig. 2): Ras/PI3K/Akt and Ras/Raf/MEK/ERK/MAP kinase (MAPK) (Atwal et al., 2000; Kaplan and Miller, 2000). TrkB activation of the MEK/ERK/MAPK pathway promotes axonal growth by phosphorylating microtubule-associated proteins (including tau; review: Atwal et al., 2000), that regulate microtubule stability and control axonal elongation (Takei et al., 2000); PI3K regulates or associates with a number of cytoskeletal proteins (review: Atwal et al., 2000). Binding of NGF or BDNF to p75 promotes neuronal survival by the NFκB pathway in the presence of trk receptor activation (review: Kaplan and Miller, 2000). When trk receptor activation is low, p75 causes cell death, principally by activating the JNK–p53–Bax system, although additional pathways involving neurotrophin receptor interacting factor, members of the TRAF family, and the zinc finger motif proteins SC-1 and NRAGE, also contribute (review: Kaplan and Miller, 2000). In peripheral neurons, neurite growth induced by trk receptor activation is inhibited by p75 signaling through the ceramide pathway, although p75 can also promote neurite growth by activating Rho (review: Kaplan and Miller, 2000). These data suggest that the actions of neurotrophins on cell survival and neurite

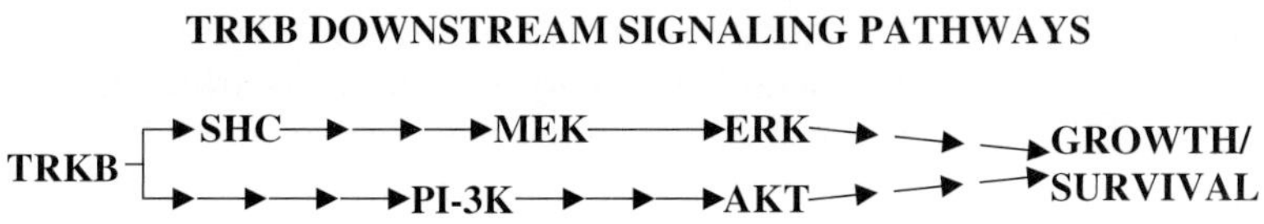

Fig. 2. Schematic diagram of trkB downstream signaling pathways that mediate neuronal growth and survival during development.

growth depend upon neuronal type, stage of development and environment (likely including the electrical activity of a neuron and its afferents).

Electrical activity shapes the development of neural circuitry

During development, the structure and function of CNS connections are modified by the level and the pattern of electrical activity in neuronal circuits (Cowan et al., 1984; Katz and Shatz, 1996). The effects of sensory development on neural circuit development are widely studied in the mammalian visual system (Sherman and Spear, 1982; Fregnac and Imbert, 1984; Frost and Innocenti, 1986). Early visual experience regulates the growth, stabilization and elimination of immature thalamocortical connections representing each eye as well as the response properties of cortical neurons (Hubel et al., 1977; Sherman and Spear, 1982; Fregnac and Imbert, 1984; Katz and Shatz, 1996). The functional changes may be due, in part, to experience-dependent modification of local cortical circuits (Callaway and Katz, 1991). In addition, rearing in constant darkness (DR) retards, but does not prevent, the attainment of a normal spine density on the apical dendrites of layer 5 pyramidal cells in mouse V1; exposure of DR mice to light while spine density is still low, rapidly accelerates the developmental increase in spine density (Valverde, 1971).

In the primary visual cortex (V1), neurons are selectively activated according to the orientation of visual contours and the direction of movement of stimuli in their receptive fields. Intracortical connections, particularly inhibitory connections, appear to participate in generating orientation and direction selectivity, although the magnitude of their contribution is controversial (Crook et al., 1996, 1997; Somers et al., 1995; Ferster et al., 1996; Sompolinsky and Shapely, 1997; Chung and Ferster, 1998; Anderson et al., 2000). Recent studies suggest that neurotrophin signaling is important in mediating the effects of sensory experience on developing of thalamocortical connections (Galuske et al., 1996; Gillespie et al., 1996).

Neural activity regulates BDNF and trkB mRNA expression and trafficking

mRNAs for BDNF and its high-affinity cognate receptor, trkB, are widely expressed in the developing and mature nervous systems and are present at relatively high levels in the mature hippocampus and cerebral cortex, regions of the adult brain notable for experience-dependent synaptic plasticity (Thoenen, 1995). (p75 is robustly expressed by neurons in the subplate (Allendoerfer et al., 1990; Meinecke and Rakic, 1993; Chen et al., 1996) and cortical plate (Dr. Phil Barker, Montreal Neurological Institute, personal communication) of the developing neocortex and is expressed at low levels in the mature cortex (Hock et al., 1998; Roux et al., 1999; Miller and Pitts, 2000). The neuronal production of BDNF mRNA is rapidly induced (1–2 h latency) by various forms of neural activity — membrane depolarization (Zafra et al., 1992; Ghosh et al., 1994), activation of excitatory neurotransmitter receptors (Zafra et al., 1990, 1992; Lindefors et al., 1992; Bessho et al., 1993; Ghosh et al., 1994; Knipper et al., 1994; Lindholm et al., 1994), seizure activity (Gall, 1993; Gall et al., 1995) and stimuli that induce long-term potentiation (LTP; Patterson et al., 1992) (Fig. 3). Manipulations that antagonize neuronal depolarization or cause hyperpolarization (Zafra et al., 1991; Lindefors et al., 1992; Lindholm et al., 1994; Knipper et al., 1994) decrease BDNF mRNA expression (Fig. 3). BDNF secretion, like BDNF mRNA expression, is positively correlated with electrical activity (Griesbeck et al., 1995, 1999; Androutsellis-Theotokis et al., 1996; Goodman et al., 1996).

Manipulations of visual experience that modulate the level or pattern of neural activity within the

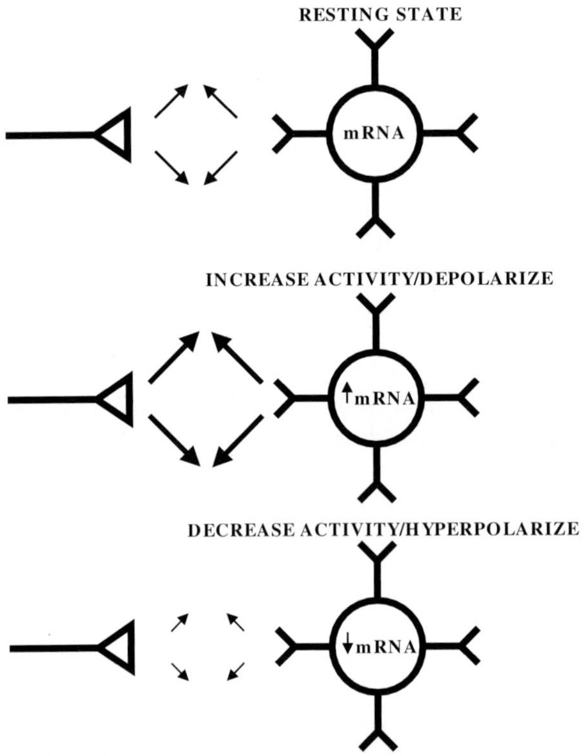

Fig. 3. Neuroelectric activity regulates the expression of BDNF mRNA and the secretion of BDNF protein. Increased activity increases BDNF mRNA levels and increases the secretion of BDNF protein, whereas decreased activity has the opposite effects.

physiological range can regulate BDNF mRNA synthesis. For instance, the production of BDNF mRNA is reduced in V1 of both rodents and carnivores following DR (Castrén et al., 1992; Schoups et al., 1995; Lein et al., 1997; Pollock et al., 2001a) or retinal impulse blockade due to intraocular injections of tetrodotoxin (TTX) (Castrén et al., 1992; Bozzi et al., 1995; Lein et al., 2000). In rodents, deprivation of pattern vision by eyelid suture reduces BDNF mRNA by about 55% (Bozzi et al., 1995), and DR reduces BDNF mRNA by 25–40% (Castrén et al., 1992; Schoups et al., 1995; Pollock et al., 2001a). (Eyelid suture also alters the spatial pattern of BDNF expression (Jones et al., 2000). The rapid increase (1 h latency) of cortical BDNF mRNA (but not NGF mRNA) induced in V1 of DR rats that are later exposed to light (Castrén et al., 1992; Schoups et al., 1995) shows that BDNF synthesis in V1 is tightly regulated by sensory experience. Because neuronal activity can also alter trkB receptor function by modulating the expression (Gall, 1993; Okazawa et al., 1994) and trafficking (Meyer-Franke et al., 1998) of trkB mRNA and the insertion of trkB protein into membranes (Meyer-Franke et al., 1998; Du et al., 2000), sensory experience could also alter the density or type (full length vs. truncated) of trkB receptors on afferent axon terminals or cortical neurons, thus modifying the capacity of these elements to bind BDNF. These complex changes may cause functionally significant alterations in the levels and trafficking of the phosphorylated BDNF/trkB complexes that initiate the intracellular signaling cascades responsible for effecting the multiple actions of BDNF. Electrical activity also modulates neurotrophin signaling by convergent regulation of the activity of downstream effector molecules, e.g. Akt (Vaillant et al., 1999), CREB (Wu et al., 2001) and Erk (Xia et al., 1996).

Comparison of the effects of neural activity on BDNF mRNA and BDNF protein

Because BDNF is a secretory protein (Mowla et al., 1999) that can be distributed by axonal transport in the retrograde (Von Bartheld et al., 1996; Ma et al., 1998) or anterograde (Zhou and Rush, 1996; Altar et al., 1997; Conner et al., 1997; Fawcett et al., 1997; Smith et al., 1997; Fawcett et al., 1998; Haubensak et al., 1998) directions, the effects of early visual experience on local levels of BDNF mRNA and BDNF protein might not be the same. This is important for understanding the role of BDNF in mediating the effects of sensory experience on neural structure and function, because protein, not mRNA, is the effector molecule. Measurements of activity-dependent changes in BDNF protein and comparisons of the effects of neural activity on BDNF mRNA and protein have been made in only a few instances (Nawa et al., 1995; Elmer et al., 1998). Therefore, our group has compared the effects of rearing in constant light (LR) and constant darkness on BDNF mRNA and BDNF protein levels in several visual and non-visual neural structures of hamsters and rats (Pollock et al., 2001a). Previous studies have demonstrated diurnal modulation of BDNF (Bova et al., 1998; Berchtold et al., 1999; Schaaf et al., 2000) and trkB (Bova

TABLE 1

Summary of changes in BDNF mRNA and BDNF protein induced in different structures by rearing in constant light (LR) or constant darkness (DR)

mRNA	Protein		
	=	+	−
=	SC/DR, V1/LR	Retina/LR Cerebellum/DR	Hippocampus/DR Hippocampus/LR
+	SC/LR	Cerebellum/LR	
−		V1/DR	Retina/DR

et al., 1998) mRNA levels. Thus, we also investigated whether these changes are sufficient to produce circadian variations in the tissue concentrations of BDNF protein (Pollock et al., 2001a).

We measured quantitatively the tissue concentration of BDNF protein using the electrochemiluminescent immunoassay (ECLIA) and the tissue concentration of BDNF mRNA using the RNase protection assay (Pollock et al., 2001a). Several important points emerge: Both LR and DR can modify the levels of BDNF mRNA and BDNF protein in the visual system and in structures that are not primarily visual, such as the hippocampus and cerebellum (Table 1). Importantly, the changes in BDNF protein and BDNF mRNA are not always correlated. Of the nine possible combinations of experience-dependent change (or constancy) of BDNF mRNA and BDNF protein, seven actually occurred. Most notably, DR increases BDNF protein levels in V1 although BDNF mRNA is reduced.

Why does BDNF protein accumulate in V1 of animals reared in constant darkness? There are several mutually compatible hypotheses: (1) DR-induced changes in neuronal activity might, by various mechanisms, reduce the removal by afferent axons of BDNF synthesized in V1; (2) BDNF might accumulate in the axon terminals of afferents to V1 as a consequence of DR-induced changes in neuronal activity; (3) DR could enhance the retention of BDNF within local cortical circuits; and (4) DR-induced alterations in neuronal activity could reduce the anterograde transport or increase the retrograde transport of BDNF by cortical efferent neurons. We are currently conducting experiments to examine these possibilities.

Why do LR and DR induce alterations in BDNF mRNA and protein in the hippocampus and cerebellum, two structures that are not primarily sensory? LR or DR might induce changes in the level or pattern of motor activity. Changes in motor activity alter BDNF mRNA levels in the hippocampus (Neeper et al., 1996; Oliff et al., 1998); similar changes might also take place in the cerebellum. LR and DR might also alter circulating hormone levels, which influence neurotrophin expression and signaling (Lindholm et al., 1994; Toran-Allerand, 1996; Gibbs, 1998; Toran-Allerand et al., 1999).

BDNF/trkB signaling mediates the activity-dependent sculpting of developing circuits in the visual cortex

An important feature of activity-mediated circuit development is that synapses can be strengthened or weakened, depending on the level and pattern of presynaptic axonal activity and post-synaptic neuronal depolarization (Bienenstock et al., 1982; Miller et al., 1989). Neurotrophins have been proposed as candidate retrograde signaling molecules that contribute to the bi-directional synaptic communication that modulates the development, efficacy and stability of connections (Domenici et al., 1991; Snider and Lichtman, 1996; Shatz, 1997; Fig. 4). BDNF is necessary for the activity-dependent establishment of GABA-mediated inhibition among visual cortical neurons in vitro (Rutherford et al., 1997) and for the in vivo expression of neuropeptide Y, calbindin and parvalbumin by cortical GABAergic neurons (Jones et al., 1994), many of which express trkB (Cellerino et al., 1996). BDNF exerts its effects on GABAergic differentiation by both activity-dependent (Marty et al., 1996a) and activity-independent (Marty et al., 1996b) means. BDNF has opposite effects on quantal amplitude at excitatory synapses on pyramidal and GABAergic neurons (Rutherford et al., 1998; Turrigiano, 1999). The activity-dependent secretion of BDNF thus provides a non-Hebbian mechanism to adjust continuously the firing rates of cortical pyramidal neurons and inhibitory interneurons and thereby maintains a dynamic balance between cortical excitation and inhibition (Rutherford et al., 1998; Turrigiano, 1999). Through its role in long-term potentiation and depression (reviews: Thoenen, 1995;

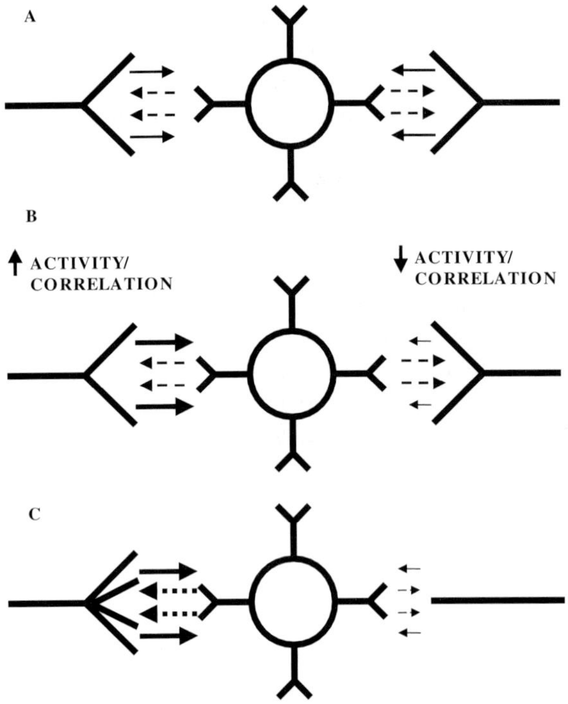

Fig. 4. BDNF can act as a retrograde signaling molecule that detects the correlation between pre- and post-synaptic activity. Thus, BDNF may be part of the mechanism by which visual experience modulates the development of thalamocortical axon arbors. Under normal conditions (A), the levels of activity (solid arrows) of the thalamocortical afferent populations representing the two eyes are comparable and the secretion of BDNF (broken arrows) at synapses made by each population of afferents is similar. When there is an imbalance in the activity of the two populations (B), the activity of common target neurons becomes more highly correlated with the activity of the more active afferents and (C) more BDNF is released at the synapses formed by those afferents. The increased BDNF levels promote the growth and synaptic efficacy of the more active afferents. Reduced BDNF levels at the synapses formed by the less active afferents cause reduced growth (or even regression) and decreased synaptic efficacy among those axons.

Schuman, 1999), BDNF has also been implicated in Hebbian plasticity of synapses between cortical neurons and their thalamic afferents. Hebbian mechanisms may also contribute to the developmental stabilization/elimination of neural connections (Goodman and Shatz, 1993).

In rats, BDNF mRNA levels in V1 are low through the time of eye opening around P14, increase rapidly to reach a peak on P21, then begin to decline on P30 and reach a plateau around 6 weeks postnatally (Castren et al., 1992; Schoups et al., 1995). The epoch during which BDNF mRNA levels are at peak or declining corresponds to the 'critical period' for vision-induced plasticity (Stafford, 1984; Fagiolini et al., 1994). In mice, the number of neurons in V1 that express BDNF protein is low prior to eye opening and increases through the 'critical period' (Jones et al., 2000). Constitutive overexpression of BDNF accelerates the maturation of visual cortical inhibitory circuitry (Hanover et al., 1999; Huang et al., 1999) and thereby advances the 'critical period' (Hanover et al., 1999; Huang et al., 1999; Fagiolini and Hensch, 2000). BDNF and NT4, signaling through trkB, modulate the effects of early monocular eyelid suture on neurophysiologically determined cortical ocular dominance (Galuske et al., 1996; Gillespie et al., 1996) and on the distribution of geniculocortical axons (Hata et al., 2000).

Dark rearing further elucidates the role of BDNF/trkB signaling in the developing visual cortex

DR reduces the eye-specific segregation of LGN axon arbors in carnivores and prolongs the critical period in rodents and carnivores (Cynader and Mitchell, 1980; Mower et al., 1985; Stryker and Harris, 1986; Swindale, 1988; Fagiolini et al., 1994). The potential mechanism by which DR-induced increases in cortical BDNF contribute to the reduced segregation of LGN axons and to changes in the visual response properties of cortical neurons depends on whether or not afferent axon terminals have access to the extra BDNF.

If the accumulated BDNF in V1 of DR animals is accessible, like infused BDNF or NT4 (Cabelli et al., 1995), it could have a direct trophic action that stabilizes afferent axon branches that are normally eliminated by competition for neurotrophins. Elevated levels of accessible BDNF could also modulate the threshold at which the effect of presynaptic activity changes from synaptic depression to potentiation (Bienenstock et al., 1982). DR reversibly diminishes this threshold, thus promoting potentiation and reducing depression (Kirkwood et al., 1995, 1996). In V1, BDNF reduces NMDA receptor-mediated synaptic depression (Akaneya et al., 1996; Huber et al., 1998; Kinoshita et al., 1999) and increases LTP (Akaneya et al., 1997; Huber et al., 1998). BDNF also scales cortical excitatory synaptic transmission by modulating AMPA and NMDA receptor-mediated post-synaptic currents and the probability of presynaptic transmitter release (Carmignoto et al., 1997; Takei et al., 1997; Rutherford et al., 1998; Sala et al., 1998; Turrigiano, 1999). BDNF regulates AMPA receptor expression (Akaneya et al., 1997) and can even act as an excitatory transmitter (Kafitz et al., 1999). Therefore, the DR-induced increase in cortical BDNF could modulate the depression/facilitation threshold change, thus potentiating (and stabilizing: Shatz, 1990; Kandel and O'Dell, 1992) LGN axon branches that would normally be depressed and eliminated.

DR could reduce the access to BDNF of afferent axons in V1, by sequestering BDNF within cortical neurons or afferent axon terminals, or diminishing receptor signaling. Reduced BDNF availability or diminished trkB signaling could have adverse trophic effects on *all* LGN axons and thereby reduce the selectivity of growth-promoting and regressive processes that cause the normal segregation of eye-specific axons. Alternatively, the sequestration of BDNF could shift the synaptic modification threshold (Bienenstock et al., 1982) upwards, thus increasing synaptic depression and elimination of LGN axons representing *both* eyes, and causing the reduced visual responsiveness of cortical neurons that is typical following DR (Fregnac and Imbert, 1984; Benevento et al., 1992; Fagiolini et al., 1994). In this instance, the reduced threshold for LTP in V1 of DR animals could be caused by the release of sequestered BDNF during experimental stimulation (a similar facilitation of LTP is induced by exogenous BDNF (Patterson et al., 1996)). DR also decreases the selectivity of V1 neurons for orientation and direction of movement (Fregnac and Imbert, 1984; Benevento et al., 1992; Fagiolini et al., 1994). One explanation of this could be that the reduced availability of BDNF causes an upward shift in the synaptic modification threshold, thus reducing the specificity of the activity-dependent focusing of immature excitatory connections that may also contribute to orientation and direction selectivity.

Changes in BDNF trafficking might explain other neurophysiological effects of DR. The DR-induced decrease in the orientation and direction selectivity of V1 neurons (Fregnac and Imbert, 1984; Benevento et al., 1992; Fagiolini et al., 1994) and the increase their spontaneous activity (Benevento et al., 1992) suggest that DR reduces the efficacy of GABAergic inhibition in V1 (Mower et al., 1985; Swindale and Cynader, 1986; Gabbott and Stewart, 1987; Ramoa et al., 1987; Tsumoto and Freeman, 1987; Swindale, 1988; Fagiolini et al., 1994). As noted above, BDNF is necessary for the activity-dependent establishment of GABA-mediated inhibition among V1 neurons. Thus, a DR-induced reduction in the availability of BDNF to GABAergic neurons could explain the reduced GABAergic tone and prolonged critical period in V1 of DR animals. As noted above, constitutive overexpression of BDNF accelerates the maturation of visual cortical inhibitory circuitry and thereby advances the critical period for vision-induced plasticity. BDNF mRNA is rapidly upregulated in V1 of DR animals that are later exposed to light (Castrén et al., 1992; Schoups et al., 1995). If this is accompanied by an increase in BDNF secretion in V1, the loss of ocular dominance plasticity (i.e. the unblocking of the functional maturation of V1) that occurs once DR animals experience normal vision (Mower et al., 1985; Asanuma et al., 1986; Swindale, 1988) is probably mediated by BDNF/trkB signaling.

Circadian changes in BDNF protein levels

In all the structures we examined, there is diurnal modulation of BDNF protein levels. In V1, the superior colliculus (SC) and retina, the tissue concentration of BDNF protein is 1.5–2.2 times greater in the middle of the light phase of the circadian cycle than in the middle of the dark phase. By contrast, in the cerebellum and hippocampus, BDNF protein levels in the middle of the light phase of the diurnal cycle were 75 and 82%, respectively, of those in the middle of the dark phase. Why do cortical BDNF protein levels decrease during the dark phase of the diurnal cycle but increase following DR? Chronic, DR-induced reductions in BDNF secretion or changes in BDNF trafficking could cause BDNF protein to accumulate in V1 (see above). The regular modulation of BDNF protein secretion and trafficking during a normal light/dark cycle would prevent such an accumulation, thus revealing the relatively small decrease in BDNF protein during the dark phase.

Our observation of elevated BDNF protein levels in the hippocampus and cerebellum during the dark phase of the diurnal cycle is consistent with previously observed increases in BDNF mRNA in the hippocampus during the dark phase (Bova et al., 1998; Berchtold et al., 1999; Schaaf et al., 2000). Hippocampal BDNF mRNA levels are increased by motor activity (see above). Thus, the diurnal modulation of BDNF protein in the hippocampus and cerebellum is probably due, in part, to the elevated nocturnal motor and cognitive activity of rodents. Diurnal changes in hormone levels might contribute to the circadian modulation of BDNF mRNA and protein (see above). Because of the profound effects of BDNF on synaptic efficacy (Thoenen, 1995; Schuman, 1999), our data suggest that circadian changes in BDNF levels could contribute to diurnal fluctuations in synaptic function in some neural circuits.

Role of BDNF/trkB signaling in the development of retinal projections

During normal development in mammals, approximately 70% of all retinal ganglion cells (RGCs) that are initially formed subsequently die (Sefton and Lam, 1984; Crespo et al., 1985; Tay et al., 1986) by pyknosis (Rehen and Linden, 1994; Cellerino et al., 2000). Developing RGC axons pass through three distinct phases — elongation of axon trunks, collateral branch formation and elaboration of terminal arbors — during which their modes of growth are qualitatively different (Bhide and Frost, 1991). During the elongation and collateralization phases, RGCs form a number of different types of transient projections, which are subsequently eliminated during the arborization phase (Frost et al., 1979; Frost, 1984; Bhide and Frost, 1991, 1992). What is the role of BDNF trkB signaling in these process?

Ontogenetic changes in BDNF protein levels in the retina and superior colliculus parallel the development of retinal projections

We used ECLIA to measure developmental changes in the tissue concentration of BDNF within the retina and SC of the Syrian hamster (Ma et al., 1997; Frost et al., 2001). Within the SC, we first detected BDNF protein (about 9 pg/mg tissue) on embryonic day 14 (E14; first 24 h following conception = E0), soon after the arrival of retinal ganglion cell (RGC) axons. BDNF protein concentration in the SC rises about 4-fold between E14 and postnatal day 4 (P4; first 24 h after birth on E15.5 = P0), remains at a plateau through P15, then declines by about one-third to attain its adult level by P18. By contrast, BDNF protein levels in the retina remain low (about 1 pg/mg tissue) through P12, then increase 4.5-fold to attain their adult values on P18. The developmental changes in retinal and collicular BDNF protein levels are temporally correlated with multiple events in the structural and functional maturation of the retinal projection system (Frost et al., 2001). This suggests a role for BDNF in the cellular mechanisms underlying some of those events.

Exogenous BDNF reduces the rate of developmental RGC death

To investigate the effect of target-derived neurotrophins on the developmental death of RGCs, we injected BDNF into the SC of neonatal hamsters (Ma et al., 1998). At the age when the rate of developmental RGC death is greatest (P4), BDNF produces, 20 h post-injection, a 13- and 15-fold reduction, respectively, in the rate of RGC pyknosis as compared to vehicle-injected and untreated hamsters. There is no effect 8 h post-injection. ECLIA measurements of BDNF protein in the retinae of normal and BDNF-treated hamsters demonstrate that there is no significant increase in BDNF protein concentration until 12 h post-injection. Cells undergoing developmental death become committed to die before pyknosis is apparent (Deckwerth and Johnson, 1993; Johnson and Deckwerth, 1993; Earnshaw, 1995). Thus, several hours are required between the arrival of retrogradely transported survival factors in their target somata and a reduction in pyknotic rate. Therefore, our data support a role for target-derived BDNF in promoting RGC survival.

Reduced trkB signaling increases the rate of developmental RGC death

Our pharmacological experiments do not address the role of trkB ligands in modulating the rate of RGC death under physiological conditions. To study this, we depleted trkB receptor ligands in the SC of hamsters by making bilateral intracollicular injections of trkB-Fc fusion proteins (Genentech) into the hamster SC 20 h prior to assaying the rate of developmental RGC death on P4 (Frost et al., 1998; Pollock et al., 2001b). This caused 1.7- and 1.5-fold increases in the rate of RGC death compared to those in normal and trkA-Fc-treated hamsters, respectively. We also compared the rate of developmental RGC death in wild-type (WT) C57Bl6/129 mice and mice that are homozygous (−/−) or heterozygous (+/−) for null mutation ('knockout') of the full-length trkB receptor (Pollock et al., 2000, 2001b) but that have normal truncated trkB receptors. On P2, the rates of RGC death are increased 2.1-fold and 1.5-fold, respectively for trkB(−/−) and trkB(+/−) mice as compared to WT. On P6, the rates of RGC death are, respectively, 7.2- and 4.3-fold more than WT. When the rates of RGC death are plotted as a function of time on P2–6, the slopes of the lines are similar for all three genotypes. Thus, the time constant of developmental changes in the rate of RGC death is not altered by trkB mutation. Immunoprecipitation combined with Western blot analysis demonstrates that the dose-dependent genetic effect on RGC death is reflected in the levels of trkB and phosphorylated trkB protein, which are reduced in trkB(+/−) mice and absent in trkB(−/−) mice. These data demonstrate that: (1) physiological concentrations of target-derived trkB ligands are survival factors for developing RGCs; and (2) these ligands exert their effects, in part, by signaling through a cascade initiated by trkB receptor activation. We are now determining the number of RGCs that survive the epoch of developmental RGC death in WT and trkB(−/−) mice. Surprisingly, homozygous knockout of BDNF does not alter the final number of murine RGCs (Cellerino et al., 1997). Therefore, we are also measuring the rate of RGC death and final number of RGCs in mice that have combined homozygous knockouts for BDNF and NT4, the high affinity ligands of trkB.

Effects of BDNF on the distribution of RGC axons

We have compared quantitatively the distribution of anterogradely labeled retinofugal projections in WT, trkB(−/−) and trkB(+/−) mice. There is no significant difference among genotypes with respect to the segregation of crossed and uncrossed retino-LGN projections. Because localized overexpression of BDNF can partially stabilize certain normally transient uncrossed retinal projections (Isenmann et al., 1999) we are currently studying the retinal projections of mice that are homozygous for knockout of the p75 receptor, to see if BDNF exerts its effects through p75 signaling.

Conclusions

During early life, the sensory environment, by modulating neural activity, contributes to the regulation of BDNF mRNA and protein levels. However the changes in BDNF mRNA and protein are not necessarily correlated, most likely due to activity-dependent changes in BDNF trafficking. This is of profound functional importance because altered trafficking potentially affects the ability of BDNF protein to bind to its receptors. BDNF/trkB signaling is likely to be altered under conditions of early abnormal visual experience due to peripheral visual defects. This change in signaling may be a mechanism for resultant structural and functional defects. Neurotrophins may be useful therapeutic agents in the treatment of these abnormalities. In addition, in normal, mature animals, there is a diurnal modulation of BDNF protein levels in the primary visual system and in motor and cognitive structures. This could induce circadian fluctuations in synaptic function in some neural circuits.

Developing RGC axons have distinctive growth behaviors at different stages and make several types of transient projections. Ontogenetic changes in BDNF protein levels in the retinal projection system are correlated with various critical steps in the development of the system. Physiological concentrations of neurotrophins (probably BDNF), signaling through full-length trkB receptors, modulate the rate of developmental RGC death. Neurotrophins may also influence the pattern of retinal projections.

Abbreviations

BDNF	brain-derived neurotrophic factor
CNS	central nervous system
DR	rearing in constant darkness
ECLIA	electrochemiluminescent immunoassay

GABA	gamma-aminobutyric acid
LGN	lateral geniculate nucleus
LR	rearing in constant light
LTP	long-term potentiation
NT4	neurotrophic factor 4
PI3K	PI3 kinase
RGC	retinal ganglion cell
SC	superior colliculus
TTX	tetrodotoxin
V1	primary visual cortex
WT	wild-type

References

Akaneya, Y., Tsumoto, T. and Hatanaka, H. (1996) Brain-derived neurotrophic factor blocks long-term depression in rat visual cortex. *J. Neurophysiol.*, 76: 4198–4201.

Akaneya, Y., Tsumoto, T., Kinoshita, S. and Hatanaka, H. (1997) Brain-derived neurotrophic factor enhances long-term potentiation in rat visual cortex. *J. Neurosci.*, 17: 6707–6716.

Alcántara, S., Frisén, J., del Rio, J.A., Soriano, E., Barbacid, M. and Silos-Santiago, I. (1997) TrkB signaling is required for postnatal survival of CNS neurons and protects hippocampal and motor neurons from axotomy-induced cell death. *J. Neurosci.*, 17: 3623–3633.

Allendoerfer, K.L., Shelton, D.L., Shooter, E.M. and Shatz, C.J. (1990) Nerve growth factor receptor immunoreactivity is transiently associated with the subplate neurons of the mammalian cerebral cortex. *Proc. Natl. Acad. Sci. USA*, 87: 187–190.

Alonso-Vanegas, M.A., Fawcett, J.P., Causing, C.G., Miller, F.D. and Sadikot, A.F. (1999) Characterization of dopaminergic midbrain neurons in a DBH:BDNF transgenic mouse. *J. Comp. Neurol.*, 413: 449–462.

Altar, C.A., Cai, N., Bliven, T., Juhasz, M., Conner, J.M., Acheson, A.L., Lindsay, R.M. and Wiegand, S.J. (1997) Anterograde transport of brain-derived neurotrophic factor and its role in the brain. *Nature*, 389: 856–860.

Anderson, J.S., Carandini, M. and Ferster, D. (2000) Orientation tuning of input conductance, excitation, and inhibition in cat primary visual cortex. *J. Neurophysiol.*, 84: 909–926.

Androutsellis-Theotokis, A., McCormack, W.J., Bradford, H.F., Stern, G.M. and Pliego-Rivero, F. (1996) The depolarisation-induced release of [^{125}I]BDNF from brain tissue. *Brain Res.*, 743: 40–48.

Asanuma, C., Ohkawa, R., Stanfield, B.B. and Cowan, W.M. (1986) Pre- and postnatal development of the medial lemniscus (ML), the brachium conjunctivum (BC) and the brachium of the inferior colliculus (BIC) in rats. *Neurosci. Abstr.*, 12: 953.

Atwal, J.K., Massie, B., Miller, F.D. and Kaplan, D.R. (2000) The trkB-Shc site signals neuronal survival and local axon growth via MEK and PI3-kinase. *Neuron*, 27: 265–277.

Bamji, S.X., Majdan, M., Pozniak, C.D., Belliveau, D.J., Aloyz, R.S., Kohn, J., Causing, C.G. and Miller, F.D. (1998) The p75 neurotrophin receptor mediates neuronal apoptosis and is essential for naturally occurring sympathetic neuron death. *J. Cell Biol.*, 140: 911–923.

Benevento, L.A., Bakkum, B.W., Port, J.D. and Cohen, R.S. (1992) The effects of dark-rearing on the electrophysiology of the rat visual cortex. *Brain Res.*, 572: 198–207.

Benevento, L.A., Bakkum, B.W. and Cohen, R.S. (1995) Gamma-aminobutyric acid and somatostatin immunoreactivity in the visual cortex in normal and dark-reared rats. *Brain Res.*, 689: 172–182.

Berchtold, N.C., Oliff, H.S., Isackson, P. and Cotman, C.W. (1999) Hippocampal BDNF mRNA shows a diurnal regulation, primarily in the exon III transcript. *Mol. Brain Res.*, 71: 11–22.

Bessho, Y., Nakanishi, S. and Nawa, H. (1993) Glutamate receptor agonists enhance the expression of BDNF mRNA in cultured cerebellar granule cells. *Mol. Brain Res.*, 18: 201–208.

Bhide, P.G. and Frost, D.O. (1991) Stages of growth of hamster retinofugal axons: implications for developing axonal pathways with multiple targets. *J. Neurosci.*, 11: 485–504.

Bhide, P.G. and Frost, D.O. (1992) Axon substitution in the reorganization of developing neural connections. *Proc. Natl. Acad. Sci. USA*, 89: 11847–11851.

Bienenstock, E.L., Cooper, L.N. and Munrow, P.W. (1982) Theory for the development of neuron selectivity: orientation specificity and binocular interaction in the visual cortex. *J. Neurosci.*, 2: 32–48.

Bova, R., Micheli, M.R., Qualadrucci, P. and Zucconi, G.G. (1998) BDNF and trkB mRNAs oscillate in rat brain during the light-dark cycle. *Mol. Brain Res.*, 57: 321–324.

Bozzi, Y., Pizzorusso, T., Cremist, F., Rossi, F.M., Barsacchi, G. and Maffei, L. (1995) Monocular deprivation decreases the expression of messenger RNA for brain-derived neurotrophic factor in the rat visual cortex. *Neuroscience*, 69: 1133–1144.

Cabelli, R.J., Hohn, A. and Shatz, C.J. (1995) Inhibition of ocular dominance column formation by infusion of NT-4/5 or BDNF. *Science*, 267: 1662–1666.

Cabelli, R.J., Shelton, D.L., Segal, R.A. and Shatz, C.J. (1997) Blockade of endogenous ligands of trkB inhibits formation of ocular dominace columns. *Neuron*, 19: 63–76.

Callaway, E.M. and Katz, L.C. (1991) Effects of binocular deprivation on the development of clustered horizontal connections in cat striate cortex. *Proc. Natl. Acad. Sci. USA*, 88: 745–749.

Carmignoto, G., Pizzorusso, T., Tia, S. and Vicini, S. (1997) Brain-derived neurotrophic factor and nerve growth factor potentiate excitatory synaptic transmission in the rat visual cortex. *J. Physiol. (Lond.)*, 498: 153–164.

Castren, E., Zafra, F., Thoenen, H. and Lindholm, D. (1992) Light regulates expression of brain-derived neurotrophic factor mRNA in rat visual cortex. *Proc. Natl. Acad. Sci. USA*, 89: 9444–9448.

Castrén, E., Zafra, F., Thoenen, H. and Lindholm, D. (1992) Light regulates expression of brain-derived neurotrophic factor mRNA in rat visual cortex. *Proc. Natl. Acad. Sci. USA*, 89: 9444–9448.

Causing, C.G., Gloster, A., Aloyz, R.S., Bamji, S.X., Chang, E., Fawcett, J.P., Kuchel, G. and Miller, F.D. (1997) Synaptic innervation density is regulated by neuron-derived BDNF. *Neuron*, 18: 257–267.

Cellerino, A., Maffei, L. and Domenici, L. (1996) The distribution of brain-derived neurotrophic factor and its receptor trkB in parvalbumin-containing neurons of the rat visual cortex. *Eur. J. Neurosci.*, 8: 1190–1197.

Cellerino, A., Carroll, P., Thoenen, H. and Barde, Y.-A. (1997) Reduced size of retinal ganglion cell axons and hypomyelination in mice lacking brain-derived neurotrophic factor. *Mol. Cell. Neurosci.*, 9: 397–408.

Cellerino, A., Pinzon-Duarte, G., Carroll, P. and Kohler, K. (1998) Brain-derived neurotrophic factor modulates the development of the dopaminergic network in the rodent retina. *J. Neurosci.*, 18(9): 3351–3362.

Cellerino, A., Galli-Resta, L. and Colombaioni, L. (2000) The dynamics of neuronal death: a time-lapse study in the retina. *J. Neurosci.*, 20(RC92): 1–5.

Chen, E.Y., Mufson, E.J. and Kordower, J.H. (1996) trk and p75 neurotrophin receptor systems in the developing human brain. *J. Comp. Neurol.*, 369: 591–618.

Chung, S. and Ferster, D. (1998) Strength and orientation tuning of the thalamic input to simple cells revealed by electrically evoked cortical suppression. *Neuron*, 20: 1177–1189.

Cohen-Cory, S. and Fraser, S.E. (1995) Effects of brain-derived neurotrophic factor on optic axon branching and remodelling in vivo. *Nature*, 378: 192–196.

Cohen-Cory, S. (1999) BDNF modulates, but does not mediate, activity-dependent branching and remodeling of optic axon arbors in vivo. *J. Neurosci.*, 22: 9996–10003.

Conner, J.M., Lauterborn, J.C., Yan, Q., Gall, C.M. and Varon, S. (1997) Distribution of brain-derived neurotrophic factor (BDNF) protein and mRNA in the normal rat CNS: evidence for anterograde axonal transport. *J. Neurosci.*, 17: 2295–2313.

Cowan, W.M., Fawcett, J.W., O'Leary, D.D.M. and Stanfield, B.B. (1984) Regressive events in neurogenesis. *Science*, 225: 1258–1265.

Crespo, D., O'Leary, D.D.M. and Cowan, W.M. (1985) Changes in the numbers of optic nerve fibers during late prenatal and postnatal development in the albino rat. *Dev. Brain Res.*, 19: 129–134.

Crook, J.M., Kisvarday, Z.F. and Eysel, U.T. (1996) GABA-induced inactivation of functionally characterized sites in cat visual cortex (area 18): effects on direction selectivity. *J. Neurophysiol.*, 75: 2071–2088.

Crook, J.M., Kisvarday, Z.F. and Eysel, U.T. (1997) GABA-induced inactivation of functionally characterized sites in cat striate cortex: effects on orientation tuning and direction selectivity. *Vis. Neurosci.*, 14: 141–158.

Cui, Q. and Harvey, A.R. (1994) NT-4/5 reduces naturally occurring retinal ganglion cell death in neonatal rats. *NeuroReport*, 5: 1882–1884.

Cynader, M.S. and Mitchell, D.E. (1980) Prolonged sensitivity to monocular deprivation in dark-reard cats. *J. Neurophysiol.*, 43: 1026–1040.

Davies, A.M. (1994) The role of neurotrophins in the developing nervous system. *J. Neurobiol.*, 25: 1334–1348.

Deckwerth, T.L. and Johnson Jr., E.M. (1993) Temporal analysis of events associated with programmed cell death (apoptosis) of sympathetic neurons deprived of nerve growth factor. *J. Cell Biol.*, 123: 1207–1222.

Domenici, L., Berardi, N., Carmignoto, G., Vantini, G. and Maffei, L. (1991) Nerve growth factor prevents the amblyopic effects of monocular deprivation. *Proc. Natl. Acad. Sci. USA*, 88: 8811–8815.

Du, J., Feng, L., Feng, Y. and Lu, B. (2000) Activity- and Ca2+-dependent modulation of surface expression of brain-derived neurotrophic factor receptors in hippocampal neurons. *J. Cell Biol.*, 150: 1423–1433.

Earnshaw, W.C. (1995) Nuclear changes in apoptosis. *Curr. Opin. Neurobiol.*, 7: 337–343.

Elmer, E., Kokaia, Z., Kokaia, M., Carnahan, J., Nawas, H. and Lindvall, O. (1998) Dynamic changes of brain derived neurotrophic factor protein levels in the rat forebrain after single and recurring kindling-induced seizures. *Neuroscience*, 83: 351–362.

Fagan, A.M., Zhang, H., Landis, S., Smeyne, R.J., Silos-Santiago, I. and Barbacid, M. (1996) trkA, but not trkC, receptors are essential for survival of sympathetic neurons in vivo. *J. Neurosci.*, 16: 6208–6218.

Fagiolini, M., Pizzorusso, Y., Berardi, N., Domenici, L. and Maffei, L. (1994) Functional postnatal development of the rat primary visual cortex and the role of visual experience: dark rearing and monocular deprivation. *Vision Res.*, 34: 709–720.

Fagiolini, M. and Hensch, T.K. (2000) Inhibitory threshold for critical-period activation in primary visual cortex. *Nature*, 404: 183–186.

Fawcett, J.P., Aloyz, R.S., McLean, J.H., Pareek, S., Miller, F.D., McPherson, P.S. and Murphy, R.A. (1997) Detection of brain-derived neurotrophic factor in a vesicular fraction of brain synaptosomes. *J. Biol. Chem.*, 272: 8837–8840.

Fawcett, J.P., Bamji, S.X., Causing, C.G., Aloyz, R.S., Ase, A.R., Reader, T.A., McLean, J.H. and Miller, F.D. (1998) Functional evidence that BDNF is an anterograde neuronal trophic factor in the CNS. *J. Neurosci.*, 18: 2808–2821.

Ferster, D., Chung, S. and Wheat, H. (1996) Orientation selectivity of thalamic input to simple cells of cat visual cortex. *Nature*, 380: 249–252.

Finkbeiner, S., Tavazoie, S.F., Maloratsky, A., Jacobs, K.M., Harris, K.M. and Greenberg, M.E. (1997) CREB: a major mediator of neuronal neurotrophin responses. *Neuron*, 19: 1031–1047.

Frade, J.M. and Barde, Y.-A. (1998) Microglia-derived nerve growth factor causes cell death in the developiong retina. *Neuron*, 20: 35–41.

Frade, J.M. and Barde, Y.-A. (1999) Genetic evidence for cell death mediated by nerve growth factor and the neurotrophin receptor p75 in the developing mouse retina and spinal cord. *Development*, 126: 683–690.

Frade, J.M., Rodriguez-Tebar, A. and Barde, Y.-A. (1996) Induction of cell death by endogenous nerve growth factor through its p75 receptor. *Nature*, 383: 166–168.

Frade, J.M., Bovolenta, P., Martinez-Morales, J.R., Arribas, A., Barbas, J.A. and Rodriguez-Tebar, A. (1997) Control of early cell death by BDNF in the chick retina. *Development*, 124: 3313–3320.

Fregnac, Y. and Imbert, M. (1984) Development of neuronal selectivity in primary visual cortex of cat. *Physiol. Rev.*, 64: 325–434.

Frost, D.O. (1984) Axonal growth and target selection during development: retinal projections to the ventrobasal complex and other 'nonvisual' structures in neonatal Syrian hamsters. *J. Comp. Neurol.*, 230: 576–592.

Frost, D.O., So, K.-F. and Schneider, G.E. (1979) Postnatal development of retinal projectins in Syrian hamsters: a study using autoradiographic and anterograde degeneration techniques. *Neuroscience*, 4: 1649–1677.

Frost, D.O. and Innocenti, G.M. (1986) Effects of sensory experience on the development of visual callosal connections. In: F. Lepore, M. Ptito and H. Jasper (Eds.), *Two Hemispheres — One Brain*. Alan Liss, New York, pp. 255–266.

Frost, D.O., Ma, Y.-T., Pollock, G., Robichon, R., Lyons, M.E., Ambalavanar, R. and Kaplan, D.R. (1998) Role of trkB ligands in the developmental death of hamster retinal ganglion cells. *Neurosci. Abstr.*, 24: 294.

Frost, D.O., Ma, Y.-T., Hsieh, T., Forbes, M.E. and Johnson, J.E. (2001) Developmental changes in BDNF protein levels in the hamster retina and superior colliculus. *J. Neurobiol.*, 49: in press.

Gabbott, P.L. and Stewart, M.G. (1987) Quantitative morphological effects of dark-rearing and light exposure on the synaptic connectivity of layer 4 in the rat visual cortex (area 17). *Exp. Brain Res.*, 68: 103–114.

Gall, C.M. (1993) Seizure-induced changes in neurotrophin expression: implications for epilepsy. *Exp. Neurol.*, 124: 150–166.

Gall, C.M., Guthrie, K. and Lauterborn, J.C. (1995) Stimulation of neurotrophic factor expression: links to different forms of brain plasticity. In: C.F. Ibanez (Ed.), *Life and Death in the Nervous System*. Elsevier, Oxford, pp. 275–295.

Galuske, R., Kim, D., Castrén, E., Thoenen, H. and Singer, W. (1996) Brain-derived neurotrophic factor reverses experience-dependent synaptic modifications in kitten visual cortex. *Eur. J. Neurosci.*, 8: 1554–1559.

Ghosh, A., Carnahan, J. and Greenberg, M.E. (1994) Requirement for BDNF in activity-dependent survival of cortical neurons. *Science*, 263: 1618–1623.

Gibbs, R.B. (1998) Levels of trkA and BDNF mRNA, but not NGF mRNA, fluctuate across the estrous cycle and increase in response to acute hormone replacement. *Brain Res.*, 787: 259–268.

Gillespie, D.C., Crair, M.C. and Stryker, M.P. (1996) NT4/5 infusion alters plasticity and responses of cat primary visual cortex during the critical period. *Neurosci. Abstr.*, 22: 276.

Goodman, C.S. and Shatz, C.J. (1993) Developmental mechanisms that generate precise patterns of neuronal connectivity. *Neuron*, 10: 77–98.

Goodman, L., Valverde, J. and Lim, F. et al. (1996) Regulated release and polarized localization of brain-derived neurotrophic factor in hippocampal neurons. *Mol. Cell. Neurosci.*, 7: 222–238.

Griesbeck, O., Blöchl, A., Carnahan, J.F., Nawa, H. and Thoenen, H. (1995) Characterization of brain-derived neurotrophic factor (BDNF) secretion from hippocampal neurons. *Neurosci. Abstr.*, 21: 1046.

Griesbeck, O., Canossa, M. and Campana, G. et al. (1999) Are there differences between the secretion characteristics of NGF and BDNF? Implications for the modulatory role of neurotrophins in activity-dependent neuronal plasticity. *Microsc. Res. Tech.*, 45: 262–275.

Hanover, J.L., Huang, Z.J., Tonegawa, S. and Stryker, M.P. (1999) Brain-derived neurotrophic factor overexpression induces precocious critical period in mouse visual cortex. *J. Neurosci.*, 19(RC40): 1–5.

Hata, Y., Ohshima, M., Ichisaka, S., Wakita, M., Fukuda, M. and Tsumoto, T. (2000) Brain-derived neurotrophic factor expands ocular dominance columns in visual cortex in monocularly deprived and non-deprived kittens but does not in adult cats. *J. Neurosci.*, 20(RC57): 1–5.

Haubensak, W., Narz, F., Heumann, R. and Lessmann, V. (1998) BDNF-GFP containing secretory granules are localized in the vicinity of synaptic junctions of cultured cortical neurons. *J. Cell Sci.*, 111: 1483–1493.

Hock, C., Heese, K., Muller-Spahn, F., Hulette, C., Rosenburg, C. and Otten, U. (1998) Decreased trkA neurotrophin receptor expression in the parietal cortex of patients with Alzheimer's disease. *Neurosci. Lett.*, 241: 151–154.

Hoyle, G.W., Mercer, E.H., Palmiter, R.D. and Brinster, R.L. (1993) Expression of NGF in sympathetic neurons leads to excessive axon outgrowth from ganglia but decreased terminal innervation within tissues. *Neuron*, 10: 1019–1034.

Huang, Z.J., Kirkwood, A., Pizzorusso, T., Porciatti, V., Morales, B., Bear, M.F., Maffei, L. and Tonegawa, S. (1999) BDNF regulates the maturation of inhibition and the critical period of plasticity in mouse visual cortex. *Cell*, 98: 739–755.

Hubel, D.H., Wiesel, T.N. and LeVay, S. (1977) Plasticity of ocular dominance columns in monkey striate cortex. *Phil. Trans. R. Soc. Lond. B*, 278: 377–409.

Huber, K.M., Sawtell, N.B. and Bear, M.F. (1998) Brain-derived neurotrophic factor alters the synaptic modification threshold in visual cortex. *Neuropharmacology*, 37: 571–579.

Isenmann, S., Cellerino, A., Gravel, C. and Baehr, M. (1999) Excess target-derived brain-derived neurotrophic factor (BDNF) preserves the transient uncrossed retinal projection in the superior colliculus. *Mol. Cell. Neurosci.*, 14: 52–65.

Johnson Jr., E.M. and Deckwerth, T.L. (1993) Molecular mechanisms of developmental neuronal death. *Annu. Rev. Neurosci.*, 16: 31–46.

Johnson, F., Hohmann, S.E., DiStefano, P.S. and Bottjer, S.W. (1997) Neurotrophins suppress apoptosis induced by deafferentation of avian motor-cortical region. *J. Neurosci.*, 17: 2101–2111.

Johnson, J.E., Barde, Y.-A., Schwab, M. and Thoenen, H. (1986) Brain-derived neurotrophic factor supports the survival of cultured rat retinal ganglion cells. *J. Neurosci.*, 6: 3031–3038.

Jones, K.R., Fariñas, I., Backus, C. and Reichardt, L.F. (1994) Targeted disruption of the BDNF gene perturbs brain and sensory neuron development but not motor neuron development. *Cell*, 76: 989–999.

Jones, K.R., Vigers, A.J., Amin, D. and Zeiler, S.R. (2000) BDNF expression in murine visual cortex is altered by monocular deprivation. *Neurosci. Abstr.*, 26: 1079.

Kafitz, K.W., Rose, C.R., Thoenen, H. and Konnerth, A. (1999) Neurotrophin-evoked rapid excitation through TrkB receptors. *Nature*, 401: 918–921.

Kandel, E.R. and O'Dell, T.J. (1992) Are adult learning mechanisms also used for development? *Science*, 258: 243–245.

Kaplan, D.R. and Miller, F.D. (2000) Neurotrophin signal transduction in the nervous system. *Curr. Opin. Neurobiol.*, 10: 381–391.

Katz, L.C. and Shatz, C.J. (1996) Synaptic activity and the construction of cortical circuits. *Science*, 274: 1133–1138.

Kinoshita, S., Yasuda, H., Taniguchi, N., Katoh-Semba, R., Hatanaka, H. and Tsumoto, T. (1999) Brain-derived neurotrophic factor prevents low-frequency inputs from inducing long-term depression in the developing visual cortex. *J. Neurosci.*, 19: 2122–2130.

Kirkwood, A., Lee, H.-K. and Bear, M.F. (1995) Co-regulation of long-term potentiation and experience-dependent synaptic plasticity in visual cortex by age and experience. *Nature*, 375: 328–331.

Kirkwood, A., Rioult, M.G. and Bear, M.F. (1996) Experience-dependent modification of synaptic plasticity in visual cortex. *Nature*, 381: 526–528.

Knipper, M., Berzaghi, M.P., Blöchl, A., Breer, H., Thoenen, H. and Lindholm, D. (1994) Positive feedback between acetylcholine and the neurotrophins nerve growth factor and brain-derived neurotrophic factor. *Eur. J. Neurosci.*, 6: 668–671.

Kohn, J., Aloyz, R.S., Toma, J.G., Haak-Frendscho, M. and Miller, F.D. (1999) Functionally antagonistic interactions between the TrkA and p75 neurotrophin receptors regulate sympathetic neuron growth and target innervation. *J. Neurosci.*, 19: 5393–5408.

Korsching, S. (1993) The neurotrophic factor concept: A reexamination. *J. Neurosci.*, 13: 2739–2748.

Lein, E., Hohn, A. and Shatz, C.J. (1997) Rapid regulation of BDNF mRNA by afferent activity in the visual system. *Neurosci. Abstr.*, 23: 47.

Lein, E.S., Finney, E.M., McQuillen, P.S. and Shatz, C.J. (1999) Subplate neuron ablation alters neurotrophin expression and ocular dominance column formation. *Proc. Natl. Acad. Sci. USA*, 96: 13491–13495.

Lein, E.S., Hohn, A. and Shatz, C.J. (2000) Dynamic regulation of BDNF and NT-3 expression during visual system development. *J. Comp. Neurol.*, 420: 1–18.

Lewin, G.R. and Barde, Y.-A. (1996) Physiology of the neurotrophins. *Annu. Rev. Neurosci.*, 19: 289–317.

Lindefors, N., Ernfors, P., Falkenberg, T. and Persson, H. (1992) Septal cholinergic afferents regulate expression of brain-derived neurotrophic factor and beta-nerve growth factor mRNA in rat hippocampus. *Exp. Brain Res.*, 88: 78–90.

Lindholm, D., Castren, E., Berzaghi, M.P., Blöchl, A. and Thoenen, H. (1994) Activity-dependent and hormonal regulation of neurotrophin mRNA levels in brain — implications for neuronal plasticity. *J. Neurobiol.*, 25: 1362–1372.

Ma, Y.-T., Hsieh, T., Forbes, M.E., Johnson, J.E. and Frost, D.O. (1997) BDNF protein levels in developing hamster visual system. *Neurosci. Abstr.*, 23: 329.

Ma, Y.-T., Hsieh, T., Forbes, M.E., Johnson, J.E. and Frost, D.O. (1998) BDNF injected into the superior colliculus reduces developmental retinal ganglion cell death. *J. Neurosci.*, 18: 2097–2107.

Majdan, M., Lachance, C., Gloster, A., Aloyz, R.S., Zeindler, C., Bamji, S.X., Bhakar, A., Belliveau, D.J., Fawcett, J.P., Miller, F.D. and Barker, P.A. (1997) Transgenic mice expressing the intracellular domain of the p75 neurotrophin receptor undergo neuronal apoptosis. *J. Neurosci.*, 17: 6988–6998.

Marty, S., Berninger, B., Carroll, P. and Thoenen, H. (1996a) GABAergic stimulation regulates the phenotype of hippocampal interneurons through the regulation of brain-derived neurotrophic factor. *Neuron*, 16: 565–570.

Marty, S., Carroll, P., Cellerino, A., Castren, E., Staiger, V., Thoenen, H. and Lindholm, D. (1996b) Brain-derived neurotrophic factor promotes the differentiation of various hippocampal nonpyramidal neurons, including Cajal–Retzius cells, in organotypic slice cultures. *J. Neurosci.*, 16: 675–687.

McAllister, A.K., Lo, D.C. and Katz, L.C. (1995) Neurotrophins regulate dendritic growth in developing visual cortex. *Neuron*, 15: 791–803.

McAllister, A.K., Katz, L.C. and Lo, D.C. (1997) Opposing roles for endogenous BDNF and NT-3 in regulating cortical dendritic growth. *Neuron*, 18: 767–778.

McAllister, A.K., Katz, L.C. and Lo, D.C. (1999) Neurotrophins and synaptic plasticity. *Annu. Rev. Neurosci.*, 22: 295–318.

Meinecke, D.L. and Rakic, P. (1993) Low-affinity p75 nerve growth factor receptor expression in monkey telencephalon: timing and localization in diverse cellular elements. *Neuroscience*, 54: 105–116.

Meyer-Franke, A., Wilkinson, G.A., Kruttgen, A., Hu, M., Munro, E., Hanson, M.G., Reichardt, L.F. and Barres, B.A. (1998) Depolarization and cAMP elevation rapidly recruit trkB to the plasma membrane of CNS neurons. *Neuron*, 21: 681–693.

Miller, K.D., Keller, J.B. and Stryker, M.P. (1989) Ocular dominance column development: analysis and simulation. *Science*, 245: 605–615.

Miller, M.W. and Pitts, A.F. (2000) Neurotrophin receptors in the somatosensory cortex of the mature rat: co-localization of p75, trk, isoforms and c-neu. *Brain Res.*, 852: 355–366.

Mower, G.D., Caplan, C.J., Christen, W.G. and Duffy, F.H. (1985) Dark rearing prolongs physiological but not anatomical plasticity of the cat visual cortex. *J. Comp. Neurol.*, 235: 448–466.

Mowla, S.J., Pareek, S., Farhadi, H.F., Petrecca, K., Fawcett, J.P., Seidah, N.G., Morris, S.J., Sossin, W.S. and Murphy, R.A. (1999) Differential sorting of nerve growth factor and brain-derived neurotrophic factor in hippocampal neurons. *J. Neurosci.*, 19: 1–12.

Nawa, H., Carnahan, J. and Gall, C.M. (1995) BDNF protein measured by a novel enzyme immunoassay in normal brain and after seizure: partial disagreement with mRNA levels. *Eur. J. Neurosci.*, 7: 1527–1535.

Neeper, S.A., Gomez-Pinilla, F., Choi, J. and Cotman, C.W. (1996) Physical activity increases mRNA for brain-derived neurotrophic factor and nerve growth factor. *Brain Res.*, 726: 49–56.

Okazawa, H., Kamei, M., Imafuku, I. and Kanazawa, I. (1994) Gene regulation of trkB and trkC in the chick retina by light/darkness exposure. *Oncogene*, 9: 1813–1818.

Oliff, H.S., Berchtold, N.C., Isackson, P. and Cotman, C.W. (1998) Exercise-induced regulation of brain-derived neurotrophic factor (BDNF) transcripts in the rat hippocampus. *Mol. Brain Res.*, 61: 147–153.

Oppenheim, R.W. (1991) Cell death during development of the nervous system. *Annu. Rev. Neurosci.*, 14: 453–501.

Palko, M.E., Coppola, V. and Tessarollo, L. (1999) Evidence for a role of truncated trkC receptor isoforms in mouse development. *J. Neurosci.*, 19: 775–782.

Patel, T.D., Jackman, A., Rice, F.L., Kucera, J. and Snider, W.D. (2000) Development of sensory neurons in the absence of NGF/trkA signaling in vivo. *Neuron*, 25: 345–357.

Patterson, S., Abel, T., Deuel, T., Martin, K., Rose, J. and Kandel, E. (1996) Recombinant BDNF rescues deficits in basal synaptic transmission and hippocampal LTP in BDNF knockout mice. *Neuron*, 16: 1137–1145.

Patterson, S.L., Grover, L.M., Schwartzkroin, P.A. and Bothwell, M. (1992) Neurotrophin expression in rat hippocampal slices: a stimulus paradigm inducing LTP in CA1 evokes increases in BDNF and NT-3 mRNAs. *Neuron*, 9: 1081–1088.

Pollock, G.S. and Frost, D.O. (2001) Complexity in the modulation of neurotrophic factor mRNA expression by visual experience. *J. Neurosci.*, submitted for publication.

Pollock, G.S., Boyd, K.A., Kerkel, K.A., Ma, Y.-T., Aloyz, R., Kaplan, D.R. and Frost, D.O. (2000) Role of trkB ligands in developmental retinal ganglion cell death. *Soc. Neurosci. Abstr.*, 26: 847.

Pollock, G.S., Vernon, E., Forbes, M.E., Yan, Q., Ma, Y.-T., Hsieh, T., Robichon, R., Frost, D.O. and Johnson, J.E. (2001a) Effects of early visual experience and diurnal rhythms on BDNF mRNA and protein levels in the visual system, hippocampus, and cerebellum. *J. Neurosci.*, 21: 3923–3931.

Pollock, G.S., Boyd, K.A., Kerkel, K.A., Lyles, J., Ma, Y.-T., Aloyz, R., Kaplan, D.R. and Frost, D.O. (2001b) Disrupted trkB receptor signaling increases developmental death of retinal ganglion cells. *J. Neurosci.*, submitted for publication.

Primi, M.-P. and Clarke, P.G.H. (1996) Retrograde neurotrophin-mediated control of neurone survival in the developing central nervous system. *Dev. Neurosci.*, 7: 473–476.

Ramoa, A.S., Shadlen, M. and Freeman, R.D. (1987) Dark-reared cats: unresponsive cells become visually responsive with microiontophoresis of an excitatory amino acid. *Exp. Brain Res.*, 65: 658–665.

Rehen, S.K. and Linden, R. (1994) Apoptosis in the developing retina: paradoxical effects of protein synthesis inhibition. *Braz. J. Med. Biol. Res.*, 27: 1647–1651.

Roux, P.P., Colicos, M.A., Barker, P.A. and Kennedy, T.E. (1999) p75 Neurotrophin receptor expression is induced by apoptotic neurons after seizure. *J. Neurosci.*, 19: 6887–6896.

Rutherford, L.C., DeWan, A., Lauer, H.M. and Turrigiano, G.G. (1997) Brain-derived neurotrophic factor mediates the activity-dependent regulation of inhibition in neocortical cultures. *J. Neurosci.*, 17: 4527–4535.

Rutherford, L.C., Nelson, B.S. and Turrigiano, G.G. (1998) BDNF has opposite effects on the quantal amplitude of pyramidal neuron and interneuron excitatory synapses. *Neuron*, 21: 521–530.

Sala, R., Viegi, A., Rossi, F.M., Pizzorusso, T., Bonanno, G., Raiteri, M. and Maffei, L. (1998) Nerve growth factor and brain-derived neurotrophic factor increase neurotransmitter release in the rat visual cortex. *Eur. J. Neurosci.*, 10: 2185–2191.

Schaaf, M.J., Duurland, R., deKloet, E.R. and Vreugdenhil, E. (2000) Circadian variation in BDNF mRNA expression in the rat hipocampus. *Mol. Brain Res.*, 75: 342–344.

Schoups, A.A., Elliott, R.C., Friedman, W.J. and Black, I.B. (1995) NGF and BDNF are differentially modulated by visual experience in the developing geniculocortical pathway. *Brain Res.*, 86: 326–334.

Schuman, E.M. (1999) Neurotrophin regulation of synaptic transmission. *Curr. Opin. Neurobiol.*, 9: 105–109.

Schwartz, P.M., Borghesani, P.R., Levy, R.L., Pomeroy, S.L. and Segal, R.A. (1997) Abnormal cerebellar development and foliation in BDNF−/− mice reveals a role for neurotrophins in CNS patterning. *Neuron*, 19: 269–281.

Sefton, A.J. and Lam, K. (1984) Quantitative and morphological studies on developing optic axons in normal and enucleated albino rats. *Exp. Brain Res.*, 57: 107–117.

Shatz, C.J. (1990) Impulse activity and the patterning of connections during CNS development. *Neuron*, 5: 745–756.

Shatz, C.J. (1997) Neurotrophins and visual system plasticity. In: M. Cowan, T. Jessell and S. Zipursky (Eds.), *Molecular and Cellular Approaches to Neural Development*. Oxford University Press, New York, pp. 509–524.

Sherman, S.M. and Spear, P.D. (1982) Organization of visual pathways in normal and visually deprived cats. *Physiol. Rev.*, 62: 738–855.

Smith, M.A., Zhang, L.-X., Lyons, W.E. and Mamounas, L.A. (1997) Anterograde transport of endogenous brain-derived neurotrophic factor in hippocampal mossy fibers. *NeuroReport*, 8: 1829–1834.

Snider, W.D. and Lichtman, J.W. (1996) Are neurotrophins synaptotrophins? *Mol. Cell. Neurosci.*, 7: 433–442.

Somers, D.C., Nelson, S.B. and Sur, M. (1995) An emergent model of orientation selectivity in cat visual cortical simple cells. *J. Neurosci.*, 15: 5448–5465.

Sompolinsky, H. and Shapely, R. (1997) New perspectives on the mechanisms for orientation selectivity. *Curr. Opin. Neurobiol.*, 7: 514–522.

Stafford, C.A. (1984) Critical period plasticity for visual function: definition in monocularly deprived rats using visually evoked potentials. *Ophthalmic Physiol. Opt.*, 4: 95–100.

Stryker, M.P. and Harris, W.A. (1986) Binocular impulse blockade prevents the formation of ocular dominance columns in cat visual cortex. *J. Neurosci.*, 6: 2117–2133.

Swindale, N.V. and Cynader, M.S. (1986) Physiological segregation of geniculo-cortical afferents in the visual cortex of dark-reared cats. *Brain Res.*, 362: 281–286.

Swindale, N.V. (1988) Role of visual experience in promoting segregation of eye dominance patches in the visual cortex of the cat. *J. Comp. Neurol.*, 267: 472–488.

Takei, N., Sasaoka, K., Inoue, K., Takahashi, M., Endo, Y. and Hatanaka, H. (1997) Brain-derived neurotrophic factor increases the stimulation-evoked release of glutamate and the levels of exocytosis-associated proteins in cultured cortical neurons from embryonic rats. *J. Neurochem.*, 68: 370–375.

Takei, Y., Teng, J., Harada, A. and Hirokawa, N. (2000) Defects in axonal elongation and neuronal migration in mice with disrupted tau and map1b genes. *J. Cell Biol.*, 150: 989–1000.

Tay, D., So, K.-F., Jen, L.S. and Lau, K.C. (1986) The postnatal development of the optic nerve in hamsters: an electron microscopic study. *Dev. Brain Res.*, 30: 268–273.

Thoenen, H. (1995) Neurotrophins and neuronal plasticity. *Science*, 270: 593–598.

Toran-Allerand, C.D. (1996) The estrogen/neurotrophin connection during neural development: is co-localization of estrogen receptors with the neurotrophins and their receptors biologically relevant? *Dev. Neurosci.*, 18: 36–48.

Toran-Allerand, C.D., Singh, M. and Setalo Jr., G. (1999) Novel mechanisms of estrogen action in the brain: new players in an old story. *Front. Neuroendocrinol.*, 20: 97–121.

Tsumoto, T. and Freeman, R.D. (1987) Dark-reared cats: responsivity of cortical cells influenced pharmacologically by an inhibitory antagonist. *Exp. Brain Res.*, 65: 666–672.

Turrigiano, G.G. (1999) Homeostatic plasticity in neuronal networks: the more things change, the more they stay the same. *Trends Neurosci.*, 22: 221–227.

Vaillant, A.R., Mazzoni, I.E., Tudan, C., Boudreau, M., Kaplan, D.R. and Miller, F.D. (1999) Depolarization and neurotrophins converge on the phosphatidylinositol 3-kinase–Akt pathway to synergistically regulate neuronal survival. *J. Cell Biol.*, 146: 955–966.

Valverde, F. (1971) Rate and extent of recovery from dark rearing in the visual cortex of the mouse. *Brain Res.*, 33: 1–11.

Vicario-Abejón, C., Collin, C., McKay, R.D.G. and Segal, M. (1998) Neurotrophins induce formation of functional excitatory and inhibitory synapses between cultured hippocampal neurons. *J. Neurosci.*, 18: 7256–7271.

Von Bartheld, C.S., Kinoshita, Y., Prevette, D., Yin, Q.-W., Oppenheim, R.W. and Bothwell, M. (1994) Positive and negative effects of neurotrophins on the isthmo-optic nucleus in chick embryos. *Neuron*, 12: 639–654.

Von Bartheld, C.S., Williams, R., Lefcort, F., Clary, D.O., Reichardt, L.F. and Bothwell, M. (1996) Retrograde transport of neurotrophins from the eye to the brain in chick embryos: roles of the p75NTR and trkB receptors. *J. Neurosci.*, 16: 2995–3008.

Wright, E.M., Vogel, K.S. and Davies, A.M. (1992) Neurotrophic factors promote the maturation of developing sensory neurons before they become dependent on these factors for survival. *Neuron*, 9: 139–150.

Wu, G.-Y., Deisseroth, K. and Tsien, R.W. (2001) Activity-dependent CREB phosphorylation: convergence of a fast, sensitive calmodulin kinase pathway and a slow, less sensitive mitogen-activated protein kinase pathway. *Proc. Nat. Acad. Sci.*, 98: 2808–2813.

Xia, Z., Dudek, H., Miranti, C.K. and Greenberg, M.E. (1996) Calcium influx by the NMDA receptor induces immediate early gene transcription by a MAP kinase/ERK-dependent mechanism. *J. Neurosci.*, 16: 5425–5436.

Xu, B., Zang, K., Ruff, N., Zhang, Y.A., McConnell, S., Stryker, M. and Reichardt, L. (2000) Cortical degeneration in the absence of neutrophin signaling: dendritic retraction and neuronal loss after removal of the receptor trkB. *Neuron*, 26: 233–245.

Zafra, F., Hengerer, B., Liebrock, J., Thoenen, H. and Lindholm, D. (1990) Activity dependent regulation of BDNF and NGF mRNAs in the rat hippocampus is mediated by non-NMDA glutamate receptors. *EMBO J.*, 9: 3545–3550.

Zafra, F., Castrén, E., Thoenen, H. and Lindholm, D. (1991) Interplay between glutamate and gamma-amino butyric acid transmitter systems in the physiological regulation of brain-derived neurotrophic factor and nerve growth factor synthesis in hippocampal neurons. *Proc. Natl. Acad. Sci. USA*, 88: 10037–10041.

Zafra, F., Castren, E., Lindholm, D., Hartikka, J. and Thoenen, H. (1992) Regulation of brain-derived neurotrophic factor and nerve growth factor mRNA in primary cultures of hippocampal neurons and astrocytes. *J. Neurosci.*, 12: 4793–4799.

Zhang, Y., Moheban, D.B., Conway, B.R., Bhattacharyya, A. and Segal, R.A. (2000) Cell surface trk receptors mediate NGF-induced survival while internalized receptors regulate NGF-induced differentiation. *J. Neurosci.*, 20: 5671–5678.

Zhou, X.-F. and Rush, R.A. (1996) Endogenous brain-derived neurotrophic factor is anterogradely transported in primary sensory neurons. *Neuroscience*, 74: 945–951.

C. Casanova and M. Ptito (Eds.)
Progress in Brain Research, Vol. 134

CHAPTER 4

Thalamic relay functions

S. Murray Sherman *

Department of Neurobiology, State University of New York, Stony Brook, NY 11794-5230, USA

Abstract: The lateral geniculate nucleus is the best understood thalamic relay. Only 5–10% of the inputs to geniculate relay cells derive from retina, which is the driving input. The rest, being modulatory, derive from local inhibitory inputs, descending inputs from visual cortex, and ascending inputs from brainstem. The nonretinal, modulatory inputs, which form the vast majority, dynamically control the nature of the geniculate relay. Among other actions, these modulatory inputs regulate membrane properties of relay cells and thereby control their mode of response to retinal inputs, and this dramatically affects the nature of information relayed to cortex. Our studies of the lateral geniculate nucleus of the cat lead to the speculation that this dynamic control depends on the animal's behavioral state and represents the neuronal substrate for many forms of visual attention. The lateral geniculate nucleus is a first-order relay, because it relays subcortical (i.e. retinal) information to cortex for the first time. In contrast, the other main thalamic relay of visual information, the pulvinar (and lateral posterior nucleus in carnivores), is largely a higher-order relay, since much of it seems to relay information from one cortical area to another. Much more corticocortical processing may involve these 're-entry' routes than has been hitherto appreciated. If so, the thalamus sits at an indispensable position for corticocortical processing.

Introduction

For a long time, the thalamus has had a bad press, particularly in studies of the visual system. The lateral geniculate nucleus, which is the thalamic relay for retinal information to visual cortex, has traditionally been seen as a passive and trivial relay (Hubel and Wiesel, 1977; Zeki, 1993). There is no significant receptive field transformation across the retinogeniculate synapse, making this relay different from all the others of the visual pathways, and in this regard, the only role it seems to play is in subtracting some retinal action potentials from information relayed. That is, it has been asserted that every action potential in a geniculate relay cell follows one in its retinal input(s) with a fixed synaptic delay, and that some retinal action potentials fail to evoke one in the relay cell (Cleland et al., 1971). Yet we know that the thalamus is an essential relay to neocortex, that it has complex patterns of synaptic interconnectivity, and its cells and circuitry display a rich array of receptors, channels, transmitters, and second-messenger systems. If the machine-like relay with some reduction in efficacy were all that the thalamus does, one would have to wonder why we even have a thalamic relay at all. What purpose is served by the lateral geniculate nucleus specifically and thalamus more generally? Why, for instance, does the retina not project directly to visual cortex?

Recent research on thalamic function will be reviewed with focus on the lateral geniculate nucleus, because this offers some answers to these questions. It seems evident now that the complex cell and circuit properties seen in thalamus have some useful functions. As a result, we can replace the above questions with some relating to what these specific functions may be and how they are carried out. One that is emphasized below is the observation that all thalamic relay cells can transmit information to cor-

* Correspondence to: S.M. Sherman, Department of Neurobiology, Department of Physiology, State University of New York, Stony Brook, NY 11794-5230, USA. Tel.: +1 (631) 632-8620; Fax: +1 (631) 632-4198;
E-mail: s.sherman@sunysb.edu

tex in two very different response modes that depend on intrinsic properties, and these different modes emphasize different aspects of the input information that is relayed to cortex. Thus the nature of these properties and how they are controlled by thalamic circuitry is of great interest. Also, once this obvious function of thalamic relays is laid out, the idea is developed that transmission of information to cortex benefits from a thalamic relay whether the information emanates from a subcortical region, like retina or brainstem, or from another cortical area. This leads to the final hypothesis that thalamus might play a critical role in corticocortical communication.

The low threshold Ca^{2+} spike

Like virtually all other neurons in the brain, thalamic relay cells do not behave like passive cables but instead display many voltage-dependent membrane conductances. A detailed review of these can be found elsewhere (McCormick and Huguenard, 1992; Sherman and Guillery, 1996, 2001). One of particular interest for thalamic function is a voltage-dependent, low threshold, transient conductance involving T (for transient) type Ca^{2+} channels. These T channels are located in the cell bodies and dendrites of relay cells, apparently being more concentrated in the latter (Zhou et al., 1997; Destexhe et al., 1998; Zhan et al., 2000). The properties of the T channels provide relay cells with the two very different response modes indicated above (see Fig. 1), and these channels are ubiquitous for relay cells: they are found for every relay cell of every thalamic nucleus of every species so far studied (reviewed in Sherman and Guillery, 1996). When these channels are open, Ca^{2+} flows into the cell, creating a current known as the *T current* or I_T, and this depolarizes the cell, producing an all-or-none Ca^{2+} spike known as the *low threshold spike* (Jahnsen and Llinás, 1984a,b; McCormick and Huguenard, 1992; Sherman and Guillery, 1996). Fig. 1D shows the all-or-none nature of this spike (Zhan et al., 1999). This spike is typically 30–50 mV in amplitude and lasts for 50–100 ms. Thus the T channels, I_T, and low threshold spike are all terms related to the same membrane property.

These T channels and I_T have 3 voltage-dependent states (see Fig. 1A–C). (1) When the membrane is more depolarized than roughly −60 to −65 mV for 50–100 ms [1], I_T becomes *inactivated* (Fig. 1A). (2) When the membrane is more hyperpolarized than about −65 to −70 mV, the inactivation of I_T is removed, and it thus becomes *de-inactivated.* (3) If I_T is de-inactivated and the membrane is then sufficiently depolarized, I_T is *activated*, leading to a low threshold spike (Fig. 1C). Thus, depolarization from more depolarized levels, when I_T is inactivated, produces no I_T or low threshold spike, but depolarization from more hyperpolarized levels, when I_T is de-inactivated, evokes I_T and a low threshold spike. Notice that qualitatively these T channels have the same voltage dependency and states of activation, inactivation and de-inactivation as the Na^+ channels underlying the conventional action potential. The main differences are quantitative: the voltage range over which the Na^+ channels operate is more depolarized, and the time constant for inactivation and de-inactivation of the Na^+ channels is roughly two orders of magnitude faster than the 50–100 ms for T channels.

The two response modes provided by the T channels are known as *tonic* [2] and *burst* (Fig. 1A–C). Tonic mode is operative when I_T is inactivated. Under these conditions, a suprathreshold depolarization (e.g. from a large EPSP) will activate a stream of unitary action potentials as long as the membrane potential is held above threshold for their firing. Burst mode is operative when I_T is de-inactivated. In this mode, a suprathreshold EPSP will activate a low threshold spike that is itself usually large enough to activate a high frequency cluster of action potentials riding its crest. It is important to emphasize here that the T channels are not found in the axon, so the low threshold spike is not conducted to cortex; only action potentials are.

Another temporal feature of the T channels involves its activation. Activation once I_T is de-inac-

[1] The degree of inactivation or de-inactivation is described by a complex function of membrane voltage and time.

[2] 'Tonic' used in this sense refers to a response mode of a thalamic relay cell, and here it is paired with 'burst'. This use of 'tonic' should not be confused with another use of 'tonic' when paired with 'phasic' to refer to a cell type in the lateral geniculate nucleus: 'tonic' for X and 'phasic' for Y cells. Throughout this chapter, the use of 'tonic' refers only to response mode and not to cell type.

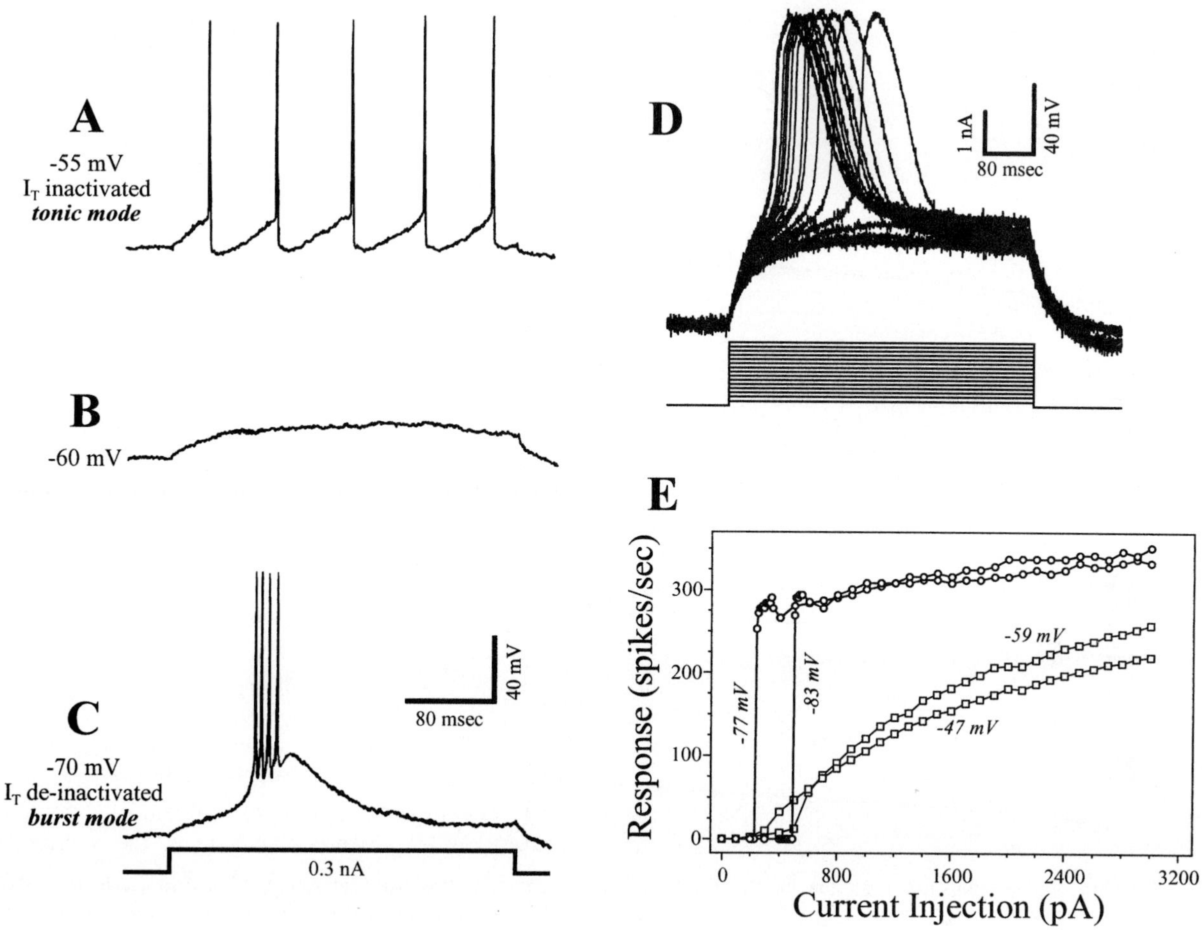

Fig. 1. Properties of I_T and the low threshold spike. All examples are from relay cells of the cat's lateral geniculate nucleus recorded intracellularly in an in vitro slice preparation. (A–C) Voltage dependency of the low threshold spike. Responses are shown to the same depolarizing current pulse delivered intracellularly but from three different initial holding potentials. When the cell is relatively depolarized (A), I_T is inactivated, and the cell responds with a stream of unitary action potentials as long as the stimulus is suprathreshold for firing. This is the tonic mode of firing. When the cell is slightly more hyperpolarized (B), I_T remains mostly inactivated, but the current pulse no longer depolarizes the cell to above threshold. Thus a simple, resistive–capacitative response is seen. When the cell is further hyperpolarized (C), I_T is de-inactivated, and the current pulse activates a low threshold spike with four action potentials riding its crest. This is the *burst mode* of firing. (D) All-or-none nature of low threshold spikes. Here, TTX is added to block conventional action potentials and reveal the low threshold spikes more clearly. The cell is held at a hyperpolarized potential to completely de-activate I_T, and current pulses were injected starting at 200 pA amplitude and incremented in 10 pA steps. Smaller (subthreshold) pulses led to pure resistive–capacitative responses, but all larger (suprathreshold) pulses led to a low threshold spike. Much like conventional action potentials, the low threshold spikes are all the same amplitude regardless of how far the depolarizing pulse exceeded activation threshold, although there is some latency variability seen for smaller suprathreshold pulses. (E) Input–output relationship for one cell. The input variable is the amplitude of the depolarizing current pulse, and the output is the firing frequency of the cell. To compare burst and tonic firing, the firing frequency was determined by the first six action potentials of the response, since this cell usually exhibited six action potentials per burst in this experiment. The initial holding potentials are shown. When in tonic mode, because the initial potentials were depolarizing (−47 and −59 mV), the input–output relationship is fairly linear. When in burst mode, because the initial potentials were hyperpolarizing (−77 and −83 mV), the input–output relationship is quite nonlinear and approximates a step function.

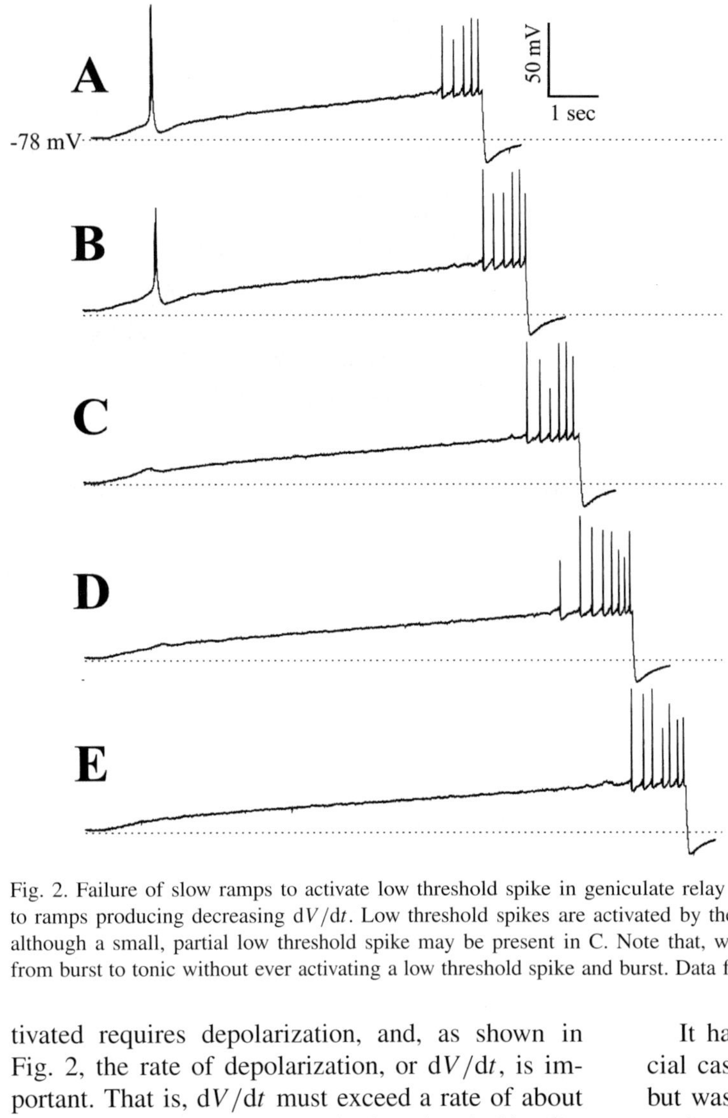

Fig. 2. Failure of slow ramps to activate low threshold spike in geniculate relay cell recorded intracellularly in vitro. (A–E) Responses to ramps producing decreasing dV/dt. Low threshold spikes are activated by the faster ramps (A,B) but not in the slower ones (C–E), although a small, partial low threshold spike may be present in C. Note that, with a sufficiently slow dV/dt, the cell can be switched from burst to tonic without ever activating a low threshold spike and burst. Data from (Gutierrez et al., 2000).

tivated requires depolarization, and, as shown in Fig. 2, the rate of depolarization, or dV/dt, is important. That is, dV/dt must exceed a rate of about 5–10 mV/s to activate I_T and a low threshold spike (Gutierrez et al., 2000). A slower rate of depolarization will not activate I_T, because, before its activation level is reached, the slower rate of depolarization allows inactivation of I_T to build up to the point that a full blown low threshold spike cannot be activated. Interestingly, it is possible with a very slow depolarization (i.e. a $dV/dt < 5$–10 mV/s) to start with a cell in burst mode with fully de-inactivated I_T and switch it to tonic mode with fully inactivated I_T without activating I_T. How this might be done under physiological conditions is considered below under *Control of response mode*.

It had been thought that burst firing was a special case not seen during the normal waking state, but was only evident during certain phases of sleep or in some pathological states, such as epilepsy (Steriade and Llinás, 1988; Steriade et al., 1993; McCormick and Bal, 1997). During these unconscious conditions, bursting is rhythmic, occurring at various rates, usually 1–10 Hz, and synchronized across large regions of thalamus. In this view, burst mode is not a true relay mode and instead represents a functional state during which the relay is disconnected. However, there is increasing evidence that, while rhythmic burst firing dominates responses during slow wave sleep, burst mode dependent on I_T is also sometimes present during alert wakefulness (Guido and Weyand, 1995; Nicolelis et al., 1995; Lenz et al., 1998; Radhakrishnan et al., 1999; Ramcharan et al., 2000; Swadlow and Gusev, 2001), although in the awake animal, bursting is usually arrhythmic, occurring at seemingly random intervals. Furthermore, geniculate relay cells in the behaving animal do respond well to visual stimuli with occasional bursts mixed among tonic firing, indicating that both tonic and burst modes are effective relay modes (Guido and Weyand, 1995; Ramcharan et al., 2000).

The obvious question, then, is: What is the functional implication of these firing modes? They represent very different ways in which the relay cell responds to the same input, indicating that the same message is relayed to cortex in one of two different ways. Thus when messages arrive at the relay cell, the level of its membrane potential, which determines the inactivation state of I_T, can strongly influence the nature of the information that is transmitted to cortex. Receptive field analysis from relay cells of the cat's lateral geniculate nucleus indicates that both response modes convey comparable levels of information in the relay to cortex (Reinagel et al., 1999), although it is also clear that the nature of that information differs between modes (Sherman, 1996). There may be many differences related to these two modes, but two that have received considerable attention are linearity of the relay process and detectability of the message that is relayed to cortex.

Linearity

From the cellular properties described above and from Fig. 1, it becomes clear that tonic mode provides a more linear relay than does burst mode. During tonic firing, an increase in amplitude of the input (e.g. EPSP size) evokes a higher rate of firing, and there is a range over which this relationship is linear (Fig. 1E). However, because the action potentials during burst firing are not evoked directly from an EPSP but instead are evoked by an all-or-none low threshold spike, the firing rate or number of action potentials in a burst tends to be fairly fixed over a wide range of EPSP amplitudes. Thus the relationship between the amplitude of the input and the response in action potentials during burst firing resembles a step function, which is highly nonlinear (Fig. 1E).

Fig. 1 shows the two firing modes in an in vitro slice preparation. Both firing modes can also be readily seen during in vivo recording, both in lightly anesthetized and in fully awake animals (Guido et al., 1992, 1995; Lu et al., 1992; Guido and Weyand, 1995; Mukherjee and Kaplan, 1995; Sherman, 1996; Ramcharan et al., 2000; Swadlow and Gusev, 2001). When the recording is intracellular in vivo, as is usual in vitro, it is possible to control the inactivation state of I_T, and thus the response mode, by injecting current into the cell to vary membrane potential. However, with extracellular recording, which is more commonly used in vivo, firing mode cannot be controlled directly. Nonetheless, relay cells then seem to switch more or less randomly between response modes every few seconds, apparently as a result of variations of synaptic input that produce fluctuations of membrane potential. It is nonetheless possible to recognize the two modes during extracellular recording because of their distinctive pattern of intervals between action potentials, and it is thus possible to divide response periods into burst or tonic modes (Lu et al., 1992; Guido and Sherman, 1998; Ramcharan et al., 2000).

One can also use more natural stimuli such as visual targets, rather than current injections, to activate the geniculate relay cells. When this is done, the same difference in linearity is seen: tonic mode reflects a higher degree of linear summation than does burst mode. Fig. 3 shows the response of a geniculate relay cell to the same visual stimulus: a drifting, sinusoidally modulated, luminance grating. During tonic firing, the shape of response resembles a sine wave and thus it faithfully or linearly reflects the contrast modulation in the visual stimulus (Fig. 3A, lower panel). During burst firing, the response no longer looks smoothly sinusoidal, because there is a nonlinear distortion between the visual input and response (Fig. 3B, lower panel). This can be demonstrated formally by Fourier analyzing the response to sinusoidal gratings, and this is shown for a population of geniculate neurons in Fig. 4A (Sherman, 1996).

There is an obvious benefit for maintaining a linear relay related to tonic firing, since the nonlinear distortions associated with the burst mode limit the ability of the cortex to faithfully reproduce the visual scene. What then is the purpose or advantage of burst mode? The answer to this question may be related to stimulus detection.

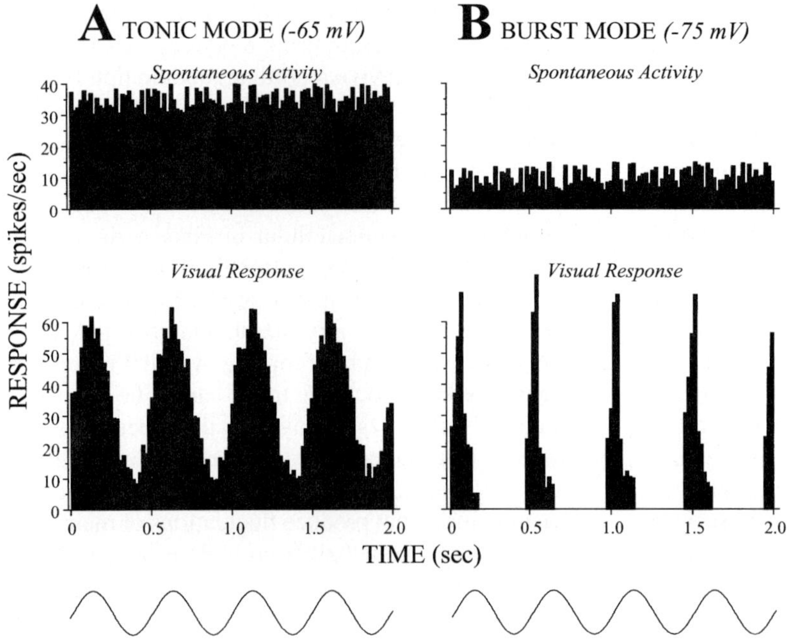

Fig. 3. Tonic and burst responses of relay cell from the cat's lateral geniculate nucleus to sinewave grating. The cell was recorded intracellularly in vivo, and current injected through the recording electrode was used to bias membrane potential to more depolarized (−65 mV), producing tonic firing, or more hyperpolarized (−75 mV), producing burst firing. The responses are shown as average response histograms. The upper histograms show spontaneous activity when the grating stimulus was removed (or, more precisely, its contrast reduced to zero), and the lower histograms show the averaged response to four cycles of the grating drifted through the receptive field. The contrast changes resulting from the drifting grating are shown below the histograms. (A) Tonic mode. The spontaneous activity is relatively high, and the response to the grating has a distinctly sinusoidal profile. (B) Burst mode. The spontaneous activity is relatively low, and the response to the grating no longer has a sinusoidal profile.

Detectability

The response profiles to a drifting sinusoidal grating shown in Fig. 3 reveal another difference between firing modes besides that of linearity. Whereas the response to the grating in both modes is vigorous, the spontaneous activity (when the grating stimulus is not present) is much lower during burst firing (Fig. 3A,B, panels)[3]. We may consider the response to the grating as the signal to be conveyed to cortex and the spontaneous activity as the noisy background against which this signal must be detected. From Fig. 3, it seems that the ratio of signal (the response to the grating) to noise (the spontaneous activity) is higher during burst than tonic mode. A higher signal-to-noise ratio is usually associated with better detectability.

Signal detectability can be formally tested by using a method from signal detection theory known as ROC (for receiver operating characteristic) analysis (Green and Swets, 1966; Macmillan and Creelman, 1991). When this is done for responses of a population of geniculate neurons to visual stimuli, the impression gained from Fig. 3 is confirmed. As summarized in Fig. 4B, all cells show better signal detectability during burst than tonic firing (Sherman, 1996).

It thus appears that each response mode has certain advantages. Tonic mode provides a more faithful, linear relay of visual information. Burst mode provides better stimulus detectability. Perhaps burst firing is preferred when stimuli must be detected or as a sort of 'wake-up call' when the relevant portion of visual field is not attended to, ensuring

[3] Interestingly, the higher spontaneous activity during tonic firing also helps preserve linearity by reducing nonlinearities associated with rectification.

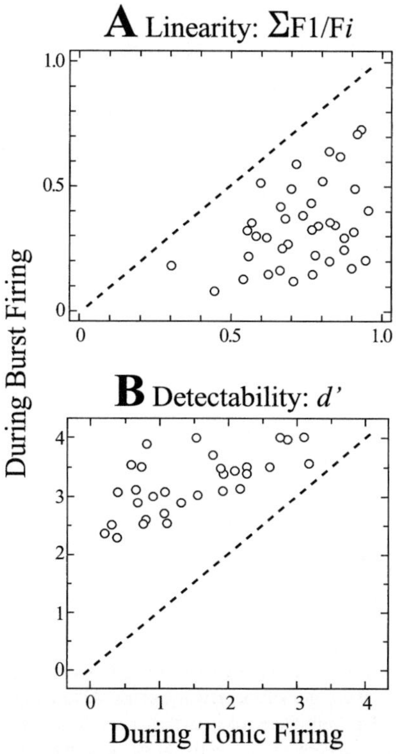

Fig. 4. Response linearity and signal detectability during tonic and burst firing. Each point in the scatter plots reflects data from one relay cell of the cat's lateral geniculate nucleus recorded in vivo during visual stimulation, and the plots compare the response during tonic firing on the abscissa versus burst firing on the ordinate. The dashed line of slope 1 is also shown in each plot. (A) Linearity. To obtain a measure of linearity, responses to sinewave gratings as in Fig. 3 were Fourier analyzed and a linearity index was computed by dividing the linear F1 component by the sum of the higher-order nonlinear components (i.e. F2, F3, etc.). The larger this index, the more linear the response. Note that every single cell shows more linearity during tonic firing. (B) Detectability. The d' values were determined from ROC analysis (for details, see Green and Swets, 1966; Swets, 1973).

that novel stimuli are detected. Once a novel stimulus is detected, the firing mode might be switched to tonic to enhance stimulus analysis by reducing nonlinear distortions in the relay (for details of this hypothesis, see Sherman, 1996; Sherman and Guillery, 2001). Consistent with this idea of bursting as a 'wake-up call' is recent evidence recording from somatosensory thalamic relay cells and their postsynaptic cortical cells in layer 4 in behaving rabbits that burst mode firing had a much higher probability of eliciting spikes in the target cortical cells than did tonic firing (Swadlow and Gusev, 2001).

There may well be many other features, besides linearity and stimulus detectability, related to these different response modes, but they are presently unexplored and undefined. By focusing on the linearity and the detectability of signal transmission, a theoretical framework for the meaning of the two response modes can be entertained. If this is to make any sense, however, there must be means of effectively controlling response mode by various afferents to relay cells. To explore this requires a consideration of geniculate circuitry.

Geniculate circuitry

If the above description of cellular properties of relay neurons were not enough to convince the reader that the thalamic relay is dynamic and consequential, then a consideration of the complex circuitry of thalamus should certainly do so.

Survey of afferents

Fig. 5 summarizes the major afferents contributing to the circuitry of the thalamus, using the lateral geniculate nucleus as an example; other thalamic nuclei have similar circuitry, although a number of details differ (Jones, 1985; Sherman and Guillery, 1996, 2001). The pattern of ionotropic and metabotropic receptors on relay cells is also shown, and the significance of this will be considered below. Relay cells receive a glutamatergic input from retina. They are also innervated by a variety of nonretinal sources. Most of the latter include GABAergic inputs from local, inhibitory cells (i.e. both intrinsic interneurons and cells of the nearby thalamic reticular nucleus), glutamatergic inputs from layer 6 of visual cortex, and cholinergic inputs from the parabrachial region of the brainstem. Synaptic terminals derived from this last input appear to contain nitric oxide as well as acetylcholine, and although the effects of nitric oxide are not well understood, several studies have suggested effects (Pape and Mager, 1992; Shaw and Salt, 1997; Cudeiro and Rivadulla, 1999).

The numbers are illuminating: only 5–10% of the synaptic inputs derive from retina, whereas about a third each derives from the local GABAergic neu-

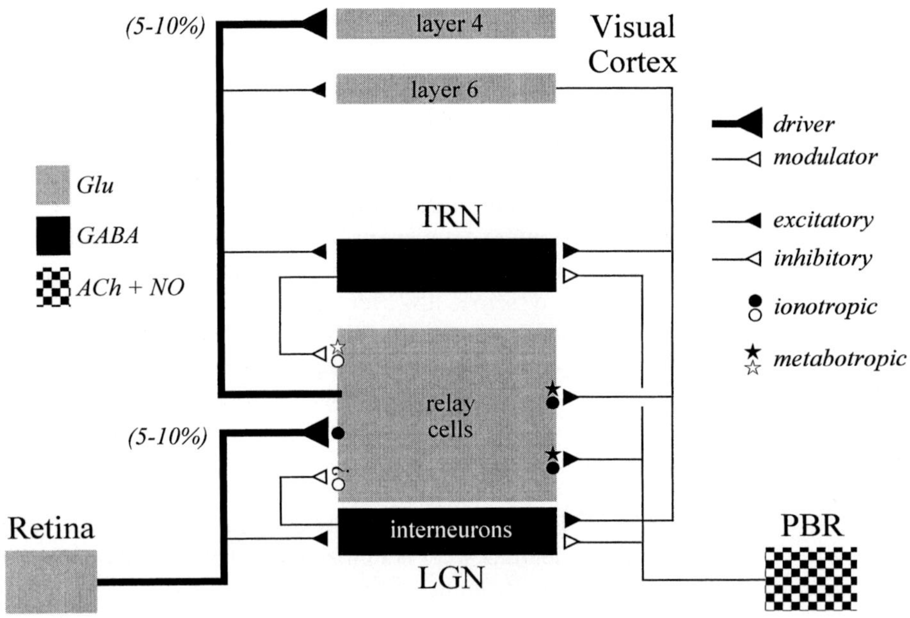

Fig. 5. Circuitry of the lateral geniculate nucleus. Shown are the various inputs to relay cells. The retinal (driver) input is distinguished from the nonretinal (modulator) inputs. Note that only about 5–10% of the synaptic inputs to relay cells derive from retinogeniculate axons, and likewise, only about 5–10% of the inputs to layer 4 cells in visual cortex derive from geniculocortical axons. Also shown are the postsynaptic receptors on relay cells associated with each of the inputs illustrated. The retinal input activates only ionotropic receptors, whereas all nonretinal inputs activate metabotropic receptors and often ionotropic receptors as well. ACh, acetylcholine; GABA, γ-aminobutyric acid; Glu, glutamate; LGN, lateral geniculate nucleus; NO, nitric oxide; PBR, parabrachial region of the brainstem; TRN, thalamic reticular nucleus. See text for further details.

rons, the corticogeniculate axons, and the cholinergic brainstem inputs (Guillery, 1969; Erişir et al., 1997; Van Horn et al., 2000). There is a remaining small input (perhaps 5% or so) not shown in Fig. 5 and not further considered here that includes noradrenergic and serotonergic inputs from the brainstem and histaminergic inputs from the tuberomamillary mamillary nucleus of the hypothalamus (for further details of other inputs, see (Sherman and Guillery, 1996, 2001). The fact that retinal input, generally regarded as providing the information to be relayed to cortex, represents such a small minority of input to relay cells, which, in turn, are embedded in such complex nonretinal circuitry, belies a simple, trivial relay function for this thalamic nucleus.

Fig. 5 also shows other details of geniculate circuitry (Sherman and Guillery, 1996, 2001). Retinal input innervates interneurons as well as relay cells, but does not innervate cells of the thalamic reticular nucleus. Geniculocortical axons branch en route to cortex to innervate reticular cells, and corticogeniculate axons do likewise in the opposite direction. Reticular cells innervate relay cells almost exclusively, with very little input to interneurons (not shown in Fig. 5). Both brainstem and corticogeniculate axons branch to innervate all of the thalamic cell types: relay cells, interneurons, and reticular cells.

The functional effects of the different inputs on relay cells are difficult to predict (see Fig. 5). Even retinal input, which excites relay cells directly, indirectly inhibits them through interneurons, so the overall, sustained effect of this input is not obvious. Likewise, cortical inputs directly excite relay cells but indirectly inhibit them via the local GABAergic cells. Cholinergic inputs from the brainstem have a less complicated excitatory effect on relay cells, because they directly excite them and also disinhibit them by inhibiting local GABAergic cells (reviewed in (McCormick, 1992; Sherman and Guillery, 1996). However, Fig. 5 shows global pathways, and individual axons may not be organized in the manner suggested. Take corticogeniculate axons for example (and this reasoning can be applied to most of the inputs). A single axon will branch to innervate reticular cells and relay cells, but if the target reticular cells do not innervate any of the cortically-targeted relay cells, there is no disynaptic inhibition of relay cells from cortex, as Fig. 5 might be misconstrued to suggest. To really interpret the functional significance of the thalamic circuitry as suggested by Fig. 5 requires knowledge of circuits entered into by individual axons, knowledge that is presently lacking.

Ionotropic and metabotropic receptors

A particularly important aspect of functional circuitry involves the nature of the postsynaptic receptors. These come in two basic flavors; *ionotropic* and *metabotropic* (see Fig. 6; for details, see Nicoll et al., 1990; Mott and Lewis, 1994; Pin and Bockaert, 1995; Pin and Duvoisin, 1995; Recasens and Vignes, 1995; Brown et al., 1997; Isaac et al., 1997). Ionotropic receptors are directly linked to the ion channels they control, and indeed, the ion channel is typically part of the receptor itself (e.g. Fig. 6, top section). Presumably because of this direct linkage, the receptor responds to its transmitter to open its ion channel quickly and transiently, with a latency of <1 ms and a duration of a few tens of millseconds. In contrast, metabotropic receptors (Fig. 6, bottom section) are linked to the affected ion channels rather indirectly. Most of these receptors are linked to a G-protein, and binding of the transmitter to the receptor releases the G-protein to initiate a cascade of biochemical reactions inside of the cell. One end result is the opening or closing of an ion channel, usually a K^+ channel in the case of thalamic neurons [4]. Presumably because of the many indirect links between receptor and ion channel, this is a slow process with a latency from transmitter binding to opening or closing of the ion channel of several ms or more and a duration of hundreds of milliseconds to several seconds, or even longer.

If we consider the nature of receptors activated by the afferents to relay cells, an interesting pattern emerges (see Fig. 5). Retinal input activates *only* ionotropic glutamate receptors (mostly AMPA and NMDA; reviewed in (Sherman and Guillery, 1996, 2001). All other inputs activate a combination of ionotropic and metabotropic receptors. Thus cortical inputs activate the same receptor types as do retinal inputs but also activate metabotropic glutamate receptors. Cholinergic brainstem inputs activate nicotinic (ionotropic) and muscarinic (metabotropic) receptors. Other inputs using noradrenaline, histamine, or serotonin as neurotransmitters (not shown in Fig. 5) seem to activate mostly only metabotropic receptors. GABAergic cells of the thalamic reticular nucleus activate $GABA_A$ (ionotropic) and $GABA_B$ (metabotropic) receptors; inputs to relay cells from interneurons activate $GABA_A$ receptors, and whether or not they also activate $GABA_B$ receptors is presently unknown. What is not clear and obviously of some importance is whether individual axons of the various nonretinal inputs activate both ionotropic and metabotropic receptors or whether some activate only one or the other type.

The importance of the distinction between receptor types is further considered below in terms of the control of response mode and for faithfully conveying information in the relay through thalamus.

Control of response mode

As suggested above, the nature of the tonic or burst response mode of a relay cell is a key parameter of thalamic relay functioning, and thus control of response mode by thalamic circuitry is of obvious importance. Such control, as noted, involves sustaining a change of membrane potential long enough (>50–100 ms) to change the inactivation state of I_T.

Consider what would be necessary to switch response mode from tonic to burst, that is, to de-inactivate I_T after the membrane had been sustained at a relatively depolarized potential sufficient to inactivate I_T. De-inactivation would now require a hyperpolarization via IPSPs to be of sufficient amplitude

---

[4] Other long-term effects of the second messenger cascade initiated by activation of a metabotropic receptor have been reported, included control of gene expression, so this can have quite extensive and long-lasting effects on the postsynaptic cell. In contrast, ionotropic receptor activation affects little other than the appropriate ion channels. However, such effects of metabotropic receptor activation beyond indirect control of ion channels have not yet been investigated in thalamic neurons.

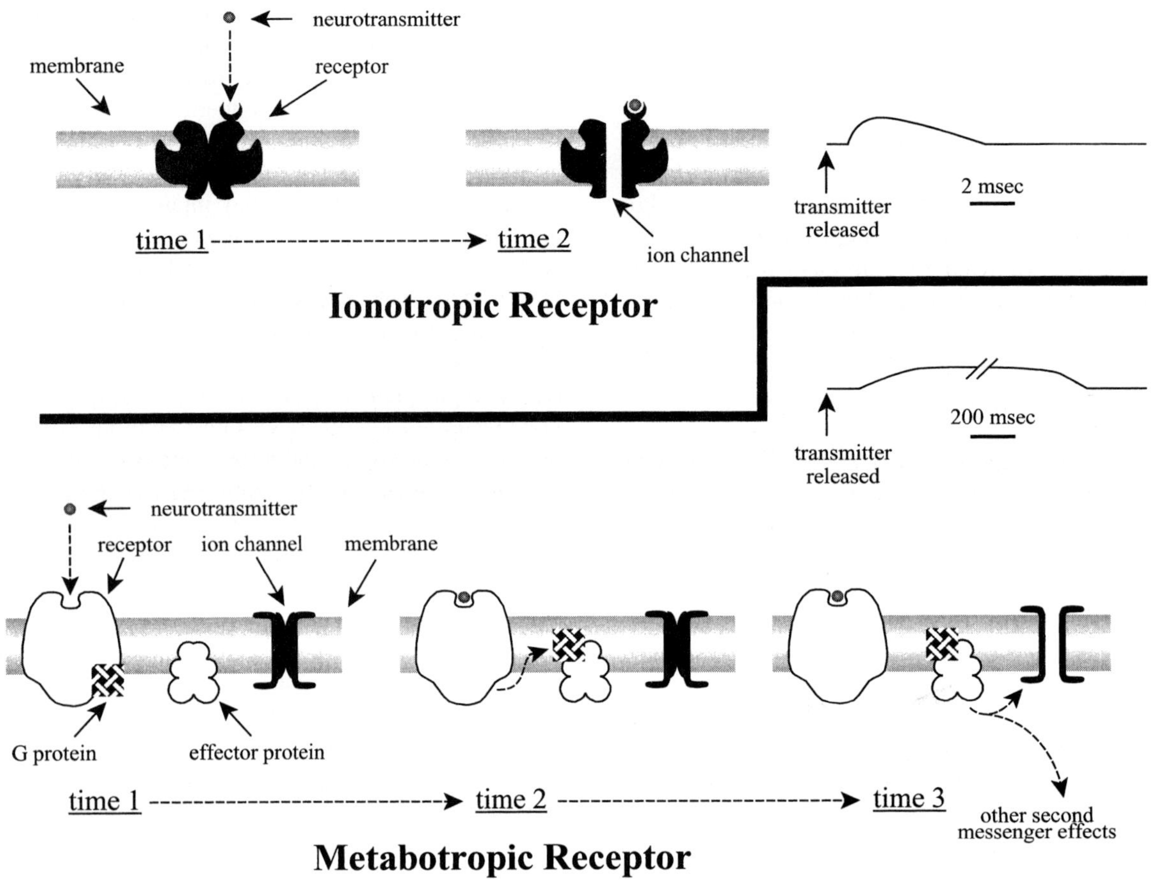

Fig. 6. Schema of ionotropic and metabotropic receptor. Upper section: ionotropic receptor. The receptor is linked directly to an ion channel, which is usually part of the receptor molecule. Binding of the receptor to the neurotransmitter quickly causes a conformational change leading to opening of the ion channel. Ions flow through the channel, creating a postsynaptic potential. This happens with a relatively short latency and duration. Lower section: metabotropic receptor. The receptor is not linked directly to an ion channel. Instead, binding of the neurotransmitter to the receptor releases a G-protein, and this produces a cascade of biochemical reactions. Occasionally the G-protein can affect the ion channel directly (not shown), but more commonly, the G-protein acts through an effector protein to eventually open or close an ion channel. Other properties of the cell can also be affected by the biochemical reactions. The end result is a slow postsynaptic potential with a relatively long latency and duration.

and duration. The obvious candidates to produce an IPSP in a relay cell are the local GABAergic neurons. If they activate ionotropic ($GABA_A$) receptors in the relay cell, this will not likely serve to change response mode, because the resultant IPSP would be over in 20–40 ms or so, which is not long enough to de-inactivate I_T. Only if there were considerable temporal summation of $GABA_A$-mediated IPSPs due to sustained, high firing rates of the GABAergic inputs could the hyperpolarization be sustained long enough to switch response mode. However, if these inputs activated metabotropic ($GABA_B$) receptors, the resulting IPSP would be sustained for >100 ms, which is long enough. Thus the $GABA_B$ receptors seem a much better tool for controlling response mode than do the $GABA_A$ receptors. Another advantage for $GABA_B$ activation in this regard is that it depends on increasing a K^+ conductance with a reversal potential of roughly -100 to -110 mV, while $GABA_A$ activation increases a Cl^- conductance with a reversal potential of about -70 mV. Thus, activation of the metabotropic, $GABA_B$ receptor produces a stronger hyperpolarization, which would also more effectively de-inactivate I_T.

A similar logic can be applied in considering inactivation of I_T to switch the firing mode from burst to tonic. Here the task is to produce a sustained depolarization. A fast EPSP via ionotropic receptors, such as retinal activation of ionotropic glutamate receptors, will not last long enough to inactivate I_T effectively. Instead, if the EPSP is large enough, it is fast enough in terms of dV/dt to activate I_T and a low threshold spike, but once this finishes, the membrane will return to its previously hyperpolarized level, and the cell will remain in burst mode. Only with temporal summation would the retinal EPSPs likely be able to switch firing modes. In contrast, the slow EPSPs evoked via metabotropic receptors (e.g. metabotropic glutamate receptors via corticogeniculate activation or muscarinic receptors via activation of brainstem inputs) can sustain the depolarization long enough to inactivate I_T and switch the response mode.

There is another potentially significant advantage of metabotropic receptors in switching response mode from burst to tonic. As noted above, activating I_T requires a minimal rate of rise of a depolarizing input. This minimum dV/dt is exceeded by EPSPs via ionotropic receptors, such as retinal EPSPs. This means that if such EPSPs through summation manage to switch firing mode to tonic from burst, they must necessarily always first activate a burst, which would be spurious if the only result wanted was a switch in firing mode. This burst signal, then, always reaches cortex, and if the ideas of burst firing as a 'wake-up call' are valid, then this serves its function before the sustained retinal inputs are then relayed via tonic firing. In other words, the switching of response mode to tonic firing with ionotropic EPSPs is a more complex event than just a mode switch. However, the very slowly rising EPSPs activated via metabotropic receptors might perform the neat trick of a clean switch in response mode to tonic firing without ever activating a spurious burst. This scenario has not yet been experimentally verified by synaptically activating only metabotropic receptors in a thalamic relay cell in burst mode, but it is a verifiable hypothesis that lends further support to the importance of metabotropic receptors in controlling response mode of these neurons. It should be noted that the appearance of a fast retinal EPSP during any slow, metabotropic depolarization before I_T is inactivated will activate a low threshold spike, but because it is initiated by a retinal input, it will not result in a spurious signal to cortex.

With this in mind, the pattern of synaptic inputs outlined in Fig. 5 can be considered further. Since retinal input activates only ionotropic receptors, it is a poor candidate to control response mode. All of the nonretinal inputs (including others not illustrated here) activate metabotropic inputs, and these could more efficiently control response mode. However, they also activate ionotropic receptors, suggesting perhaps that these inputs have functions other than controlling response mode. As noted above, what is not clear from Fig. 5 is whether subsets of nonretinal inputs exclusively activate one or the other receptor type, which would clearly provide these pathways with more flexibility and diversity of function. If, for example, every cortical axon activated both ionotropic and metabotropic glutamate receptors, it is difficult to see how this pathway could switch response mode from burst to tonic without activating a burst. Nonetheless, with this proviso and the need to learn the pattern of postsynaptic receptors activated by individual afferents, one can suggest that one important function of nonretinal inputs to the lateral geniculate nucleus is to control response mode of the relay cells.

Drivers and modulators

The point has been made in detail elsewhere (Sherman and Guillery, 1998) that afferent inputs to thalamic relay cells are not all the same but can be divided into at least two functionally distinct groups: *drivers* and *modulators*. Drivers are the inputs that covey the basic information to be relayed to cortex. In the lateral geniculate nucleus, this is the retinal input, and in other sensory relays, drivers can also be clearly defined as the medial lemniscal afferents for the ventrobasal nuclei (or, the ventral posterolateral and ventral posteromedial nuclei, which are the somatosensory relays) and the lateral lemniscal afferents for the ventral part of the medial geniculate nucleus (i.e. the auditory relay). Drivers can also be clearly recognized for some other thalamic relays, but in some nuclei, the identity of the drivers is not yet obvious. By definition, any afferents that are not drivers are modulators. Their job is to provide modulation of the thalamic relay. An example of modulation is the control of response mode.

As is indicated in Fig. 5, one distinction between the driver (retinal) and modulator (nonretinal) inputs is the nature of postsynaptic receptors they can activate: the drivers activate only ionotropic receptors, whereas the modulators can also activate metabotropic receptors. The fact that drivers such as retinal inputs activate only ionotropic receptors implies that the EPSPs they evoke are relatively fast in terms of latency and duration. The short latency is clearly important if the information is to be relayed to cortex in a timely fashion, and the long latencies associated with metabotropic receptors would be an obvious disadvantage. Also the short duration of the EPSP helps ensure that the pattern of two events, or action potentials, closely spaced in time will be relayed to cortex. If the EPSPs were very long-lasting, as would happen with metabotropic receptors, action potentials occurring with short intervals in the input would no longer be resolved as individual signatures in the relay to cortex. Another way of stating this is that a postsynaptic potential via metabotropic receptor activation acts like a low pass temporal filter that results in a loss of high frequency information. This loss is minimized via ionotropic receptors. Thus there seems to be an obvious advantage to assigning only ionotropic receptors to driver inputs that carry the information to be relayed.

There is also a potential advantage to the slow time course of metabotropic receptor activation for modulators. Generally, the long, sustained postsynaptic potentials will lead to overall excitability changes in relay cells, which is one obvious task for modulator input. More specifically, thalamic relay cells have many voltage- and time-dependent ionic conductances in addition to those underlying action potentials and I_T: these include other K^+, Na^+, and Ca^{2+} conductances (for details, see McCormick and Huguenard, 1992; Sherman and Guillery, 1996, 2001), all of which are voltage- and time-dependent, meaning that, like I_T, they are activated by a change in membrane potential that must be sustained usually for tens of millseconds or longer. These conductances together play important roles in how a relay cell responds to its driver input. As with I_T, activation of ionotropic receptors is poorly matched temporally to control these conductances, but activation of metabotropic receptors suits admirably. It thus makes as much sense for modulators to activate metabotropic receptors as for drivers not to do so.

Furthermore, note that, in the lateral geniculate nucleus, the driver (retinal) input represents a small minority of synaptic input to relay cells (5–10%). Limited evidence from other sensory thalamic relays also indicates that the driver inputs provide a small minority of synapses onto the relay cells. It has been argued elsewhere (Sherman and Guillery, 1998, 2001) that this makes sense, because bringing the basic information to a thalamic nucleus does not require as many synaptic inputs as would be required for fine modulation of the relay. This idea of driver inputs to an area is probably not limited to thalamus. For example, it now seems clear that the main information is brought to layer 4 cells in visual cortex by geniculocortical axons (Reid and Alonso, 1995, 1996; Ferster et al., 1996; Chung and Ferster, 1998), yet these provide only about 5–10% of the synaptic inputs to these cells (Ahmed et al., 1994; Latawiec et al., 2000). Also, an analysis of synaptic counts on spinal motoneurons indicates that Ia afferents, which constitute a major driver input, provide <5% of the synaptic terminals to these cells (reviewed on p. 462 of Henneman and Mendell, 1981). It will be interesting to see how general beyond the sensory thalamic relays this finding is that driver inputs constitute a small minority of synapses.

An important point that is reiterated below is that in many areas of the brain there is a tendency to equate functional importance with the size of the input to an area. This, of course, completely ignores the fact that different inputs may be functionally quite different and thus cannot be compared anatomically. If that strategy were applied to the lateral geniculate nucleus, one would come to the silly conclusion that retinal input is of minor importance to a thalamic nucleus that relays brainstem information to cortex.

How, then, do we distinguish between driver and modulator inputs? If we use the lateral geniculate nucleus as a template, we can begin to enumerate some of the differences between drivers and modulators that may be generalized to other thalamic nuclei (see Figs. 5 and 7 for some of these differences and Sherman and Guillery, 1996, 1998, 2001 for others):

- The driver (retinal) afferents innervate relay cells and interneurons, but fail to innervate the tha-

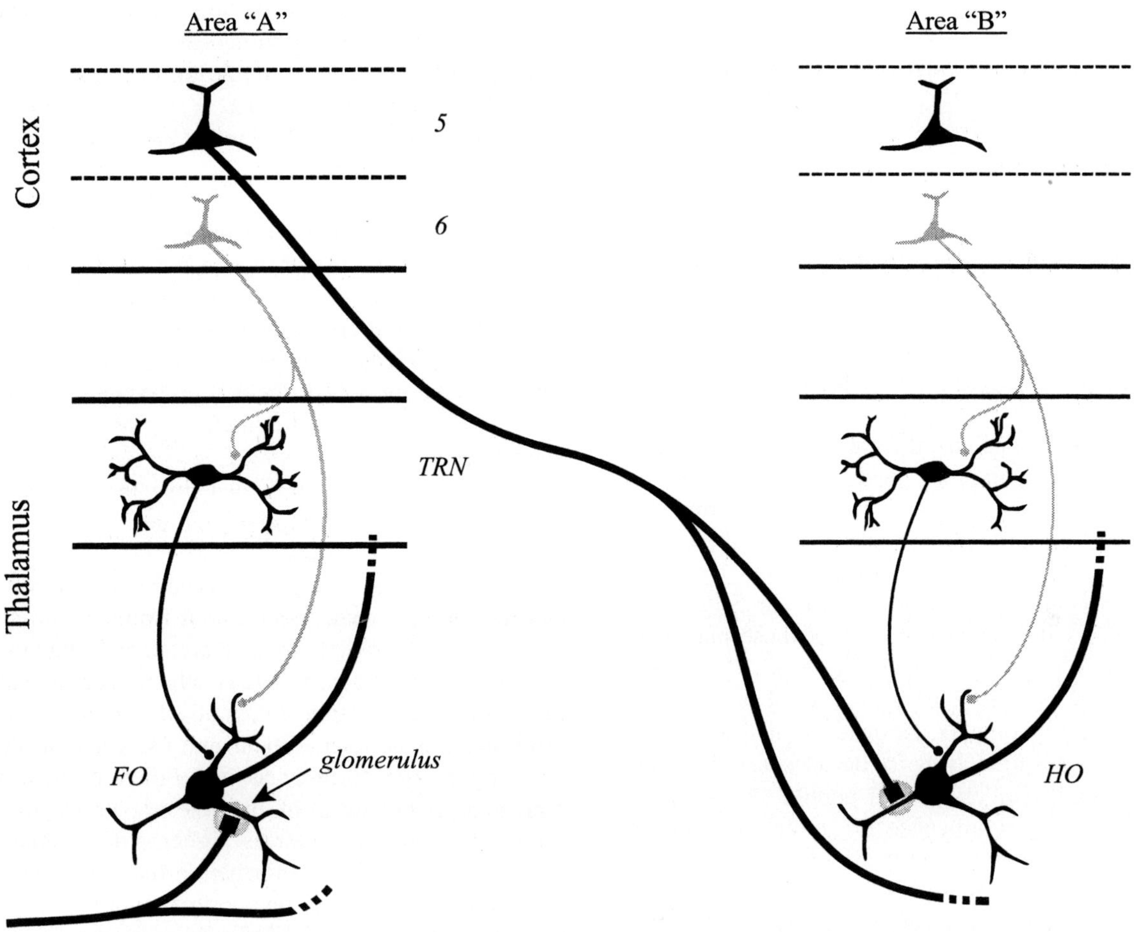

Fig. 7. Comparison of corticothalamic axons from layer 6 versus layer 5. First-order (FO) thalamic regions receive driver inputs from subcortical sources, whereas higher-order (HO) thalamic regions receive driver inputs from cortical layer 5. See text for details.

lamic reticular nucleus, whereas the modulator (nonretinal) afferents innervate the thalamic reticular nucleus as well.

- Driver inputs activate only ionotropic receptors, whereas modulator inputs activate metabotropic receptors as well and sometimes do so exclusively.
- Driver axons exhibit a morphology known as type II (Guillery, 1966), having thick axons with richly branched, flowery, dense terminal arbors. Most modulatory inputs have type I axons (Guillery, 1966), which involve thin axons with few preterminal branches and terminals en passant or on short side branches.
- Driver synaptic terminals are larger than any others in the geniculate neuropil, and they contact proximal dendrites, often in glomeruli and having triadic arrangements with terminals from interneurons.
- Driver axons often (perhaps always, as is the case for retinal axons) branch to innervate extrathalamic structures. At least some modulatory afferents (i.e. from cortex and the thalamic reticular nucleus) innervate only thalamic structures; whether brainstem modulatory afferents branch to innervate extrathalamic targets is not presently known.

In the following section, many of these criteria are used to help identify drivers to many thalamic nuclei and in the process demonstrate that two very different sorts of thalamic relays can be defined.

First and higher order relays

Layer 6 versus layer 5 corticothalamic inputs

It appears that a layer 6 modulatory input is a general property for all thalamic nuclei, and if the sensory relays are typical, this layer 6 corticothalamic pathway is roughly reciprocal in that it derives mostly, but not exclusively, from cortical areas to which the thalamic nucleus in question projects. It has been known for some time that some thalamic nuclei, in addition, receive a layer 5 input from some cortical areas (Guillery, 1995). Examples of nuclei that receive layer 5 afferents are the pulvinar[5], the posterior medial nucleus, the magnocellular division of the medial geniculate nucleus (as opposed to the ventral division, which receives lateral lemniscal input), the medial dorsal nucleus, and others (for details, see Guillery, 1995; Sherman and Guillery, 1996, 2001). It is not clear if the layer 5 innervation supplies the entirety of each of these nuclei or only certain as yet undefined segments. Also, there may be sparse layer 5 input to certain nuclei, like the ventrobasal complex. Knowledge of this layer 5 innervation was filed away for decades as a thalamic curiosity until Guillery (1995) pointed out the possible functional significance of certain differences between layer 5 and layer 6 afferents to thalamus. Fig. 7 summarizes some of the evidence accumulated so far, from which it is clear that the layer 5 afferents are quite unlike layer 6 afferents but bear a striking anatomical resemblance to driver afferents as described for the main sensory relays (compare with the driver/modulator bulleted list above; for details, see (Sherman and Guillery, 1996, 1998; Vidnyánszky et al., 1996):

- They innervate dorsal thalamic nuclei but fail to innervate the thalamic reticular nucleus with collateral branches even though they pass through this region en route to their dorsal thalamic target.
- Where studied, layer 5 inputs activate only ionotropic receptors on relay cells, whereas layer 6 inputs activate metabotropic receptors as well.
- Their axons are thick, with type II morphology and terminal fields.
- Their synaptic terminals are quite large and seem to innervate proximal dendrites, often in glomeruli and having triadic arrangements with terminals from interneurons.
- Many, if not all, branch to innervate extrathalamic targets.

Indeed the above list matches point-for-point the earlier list that distinguishes drivers from modulators. It thus seems reasonable to regard these layer 5 afferents as drivers in the same sense that we consider retinal afferents as the driver for the lateral geniculate nucleus. This is of further interest, because, for the most part, there is no obvious subcortical driver input to most thalamic regions receiving layer 5 innervation[6].

First and higher order thalamic relays

To extend this idea, it appears that some thalamic nuclei receive their main driver input from subcortical sources, like the retina, brainstem etc., and relay this information to cortex, whereas others receive their main driver input from cortex itself and relay this information to another cortical area. We can consider the former type of relay as first order, because it represents a first pass of the relevant information into cortex, and the latter as higher order, because it represents a relay of information that has already reached cortex but from one cortical area to another (see Fig. 7 and Guillery, 1995). Because some thalamic nuclei may get driver input from both subcortical and layer 5 sources, it may be more appropriate to consider first order versus higher order circuitry for thalamic relays rather than for entire thalamic nuclei.

It is interesting that, when thought of this way, each of the main sensory systems has both types of relay for vision, the lateral geniculate nucleus is the first order relay, and most of the pulvinar is the higher order relay; for somatosensation, the ventrobasal nuclei are the first order relay, and the me-

[5] For simplicity, the term 'pulvinar' includes the lateral posterior nucleus in carnivores.

[6] There is a projection from the midbrain to parts of the pulvinar that is often treated implicitly as a driver. Perhaps it is, but it is also possible that it is a modulatory input. Also, it may be that the pulvinar can be divided into one sector that receives driver input from midbrain and another that receives its driver input from layer 5 of cortex.

dial portion of the posterior complex[7] is the higher order relay; and for audition, the ventral part of the medial geniculate nucleus is the first order relay, and the magnocellular part of this nucleus is the higher order relay. (Olfactory information reaches cortex in an unusual way that makes it difficult to fit into this duality.) Whether there is such a neat duality for other types of information relayed through thalamus remains to be determined.

Implications for corticocortical communication

Cortex is comprised of many distinct areas that obviously communicate prolifically amongst themselves. Just how this is done is one of the major problems facing neuroscientists. A consideration of the many areas of visual cortex help to frame the problem and a different approach to it that is suggested here.

We know from many anatomical and electrophysiological studies over the past four decades that the visual world in carnivores and primates is analyzed by many different areas (more than 30 in monkeys) in the occipital, parietal, and temporal lobes (for reviews, see Van Essen, 1985; Felleman and Van Essen, 1991; Van Essen et al., 1992). Attempts to make sense of how these areas cooperate and communicate with one another in visual analysis has focused largely on direct corticocortical connections. Fig. 2 of Van Essen et al. (1992), which is a much copied schema, shows the rich and often reciprocal connectivity among these areas. Strategies have been offered to distinguish feedforward from feedback pathways among these connections (Felleman and Van Essen, 1991). The basic notion in this scheme, a notion challenged below, remains constant: visual information enters striate cortex from the lateral geniculate nucleus, and in a more or less hierarchical set of feedforward connections, the information is passed from striate cortex to higher and higher areas, with many feedback connections present as well. Note that, according to this view, once the information reaches cortex from the lateral geniculate nucleus, it stays within cortex, being routed effectively only amongst cortical areas. Among other drawbacks, this view of visual processing has little regard for the pulvinar, which is a much larger thalamic structure than is the lateral geniculate nucleus.

One of the reasons this view is so widely held is the very massive nature of direct corticocortical connections. Any cortical area receives the vast majority of its extrinsic afferents from other cortical areas and rather little from subcortical structures, like the thalamus. But this linking of functional importance of a pathway with its size is the very thinking that, as suggested above, would lead one to conclude that retinal input to the lateral geniculate nucleus is functionally of little consequence.

To frame our alternative view versus the traditional one for corticocortical communication, it is helpful to consider the extreme alternative first. For cortical afferents, just as in those of the thalamus, it may be that drivers and modulators exist. The drivers carry the main information, and identifying them among afferents to a cortical area becomes supremely important. If, as in thalamus, the driver inputs are a small minority, then concentrating on large pathways, such as most of the direct corticocortical connections, may be misleading. Perhaps only a small minority of these direct pathways are drivers, with the rest being modulators.

The most extreme view, offered for clarity, is that *none* of the direct corticocortical projections are drivers, and instead they are all modulators. The drivers, then, are limited to thalamocortical afferents. By this extreme version of our hypothesis, the information route for corticocortical communication travels from layer 5 of one area down to a higher order thalamic relay (i.e. pulvinar for visual cortical communication) and then back up to the target cortical area (see Fig. 8). Another way of thinking about this is to consider the benefits of relaying retinal information through the lateral geniculate nucleus to cortex instead of having a direct retino-cortical pathway: it may be that *any* new information coming into a cortical area, whether originating subcortically or in a another cortical area, benefits from a thalamic relay.

[7] Terminology across species can often be confusing. The primate equivalent to the medial portion of the posterior complex in rodents and carnivores is the anterior or 'oral' part of pulvinar. The nonprimate terminology is used here, and so the pulvinar (which includes what is sometimes called the lateral posterior nucleus) is a structure associated essentially only with vision.

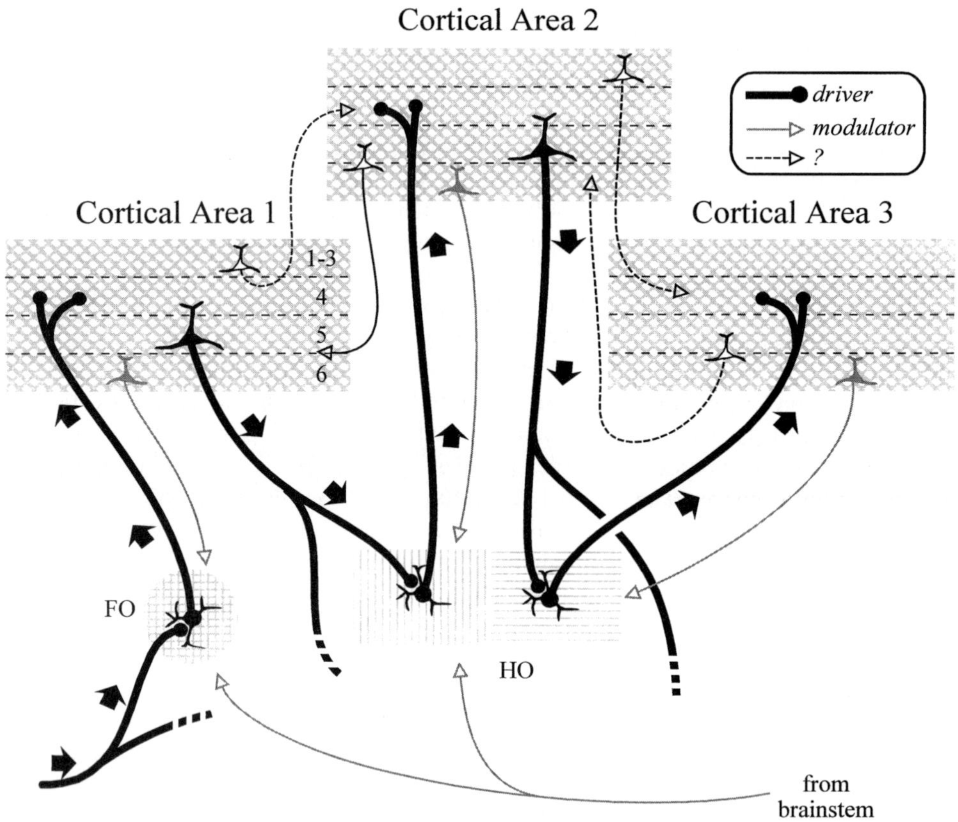

Fig. 8. Schema of hypothesis that corticocortical information flow involves a relay through a higher-order thalamic region. The first-order (FO) relay (e.g. lateral geniculate nucleus) relays a driver (e.g. retinal) input to primary cortex (e.g. V1). From here, information is relayed among cortical areas via cortico–thalamo–cortical paths involving different regions of a higher-order (HO) thalamic nucleus (e.g. the pulvinar) routes. Thick, dark pathways represent the drivers, and thin, lighter pathways with solid lines represent the modulators. The nature of direct corticocortical projections (dashed lines) is ambiguous as to identity as driver or modulator.

A less extreme hypothesis would maintain that one important route for corticocortical communication involves a relay through higher order thalamic nuclei, but that another route involves a minority of corticocortical connections, the rest being modulatory. However, even here it is possible to point out an important difference between corticocortical drivers and those involving cortico–thalamo–cortical routes. Information carried by the former stays strictly within cortex, but that carried by the latter pathway also informs other regions of the neuroaxis.

Even if our hypothesis proves wrong, it does draw attention to the need to avoid treating all connections among cortical areas as functionally equivalent. Just knowing, for instance, which corticocortical afferents activate ionotropic and/or metabotropic receptors would be a useful step in functionally classifying these pathways.

Conclusions

The complex cell and circuit properties of thalamic nuclei leave little doubt that the relay of information to cortex is an active and mutable process. The question should no longer be why we have thalamic relays but rather how these relays affect the nature of information arriving in cortex and how their different relay properties are controlled. Some specific suggestions have been made here about how circuit properties control a voltage-dependent conductance, I_T, in relay cells to control responsiveness, and how this could affect the nature of information relayed to cortex. However, it should be appreciated that this property related to tonic and burst response modes may be one of many mechanisms by which thalamic relays can control the flow of information to cortex.

Nonetheless, once we appreciate that the insertion of a thalamic relay in the information pathway to cortex has great functional significance, we can also re-investigate the role of thalamus in corticocortical communication. The discovery that many thalamic regions seem to receive their driving input from layer 5 of cortex itself leads to the suggestion that much of corticocortical communication involves a route through thalamus, with the same advantages of having a thalamic relay for this route as exists for relaying, say, retinal information to cortex. The alternate route for corticocortical communication — direct connections among areas — needs to be reconsidered with regard to the nature of these pathways and the possibility that many, and perhaps all, are modulatory in nature. Thus the full impact of thalamus may be much more than simply controlling flow of information to cortex: it may remain an active partner in all cortical computations.

Acknowledgements

The author's laboratory during the preparation of this manuscript was supported by USPHS Grants EY03038 and EY11409. The author thanks R.W. Guillery for invaluable discussion and initiation of many of the ideas contained in this chapter.

References

Ahmed, B., Anderson, J.C., Douglas, R.J., Martin, K.A.C. and Nelson, J.C. (1994) Polyneuronal innervation of spiny stellate neurons in cat visual cortex. *J. Comp. Neurol.*, 341: 39–49.

Brown, D.A., Abogadie, F.C., Allen, T.G., Buckley, N.J., Caulfield, M.P., Delmas, P., Haley, J.E., Lamas, J.A. and Selyanko, A.A. (1997) Muscarinic mechanisms in nerve cells. *Life Sci.*, 60: 1137–1144.

Chung, S. and Ferster, D. (1998) Strength and orientation tuning of the thalamic input to simple cells revealed by electrically evoked cortical suppression. *Neuron*, 20: 1177–1189.

Cleland, B.G., Dubin, M.W. and Levick, W.R. (1971) Sustained and transient neurones in the cat's retina and lateral geniculate nucleus. *J. Physiol. (Lond.)*, 217: 473–496.

Cudeiro, J. and Rivadulla, C. (1999) Sight and insight — on the physiological role of nitric oxide in the visual system. *Trends Neurosci.*, 22: 109–116.

Destexhe, A., Neubig, M., Ulrich, D. and Huguenard, J. (1998) Dendritic low-threshold calcium currents in thalamic relay cells. *J. Neurosci.*, 18: 3574–3588.

Erişir, A., Van Horn, S.C. and Sherman, S.M. (1997) Relative numbers of cortical and brainstem inputs to the lateral geniculate nucleus. *Proc. Natl. Acad. Sci. USA*, 94: 1517–1520.

Felleman, D.J. and Van Essen, D.C. (1991) Distributed hierarchical processing in the primate cerebral cortex. *Cerebral Cortex*, 1: 1–47.

Ferster, D., Chung, S. and Wheat, H. (1996) Orientation selectivity of thalamic input to simple cells of cat visual cortex. *Nature*, 380: 249–252.

Green, D.M. and Swets, J.A. (1966) *Signal Detection Theory and Psychophysics*. Wiley, New York.

Guido, W. and Sherman, S.M. (1998) Response latencies of cells in the cat's lateral geniculate nucleus are less variable during burst than tonic firing. *Vis. Neurosci.*, 15: 231–237.

Guido, W. and Weyand, T. (1995) Burst responses in thalamic relay cells of the awake behaving cat. *J. Neurophysiol.*, 74: 1782–1786.

Guido, W., Lu, S.-M. and Sherman, S.M. (1992) Relative contributions of burst and tonic responses to the receptive field properties of lateral geniculate neurons in the cat. *J. Neurophysiol.*, 68: 2199–2211.

Guido, W., Lu, S.-M., Vaughan, J.W., Godwin, D.W. and Sherman, S.M. (1995) Receiver operating characteristic (ROC) analysis of neurons in the cat's lateral geniculate nucleus during tonic and burst response mode. *Vis. Neurosci.*, 12: 723–741.

Guillery, R.W. (1966) A study of Golgi preparations from the dorsal lateral geniculate nucleus of the adult cat. *J. Comp. Neurol.*, 128: 21–50.

Guillery, R.W. (1969) The organization of synaptic interconnections in the laminae of the dorsal lateral geniculate nucleus of the cat. *Z. Zellforsch.*, 96: 1–38.

Guillery, R.W. (1995) Anatomical evidence concerning the role of the thalamus in corticocortical communication: a brief review. *J. Anat.*, 187: 583–592.

Gutierrez, C., Cox, C.L. and Sherman, S.M. (2000) Dynamics of low threshold spike activation in relay neurons of the cat lateral geniculate nucleus, submitted for publication.

Henneman, E. and Mendell, L.M. (1981) Functional organization of motoneuron pool and its inputs. In: V.B. Brooks (Ed.), *Handbook of Physiology. Section 1: The Nervous System. Volume II. Motor Control, Part 1*. American Physiological Society, Bethesda, MD, pp. 423–507.

Hubel, D.H. and Wiesel, T.N. (1977) Functional architecture of macaque monkey visual cortex. *Proc. R. Soc. Lond. B*, 198: 1–59.

Isaac, J.T.R., Crair, M.C., Nicoll, R.A. and Malenka, R.C. (1997) Silent synapses during development of thalamocortical inputs. *Neuron*, 18: 269–280.

Jahnsen, H. and Llinás, R. (1984a) Electrophysiological properties of guinea-pig thalamic neurones: an in vitro study. *J. Physiol. (Lond.)*, 349: 205–226.

Jahnsen, H. and Llinás, R. (1984b) Ionic basis for the electroresponsiveness and oscillatory properties of guinea-pig thalamic neurones in vitro. *J. Physiol. (Lond.)*, 349: 227–247.

Jones, E.G. (1985) *The Thalamus*. Plenum Press, New York.

Latawiec, D., Martin, K.A.C. and Meskenaite, V. (2000) Termination of the geniculocortical projection in the striate cortex of macaque monkey: a quantitative immunoelectron microscopic study. *J. Comp. Neurol.*, 419: 306–319.

Lenz, F.A., Garonzik, I.M., Zirh, T.A. and Dougherty, P.M. (1998) Neuronal activity in the region of the thalamic principal sensory nucleus (ventralis caudalis) in patients with pain following amputations. *Neuroscience*, 86: 1065–1081.

Lu, S.-M., Guido, W. and Sherman, S.M. (1992) Effects of membrane voltage on receptive field properties of lateral geniculate neurons in the cat: contributions of the low threshold Ca^{++} conductance. *J. Neurophysiol.*, 68: 2185–2198.

Macmillan, N.A. and Creelman, C.D. (1991) *Detection Theory: A User's Guide*. Cambridge University Press, Cambridge.

McCormick, D.A. (1992) Neurotransmitter actions in the thalamus and cerebral cortex and their role in neuromodulation of thalamocortical activity. *Prog. Neurobiol.*, 39: 337–388.

McCormick, D.A. and Bal, T. (1997) Sleep and arousal: thalamocortical mechanisms. *Annu. Rev. Neurosci.*, 20: 185–215.

McCormick, D.A. and Huguenard, J.R. (1992) A model of the electrophysiological properties of thalamocortical relay neurons. *J. Neurophysiol.*, 68: 1384–1400.

Mott, D.D. and Lewis, D.V. (1994) The pharmacology and function of central GABAB receptors. *Int. Rev. Neurobiol.*, 36: 97–223.

Mukherjee, P. and Kaplan, E. (1995) Dynamics of neurons in the cat lateral geniculate nucleus: in vivo electrophysiology and computational modeling. *J. Neurophysiol.*, 74: 1222–1243.

Nicolelis, M.A., Baccala, L.A., Lin, R.C. and Chapin, J.K. (1995) Sensorimotor encoding by synchronous neural ensemble activity at multiple levels of the somatosensory system. *Science*, 268: 1353–1358.

Nicoll, R.A., Malenka, R.C. and Kauer, J.A. (1990) Functional comparison of neurotransmitter receptor subtypes in mammalian central nervous system. *Physiol. Rev.*, 70: 513–565.

Pape, H.-C. and Mager, R. (1992) Nitric oxide controls oscillatory activity in thalamocortical neurons. *Neuron*, 9: 441–448.

Pin, J.P. and Bockaert, J. (1995) Get receptive to metabotropic glutamate receptors. *Curr. Opin. Neurobiol.*, 5: 342–349.

Pin, J.P. and Duvoisin, R. (1995) The metabotropic glutamate receptors: structure and functions. *Neuropharmacology*, 34: 1–26.

Radhakrishnan, V., Tsoukatos, J., Davis, K.D., Tasker, R.R., Lozano, A.M. and Dostrovsky, J.O. (1999) A comparison of the burst activity of lateral thalamic neurons in chronic pain and non-pain patients. *Pain*, 80: 567–575.

Ramcharan, E.J., Gnadt, J.W. and Sherman, S.M. (2000) Burst and tonic firing in thalamic cells of unanesthetized, behaving monkeys. *Vis. Neurosci.*, 17: 55–62.

Recasens, M. and Vignes, M. (1995) Excitatory amino acid metabotropic receptor subtypes and calcium regulation. *Ann. New York Acad. Sci.*, 757: 418–429.

Reid, R.C. and Alonso, J.M. (1995) Specificity of monosynaptic connections from thalamus to visual cortex. *Nature*, 378: 281–284.

Reid, R.C. and Alonso, J.M. (1996) The processing and encoding of information in the visual cortex. *Curr. Opin. Neurobiol.*, 6: 475–480.

Reinagel, P., Godwin, D.W., Sherman, S.M. and Koch, C. (1999) Encoding of visual information by LGN bursts. *J. Neurophysiol.*, 81: 2558–2569.

Shaw, P.J. and Salt, T.E. (1997) Modulation of sensory and excitatory amino acid responses by nitric oxide donors and glutathione in the ventrobasal thalamus of the rat. *Eur. J. Neurosci.*, 9: 1507–1513.

Sherman, S.M. (1996) Dual response modes in lateral geniculate neurons: mechanisms and functions. *Vis. Neurosci.*, 13: 205–213.

Sherman, S.M. and Guillery, R.W. (1996) The functional organization of thalamocortical relays. *J. Neurophysiol.*, 76: 1367–1395.

Sherman, S.M. and Guillery, R.W. (1998) On the actions that one nerve cell can have on another: distinguishing 'drivers' from 'modulators'. *Proc. Natl. Acad. Sci. USA*, 95: 7121–7126.

Sherman, S.M. and Guillery, R.W. (2001) *Exploring the Thalamus*. Academic Press, San Diego.

Steriade, M. and Llinás, R. (1988) The functional states of the thalamus and the associated neuronal interplay. *Physiol. Rev.*, 68: 649–742.

Steriade, M., McCormick, D.A. and Sejnowski, T.J. (1993) Thalamocortical oscillations in the sleeping and aroused brain. *Science*, 262: 679–685.

Swadlow, H.A. and Gusev, A.G. (2001) The impact of 'bursting' thalamic impulses at a neocortical synapse. *Nat. Neurosci.*, 4: 402–408.

Swets, J.A. (1973) The relative operating characteristic in psychology. *Science*, 182: 990–1000.

Van Essen, D.C. (1985) Functional organization of primate visual cortex. In: A. Peters and E.G. Jones (Eds.), *Cerebral Cortex*, Vol. 3. Plenum, New York, pp. 259–329.

Van Essen, D.C., Anderson, C.H. and Felleman, D.J. (1992) Information processing in the primate visual system: an integrated systems perspective. *Science*, 255: 419–423.

Van Horn, S.C., Erişir, A. and Sherman, S.M. (2000) The relative distribution of synapses in the A-laminae of the lateral geniculate nucleus of the cat. *J. Comp. Neurol.*, 416: 509–520.

Vidnyánszky, Z., Görcs, T.J., Négyessy, L., Borostyánkoi, Z., Kuhn, R., Knöpfel, T. and Hámori, J. (1996) Immunocytochemical visualization of the mGluR1a metabotropic glutamate receptor at synapses of corticothalamic terminals originating from area 17 of the rat. *Eur. J. Neurosci.*, 8: 1061–1071.

Zeki, S. (1993) *A Vision of the Brain*. Blackwell Scientific Publications, Oxford, pp. 1–366.

Zhan, X.J., Cox, C.L., Rinzel, J. and Sherman, S.M. (1999) Current clamp and modeling studies of low threshold calcium spikes in cells of the cat's lateral geniculate nucleus. *J. Neurophysiol.*, 81: 2360–2373.

Zhan, X.J., Cox, C.L. and Sherman, S.M. (2000) Dendritic de-

polarization efficiently attenuates low threshold calcium spikes in thalamic relay cells. *J. Neurosci.*, 20: 3909–3914.
Zhou, Q., Godwin, D.W., O'Malley, D.M. and Adams, P.R. (1997) Visualization of calcium influx through channels that shape size burst and tonic firing modes of thalamic relay cells. *J. Neurophysiol.*, 77: 2816–2825.

C. Casanova and M. Ptito (Eds.)
Progress in Brain Research, Vol. 134

CHAPTER 5

Higher-order motion processing in the pulvinar

C. Casanova [1,*], L. Merabet [1], A. Desautels [2] and K. Minville [2]

[1] *Laboratoire des Neurosciences de la Vision, École d'Optométrie, Université de Montréal, Montréal, PQ, Canada*
[2] *Centre de Recherche en Sciences Neurologiques, Université de Montréal, Montréal, PQ, Canada*

Abstract: Thalamic nuclei have long been considered as passive relay stations for sensory signals en route to the cerebral cortex, where higher level processing occurs. In recent years, it has been proposed that thalamic nuclei may actively participate in the processing of specific information in conjunction with cortical areas. In support of this hypothesis, we recently discovered that neurons in the main extrageniculate visual nucleus, *the pulvinar*, exhibit higher-order visual properties that were, until now, only associated with higher-order cortical areas. Pulvinar neurons can indeed code the veridical direction of a moving plaid pattern, indicating that these cells can integrate ambiguous signals into a coherent percept. This finding as well as our demonstration that there are cortico-thalamo-cortical loops involved in complex motion analysis open promising avenues in unraveling the function of the pulvinar complex in normal vision.

Introduction

For many years most physiologists have regarded thalamic nuclei as stations that passively relay sensory information to the cortex, dependent on the animal's state of arousal, and in which minimal sub-cortical processing takes place (Macchi et al., 1996; Sherman and Guillery, 1996; Sillito and Jones, 1997). This conventional view does not stand when one considers the extensive reciprocal connectivity between the thalamus and the visual cortex. Both first- and second-order thalamic nuclei (see Sherman, 2001, this volume) are closely linked to the cortex through cortico-thalamo-cortical loops, and it has been proposed in recent years, that thalamic nuclei may actively participate in the processing of specific information in conjunction with cortical areas (Mumford, 1991; Macchi et al., 1996; Miller, 1996; Sherman and Guillery, 1996; Grieve et al., 2000; Miller and Schreiner, 2000). In support of this proposal, we recently discovered that neurons in the main extrageniculate visual nucleus, *the pulvinar*, exhibit higher-order visual properties that were, until recently, only associated with higher-order cortical areas (Merabet et al., 1998). This chapter will summarize these findings and further demonstrates the involvement of the pulvinar complex in higher-order motion processing. Motion processing represents an *essential* aspect of vision and is characterized by at least two known levels of analysis (Derrington and Badcock, 1985; Movshon et al., 1986; Newsome et al., 1986; Vaina and Cowey, 1996; Greenlee and Smith, 1997). The first level is involved in local motion measurement and the comprising *first-order* neurons provide only partial information about image motion. A second level is therefore needed in which *second-order* neurons integrate the signals from image components and provide information on the 'veridical' motion of a scene (Adelson and Movshon, 1982; Movshon et al., 1986). Until recently, neurons with such higher-order properties were only found in higher-order cortical areas (the middle temporal (MT) area in primates, and

* Corresponding author: C. Casanova, Laboratoire des neurosciences de la vision, École d'optométrie, Université de Montréal, C.P. 6128, Succ. Centre-Ville, Montréal, PQ, H3C 3J7 Canada. Tel.: +1-514-343-2407; Fax: +1-514-343-2382;
E-mail: christian.casanova@umontreal.ca

the visual part of the ectosylvian cortex in cats (Movshon et al., 1986; Rodman and Albright, 1989 in primates; Scannell et al., 1996 in cats) when tested with plaid patterns and/or complex random dot kinematograms (RDKs) (see Zhou and Baker, 1993; Mareschal and Baker, 1998; Baker, 1999 for reports of second-order processing in the primary visual cortex).

The lateral posterior-pulvinar complex: a thalamic candidate for a sub-cortical counterpart to the cortex for the analysis of moving objects

In higher mammals, the pulvinar is the main extrageniculate visual thalamic complex and has considerably developed during evolution in parallel with the expansion of the neocortex (see Jones, 1985). This thalamic region has often been associated with visual salience (Petersen et al., 1985; Robinson and Petersen, 1992; Robinson and Cowie, 1997) and visually guided movement (Grieve et al., 2000), but for the most part its function has not been elucidated (Casanova et al., 1989; Chalupa, 1991; Grieve et al., 2000). In cats, our animal model, the lateral posterior-pulvinar (LP-pulvinar) complex can be subdivided into at least three main regions, each containing a complete representation of the contralateral visual field (Hutchins and Updyke, 1989; Chalupa, 1991). These areas include the lateral (LPl) and medial (LPm) parts of LP, and the pulvinar, which are considered respectively as the striate-, tecto-, and retino-recipient zones of the complex (Graybiel and Berson, 1980; Updyke, 1983 Chalupa and Abramson, 1988; Hutchins and Updyke, 1989). The LP-pulvinar receives prominent signals from both the mesencephalon and the primary visual cortex, and establishes reciprocal connections with virtually all visual cortical areas (Raczkowski and Rosenquist, 1983; Abramson and Chalupa, 1985, 1988). Thus, the LP-pulvinar represents a thalamic structure with great strategic potential for processing visual information, and a unique platform for study because it receives neural signals from the two main retinofugal pathways and may integrate them (Benedek et al., 1983; Casanova et al., 1991). Given that the LP nucleus receives its primary afferents from descending pathways from layer V of the cortex, it is considered to be a higher order nucleus (Guillery, 1995).

Neurons in the LP-pulvinar have large receptive fields (RFs) of low acuity (Casanova et al., 1989) and recent data from our laboratory and others suggest that this structure is involved in several aspects of motion analysis. For example, most cells are direction selective (Casanova et al., 1989; Chalupa and Abramson, 1989), practically all LPl cells respond to the motion of textured patterns (Casanova and Savard, 1996a); these patterns, when presented as a background, can modulate the responses evoked by a sine-wave grating drifting across the RF (Casanova and Savard, 1996b). Moreover, the LP-pulvinar complex is in reciprocal communication with areas specialized in motion processing (Raczkowski and Rosenquist, 1983; Abramson and Chalupa, 1985). In cats, two cortical areas are believed to be crucial in the analysis of motion: the posteromedial part of the lateral suprasylvian (PMLS) cortex and the anterior ectosylvian visual (AEV) cortex (see Mucke et al., 1982; Benedek et al., 1983; Pasternak et al., 1989; Spear, 1991; Lomber et al., 1994; Rudolph and Pasternak, 1996; Merabet et al., 2000 for a detailed description of response properties in those areas and the effects of specific lesions on cat behavior). Neuroanatomical studies have shown that most PMLS neurons projecting to the LP-pulvinar are located in layer V (Updyke, 1981; Abramson and Chalupa, 1985). LP-pulvinar cells project to PMLS neurons lying in layer IV (and to a lesser extent, in layer I) (Abramson and Chalupa, 1985) and double-labeling techniques demonstrated that a subset of LP neurons projects to both the PMLS and the primary visual cortex (Miceli et al., 1991). AEV neurons project only to the LPm and most of them are located in layers V and VI. LPm cells projecting to AEV cortex end for the most part in layer IV (Norita et al., 1986; Olson and Graybiel, 1987). Some LPm neurons project to both the posterolateral part of the LS (but not the PMLS) and the AEV cortex (Miceli et al., 1991). Fig. 1 summarizes some of these projections and illustrates the fact that the LP-pulvinar complex is in a unique position to inform multiple cortical areas about the processing occurring in lower or higher level areas and/or to increase the effectiveness of the processing taking place in a given cortical area.

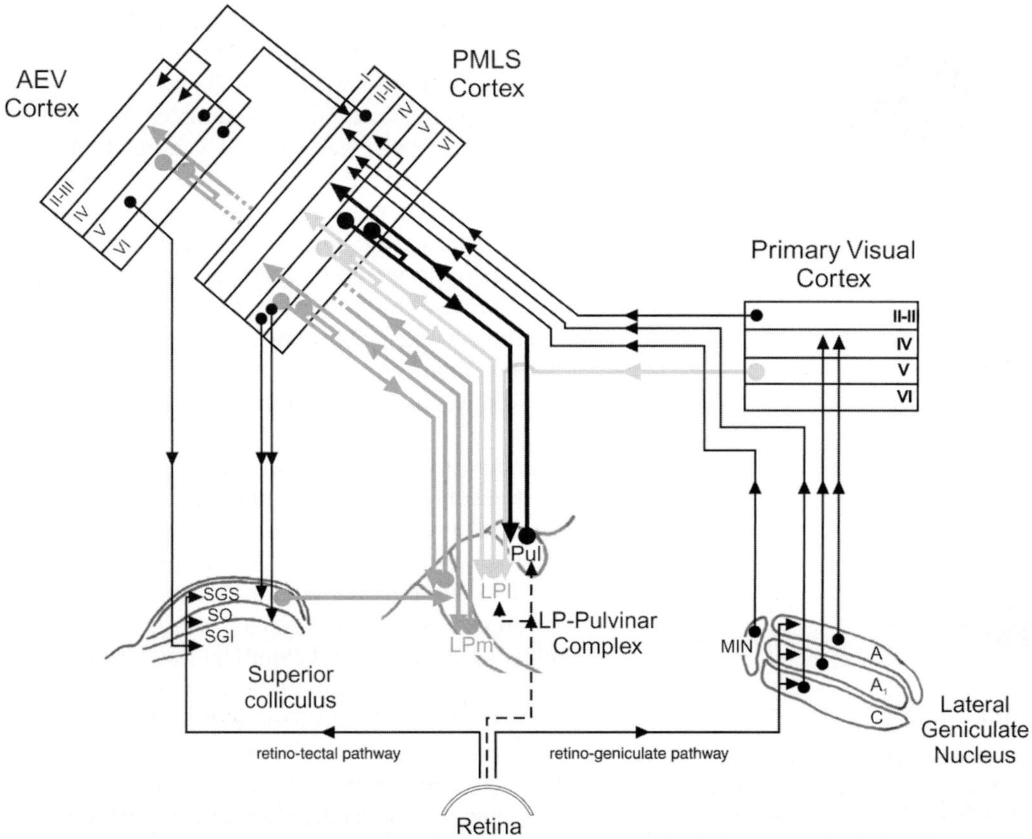

Fig. 1. Schematic representation of major visual pathways implicating subcortical–cortical interrelationships in the cat. The connections involving the LP-pulvinar complex are represented by thick lines of different gray levels. Note that some projections are not shown in order to clarify the diagram (e.g. area 17 to LGN).

General methods

Moving plaid patterns were used to investigate the higher-order motion sensitivity of neurons in the anesthetized cat (see Casanova et al. (1997) and Merabet et al. (1998) for details on procedures). All animals were treated in accordance with the guidelines of the Canadian Council on Animal Care. The plaid pattern is shown in Fig. 2 and is composed of two superimposed drifting gratings differing only in orientation (Fig. 2A). At the perceptual level, one sees a single rigid pattern moving unambiguously with a direction and velocity that are uniquely consistent with the constraints imposed by the motion of the individual components (Fig. 2B) (Adelson and Movshon, 1982; Movshon et al., 1985; Stoner and Albright, 1992). At the neuronal level, a cell that is selective for the global motion of the plaid pattern responds with a profile similar to that of a single grating moving in the integrated direction ('pattern' motion selectivity; Fig. 2B) rather than in the directions of the oriented components comprising the pattern ('component' motion selectivity; Fig. 2C) (Adelson and Movshon, 1982; Scannell et al., 1996). To demonstrate the contribution of the visual cortex on complex motion responses in the LP-pulvinar complex, we performed two sets of experiments. In the first series, the AEV cortex was deactivated by restricted injections of γ-aminobutyric acid (GABA, 200 μM, stained with 1% Chicago Sky Blue). In the second series of experiments, plaid responses in the LP-pulvinar were characterized after the acute bilateral ablation (by aspiration) of the anterior ectosylvian sulcus, including the entire visual area (i.e. the AEV), with or without the PMLS cortex or the whole LS cortices i.e. the regions located in the

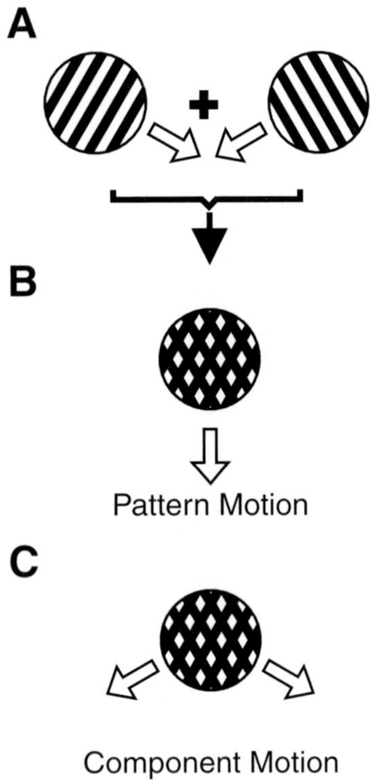

Fig. 2. Diagram illustrating a plaid pattern. (A) A plaid is composed of two superimposed drifting gratings differing only in orientation. (B) Pattern motion: only a single, coherent, direction of motion is seen. (C) Component motion: the motion of both components is perceived. See explanations in text.

medial and lateral banks of the suprasylvian sulcus (Palmer et al., 1978). Details of these procedures are given in Casanova et al. (1997) and Minville and Casanova (1998).

Results

Pattern motion selectivity of LP-pulvinar neurons

Twenty-six direction-selective neurons in the LP-pulvinar out of 89 responded to moving plaids with pattern-motion (PM) responses, indicating that these thalamic cells can integrate separate motion signals into a coherent moving percept. Fig. 3 shows a representative example that illustrates the close correspondence between the directional tuning functions computed from responses to moving gratings and plaids. Other examples of PM responses are shown in Fig. 4. It was noted that PM selective responses strongly depend on the coherence of the stimulus, and that changing the parameters of one of the two gratings yielded a reduction in the cell's discharges, down to spontaneous levels. Examples in which the responses to plaids were studied as a function of the spatial and temporal frequencies of the constituent gratings are shown in Fig. 5. Maximum discharges for both cells (Fig. 5A,B) were clearly elicited by the plaid, only when the spatiotemporal characteristics of the two stimulus components (non-transparent condition) were perfectly matched.

The remaining 63 LP-pulvinar cells did not code the veridical direction of the plaid pattern. A first subset of 12 LP cells exhibited bi-lobed tuning curves with peaks approximately symmetrical to the peak obtained in the single grating experiment. These responses matched the predicted tuning curve for component-motion (CM) responses, implying that these LP-pulvinar neurons can only process the one-dimensional motion signals making up the plaid pattern. Therefore, the LP-pulvinar complex is a region where PM as well as CM responses are present, indicating that both local and global information are processed at this thalamic level. The remaining 51 units could not be grouped in either of the two categories and were considered as 'unclassified direction selective cells'.

Receptive field characteristics

Examination of cell properties revealed that the receptive fields of PM selective LP-pulvinar neurons (480 ± 234 deg^2) tended to be larger than that of CM selective (371.5 ± 177 deg^2) and of unclassified direction selective units (402 ± 260 deg^2), but these differences were not statistically significant (One sample normality test, Kolmogorov–Smirnov.) Fig. 6B–D shows the distribution of the receptive field size for the three cell groups. We did not find any significant differences between the selectivity for plaid patterns and drifting gratings (mean bandwidths of $52.4 \pm 32°$ and $54.7 \pm 31°$, respectively). The relationship between direction bandwidths is shown in Fig. 6A: most data are located close to either side of the perfect regression line, indicating that selectivity of LP cells is comparable for the two stimuli. Other properties such as orientation, spatial, and temporal selectivity were similar between groups.

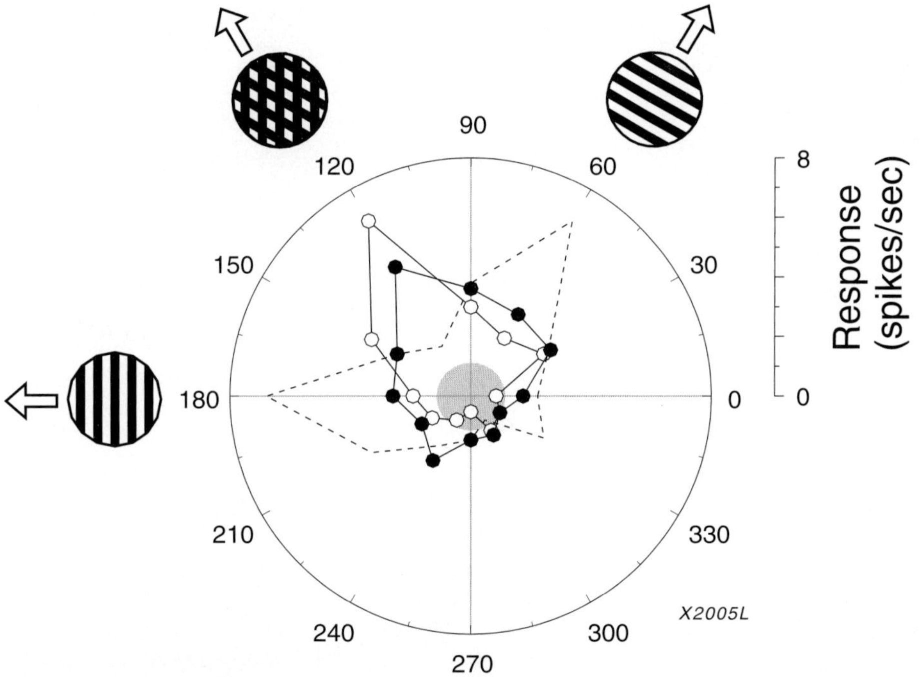

Fig. 3. Polar graph illustrating the responses of a pattern-motion selective LP-pulvinar neuron to gratings (open symbols) and plaid patterns (filled symbols) drifted in 12 directions of motion. The response to gratings alone is considered as the predicted profile for a truly pattern direction selective unit. The dashed line represents the predicted response to plaids for a component-direction selective unit. The grey central circle represents spontaneous activity level.

Cell localization

The majority of pattern motion selective LP-pulvinar cells (around 70%) were located in the medial part of the LP nucleus (LPm), whereas the remaining units were found in the lateral section (LPl) of this nucleus. Three PM selective units were located at the border or in the suprageniculate nucleus. The LPm corresponds to the tecto-recipient zone of the LP-pulvinar, which receives a major input from the superior colliculus (SC) and establishes reciprocal connections with the anterior ectosylvian visual (AEV) cortex (Norita et al., 1986; Olson and Graybiel, 1987).

Influence of the visual cortex

Pharmacological deactivation of the AEV cortex revealed that the PM sensitivity of LP-pulvinar cells might strongly depend on descending pathways from this cortical area. Fig. 7 shows an example in which the response of a LPm cell was dramatically reduced by the reversible deactivation of a visuotopically corresponding region of the AEV cortex (see Merabet et al., 1998). However, responses of a number of cells were not affected by the cortical deactivation, suggesting that PM selectivity comes from other cortical areas, and one cannot exclude that there may be a sub-population of LS neurons which can code the true direction of moving objects, as proposed by Scannell et al. (1997).

To further investigate the contribution of the cortical areas known to be involved in motion processing to the PM responses of LP-pulvinar units, we bilaterally destroyed the AEV cortex alone, and in conjunction with either the PMLS cortex or the whole LS cortex. Destruction of the AEV cortex, which represents the cat's only cortical area known to contain PM selective neurons (Scannell et al., 1996), did not prevent LP-pulvinar cells from coding the true direction of a plaid (Merabet et al., 1998), supporting then the pharmacological deactivation experiments. The remaining cells were, as for intact animals, CM selective or unclassified direction selective. Destruc-

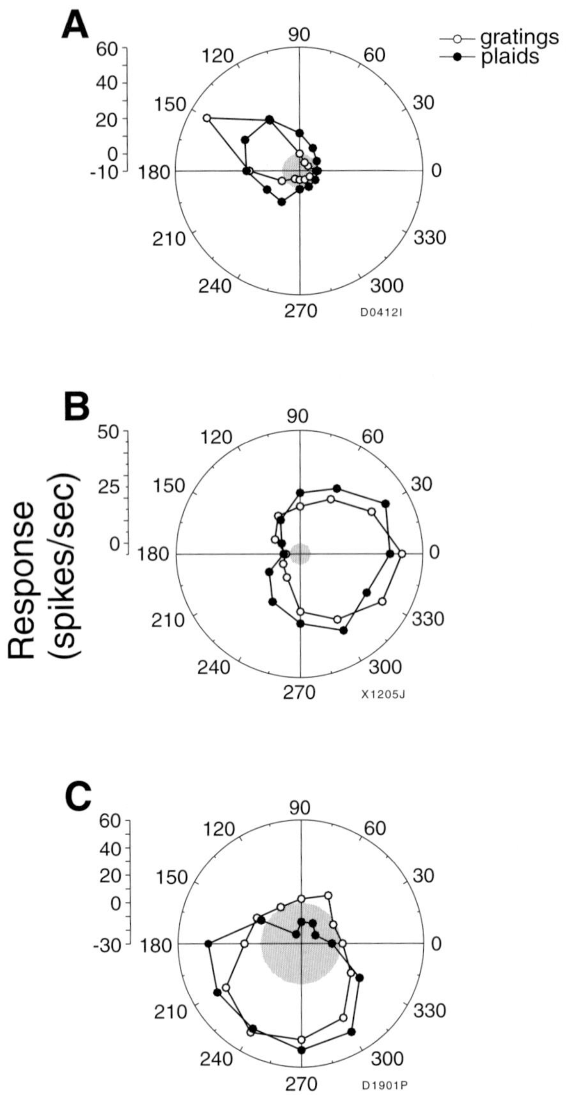

Fig. 4. Additional examples of pattern motion responses in the LP-pulvinar complex. A, B, and C illustrate the activity of three distinct neurons. Conventions are as in Fig. 3.

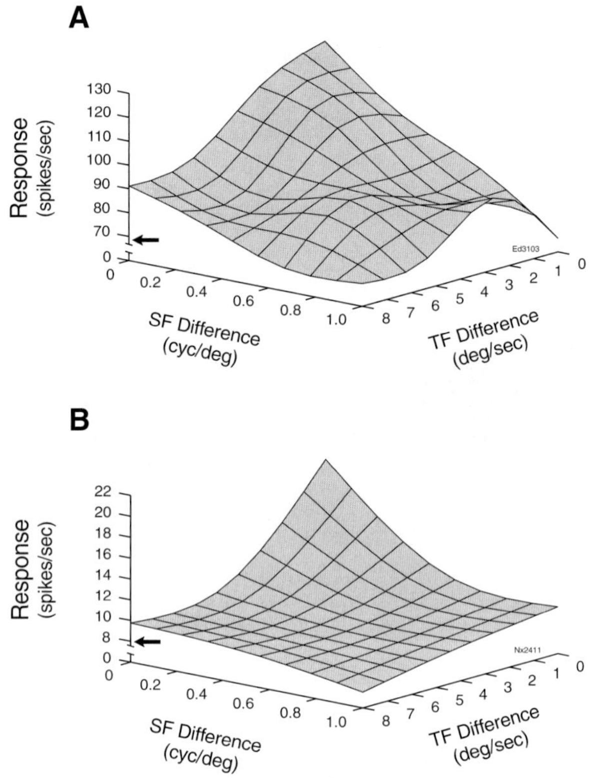

Fig. 5. Responses of two pattern-motion selective LP-pulvinar cells (A and B) as a function of the coherence of the plaid pattern. The response of the two neurons is maximal when the components of the plaid are identical (coherent condition) and decrease when both component gratings are differing in temporal (TF) and/or spatial frequencies (SF). The arrows represent spontaneous activity levels.

tion of the AEV in conjunction with the PMLS cortex, while reducing the overall number of direction selective units in the LP-pulvinar, yielded comparable findings. The persistence of PM selectivity after such lesions may indicate that intrinsic computations are taking place within the thalamus (e.g. integration of multiple component signals). Finally, ablating the entire LS cortex yielded a profound reduction in the number of PM selective cells as well as other direction selective units. This decrease of LP-pulvinar responsiveness may be related to the surgical trauma and therefore may not accurately reflect the real functional impact of the lesioned corticofugal projections.

Discussion

The present study indicates that neurons in the LP-pulvinar complex can signal the true direction of motion of a plaid pattern, implying that thalamic cells can integrate separate motion signals into a coherent moving percept. Pattern-motion selective neurons were distinguished by large receptive fields, suitable to perform spatial integration, and were mostly located in the medial part of the LP nucleus.

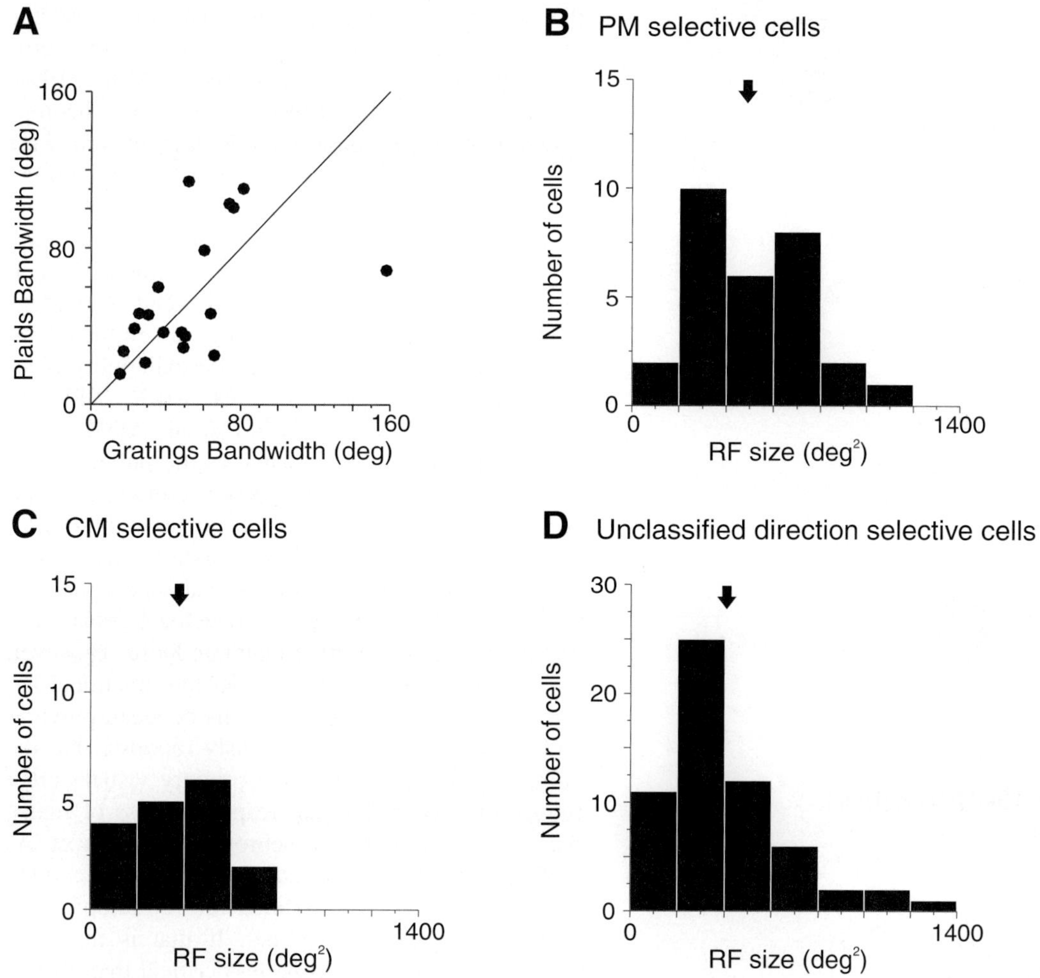

Fig. 6. (A) Relationship between the direction bandwidths of PM selective neurons computed from their responses to gratings and plaids. (B–D) Distribution of receptive field size for PM and CM selective, and direction unclassified LP-pulvinar cells. The arrows represent mean values.

Until now, this plaid-defined higher level neuronal operation was only reported in higher-order visual areas: PM responses were described in the primate area MT (Movshon et al., 1985) and subsequently in the cat's AEV cortex (Scannell et al., 1996), both regions being reciprocally connected to the pulvinar.

The presence of PM selectivity in the LP-pulvinar in anaesthetized cats provides evidence that the function of thalamic nuclei goes beyond the relaying of sensory information in relation to the state of vigilance. Moreover, the fact that thalamic neurons can perform complex neuronal operations [1] is of fundamental importance in the renewed effort by

[1] In support of this assumption, we recently reported that cells in the cat's LP-pulvinar can code the displacement of complex random dot kinematograms whose comprising elements do not signal locally the direction of motion (Dumbrava et al., 2001). Signaling the direction of motion of such patterns requires the integration of local motion signals over space and time. In addition, it appears that LGN cells may also respond to stimuli defined by second-order characteristics (Barraclough et al., 2000).

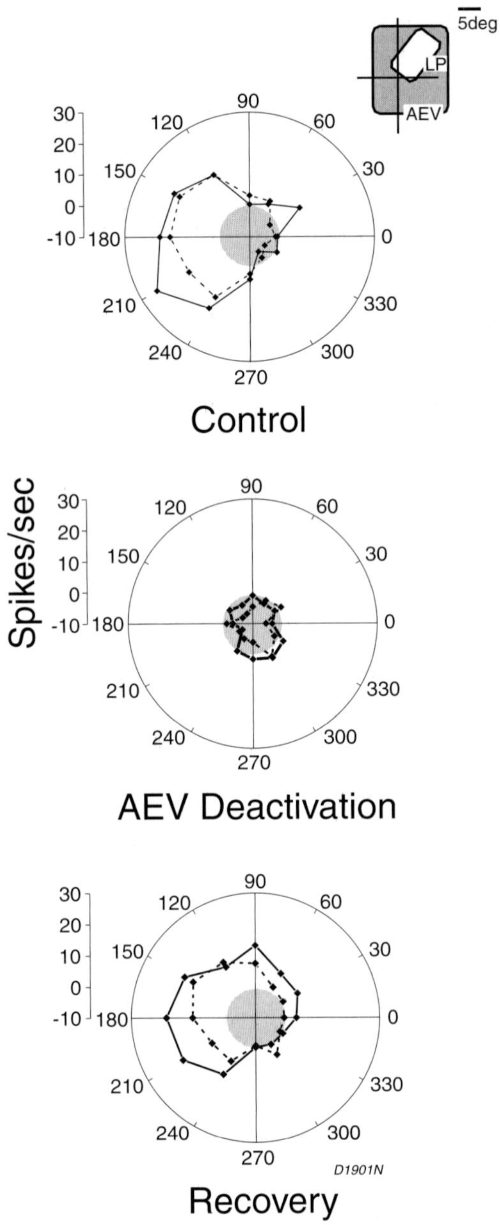

Fig. 7. Effect of deactivating the AEV cortex on a LP-pulvinar pattern motion selective neuron. During the deactivation, a robust suppression of the cell's response and a concomitant loss of its ability to signal the direction of the drifting grating (solid line) and plaid pattern (dashed line) were observed. In each polar graph, data points within the shaded region represent cell discharges below spontaneous activity levels. The inset shows the location of the thalamic neuron's RF in reference to the AEV scotoma. (Reproduced with permission from Merabet et al., 1998.)

theoreticians and neurophysiologists to assess the role of the thalamus and of cortico-thalamo-cortical loops in *specific* visual processing (Miller, 1996; Sherman and Guillery, 1996). For example, theoretical studies have proposed that the thalamus may act as an active blackboard where signals from cortical areas are compared and used to refine processing at higher levels (Mumford, 1991). To experimentally reveal such a function will not be simple since it has already proved remarkably difficult to demonstrate corticofugal effects on relay cells in the lateral geniculate nucleus even if cortico-thalamic projections outnumber retinal afferents (Koch, 1987, but see the experiments of Sillito et al., 1994). Second-order thalamic nuclei such as the pulvinar may represent a better model to study cortico-thalamo-cortical loops given that, in contrast to first-order nuclei (such as the lateral geniculate nucleus), they do not receive powerful subcortical inputs that can mask the subtler role of cortical feedback projections and corresponding cortico-thalamic loops. However, at this time, little is known about the functional nature of the reciprocal connections between pulvinar and cortical areas. We previously reported that the cooling or destruction of the primary visual cortex reduced the overall visual responsiveness of many, but not all, LP-pulvinar neurons (Casanova et al., 1997). These data suggest that the striate cortex may be necessary to establish the retinotopic map found in the cat LP-pulvinar. If that is the case, this cortical input would be less critical than that in primates because the removal of the primary visual cortex in the latter yielded a virtually total loss of visual responses in the pulvinar (Bender, 1983). We also studied the projections from the LP-pulvinar to the PMLS cortex because these afferents represent the main thalamic input to PMLS. Deactivating the LPl had little impact on spatial and temporal frequency tuning functions and on direction selectivity of PMLS neurons (Minville and Casanova, 1998). This lack of effect may indicate that the LPl projections are not used to drive most PMLS cells but are rather used for more subtle functions (including a modulatory action).

As previously mentioned, the pulvinar is in a unique position to either influence or inform multiple cortical areas about processing occurring in lower or higher level areas and/or to increase the

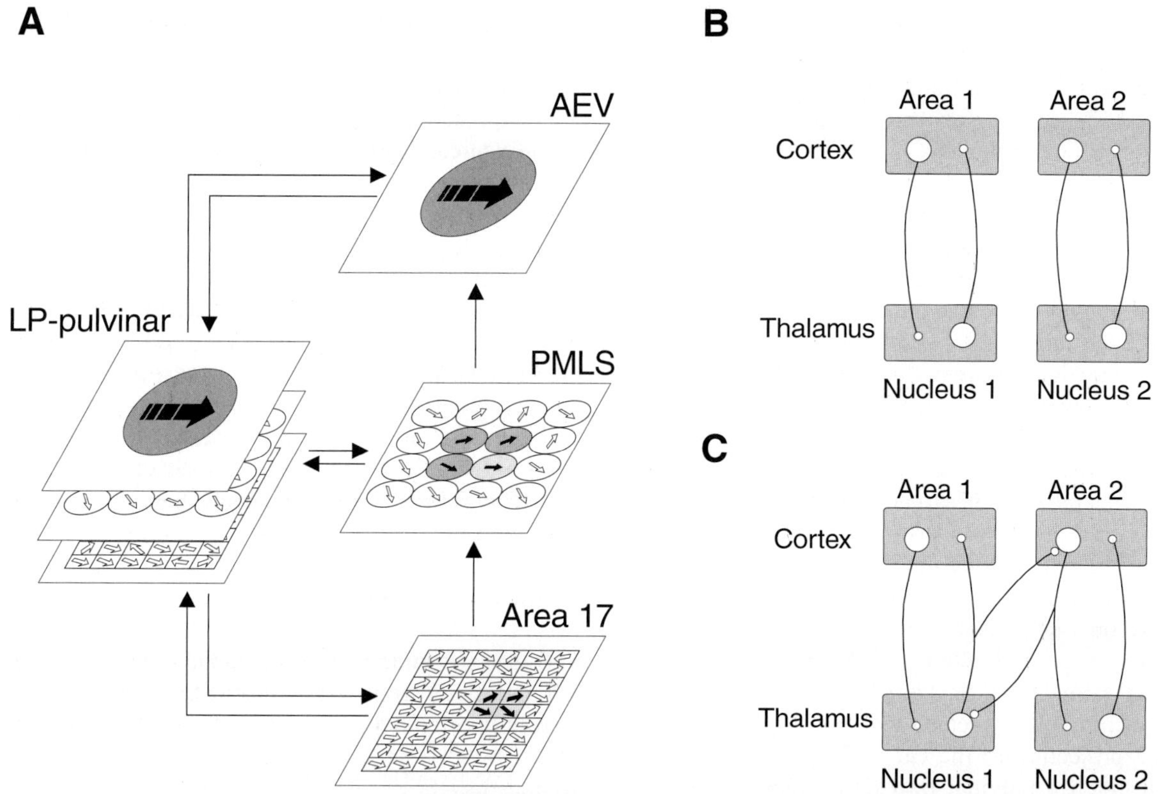

Fig. 8. A shows a hypothetical schematic for integration of motion signals based on the two-stage model proposed in primates (e.g. Nowlan and Sejnowski, 1995), now taking into consideration the LP-pulvinar complex. Local signals are processed in area 17, and then integrated at a second (that may be the PMLS, based on our most recent (unpublished) findings on complex motion sensitivity), and third cortical level. The pulvinar complex in cats is reciprocally connected with these three areas and contains all cell types that were characterized in cortical areas. One fundamental question is whether the projection cells are preferentially connected to neurons of similar properties (yielding specific cortico-thalamic loops that may be used to increase salience (B)) or if the projection neurons are also linked to cells having lower or higher-order motion properties (C). In the latter case, activity within a loop (e.g. PMLS-LPl) could be compared with incoming (e.g. area 17) and outgoing (e.g. AEV) signals, and modified accordingly.

effectiveness of the processing taking place in a given cortical area (Fig. 1). We proposed that the pulvinar may, through successive iterations within a given cortico-thalamo-cortical loop (e.g. involving the AEV cortex), help to refine the cortical image (e.g. segmentation from motion) or its saliency (Merabet et al., 1998). In this context, it is possible that extra-geniculate cortico-thalamo-cortical loops may represent basic computational modules involved in the analysis of specific features of complex visual scenes (Merabet et al., 1998; see also Grieve et al., 2000). In parallel or as an alternative, given its extensive reciprocal connections with virtually all visual cortical areas, the LP-pulvinar may provide an indirect route for cortico-cortical communication (Crick and Koch, 1998). Most importantly, it may also be a site where higher-order cortical information can be instantly compared, and redirected to refine computations taking place in given areas (Mumford, 1991). For instance, in our animal model, it is possible that the sensory maps in the AEV and PMLS cortex are used to establish a 'global' template in the LP-pulvinar. Through feedback loops, these maps could be dynamically used to compare the first, second, and third stages of motion processing for an image encoded at cortical levels with the information stored at the thalamic level (Merabet et al., 1998). Such organization could also be used to enhance stimulus saliency (Grieve et al., 2000). Fig. 8 illustrates the fact that the pulvinar may not only interact with a given cortical area through reciprocal connections, but may also inform higher-order cortical areas about incoming signals while notifying primary visual areas about higher-order analysis taking place further along the cortical pathways.

Paraphrasing Sillito and Jones (1997), we believe that pulvinar and cortical levels of visual processing cannot be easily separated: they form a circuit not a sequence. As such, the understanding of pulvinar function largely depends on our ability to clearly establish the functional significance of the bi-directional connections between this large extrageniculate nucleus and the visual cortex. To achieve this goal, the morphology, extent, and associated receptors of all major pulvino-cortical and cortico-pulvinar terminals, as well as their axonal branching, must first be determined using modern neuroanatomical techniques. This will, among other things, help to determine whether the nature of the action that a neuron can have on another is of a 'modulatory' or 'driving' type (Sherman and Guillery, 1998). Such studies in cats and primates (Vidnyánszky et al., 1996; Feig and Harting, 1998) revealed that layer V neurons in area 17 projecting to the cat's LP nucleus and the primate inferior pulvinar provide a functional drive for many thalamic cells, in accordance with electrophysiological observations (Bender, 1983; Casanova et al., 1997). Many questions need to be answered. For instance, are the cortico-thalamo-cortical loops independent from each other (Fig. 8B)? This seems unlikely given the complexity of the pulvinar connectivity described in cats and primates (Vidnyánszky et al., 1996; Rockland, 1996, 1998; Rockland et al., 1999). There is also evidence that cat LP cells can project to both the PMLS and the primary visual cortex (Miceli et al., 1991). Having a given LP-pulvinar neuron that projects to multiple areas via axon collaterals will not only permit computations along a given loop, but will also allow other cortical areas to be informed about the computations taking place along the loop, and by extension in the cortex connected to it. It thus becomes possible to compare first- and second-order processing (see Fig. 8A,C). In addition, the possibility that the subdivisions within the pulvinar (e.g. LPm, LPl, and pulvinar in cats) are linked by intrinsic connections cannot be ruled out. Another important task is obviously to determine whether neurons in two or more cortical areas can project to a single locus in a pulvinar subdivision.

To further reveal the role of the pulvinar and its reciprocal connections, first- and second-order receptive field properties of pulvino-cortical and cortico-pulvinar neurons must be determined in great detail. Our laboratory had previously characterized the properties of area 17 complex cells projecting to the LPl (Casanova, 1993); however, this study was completed before we knew that thalamic cells could perform higher-order computations and a re-evaluation of these properties might be necessary. Knowing the nature of the signals leaving the cortex to the thalamus and vice versa is a prerequisite for studying cortico-thalamo-cortical loops (e.g. by cross-correlation techniques) and for unveiling their function in normal vision.

Acknowledgements

MT-14825 from the CIHR of Canada to C.C. Part of C.C.'s salary was provided by FRSQ. L.M. and A.D. were supported in part by FCAR-FRSQ studentships.

References

Abramson, B.P. and Chalupa, L.M. (1985) The laminar distribution of cortical connections with the tecto- and cortico-recipient zones in the cat's lateral posterior nucleus. *Neuroscience*, 15: 81–95.

Abramson, B.P. and Chalupa, L.M. (1988) Multiple pathways from the superior colliculus to the extrageniculate visual thalamus of the cat. *J. Comp. Neurol.*, 271: 397–418.

Adelson, E.H. and Movshon, J.A. (1982) Phenomenal coherence of moving visual patterns. *Nature*, 300: 523–525.

Baker, C.L.J. (1999) Central neural mechanisms for detecting second-order motion. *Curr. Opin. Neurobiol.*, 9: 461–466.

Barraclough, N.E., Derrington, A.M. and Felisberti, F.M. (2000) Responses to second-order patterns in primate lateral geniculate nucleus. *Soc. Neurosci. Abstr.*, 26: 1196.

Bender, D.B. (1983) Visual activation of neurons in the primate pulvinar depends on cortex but not colliculus. *Brain Res.*, 279: 258–261.

Benedek, G., Norita, M. and Creutzfeldt, O.D. (1983) Electrophysiological and anatomical demonstration of an overlapping striate and tectal projection to the lateral posterior-pulvinar complex of the cat. *Exp. Brain Res.*, 52: 157–169.

Casanova, C. (1993) Response properties of neurons in area 17 projecting to the striate-recipient zone of the cat's lateralis posterior-pulvinar complex: comparison with cortico-tectal cells. *Exp. Brain Res.*, 96: 247–259.

Casanova, C. and Savard, T. (1996a) Responses to moving texture patterns of cells in the striate-recipient zone of the cat's lateral posterior-pulvinar complex. *Neuroscience*, 70: 439–447.

Casanova, C. and Savard, T. (1996b) Motion sensitivity and stimulus interactions in the striate-recipient zone of the cat's lateral posterior-pulvinar complex. *Prog. Brain Res.*, 112: 277–287.

Casanova, C., Freeman, R.D. and Nordmann, J.P. (1989) Monocular and binocular response properties of cells in the striate-recipient zone of the cat's lateral posterior-pulvinar complex. *J. Neurophysiol.*, 62: 544–557.

Casanova, C., Nordmann, J.P. and Molotchnikoff, S. (1991) Pulvinar-lateralis posterior nucleus complex of mammals and the visual function. *J. Physiol. (Paris)*, 85: 44–57.

Casanova, C., Savard, T. and Darveau, S. (1997) Contribution of area 17 to cell responses in the striate-recipient zone of the cat's lateral posterior-pulvinar complex. *Eur. J. Neurosci.*, 9: 1026–1036.

Chalupa, L.M. (1991) Vision function of the pulvinar. In: A.G. Leventhal (Ed.), *Vision and Visual Dysfunction. The Neural Basis of Visual Function*, Vol. 4, CRC Press, Boca Raton, FL, pp. 140–159.

Chalupa, L.M. and Abramson, B.P. (1988) Receptive-field properties in the tecto- and striate-recipient zones of the cat's lateral posterior nucleus. *Prog. Brain Res.*, 75: 85–94.

Chalupa, L.M. and Abramson, B.P. (1989) Visual receptive fields in the striate-recipient zone of the lateral posterior-pulvinar complex. *J. Neurosci.*, 1: 347–357.

Crick, F. and Koch, C. (1998) Constraints on cortical and thalamic projections: the no-strong-loops hypothesis. *Nature*, 391: 245–250.

Derrington, A.M. and Badcock, D.R. (1985) The low level motion system has both chromatic and luminance inputs. *Vision Res.*, 25: 1879–1884.

Dumbrava, D., Faubert, J. and Casanova, C. (2001) Global motion integration in the cat's lateral posterior-pulvinar complex. *Eur. J. Neurosci.*, in press.

Feig, S. and Harting, J.K. (1998) Corticocortical communication via the thalamus: ultrastructural studies of corticothalamic projections from area 17 to the lateral posterior nucleus of the cat and inferior pulvinar nucleus of the owl monkey. *J. Comp. Neurol.*, 395: 281–295.

Graybiel, A.M. and Berson, D.M. (1980) Histochemical identification and afferent connections of subdivisions in the lateralis posterior-pulvinar complex and related thalamic nuclei in the cat. *Neuroscience*, 5: 1175–1238.

Greenlee, M.W. and Smith, A.T. (1997) Detection and discrimination of first- and second-order motion in patients with unilateral brain damage. *J. Neurosci.*, 17: 804–818.

Grieve, K.L., Acuna, C. and Cudeiro, J. (2000) The primate pulvinar nuclei: vision and action. *Trends Neurosci.*, 23: 35–39.

Guillery, R.W. (1995) Anatomical evidence concerning the role of the thalamus in corticocortical communication: a brief review. *J. Anat.*, 187(Pt 3): 583–592.

Hutchins, B. and Updyke, B.V. (1989) Retinotopic organization within the lateral posterior complex of the cat. *J. Comp. Neurol.*, 285: 350–398.

Jones, E.G. (1985) *The Thalamus*, Plenum, New York.

Koch, C. (1987) The action of the corticofugal pathway on sensory thalamic nuclei: a hypothesis. *Neuroscience*, 23: 399–406.

Lomber, S.G., Cornwell, P., Sun, J.S., MacNeil, M.A. and Payne, B.R. (1994) Reversible inactivation of visual processing operations in middle suprasylvian cortex of the behaving cat. *Proc. Natl. Acad. Sci. USA*, 91: 2999–3003.

Macchi, G., Bentivoglio, M., Minciacchi, D. and Molinari, M. (1996) Trends in the anatomical organization and functional significance of the mammalian thalamus. *Ital. J. Neurol. Sci.*, 17: 105–129.

Mareschal, I. and Baker, C.L.J. (1998) Temporal and spatial response to second-order stimuli in cat area 18. *J. Neurophysiol.*, 80: 2811–2823.

Merabet, L., Desautels, A., Minville, K. and Casanova, C. (1998) Motion integration in a thalamic visual nucleus. *Nature*, 396: 265–268.

Merabet, L., Minville, K., Ptito, M. and Casanova, C. (2000) Responses of neurons in the cat posteromedial lateral suprasylvian cortex to moving texture patterns. *Neuroscience*, 97: 611–623.

Miceli, D., Reperant, J., Marchand, L., Ward, R. and Vesselkin, N. (1991) Divergence and collateral axon branching in subsystems of visual cortical projections from the cat lateral posterior nucleus. *J. Hirnforsch.*, 32: 165–173.

Miller, R. (1996) Cortico-thalamic interplay and the security of operation of neural assemblies and temporal chains in the cerebral cortex. *Biol. Cybern.*, 75: 263–275.

Miller, L.M. and Schreiner, C.E. (2000) Stimulus-based state control in the thalamocortical system. *J. Neurosci.*, 20: 7011–7016.

Minville, K. and Casanova, C. (1998) Spatial frequency processing in posteromedial lateral suprasylvian cortex does not depend on the projections from the striate-recipient zone of the cat's lateral posterior-pulvinar complex. *Neuroscience*, 84: 699–711.

Movshon, J.A., Adelson, E.H., Gizzi, M.S. and Newsome, W.T. (1985) The analysis of moving visual patterns. *Pont. Acad. Sci. Varia.*, 54: 117–151.

Movshon, J.A., Adelson, E.H., Gizzi, M.S. and Newsome, W.T. (1986) The analysis of moving visual patterns. In: *Pattern Recognition Mechanisms*, New York, pp. 148–164.

Mucke, L., Norita, M., Benedek, G. and Creutzfeldt, O. (1982) Physiologic and anatomic investigation of a visual cortical area situated in the ventral bank of the anterior ectosylvian sulcus of the cat. *Exp. Brain Res.*, 46: 1–11.

Mumford, D. (1991) On the computational architecture of the neocortex. I. The role of the thalamo-cortical loop. *Biol. Cybern.*, 65: 135–145.

Newsome, W.T., Mikami, A. and Wurtz, R.H. (1986) Motion selectivity in macaque visual cortex. III. Psychophysics and physiology of apparent motion. *J. Neurophysiol.*, 55: 1340–1351.

Norita, M., Mucke, L., Benedek, G., Albowitz, B., Katoh, Y. and Creutzfeldt, O.D. (1986) Connections of the anterior ectosylvian visual area (AEV). *Exp. Brain Res.*, 62: 225–240.

Nowlan, S.J. and Sejnowski, T.J. (1995) A selection model for motion processing in area MT of primates. *J. Neurosci.*, 15: 1195–1214.

Olson, C.R. and Graybiel, A.M. (1987) Ectosylvian visual area of the cat: location, retinotopic organization, and connections. *J. Comp. Neurol.*, 261: 277–294.

Palmer, L.A., Rosenquist, A.C. and Tusa, R.J. (1978) The retinotopic organization of lateral suprasylvian visual areas in the cat. *J. Comp. Neurol.*, 177: 237–256.

Pasternak, T., Horn, K.M. and Maunsell, J.H. (1989) Deficits in speed discrimination following lesions of the lateral suprasylvian cortex in the cat. *Vis. Neurosci.*, 3: 365–375.

Petersen, S.E., Robinson, D.L. and Keys, W. (1985) Pulvinar nuclei of the behaving rhesus monkey: visual responses and their modulation. *J. Neurophysiol.*, 54: 867–886.

Raczkowski, D. and Rosenquist, A.C. (1983) Connections of the multiple visual cortical areas with the lateral posterior-pulvinar complex and adjacent thalamic nuclei in the cat. *J. Neurosci.*, 3: 1912–1942.

Robinson, D.L. and Cowie, R.J. (1997) The primate pulvinar: structural, functional, and behavioral components of visual salience. In: M. Steriade, E.G. Jones and D.A. McCormick (Eds.), *Thalamus*, Vol. 2, Elsevier Science, Oxford, pp. 53–92.

Robinson, D.L. and Petersen, S.E. (1992) The pulvinar and visual salience. *Trends Neurosci.*, 15: 127–132.

Rockland, K.S. (1996) Two types of corticopulvinar terminations: round (type 2) and elongate (type 1). *J. Comp. Neurol.*, 368: 57–87.

Rockland, K.S. (1998) Convergence and branching patterns of round, type 2 corticopulvinar axons. *J. Comp. Neurol.*, 390: 515–536.

Rockland, K.S., Andresen, J., Cowie, R.J. and Robinson, D.L. (1999) Single axon analysis of pulvinocortical connections to several visual areas in the macaque. *J. Comp. Neurol.*, 406: 221–250.

Rodman, H.R. and Albright, T.D. (1989) Single-unit analysis of pattern-motion selective properties in the middle temporal visual area (MT). *Exp. Brain Res.*, 75: 53–64.

Rudolph, K.K. and Pasternak, T. (1996) Lesions in cat lateral suprasylvian cortex affect the perception of complex motion. *Cereb. Cortex*, 6: 814–822.

Scannell, J.W., Sengpiel, F., Tovee, M.J., Benson, P.J., Blakemore, C. and Young, M.P. (1996) Visual motion processing in the anterior ectosylvian sulcus of the cat. *J. Neurophysiol.*, 76: 895–907.

Scannell, J.W., Burns, J.A.P.C., O'Neill, M.A., Hilgetag, C.C. and Young, M.P. (1997) The organisation of the thalamo-cortical network of the cat. *Soc. Neurosci. Abstr.*, 23: 1306.

Scannell, J.W., Burns, G.A., Hilgetag, C.C., O'Neil, M.A. and Young, M.P. (1999) The connectional organization of the cortico-thalamic system of the cat. *Cereb. Cortex*, 9: 277–299.

Sherman, S.M. (2001) Thalamic relay functions. In: C. Casanova and M. Ptito (Eds.), *Vision: From Neurons to Cognition. Progress in Brain Research*, Vol. 134. Elsevier, Amsterdam, pp. 51–69.

Sherman, S.M. and Guillery, R.W. (1996) Functional organization of thalamocortical relays. *J. Neurophysiol.*, 76: 1367–1395.

Sherman, S.M. and Guillery, R.W. (1998) On the actions that one nerve cell can have on another: Distinguishing 'drivers' from 'modulators'. *Proc. Natl. Acad. Sci. USA*, 95: 7121–7126.

Sillito, A. and Jones, H.E. (1997) Functional organization influencing neurotransmission in the lateral geniculate nucleus. In: *Thalamus*, Vol. II. *Experimental and Clinical Aspects*, Elsevier Science, Oxford.

Sillito, A.M., Jones, H.E., Gerstein, G.L. and West, D.C. (1994) Feature-linked synchronization of thalamic relay cell firing induced by feedback from the visual cortex. *Nature*, 369: 479–482.

Spear, P.D. (1991) Functions of extrastriate visual cortex in non-primate species. In: A.G. Leventhal (Ed.), *Vision and Visual Dysfunctions. The Neural Basis of Visual Function*, Vol. 4. CRC Press, Boca Raton, FL, pp. 339–370.

Stoner, G.R. and Albright, T.D. (1992) Neural correlates of perceptual motion coherence. *Nature*, 358: 412–414.

Updyke, B.V. (1981) Projections from visual areas of the middle suprasylvian sulcus onto the lateral posterior complex and adjacent thalamic nuclei in cat. *J. Comp. Neurol.*, 201: 477–506.

Updyke, B.V. (1983) A reevaluation of the functional organization and cytoarchitecture of the feline lateral posterior complex, with observations on adjoining cell groups. *J. Comp. Neurol.*, 219: 143–181.

Vaina, L.M. and Cowey, A. (1996) Impairment of the perception of second order motion but not first order motion in a patient with unilateral focal brain damage. *Proc. R. Soc. Lond. B. Biol. Sci.*, 263: 1225–1232.

Vidnyánszky, Z., Borostyankoi, Z., Gorcs, T.J. and Hamori, J. (1996) Light and electron microscopic analysis of synaptic input from cortical area 17 to the lateral posterior nucleus in cats. *Exp. Brain Res.*, 109: 63–70.

Zhou, Y.X. and Baker Jr., C.L. (1993) A processing stream in mammalian visual cortex neurons for non-Fourier responses. *Science*, 261: 98–101.

C. Casanova and M. Ptito (Eds.)
Progress in Brain Research, Vol. 134

CHAPTER 6

Response properties in the pulvinar complex after neonatal ablation of the primary visual cortex

Alex Desautels and Christian Casanova *

Laboratoire des Neurosciences de la Vision, École d'Optométrie, Université de Montréal, Montréal, PQ, Canada

Abstract: Injuries to specific areas of the brain (such as cerebrovascular accidents or surgical procedures) and particularly to the primary visual cortex, yield profound visual defects. The level of spared visual functions or *residual vision* [1] depends on the extent and location of the lesion as well as the age at which the trauma occurs. For instance, in primate as well as non-primate species, it is well established that lesions in adulthood have a more profound effect than those occurring in young animals. The recovery of visually guided behavior observed after massive destruction of the occipital cortex in young animals across many species has been generally associated with the reorganization of the pathways from the extrageniculate thalamus to the spared visual cortex, i.e. the extrastriate areas. In this chapter, we present some evidence that the lateral posterior-pulvinar (LP-pulvinar) complex may contribute to maintaining visual capacities in brain-damaged cats. Our data indicate that the overall visual responsiveness of the lateral part of the LP (LPl) cells is not altered by the early removal of the visual cortex. However, some specific properties differ from those of intact animals: on average, LPl neurons in brain-damaged animals are more broadly tuned for orientation than that in intact cats. Spatial frequency tuning functions are also affected since most units in lesioned animals are of the low-pass type. Moreover, most LPl cells of lesioned cats responded to drifting gratings with modulated discharges and a linear spatial summation within their receptive field, a characteristic that is infrequently observed in intact animals. The change in LPl response properties observed in the present study is likely to come from the reorganization of cortical and retinal fibers reaching this extrageniculate nucleus.

Introduction

The partial or total destruction of the primary visual cortex yields, both in cats and primates, a reduction or even a loss of visual capacities whose severity depends on the age of the animal, the extent of the lesion, and the nature of the experimental test used (Blythe et al., 1986; Cornwell and Payne, 1989; Fendrich et al., 1992; Schupert et al., 1993; Greenlee et al., 1995; Moore et al., 1995; Pasternak et al., 1995). The visual deficit is generally more pronounced when the lesions occur in adulthood rather then in young developing animals (Mitchell, 1990; Schupert et al., 1993; Lomber et al., 1995). The residual visual functions of the brain-damaged animals may be related to the persistence and activation of the retino-collicular and/or the extrageniculate pathways (Schupert et al., 1993; Williams et al., 1995). In the adult cat, the ablation of area 17 in conjunction with areas 18 and 19 provokes an important deficit in single or multiple form discrimination tasks (Pasternak et al., 1989, 1995; Schupert et al., 1993) and in stereoperception (Ptito and Lepore, 1983; Ptito et al., 1992; Schupert et al., 1993). These behavioral deficits are much more dramatic when

* Corresponding author: C. Casanova, Laboratoire des Neurosciences de la Vision, École d'Optométrie, Université de Montréal, C.P. 6128, Succ. Centre-Ville, Montréal, PQ, H3C 3J7 Canada. Tel.: +1-514-343-2407; Fax: +1-514-343-2382;
E-mail: christian.casanova@umontreal.ca

[1] In this text, the term residual vision is used in a general sense and defines the residual visual capacities observed after damage of one or several visual structures (see Weiskrantz et al., 1995; Payne et al., 1996, for details).

the ablation is not restricted to the primary visual cortex but also includes the lateral suprasylvian (LS) cortex (Spear, 1988; Livingston, 1990; Spear, 1991; Schupert et al., 1993), suggesting that the LS cortex is necessary to preserve visual capacities, albeit reduced, in an animal sustaining occipital brain damage at adulthood.

A different picture emerges when cerebral lesions are induced during the course of development, i.e. in neonates and young animals. Indeed, these animals exhibit, when subjected as adult animals to identical discrimination and orientation tests, a visually guided behavior often described as *quasi-normal* or, at least, significantly better than that observed in cats which sustained cortical ablation during adulthood (Spear, 1979; Schupert et al., 1993). Again, the LS cortex, and particularly the postero-medial part of the LS (PMLS) cortex, would be essential to preserve visual functions in these animals. Two observations support this hypothesis. First, the receptive field properties of PMLS neurons in animals sustaining early visual cortex damage (first postnatal month) are virtually identical to those characterized in intact animals (Spear et al., 1980; Guido et al., 1990). Second, when neonatal lesions extend beyond the primary visual cortex to include the LS cortex, there is no functional recovery and the animal displays substantial visual deficits (Schupert et al., 1993). It is thus likely that the sparing of visual integrity of cells in PMLS cortex in an animal sustaining early cortical ablations results from the reorganization of the sub-cortical pathways that generally include the LP-pulvinar complex. Labeling techniques have indeed shown that there is an expansion of the retino-pulvinar projections (type ε or W cells) at the level of the ipsilateral hemisphere (Labar et al., 1981). The apparition of a novel projection (bilateral) from the retina to the LPl was reported (Payne et al., 1993, but see Discussion). In addition, neuroanatomical studies (Kato et al., 1993; Lomber et al., 1995) have shown that there is a change at the level of the thalamo-PMLS projections: in addition to a degeneration of the geniculate layers A–A1, one observed: (1) an expansion of the projections of the medial part of the LP (by a factor of 2) to the LS cortex, especially when the lesion is incurred at PND 1–7; (2) an expansion of the projections of layer C (by a factor of 3), particularly when the lesion was carried out at PND 21–28; (3) the apparition of a *new* direct pathway from layers A–A1 towards the PMLS was observed. Finally, there is an expansion of the projections of the PMLS towards the stratum griseum superficiale of the superior colliculus (Sun et al., 1994). These compensatory mechanisms do not manifest themselves in the adult lesioned animal (Tong et al., 1984; Cornwell and Payne, 1989). On the basis of these neuroanatomical observations, it may be suggested that the LP-pulvinar, through its extensive reciprocal connections with sub-cortical and cortical areas, contributes to maintaining neuronal properties in extrastriate cortices and visual capacities in animals sustaining early ablation of the visual cortex (Spear et al., 1980; Cornwell and Payne, 1989; Guido et al., 1992; Schupert et al., 1993). This study will show that the receptive field properties of neurons in the LPl of 'chronic' brain-damaged animals are, to some extent, consistent with this last assumption.

General methods

Subjects

Ten kittens, from seven different litters sustained unilateral ($n = 8$) or bilateral ($n = 2$) lesions of the primary visual cortex. The age at which the lesion occurred varied from 7 to 30 postnatal days (Table 1). Kittens were born in the Université de Sherbrooke breeding colony and remained with their mother until they were weaned. Eleven additional normal adult cats served as controls.

Recording procedures

Recording sessions were performed when the animals reached adulthood (2.5–3.5 kg). The anesthesia and surgical procedures are described in detail in our previous papers (e.g. Casanova et al., 1997). All animals were treated in accordance with the guidelines of the Canadian Council on Animal Care. Extracellular single-unit recordings were made in the LP-pulvinar complex ipsilateral to the cortical lesion. General properties of LP-pulvinar neurons were assessed using manually controlled stimuli projected on a translucent screen facing the animal. For quantitative analysis, this tangent screen was

TABLE 1

Experimental subjects that sustained chronic ablation of the primary visual cortex at an early age

Animal	Age at ablation (days)	Age at recording (months)	Extent of the cortical lesion
X2801	25	35	17–(18)–(19)
X1702	30	19	17–(18)–(19)
X0403	30	20	17
X2503	22	23	17–(18)
X1205	22	25	LH: 17–(18) RH: 17
X1606	11	25	LH: 17 RH: 17
X1111	30	28	17–(18)–(19)
X0912	7	30	17–18–(19)
W0701	7	31	17
D2601	21	34	17

Numbers in brackets indicate a partial lesion. LH, left hemisphere; RH, right hemisphere.

replaced with a cathode ray tube (CRT, Datacheck 5117; mean luminance of 14 cd/m^2) displaying full-screen sinusoidal drifting gratings at 50% contrast. Orientation was varied over 360º in 12 steps of 30º. The cell's direction selectivity was determined and quantified as follows: Direction index (DI) = 1 − (response in the non-preferred direction/response in the preferred direction). Cells with DI > 0.5 were regarded as selective to the direction of the stimulus motion. Cell responses at optimal orientation were also studied as a function of spatial and temporal frequencies and of grating contrast. Each neuron was classified on the basis of the unit's modulation index (MI) derived from its response to drifting sine-wave gratings (Skottun et al., 1991). The MI was calculated by dividing the response at the first harmonic (a.c. component) by the mean firing rate (d.c. component) from which the spontaneous level was subtracted. Responses of LP-pulvinar units were also classified on the basis of spatial summation linearity or non-linearity (phase sensitivity) using counter-phased sine-wave gratings. Cells with linear spatial summation (LSS) are characterized by the presence of a phase position in their RF at which the cell ceases to respond (a null position). Cells with non-linear spatial summation (NLSS) have no null position, but rather, show a temporal distortion at all spatial-phase positions (Enroth-Cugell and Robson, 1966). The maximum of the 2nd/1st harmonic ratio was taken as an index of non-linearity (Hochstein and Shapley, 1976).

Cortical lesions

Visual cortex lesions were performed under deep anesthesia and sterile conditions. The scalp was incised, the muscles were retracted and a craniotomy was performed. The dura was incised, the blood vessels were cauterized and the visual cortex was ablated by aspiration as described in Merabet et al. (1998). When the ablation was completed, the cranial cavity was filled with sterile gelatin sponge. The excised bone segment and retracted muscle fascia were then replaced and the wound was sutured. Kittens were maintained under observation until they recovered from anesthesia and could then be returned with their mother. Animals received a postoperative antibiotic (Trimethoprime and sulfadiazine: Tribrissen® 24%, 15 mg/kg s.c. b.i.d.) and analgesic (Buprenorphine: Temgesic®, 0.005 mg/kg s.c. b.i.d.) treatment for 5 and 3 days, respectively. None of the animals exhibited abnormal visual behavior based on observations by the experimenters and the animal facilities staff, including the veterinarian.

Ablation assessment

The extent of the cortical lesion was initially assessed during the surgical procedure, and later by direct inspection of the adult brain, and in photographs taken from three different plans (dorsal, postero-median, dorso-posterior). The ablated area was then charted onto a gross drawing of the cat cerebral cortex (Reinoso-Suarez, 1961). The location and size of the lesion were also determined by examining serial frozen coronal sections through the cortex (Otsuka and Hassler, 1962; Sanides and Hoffmann, 1969). The *minimum* ablated area was then plotted using the visual field maps of Tusa et al. (1978, 1979) to estimate the extent of the visual-field representation that was removed. Subsequently, the boundaries of the dLGN and medial interlaminar nucleus (MIN) were determined using a computer-assisted microscopy system, and the degree of retrograde degeneration was plotted onto visuotopic maps of the dLGN (Sanderson, 1971).

Extent of the lesions

Lesion reconstruction shows that the anterior posterolateral gyrus and part of the splenial gyrus on the medial wall of the hemisphere were removed. In a few brains, some sparing occurred. The most frequent location of spared tissue was the caudal pole of the posterolateral gyrus and the upper part of the splenial sulcus. The pattern of retrograde degeneration of the dLGN and MIN, as well as comparison of the lesions with the visuotopic maps of Tusa et al. (1978) indicate that in all cases, damage to area 17 included the cortical representation of the central visual field.

Results

General observations

A total of 234 neurons were recorded in the striate-recipient zone of the LP-pulvinar of lesioned animals and 82 of those exhibited clear visual responses to drifting gratings. The proportion of visual cells was similar to that observed in the control group (55 out of 153 cells). These proportions should not be considered as representative values of the absolute number of visual cells in the LPl since, in both groups, we deliberately quantified only the units showing robust and reliable visual responses to sine-wave gratings (no other stimuli such as bars and noise were used). The mean spatial location for the characterized cells was $-15.2 \pm 9.7°$ to $19.8 \pm 9.6°$ for azimuth, and $-13.8 \pm 7.9°$ to $25.4 \pm 7.7°$ for elevation. It was not more difficult than usual to find and characterize cells in the LPl of the animals that sustained early ablation of the visual cortex. In fact, their optimal visual discharge rate tended to be greater than that of normal cats, but this difference was not statistically significant (mean of 28.9 ± 28 and 33.4 ± 22.8 spikes/s for intact and lesioned animals, respectively. Mann–Whitney, $P = 0.053$). The same observation stands for the spontaneous discharge level (mean of 7.7 ± 8.3 and 11.7 ± 14.6 spikes/s for intact and lesioned animals, respectively. Mann–Whitney, $P = 0.09$). In general, receptive fields in lesioned animals could be mapped with confidence and their size and eccentricity were not different from those studied in normal cats (Mann–Whitney, $P = 0.433$ and $P = 0.117$, respectively). We did not investigate the possibility that the visuotopic organization of the LP nucleus was altered by the early removal of the visual cortex. The visual map in the LP is complex and repeated systematic successful recordings are necessary to clearly unveil its retinotopic organization (Hutchins and Updyke, 1989). However, no obvious differences were noted by the experimenters between the two groups regarding the progression of the receptive field location as the electrode descended in the LP nucleus. Finally, no difference was observed between the distribution of LPl cells ocular dominance in intact and lesioned animals ($\chi^2 = 1.7$, $P = 0.4$).

Orientation and direction selectivity

The majority of the LPl cells studied were selective for the orientation of the drifting grating. An example is shown in Fig. 1A. The cell responded optimally to stimulus orientations of 30–60° with a bandwidth of 44°. The distribution of orientation tuning widths for all cells in both animal groups is presented in Fig. 1B. Clearly, the overall selectivity for orientation of LPl cells in lesioned animals was decreased as their mean tuning function was broader than that in normal cats ($64.2 \pm 38.6°$ and $41.9 \pm 21°$, respectively; Mann–Whitney, $P = 0.002$). For a number of cells, the orientation selectivity was only apparent when one considered the cell discharges at the first (1 and 11 in intact and lesioned animals, respectively) or second harmonic (2 and 7 in intact and lesioned cats) of the drifting grating. This cell behavior was previously reported in normal animals by Casanova et al. (1989) and was attributed to converging cortical inputs. The proportion of direction selective cells in lesioned animals was not significantly different from that of intact cats ($\chi^2 = 2.13$, $P = 0.14$) despite the fact that we observed a difference in the distribution of direction selective units between the two groups (t-test; $P = 0.036$, see Fig. 1C).

Spatial and temporal frequency processing

Removal of the primary visual cortex in kittens yielded a change in the response profile of LPl cells as a function of stimulus spatial frequency. In lesioned animals, most units (70.5%) exhibited a low-pass tuning function (Fig. 2A); this proportion is

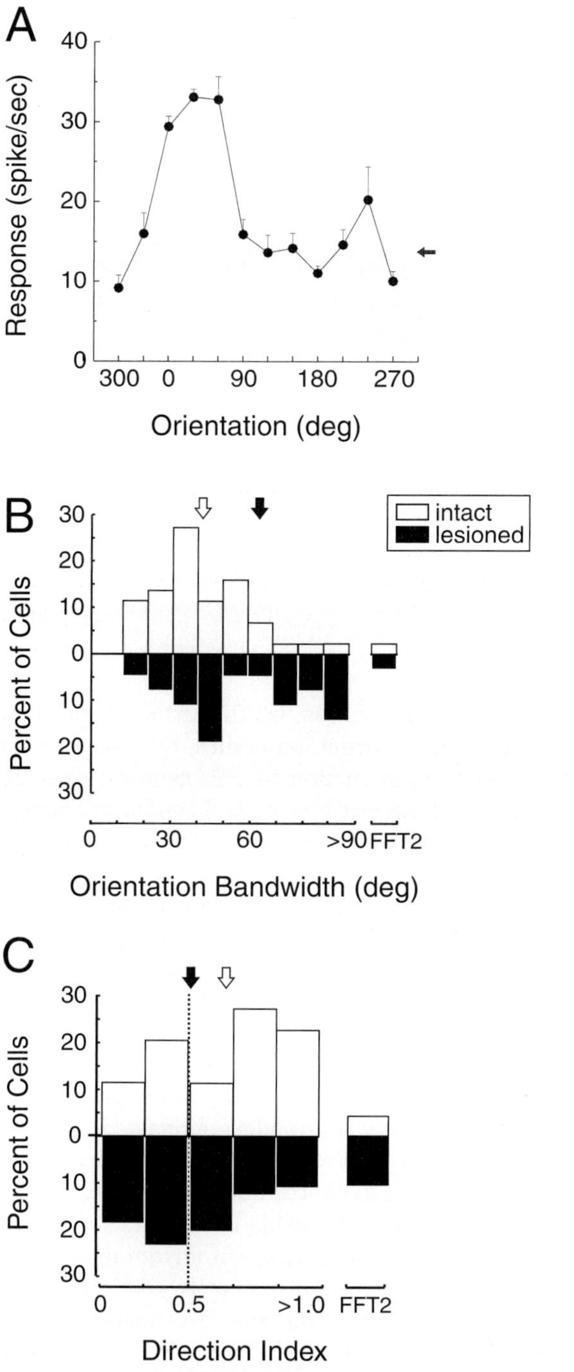

Fig. 1. Orientation and direction selectivity. (A) Orientation tuning curve for one LPl cell recorded in a lesioned cat. Arrow on the right indicates the spontaneous discharge rate of the cell. Distribution of the orientation tuning widths (B) and direction index (C) for lesioned and intact animals. In B and C, arrows indicate mean values.

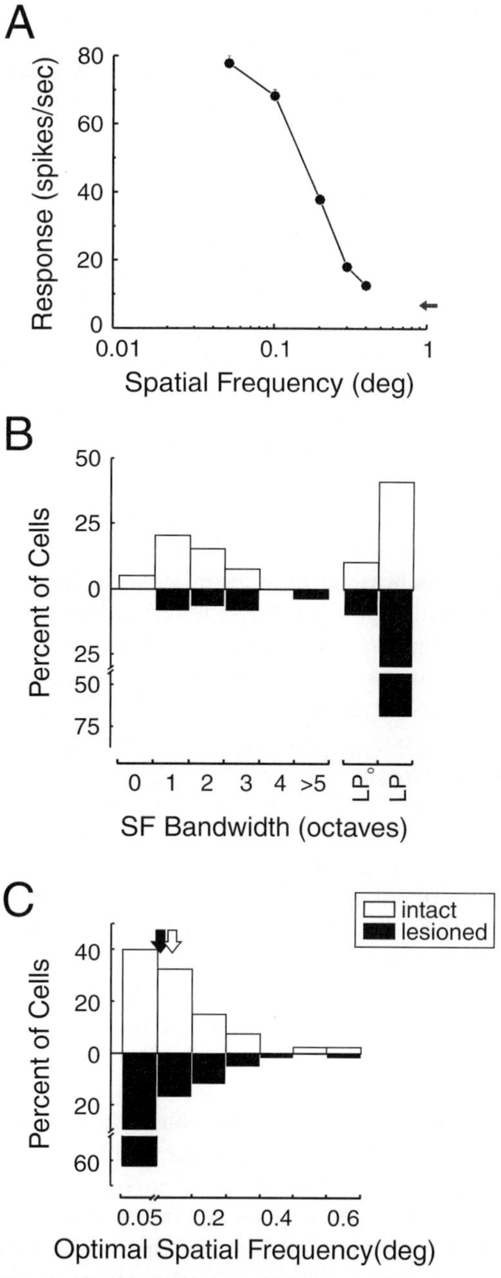

Fig. 2. Spatial frequency sensitivity. (A) Example of spatial frequency response functions for LPl neurons in the lesioned cat (PND = 25). Spontaneous discharge rate is represented by the arrow on the right. Distribution of bandwidth of spatial turning curves (B) and preferred spatial frequencies (C) for both groups, lesioned and intact animals. LP, cells that displayed low pass response profiles; LP_o, neurons that showed low-pass response profiles with an optimal spatial frequency higher than 0.05 c/deg. In C, arrows indicate the mean spatial frequency for each group.

greater than that observed in intact animals (47.6%). This difference is illustrated in Fig. 2B showing LPl neuron spatial frequency bandwidth distributions recorded in normal and lesioned animal groups ($\chi^2 = 5.4$, $P = 0.02$). In the two groups, almost all units preferred spatial frequencies less than 0.5 c/deg (Fig. 2C). Statistical comparison of the optimal frequency in the two cat populations revealed that a greater proportion of cells in lesioned animals responded to the lowest frequency used in the study (i.e. 0.05 c/deg; $\chi^2 = 0.03$), in agreement with the finding that more units in lesioned cats showed a low-pass tuning function. Despite these differences, there was no significant change in the neurons' spatial resolution and an identical mean higher cut-off was computed in both groups (0.53 c/deg).

The temporal frequency characteristics of 55 LPl neurons in operated and 37 in intact animals were studied. There was no difference between the two groups with respect to the cells' preferred frequency (Mann–Whitney, $P = 0.28$), bandwidth (t-test, $P = 0.587$) as well as their mean temporal frequency high-cut off (t-test, $P = 0.517$).

Modulation index

As expected from previous findings (Casanova et al., 1989), the majority of cells (80%) in the LPl of intact cats did not exhibit a strong modulation of their discharges to drifting gratings, a behavior that goes along with the organization of the receptive field (overlapping On and Off sub-regions). A different picture emerged in lesioned animals: almost half of the LPl cells responded to drifting gratings with modulated discharges. The level of modulation of each neuron was quantified by computing a modulation index (MI, see Methods). The distribution of the MIs for both groups is shown in Fig. 3. One may clearly see that a substantial number of cells in lesioned animals have a MI greater than 1, i.e. that these cells showed a clear response modulation. The proportion of these cells in lesioned animals outnumbers that in intact cats ($\chi^2 = 10.32$, $P = 0.001$).

Linear spatial summation

Given the possible change in the receptive field organization revealed by the modification in the level

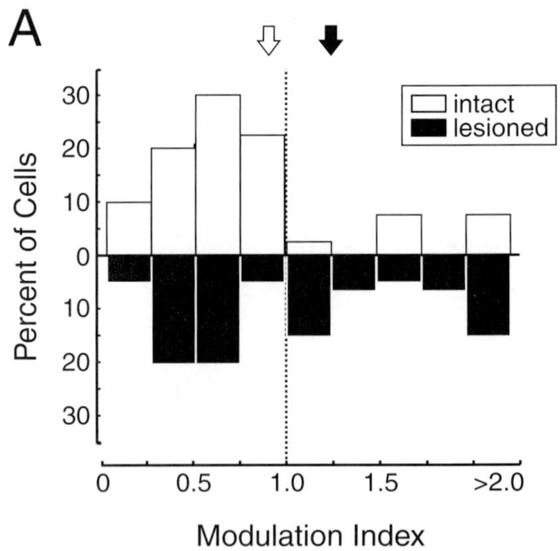

Fig. 3. Distribution of the modulation index of LPl neurons for intact cats compared to lesioned animals. An index >1 (dotted line) indicates that the cell's discharge is clearly modulated. Arrows indicate the mean MI value for each group.

of discharge modulation, we further investigated the receptive field spatial properties by studying the linear spatial summation of LPl neurons. Two examples of phase sensitive cells recorded in lesioned animal are presented in Fig. 4. Varying the grating spatial phase in intact animals revealed, by direct observation of the tuning curves, that 35% of the units ($n = 20$) exhibited a clear null position, while 40% did not show this behavior (Fig. 5A). The remaining 25% of units did not respond to counter-phased gratings. We quantified the phase sensitivity by computing a non-linearity index (see methods). Examination of the distribution presented in Fig. 5B shows that, in intact animals, 33% of the units were characterized by an index greater than 1, i.e. they did not exhibit a linear spatial summation within their receptive field. Different results were obtained in lesioned animals. In this group, approximately three-quarters of the cells (71%; $n = 45$) exhibited a null position (Fig. 5A) and a non-linearity index inferior to 1 (Fig. 5B). The proportion of phase-sensitive units and cells that present a non-linearity index inferior to 1 is significantly different in the two groups (Fisher, $P = 0.013$; Fisher, $P = 0.025$, respectively), indicating that most receptive fields of LPl neurons in the lesioned

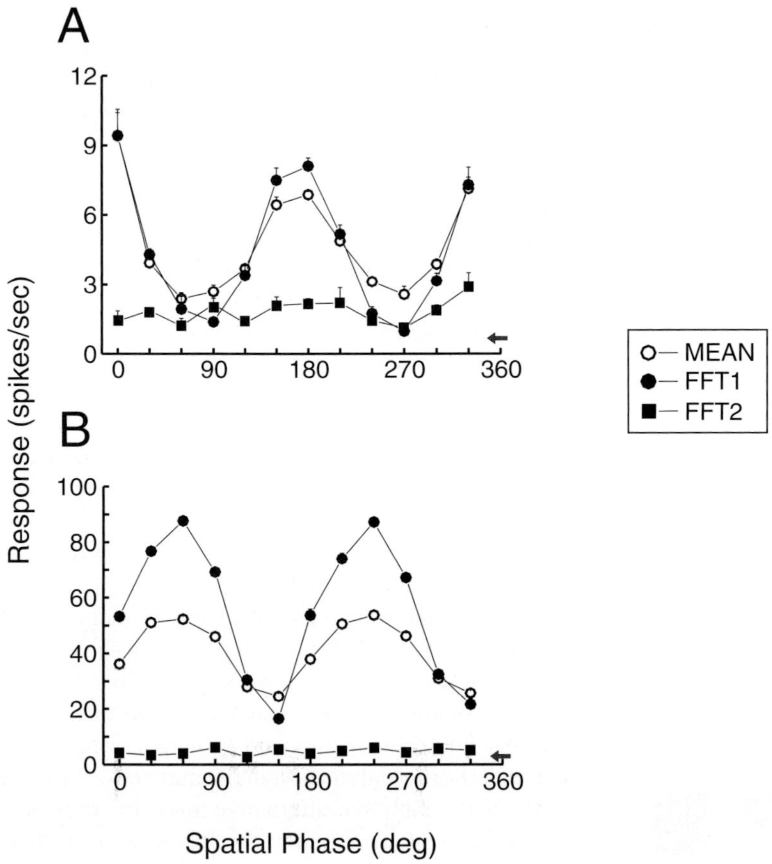

Fig. 4. Average discharge rate (mean) and the responses at the 1st and 2nd harmonics (FFT1, FFT2) as a function of orientation for two LP-pulvinar cells in lesioned cats. Note that cells exhibit linear spatial summation. Spontaneous activity is indicated by an arrow.

group are characterized by a linear spatial summation.

Long-lasting visual responses

Three units recorded in the lesion group behaved in an unusual manner. These cells exhibited very long-lasting discharges initiated by short duration visual stimuli. An example is shown in Fig. 6. In the absence of external stimulation, the LPl neuron was not spontaneously active. After the appearance of a brief visual stimulus within the receptive field, one can clearly see an increase in the discharge rate that lasted 182 s before decreasing progressively. While the number of cells behaving that way was rather small, their presence may be of significant importance since we never recorded from such neurons in intact animals. Similar cells have been previously reported in normal animals by Bender (1982) and Chalupa and Fish (1978). It has been proposed that such cellular activity is likely to be associated with short-term mnemonic processing (Chalupa, 1991). In the context of this study, the presence of this singular pattern of responses may be reminiscent of the destruction of a major cortical input and may represent a compensatory mechanism to reinforce the functional connectivity between the LP-pulvinar and the spared extrastriate visual cortical areas.

Discussion

The first conclusion of the present study is that the overall visual responsiveness of cat LPl neurons that sustained the ablation of the primary visual cortex

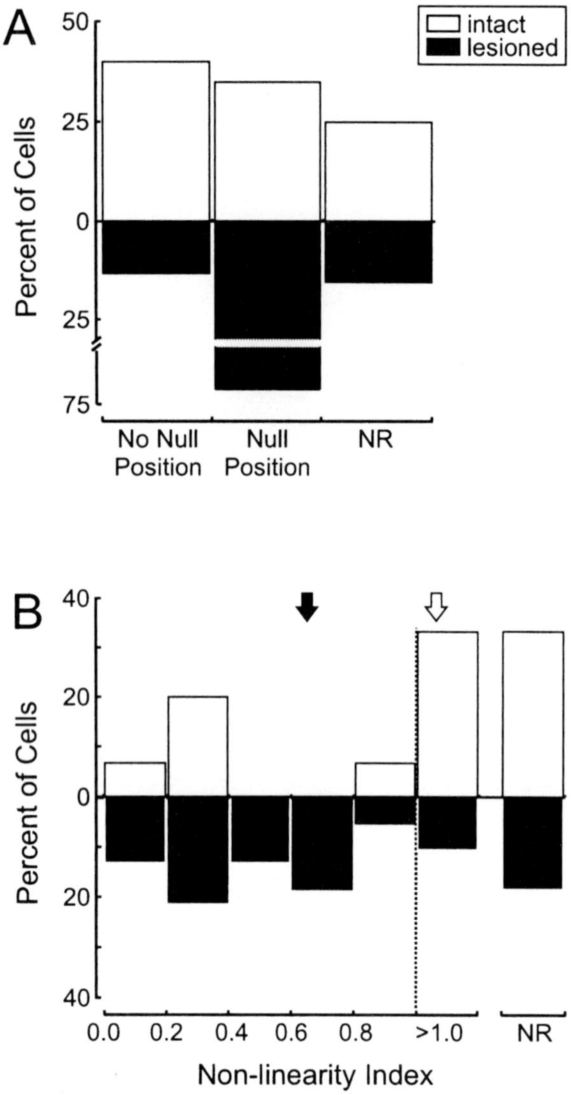

Fig. 5. Linear spatial summation. Quantitative evaluation of the phase sensitivity (A) and non-linearity index (B) for intact and operated animals. In B, cells with a non-linearity index >1 (dotted line) exhibit linear spatial summation within their receptive field. Arrows indicate the mean non-linearity index for each group. NR, cells that failed to respond to the counter-phased grating at any spatial location.

during the first postnatal month is comparable to that of intact animals: a similar number of cells could be driven by drifting gratings and the optimal responses were as robust. Given that the acute ablation of area 17 in the adult reduces the number of visual cells, as well as the responsiveness of the remaining visual LPl units (Casanova et al., 1997), it is likely that the maintained activity in LPl of early lesioned animals comes from the reorganization of its afferent and efferent connections. It has been shown that the destruction of the primary visual areas in kittens yielded an increase in the projections from the medial part of the LP nucleus to the lateral suprasylvian cortex (Lomber et al., 1995). To our knowledge, no studies have investigated the reciprocal projections (i.e. from cortex to LP-pulvinar complex), as well as the projections from the superior colliculus (SC); these two pathways may represent the main substrate for the maintenance of visual activity in the extrageniculate thalamus. However, Mize and Murphy (1976) did not observe any evidence that neurons in SC are functionally involved in the recovery of the visual capacities following ablation in infant cats. It is also possible that part of the visual properties come from direct retinal projections. Labar et al. (1981) reported that removal of the primary visual cortex early in life leads to an increase in the density of retino-pulvinar projections. It is possible that the neurons' dendrites of a given sub-region of the LP-pulvinar complex may extend to neighboring areas, and that retino-pulvinar signals may be conveyed to the LPl. Another alternative may be proposed on the basis of the findings by Payne et al. (1993) stating that the total or partial ablation of the visual cortex in immature animals provokes, in some cases, the appearance of a novel retinal projection to the LPl. If present, such novel retino-LP pathways may certainly participate in establishing the response properties of LPl cells that we reported in the lesion group. However, recent findings from our group (Boire et al., 2000) suggest that this is most likely not the case (see below).

The nature of the visual properties of LPl cells brings us to the second main outcome of the present experiments: we found that there are significant differences in the receptive field properties between intact and lesioned animals. The first finding is that LPl neurons in early lesioned cats are more broadly tuned for orientation than that in normal ones. This loss of sensitivity could be related to the absence of cortical afferents from area 17. It is well known that orientation selectivity first appears in area 17 and that, overall, neurons in this area are more finely tuned for orientation than their counterparts in ex-

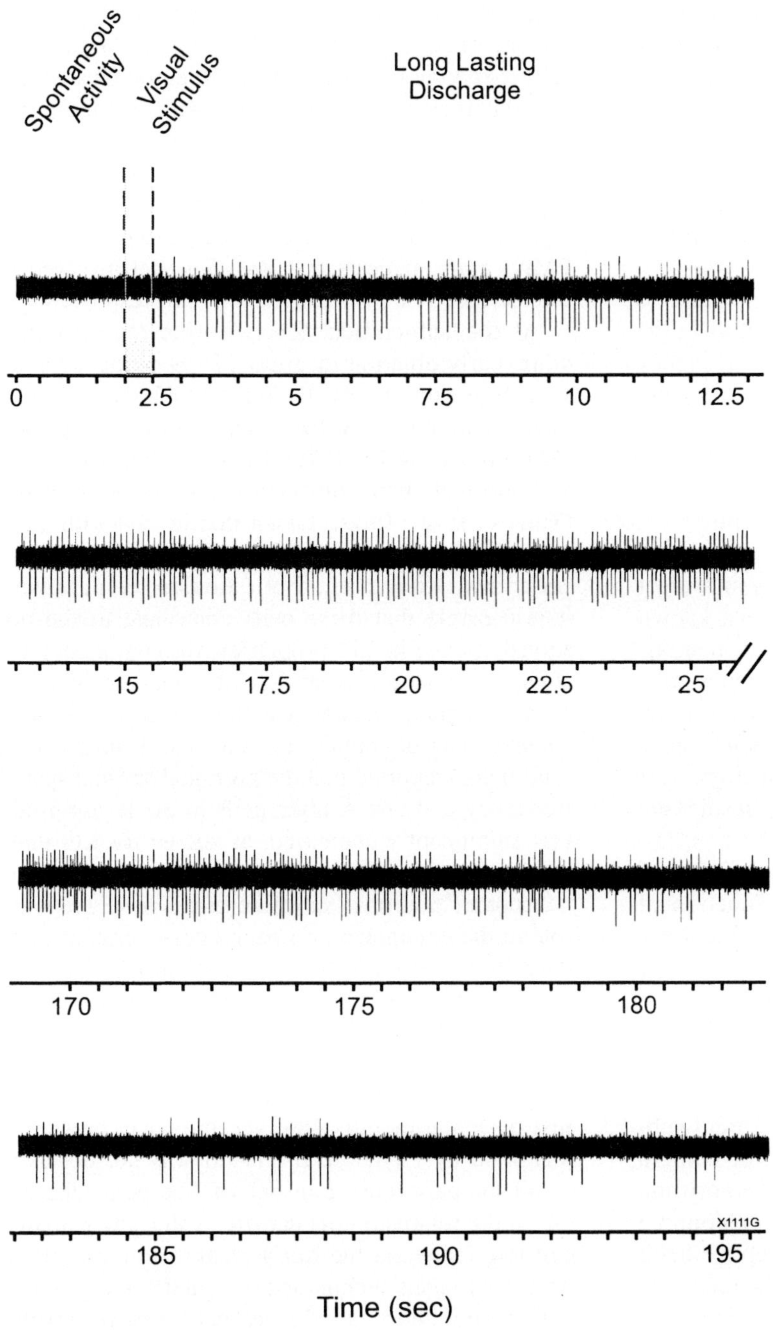

Fig. 6. Example of a LP-pulvinar cell recorded in lesioned cat showing long lasting discharges following a brief visual stimulation in its receptive field.

tra-striate areas (Orban et al., 1990; Hammond and Andrews, 1978). The broad selectivity in LPl may therefore not only reflect the lack of striate projections, but also the selectivity found in spared cortical areas projecting to the extrageniculate thalamus. In this context, it is worth pointing out that cats that sustained acute ablation of area 17 can still behaviorally discriminate the orientation of a target (Pasternak et al., 1995). In addition, LPl cells in lesioned cats retain their capacity to selectively code for direction. Interestingly, this was not the case when similar chronic ablations were performed at adulthood (preliminary unpublished observations), suggesting again that compensatory mechanisms occur in young animals.

The second finding is that, when compared to intact animals, a higher proportion of neurons in the lesion group exhibited low-pass spatial frequency tuning functions and therefore responded optimally to very low spatial frequency. No improvement in spatial processing was observed in LP, making it thus unlikely that this structure is involved in high spatial frequency analysis in operated animals. It may be proposed once more that the reduction in the number of band-pass units comes from removal of the primary visual cortex, which is the sole known cortical region in cat, in which almost all neurons are band-pass tuned for the spatial frequency of a grating (Movshon et al., 1978). In all other cortical areas projecting to the LP-pulvinar complex, cells are characterized by low-pass tuning functions (for a review, see Spear, 1991). The present results are in agreement with some of our early observations. For instance, we have shown that cooling area 17 may alter the spatial frequency tuning function of some cells in LPl; in particular, spatial frequency band-pass units exhibited a low-pass profile after the reversible inactivation of area 17 (see Fig. 6D in Casanova et al., 1997).

The last, and perhaps most interesting finding, is that removal of the primary visual cortex yielded a change in the organization of receptive field subregions. Indeed, a significant proportion of cells in the LPl of brain-damaged cats responded to drifting gratings with modulated discharges and exhibited a linear spatial summation within their receptive field; this last property may allow LPl cells to be more implicated in spatial coding. Since these two characteristics are not frequently observed in intact animals, it is likely that they reflect a change in the nature of the signals reaching the LP-pulvinar complex. At the cortical level, only the properties in PMLS cortex have been investigated in cats that sustained early ablation of areas 17–19 (Spear et al., 1980; Guido et al., 1992). None of these studies specifically addressed these properties, even though Guido et al. (1992) reported that most PMLS neurons responded with an increase in both mean and first harmonic amplitudes, but that the difference in the maximum FFT1 response rate between their normal and lesion groups was not significant. Therefore, the lack of significant changes in the discharge modulation of PMLS cells suggests that PMLS is not involved in the increased FFT1 component of LPl responses.

At the sub-cortical level, it was reported that, while early ablation of areas 17–19 produces a severe degeneration of cells in the LGN, the surviving neurons in layers A have quasi-normal properties (Murphy and Kalil, 1979; Tumosa et al., 1989) and that some of them exhibit linear spatial summation (Tumosa et al., 1989). Given that in cats with early cortical damage, layer A neurons now project to the LS cortex (Kalil et al., 1991; Lomber et al., 1995), it is possible that these cells contribute to the observed change in LPl properties, through geniculate signals originating from X cells, and reaching the extrageniculate nucleus via the LS cortex. In this context, it is of interest to note that Tumosa et al. (1989) also reported that the averaged optimal spatial frequency of LGN A-layer cells in the lesion group was significantly decreased, as shown for LPl units in the present study.

Another neuronal substrate could have played a role in the emergence of linear spatial summation in the LPl, in response to early cortical injury. Payne et al. (1993) reported the existence of novel retinal projections to the LPl (normally absent in intact animals) in cats that sustained total or partial ablation of the primary visual cortex during and after the first postnatal month. However, the novel projection identified by Payne et al. (1993) was not observed in all animals (only one out of five hemispheres). Given the relatively low density of the new ganglion cell terminals and the fairly weak resolution of the neuroanatomical technique used (HRP), it is possible that these authors failed to reveal the novel projection in most lesioned subjects, and in intact cats. A previous study (Itoh et al., 1983) did report the presence of similar retinal axonal patches in normal cats. These findings were recently corroborated by our group (Boire et al., 2000) as intraocular injection of the B fragment of cholera toxin revealed that the LPl in both intact and lesioned cats receives direct retinal projections. Altogether these findings do not support reports that ablation of the visual cortex leads to the appearance of a novel retinal projection to LPl[2] (Payne et al., 1993). However, it indicates that the LP-pulvinar complex of operated cats receives direct signals from ganglion cells. It remains to be determined whether there are some functional changes between retinal projections in both groups.

The retinal projections identified in lesioned cats could mediate the linear spatial summation observed in the present study. It is known that X cell receptive fields are characterized by a linear spatial summation (Enroth-Cugell and Robson, 1966). However, it is difficult to reconcile the properties of LPl neurons as described in this study (large receptive fields, low optimal spatial frequencies) with those of X cells, despite the fact that Tumosa et al. (1989) reported an increase in receptive field size, and a decrease in the optimal spatial frequency of X LGN cells in their early lesion group. On the basis of our physiological findings, a more likely (or at least contributing) candidate would be the γ cells (phasic W units). These neurons are less affected than β cells by the ablation of the primary visual cortex (Tong et al., 1982; Kalil, 1984; Payne et al., 1984; Kalil et al., 1991; Payne and Lomber, 1998) and have similar properties to those LPl cells described in this study, namely large receptive fields and linear spatial summation (Stanford et al., 1983; Sherman, 1985; Rowe and Palmer, 1995). W cells may also contribute, through the increase of the retino-pulvinar projections, to the maintaining of visual activity in the LP-pulvinar complex (Labar et al., 1981; Mason, 1981).

While all the above explanations can be proposed to understand the origin of the changes in LPl cell response properties, it is also possible that this functional reorganization comes from intrinsic changes in the LPl circuitry that may occur after an early cortical lesion.

In conclusion, we have shown that the destruction of the primary visual cortex does not alter the overall visual responsiveness of LPl neurons. However, there are significant changes in specific properties, that may result from the reorganization of the neuronal pathways projecting to the LP-pulvinar complex, which have yet to be fully explored at the neuroanatomical and physiological levels. Whether this functional compensation comes from sub-cortical areas or extrastriate cortical areas, the maintenance of visual activity in the LPl described here suggests that the LP-pulvinar complex may contribute to the behaviorally defined residual visual functions in animals (Cunningham et al., 1979; Perry and Cowey, 1979) and humans (Ptito et al., 1999) who sustained early damage of the primary visual cortex.

[2] Thus, one should not consider these 'novel' projections in general schemes describing the reorganization of neuronal pathways in cats sustaining early ablation of areas 17–19 (such as in Payne et al., 1996).

Acknowledgements

We thank B. Plaziac and J. Brûlé for their help in neuroanatomical analysis. We are also grateful to D. Boire for comments on the manuscript. This work was supported by a E.A. Baker Foundation grant to C.C. Part of C.C.'s salary was supported by FRSQ (Chercheur-boursier). A.D. was supported in part by a FCAR-FRSQ-Santé studentship.

References

Bender, D.B. (1982) Receptive-field properties of neurons in the macaque inferior pulvinar. *J. Neurophysiol.*, 48: 1–17.

Blythe, I.M., Bromley, J.M., Kennard, C. and Ruddock, K.H. (1986) Visual discrimination of target displacement remains after damage to the striate cortex in humans. *Nature*, 320: 619–621.

Boire, D., Casanova, C. and Ptito, M. (2000) Retinal projections to the lateral posterior-pulvinar in normal and striate ablated cats: a cholera toxin B fragment study. *Soc. Neurosci. Abstr.*, 26: 1471.

Casanova, C., Freeman, R.D. and Nordmann, J.P. (1989) Monocular and binocular response properties of cells in the striate-recipient zone of the cat's lateral posterior-pulvinar complex. *J. Neurophysiol.*, 62: 544–557.

Casanova, C., Savard, T. and Darveau, S. (1997) Contribution of area 17 to cell responses in the striate-recipient zone of the cat's lateral posterior-pulvinar complex. *Eur. J. Neurosci.*, 9: 101–111.

Chalupa, L.M. and Fish, S.E. (1978) Response characteristics of visual and extravisual neurons in the pulvinar and lateral posterior nuclei of the cat. *Exp. Neurol.*, 36: 96–120.

Chalupa, L.M. (1991) Visual function of the pulvinar. In: A.G. Leventhal (Ed.), *Vision and Visual Dysfunction. The Neural Basis of Visual Function*, Vol. 4. CRC Press, Boca Raton, FL, pp. 140–159.

Cornwell, P. and Payne, B.R. (1989) Visual discrimination by cats with adult or one- or two-stage neonatal lesions of visual cortex. *Behav. Neurosci.*, 103: 1191–1199.

Cunningham, T.J., Huddleston, C. and Murray, M. (1979) Modification of neuron numbers in the visual system of the rat. *J. Comp. Neurol.*, 184: 423–434.

Enroth-Cugell, C. and Robson, J.G. (1966) The contrast sensitivity of retinal ganglion cells of the cat. *J. Physiol.*, 187: 517–552.

Fendrich, R., Wessinger, C.M. and Gazzaniga, M.S. (1992) Residual vision in a scotoma: implications for blindsight. *Science*, 258: 1489–1491.

Guido, W., Spear, P.D. and Tong, L. (1990) Functional compensation in the lateral suprasylvian visual area following bilateral visual cortex damage in kittens. *Exp. Brain Res.*, 83: 219–224.

Guido, W., Spear, P.D. and Tong, L. (1992) How complete is physiological compensation in extrastriate after visual cortex damage in kittens? *Exp. Brain Res.*, 91: 455–466.

Greenlee, M.W., Lang, H.J., Mergner, T. and Seeger, W. (1995) Visual short-term memory of stimulus velocity in patients with unilateral posterior brain damage. *J. Neurosci.*, 15: 2287–2300.

Hammond, P. and Andrews, D.P. (1978) Orientation tuning of cells in areas 17 and 18 of the cat's visual cortex. *Exp. Brain Res.*, 31: 341–351.

Hochstein, S. and Shapley, R.M. (1976) Quantitative analysis of retinal ganglion cell classifications. *J. Physiol.*, 262: 237–264.

Hutchins, B. and Updyke, B.V. (1989) Retinotopic organization within the lateral posterior complex of the cat. *J. Comp. Neurol.*, 285: 350–398.

Itoh, K., Mizuno, N. and Kudo, M. (1983) Direct retinal projections to the latero-posterior and pulvinar nuclear complex (LP-PUL) in the cat, as revealed by the anterograde HRP method. *Brain Res.*, 276: 325–328.

Kalil, R.E. (1984) Removal of visual cortex in the cat: effects on the morphological development of the retino-geniculo-cortical pathway. In: J. Stone, B. Dreher and D.H. Rapaport (Eds.), *Development of Visual Pathways in Mammals*. Liss, New York, pp. 257–274.

Kalil, R.E., Tong, L.L. and Spear, P.D. (1991) Thalamic projections to the lateral suprasylvian visual area in cats with neonatal or adult visual cortex damage. *J. Comp. Neurol.*, 314: 512–525.

Kato, N., Price, D.J., Ferrer, J.M. and Blakemore, C. (1993) Plasticity of an aberrant geniculocortical pathway in neonatally lesioned cats. *NeuroReport*, 4: 915–918.

Labar, D.R., Berman, N.E. and Murphy, E.H. (1981) Short- and long-term effects of neonatal and adult visual cortex lesions on the retinal projection to the pulvinar. *J. Comp. Neurol.*, 197: 639–659.

Livingston, M. (1990) Segregation of form, color, movement, and depth processing in the visual system: anatomy, physiology, art, and illusion. In: B. Cohen and I. Bodis-Wollner (Eds.), *Vision and the Brain. The Organisation of the Central Visual System*, Vol. 67. Raven Press, New York, pp. 119–138.

Lomber, S.G., MacNeil, M.A. and Payne, B.R. (1995) Amplification of thalamic projections to middle suprasylvian cortex following ablation of immature primary visual cortex in the cat. *Cereb. Cortex*, 5: 166–191.

Mason, R. (1981) Differential responsiveness of cells in the visual zones of the cat's LP-pulvinar complex to visual stimuli. *Exp. Brain Res.*, 43: 25–33.

Merabet, L., Desautels, A., Minville, K. and Casanova, C. (1998) Motion integration in a thalamic visual nucleus. *Nature*, 396: 265–268.

Mitchell, D.E. (1990) Sensitive periods in visual development: insights gained from studies of recovery of visual function in cats following early monocular deprivation or cortical lesions. In: C. Blakemore (Ed.), *Vision: Coding and Efficiency*. Cambridge University Press, Cambridge, pp. 234–246.

Mize, R.R. and Murphy, E.H. (1976) Alterations in receptive field properties of superior colliculus cells produced by visual cortex ablation in infant and adult cats. *J. Comp. Neurol.*, 168: 393–424.

Moore, T., Rodman, H.R., Repp, A.B. and Gross, C.G. (1995) Localization of visual stimuli after striate cortex damage in monkeys: parallels with human blindsight. *Proc. Natl. Acad. Sci. USA*, 92: 8215–8218.

Movshon, J.A., Thompson, I.D. and Tolhurst, D.J. (1978) Spatial and temporal contrast sensitivity of neurones in areas 17 and 18 of the cat's visual cortex. *J. Physiol. Lond.*, 283: 101–120.

Murphy, E.H. and Kalil, R. (1979) Functional organization of lateral geniculate cells following removal of visual cortex in the newborn kitten. *Science*, 206: 713–716.

Orban, G.A., Vandenbussche, E., Sprague, J.M. and DeWeerd, P. (1990) Orientation discrimination in the cat: a distributed function. *Proc. Natl. Acad. Sci. USA*, 87: 1134–1138.

Otsuka, R. and Hassler, R. (1962) Uber aufbau und gliederung der corticalen sehesphäre bei der katze. *Archiv. Psychiatr. Z. Neurol.*, 203: 212–234.

Pasternak, T. Horn, K.M. and Maunsell, J.H. (1989) Deficits in speed discrimination following lesions of the lateral suprasylvian cortex in the cat. *Vis. Neurosci.*, 3: 365–375.

Pasternak, T., Tompkins, J. and Olson, C.R. (1995) The role of striate cortex in visual function of the cat. *J. Neurosci.*, 15: 1940–1950.

Payne, B.R. and Lomber, S.G. (1998) Neuroplasticity in the cat's visual system, origin, termination, expansion and increased coupling of the retino-geniculo-middle suprasylvian visual pathway following early ablations of areas 17 and 18. *Exp. Brain Res.*, 121: 334–349.

Payne, B.R., Pearson, H.E. and Cornwell, P. (1984) Transneuronal degeneration of beta retinal ganglion cells in the cat. *Proc. R. Soc. Lond. B*, 222: 15–32.

Payne, B.R., Foley, H. and Lomber, S.G. (1993) Visual cortex damage-induced growth of retinal axons into the lateral posterior nucleus of the cat. *Vis. Neurosci.*, 10: 727–752.

Payne, B.R., Lomber, S.G., Macneil, M.A. and Cornwell, P. (1996) Evidence for greater sight in blindsight following damage of primary visual cortex early in life. *Neuropsychologia*, 34: 741–774.

Perry, V.H. and Cowey, A. (1979) Changes in the retino-fugal pathways following cortical and tectal lesions in neonatal and adult rats. *Exp. Brain Res.*, 35: 97–108.

Ptito, M. and Lepore, F. (1983) Effects of unilateral and bilateral lesions of the lateral suprasylvian area on learning and interhemispheric transfer of pattern discrimination in the cat. *Behav. Brain Res.*, 7: 211–227.

Ptito, M., Lepore, F. and Guillemot, J.P. (1992) Loss of stereopsis following lesions of cortical areas 17–18 in the cat. *Exp. Brain Res.*, 89: 521–530.

Ptito, M., Johannsen, P., Faubert, J. and Gjendde, A. (1999) Activation of human extrageniculostriate pathways after damage to area V1. *NeuroImage*, 9: 97–107.

Reinoso-Suarez, F. (1961) *Topographischer Hirnatlas der Katze fur experimentale physiologische Untersuchungen* [Topographical atlas of the cat brain for experimental-physiological research]. Merk, Darmstad, Germany.

Rowe, M.H. and Palmer, L.A. (1995) Spatio-temporal receptive-field structure of phasic W cells in the cat retina. *Vis. Neurosci.*, 12: 117–139.

Sanderson, K.J. (1971) The projection of the visual field to the lateral geniculate and medial interlaminar nuclei in the cat. *J. Comp. Neurol.*, 143: 101–118.

Sanides, F. and Hoffmann, J. (1969) Cyto- and myeloarchitecture of the visual cortex of the cat and the surrounding integration cortices. *J. Hirnforsch.*, 11: 79–104.

Schupert, C., Cornwell, P. and Payne, B.R. (1993) Differential sparing of depth perception, orienting and optokinetic nystagmus after neonatal versus adult lesions of cortical areas 17, 18, 19 in the cat. *Behav. Neurosci.*, 107: 633–650.

Sherman, M.S. (1985) Functional organization of the W-, X- and Y-cell pathways in the cat: A review and hypothesis. In: J.M. Sprague and A.N. Epstein (Eds.), *Progress in Psychobiology and Physiological Psychology*, Vol. 11, Academic Press, New York, pp. 233–314.

Skottun, B.C., De Valois, R.L., Grosof, D.H., Movshon, J.A., Albrecht, D.G. and Bonds, A.B. (1991) Classifying simple and complex cells on the basis of response modulation. *Vision Res.*, 31: 1079–1086.

Spear, P.D. (1979) Behavioural and neurophysiological consequences of visual cortex damage. In: J.M. Sprague and A.N. Epstein (Eds.), *Progress in Psychobiology and Physiological Psychology*. Academic Press, New York, pp. 45–90.

Spear, P.D. (1988) Influence of areas 17, 18, and 19 on receptive-field properties of neurons in the cat's posteromedial lateral suprasylvian visual cortex. *Prog. Brain Res.*, 75: 197–210.

Spear, P.D. (1991) Functions of extrastriate visual cortex in non-primate species. In: *Vision and Visual Dysfunction. The Neural Basis of Visual Function*, Vol. 4. CRC Press Boca Raton, FL, pp. 339–370.

Spear, P.D., Kalil, R.E. and Tong, L. (1980) Functional compensation in lateral suprasylvian visual area following neonatal visual cortex removal in cats. *J. Neurophysiol.*, 43: 851–869.

Stanford, L.R., Friedlander, M.J. and Sherman, S.M. (1983) Morphological and physiological properties of geniculate W-cells of the cat: A comparison with X- and Y- cells. *J. Neurophysiol.*, 50: 582–608.

Sun, J.S., Lomber, S.G. and Payne, B.R. (1994) Expansion of suprasylvian cortex projection in the superficial layers of the superior colliculus following damage of areas 17 and 18 in developing cats. *Vis. Neurosci.*, 11: 13–22.

Tong, L., Kalil, R.E. and Spear, P.D. (1984) Critical periods for functional and anatomical compensation in the lateral suprasylvian visual area following removal of visual cortex in cats. *J. Neurophysiol.*, 52: 941–960.

Tong, L., Spear, P.D., Kalil, R.E. and Callahan, E.C. (1982) Loss of retinal X cells in cats with neonatal or adult visual cortex damage. *Science*, 217: 72–75.

Tumosa, N., McCall, M.A., Guido, W. and Spear, P.D. (1989) Responses of lateral geniculate neurons that survive long-term visual cortex damage in kittens and adult cats. *J. Neurosci.*, 9: 280–298.

Tusa, R.J., Palmer, L.A. and Rosenquist, A.C. (1978) Retinotopic organization of area 17 (striate cortex) in the cat. *J. Comp. Neurol.*, 177: 213–236.

Tusa, R.J., Rosenquist, A.C. and Palmer, L.A. (1979) Retinotopic organization of areas 18 and 19 in the cat. *J. Comp. Neurol.*, 185: 657–678.

Weiskrantz, L., Barbur, J.L. and Sahraie, A. (1995) Parameters affecting conscious versus unconscious visual discrimination with damage to the visual cortex (V1). *Proc. Natl. Acad. Sci. USA*, 92: 6122–6126.

Williams, C., Azzopardi, P. and Cowey, A. (1995) Nasal and temporal retinal ganglion cells projecting to the midbrain: implications for 'blindsight'. *Neuroscience*, 65: 577–586.

C. Casanova and M. Ptito (Eds.)
Progress in Brain Research, Vol. 134

CHAPTER 7

The superior colliculus and its control of fixation behavior via projections to brainstem omnipause neurons

André Bergeron and Daniel Guitton *

Department of Neurology and Neurosurgery, and Montreal Neurological Institute, McGill University, Montreal, PQ, H3A2B4 Canada

Abstract: Evidence, obtained in the animal whose head is unrestrained, has shown that the superior colliculus (SC) controls, not specifically eye-in-head motion, but rather saccadic shifts of the visual axis (gaze) composed of coordinated eye and head movements. The SC has also been implicated in fixation control. In a current hypothesis, activity on the SC motor map reflects two conflictual behavioral states: 'Orient!' versus 'Don't orient!' The latter behavior is thought to be commanded from a 'fixation zone' in the rostral SC that includes the foveal representation of the retinotopic map. 'Fixation neurons' (SCFNs) in this zone project to brainstem 'omnipause neurons' (OPNs) that inhibit the gaze–saccade generating circuits. It has been proposed that activity in SCFNs during active fixation, drives OPNs which in turn inhibit the gaze saccade generator, thereby maintaining the visual axis stable on a target of interest. Cats with head unrestrained frequently orient in the dark, to a briefly visible target, using multiple-step gaze shifts with a variable number of gaze saccades interspersed with periods of steady fixation. We found that SCFNs are not always active during the inter-step fixation periods when the visual axis is immobile — whereas OPNs are tonically active — thereby implying that activity in FNs and OPNs can be decoupled. In cats with head unrestrained, SCFNs encode the error between desired and actual gaze positions, not necessarily that the visual axis is immobile. By comparison, OPNs are tonically active when the visual axis is immobile, but some also encode gaze position error. Thus, the discharge of an OPN may reflect combined inputs from SCFNs combined with a steady bias.

Introduction

The superior colliculus (SC) and its homologue, the optic tectum of non-mammalian vertebrates, is a laminated structure consisting of alternating fiber and cell body layers that are oriented parallel to its surface. The deeper layers are organized into a motor map that has long been known to be involved in the sensory-motor processes leading to orienting behavior. It is generally agreed upon that, in species as different as barn owl, cat and monkey, the SC is strongly implicated in the control of rapid saccade-like orienting movements of the visual axis (gaze) composed of species-specific combinations of eye and head movements (reviewed in: Sparks and Hartwich-Young, 1989; Guitton and Munoz, 1991; Guitton, 1992; Moschovakis et al., 1996; Freedman and Sparks, 1997). Although neurons in the collicular motor-map discharge prior to both sensory and cognitively triggered eye or gaze saccades, the fundamental orienting behavior controlled by the SC may be of the primitive reflex type. Indeed, without cortical 'executive' control on eye saccade generation, patients with lesions of a frontal lobe are prisoners of irrepressible reflex orienting behavior attributed to an unchecked parieto–SC–brainstem pathway (Guitton et al., 1985).

In the last decade, this historically appealing role of the SC as a cross-species motor controller of 'reflexive' gaze saccades in two-dimensional space is being extended. Recordings in the superior collicu-

* Corresponding author: D. Guitton, Montreal Neurological Institute, 3801 University St., Montreal, PQ, H3A2B4 Canada. E-mail: dguitt@mni.mcgill.ca

lus (SC) of the alert cat and monkey suggest that anatomically separate neural systems respectively generate and suppress saccadic movements of the visual axis (gaze, see Methods; Munoz and Guitton, 1989; Munoz et al., 1991; Paré and Guitton, 1994; Paré et al., 1994). Recall that a visual 'map' of one-half the visual field, is represented retinotopically in the superficial layers of the contralateral SC. In particular, in the rostral SC, a 'fixation zone', coextensive with the representation of the fovea or area centralis, may be involved in the active control of fixation behavior and in the process of suppressing saccadic eye or gaze shifts.

A simple schema of a possible organization is shown in Fig. 1a. Tecto-reticular neurons (TRNs) in the SC's motor map generate saccadic gaze shifts via projections to brainstem reticular motor circuits (Grantyn and Grantyn, 1982; Grantyn and Berthoz, 1985; Munoz et al., 1991). By comparison, a 'fixation zone' in the SC's rostral pole contributes to suppressing gaze shifts (Munoz and Guitton, 1989; Munoz et al., 1991; Munoz and Wurtz, 1993a,b, 1995; Paré and Guitton, 1994; Paré et al., 1994; Peck and Baro, 1997; Everling et al., 1998) via putative inhibitory influences on the motor map (Munoz and Istvan, 1998) in concert with projections of 'fixation-TRNs' (superior colliculus fixation neurons, SCFNs) to brainstem 'omnipause neurons' (OPNs; Paré and Guitton, 1994; Büttner-Ennever and Horn, 1995; Gandhi and Keller, 1997, 1999a,b; Paré and Guitton, 1998; Büttner-Ennever et al., 1999). Electrical stimulation of either OPNs or the rostral SC suppresses eye/gaze (monkey/cat) saccades (Evinger et al., 1982; Paré and Guitton, 1994; Paré et al., 1994) and pharmacologically induced deactivation of the rostral SC leads to difficulty in maintaining fixation (Munoz and Wurtz, 1993b).

Although SCFNs project onto OPNs the question of how SCFNs influence OPN discharges during gaze shifts is still unclear. Recently, Everling et al. (1998) found differences between the patterns of activity of SCFNs and OPNs in monkeys performing the 'gap' saccade task. They observed that the discharge frequency of SCFNs diminished during the gap period, whereas that of OPNs did not change. Furthermore, although the tonic discharges of both SCFNs and OPNs pause during saccades, the onset and offset of OPN pauses are better synchronized with saccade onset and offset, respectively, than that of SCFNs. Finally, OPNs present a more regular and higher frequency tonic discharge than SCFNs. From these data, Everling et al. (1998) conclude that SCFN inputs alone do not determine OPN discharges.

To better understand the respective role of SCFNs and OPNs in the generation of gaze shifts and in fixation behavior, we have studied the activity of both cells during multiple-step gaze shifts in cats. Multiple-step gaze shifts are composed of a variable number of gaze saccades interspersed with periods of steady fixation. The interesting particularity of this orienting behavior is that, during a saccade task, the gaze axis becomes immobile at a number of locations prior to reaching the target. In a previous study (Bergeron and Guitton, 2000), we showed that SCFNs encode the distance between the visual axis and the target (gaze-position error) and are not concerned with the occurrence of saccades and fixation periods in the gaze trajectory. By comparison, OPNs are thought to gate the saccade burst generator. This would suggest that SCFNs and OPNs have very different discharge properties during multiple-step gaze shifts, a fact that we confirm in this study. Indeed, unlike SCFNs, OPNs encode the occurrence of gaze-steps and fixation periods during multiple-step gaze shifts. However, in some OPNs the tonic discharge additionally encodes gaze-position error, thereby reflecting an SCFN input.

Methods

Behavioral techniques and paradigms

Four cats were prepared for chronic single unit recordings in the brainstem: three for the study of 'fixation neurons' (SCFNs) of the rostral superior colliculus (SC), and two different animals for the study of 'omnipause neurons' (OPNs) in the nucleus raphe interpositus (Paré and Guitton, 1994; Büttner-Ennever and Horn, 1995; Gandhi and Keller, 1997). Eye and head movements were recorded using the search coil in magnetic field technique (Robinson, 1963). All surgical and experimental protocols were approved by the Animal Care Committee of the Montreal Neurological Institute and complied with the Canadian Council on Animal Care policy on the use of laboratory animals. All animals were

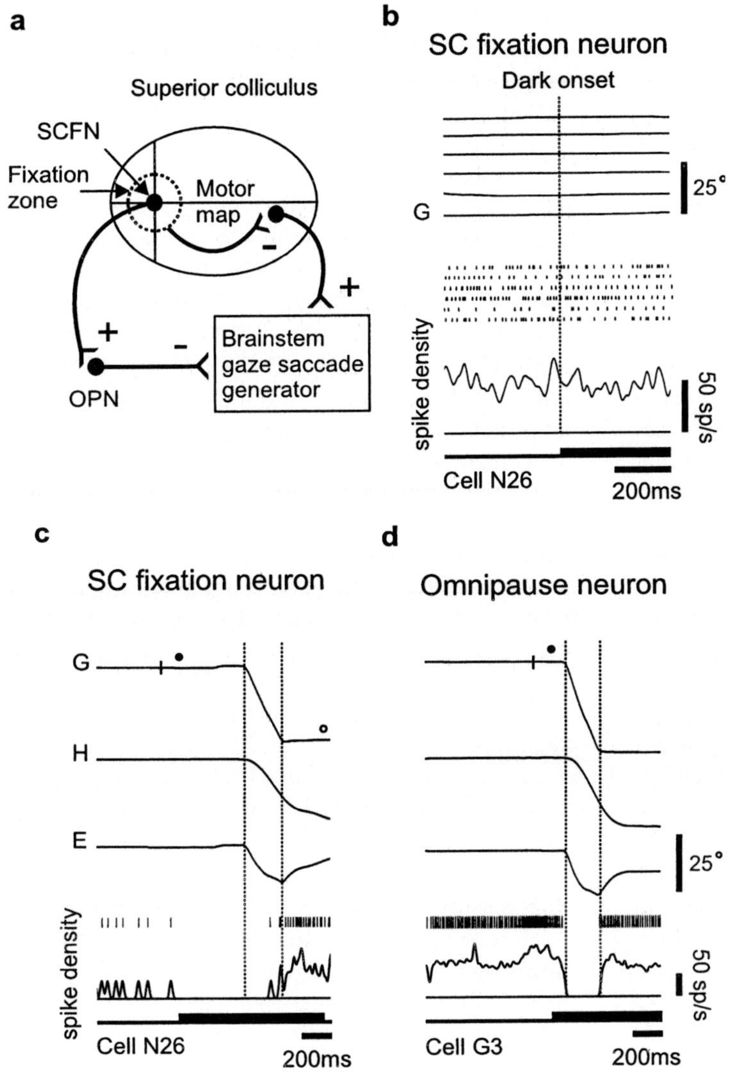

Fig. 1. Overview of connectivity and discharge patterns of a SCFN and an OPN. (a) The large oval represents a dorsal view of the SC. The dotted circle in the rostral SC identifies a fixation zone whose precise boundaries are unknown. The vertical and horizontal lines indicate locations where, respectively, horizontal and vertical saccades are encoded. Small dark circles and attached curved lines indicate TRNs, cells whose axons project to the brainstem reticular formation. Those emanating from the fixation zone are SCFNs which project to OPNs, which in turn inhibit the saccade generator. (b) Cat steadily fixated a food target and at the vertical dotted line the ambient lighting was extinguished. This was repeated six times. At the top are the six horizontal gaze traces, and below the associated discharges of SCFN, cell N26 in the right SC. Below is the averaged discharge, the spike density histogram. (c) Vertical tic-marks below eye position trace (E) show action potentials of cell N26, during a single-step gaze position (G) shift (see text). H, head position. (d) Discharge pattern of OPN during single-step gaze shift (see text). The thicker horizontal line in the bottom trace of each panel indicates when cat was in complete darkness. This is also shown by circles above G traces: dark circle, light off; open circle, light on. Vertical tic-mark on G trace indicates when target was shown to cat. In all traces, down means leftward movement.

enveloped in a loosely fitting bag and then placed in an open-top box that allowed full ranges in horizontal and vertical-up head motion. Downward head motion was restricted to about 35° below normal head posture. We restricted our study to horizontal gaze shifts. The animals faced an opaque barrier of variable width (10–60°) directly in front of them at a distance of about 35 cm. The head of each cat was attached, via two universal joints, to a vertical shaft rotating in low-friction bearings. This minimized constraint on the animal's orienting behavior. In our 'barrier paradigm' a small food target was hidden behind the barrier and suddenly appeared on one of the two vertical sides. The hungry cats naturally redirected their visual axis to the target and were fed. The amplitude of the overall gaze shift required to fixate the target depended on the initial gaze position which varied from trial to trial. With practice, the timing of a cat's orienting behavior became very reliable. A fluorescent light with very fast decay time (~100 μs) provided ambient lighting. Some trials were performed in the light; in others, the light was extinguished for 1 s beginning 120 ms after target appearance, such that gaze shifts were made in complete darkness.

Before recording neurons, we first confirmed that our electrodes were in the rostral SC by exploring the SC's motor map using electrical stimulation. The map's organization was deduced based on the amplitude and direction of the gaze shifts evoked at different electrode positions (Paré et al., 1994). We were able to predict the stereotaxic location of the rostral SC's fixation zone. A histological reconstruction of the recording site was made in two of the cats. We also placed stimulating electrodes in the predorsal bundle of all cats so as to determine by antidromic stimulation whether a SCFN was a tecto-reticular neuron (TRN).

SCFNs are very difficult to record in the head-unrestrained condition because head movements cause small displacements of the brainstem relative to the microelectrode tip and contact with the cell is easily lost. Nevertheless, we recorded in three cats the activity of 14 cells in the rostral SC that we classified as SCFNs according to criteria which conform to prior descriptions of SCFNs in cat and monkey (Fig. 1b,c; Munoz and Guitton, 1989; Munoz et al., 1991; Munoz and Wurtz, 1993a; Peck and Baro, 1997; Everling et al., 1998). Six of these cells were identified as TRNs. The lack of identification of the remaining SCFNs does not imply that they were not TRNs; with time, the reliability of the stimulating electrodes waned. To compare with SCFNs, we recorded the activity of 16 OPNs. For each SCFN and OPN that we analyzed, we had between 5 and 60 (average about 20) multiple-step gaze shifts from which we could reliably assess a cell's discharge pattern.

Data analysis

The eye and head coils gave eye position in space. Gaze (G) = eye position in space = eye-in-head (E) + head-in-space (H). We also recorded target position and light offset and duration of dark period. Data were stored on DAT tape. In off-line analysis, E was calculated from G and H. Action potentials were converted to logic pulses via a time-amplitude window discriminator (BAK Electronics). Movement and pulse traces were digitized at 2 kHz with data acquisition software and analyzed with Matlab. Spike density histograms were generated by substituting for each spike a Gaussian function with a width of 10 ms (MacPherson and Aldridge, 1979; Richmond et al., 1987) and then summing all of the Gaussians together to generate a continuous function in time.

Results

SCFN and OPN discharges during single-step gaze shifts

Suppressing saccades is important for maintaining fixation on a target of interest and in this context the discharges of SCFNs have been interpreted as essentially motor. Our results point to a more complex role, but before considering this we will overview briefly some basic SCFN and OPN discharge characteristics. When the animal fixated the food target in the light, SCFNs discharged tonically (Fig. 1b; for all cells, firing frequency was >10 spikes/s). When ambient illumination was extinguished and the animal was suddenly in complete darkness, tonic discharge in all cells continued for at least 400 ms. In some cells, as shown in Fig. 1b, the rate in the dark was similar to that in light. In others, the rate in the dark decreased, but never below 10 spikes/s. In general, our observations conformed totally to previous findings in head-fixed monkey (Munoz and Wurtz, 1993a,b) that have been taken as evidence that SCFN tonic discharges during fixation are not solely visually induced.

Fig. 1c illustrates the typical discharge of a SCFN in relation to a single-step gaze shift in our barrier paradigm (see Methods). Before a gaze shift, the cat faced the plain opaque barrier on which there was no target of significance. In this experimental context, the cat undoubtedly anticipated target appearance to one or the other side of the barrier (Munoz and Guitton, 1991; Munoz et al., 1991). The neuron had a characteristically low tonic discharge (Munoz and Wurtz, 1993a), due perhaps to either or both the lack of a significant fixation target and to motor preparation for the next orienting gaze shift (Munoz and Guitton, 1991; Munoz et al., 1991). The early tonic discharge ceased shortly after the food target was presented to one side of the barrier and the pause continued, in the dark, throughout most of the gaze saccade directed contralateral to the recording site. At the end of the gaze shift, the visual axis was immobile on the invisible but remembered location of the target. Discharge resumed just before the end of the gaze shift, and firing rate peaked just after the end. This overall discharge pattern is expected from prior studies of SCFNs in head-fixed monkeys and head-unrestrained cats (Munoz and Guitton, 1989, 1991; Munoz et al., 1991; Munoz and Wurtz, 1993a; Peck and Baro, 1997; Everling et al., 1998).

The discharge of a typical OPN in the same experimental paradigm is shown in Fig. 1d. The OPN discharged tonically when the visual axis was immobile and activity paused during the gaze saccade. Note that, compared to the SCFN, the discharge pattern of the OPN was modulated in much closer synchrony with the motor phases of fixation and gaze saccades. This also has been reported during saccades in the head-fixed monkey (Everling et al., 1998). The difference between the discharge patterns of SCFNs and OPNs is even more vivid during gaze shifts that have complex trajectories, as we will now show.

SCFN and OPN discharges during multiple-step gaze shifts

The cat has eye motion restricted to about ±15° from center. Thus, head motion in this animal is indispensable for the generation of large orienting gaze shifts which makes the cat an ideal model to study eye–head gaze control. Large gaze shifts in this animal are frequently generated with multiple steps. Fig. 2a shows the typical pattern of discharge of an OPN during multiple-step gaze shifts made by a cat as it oriented to a target situated at distances varying from about 50° (top gaze trace) to 25° (bottom trace) from the initial fixation position. Note that no two movement trajectories are identical: they could differ in the size and number of gaze steps and in the duration of inter-step plateaus. In Fig. 2a, the movements are aligned on the onset of the first gaze step. The tonic activity of this typical OPN paused just before, and silence continued during, this first gaze saccade. Activity resumed at the end of the saccade and continued during the following plateau phase. This pattern repeated itself during all subsequent saccades and plateaus. In Fig. 2b the traces are aligned on the end of the first plateau that followed the first saccade. Note the strong link between plateau duration and discharge duration. This relationship is also evident in Fig. 2c where the traces have been aligned on the end of the multiple-step gaze trajectories. Fig. 2b shows also that during many plateaus, OPN firing frequency was less than before the onset of multiple-step sequences (Paré and Guitton, 1998). Note also, by comparing Fig. 2c and a, that OPN firing rate at the end of multiple-step sequences was greater than at the start.

Fig. 2d–f show the discharge pattern of a typical SCFN during multiple-step sequences directed contralateral to the recording site. In each panel, the traces have been aligned on the same feature of a gaze trajectory as in the OPN panel directly above. A comparison of the panels in each column shows a clear difference between the patterns of activity of SCFNs and OPNs. For example, the tonic discharge of this typical SCFN ceased shortly after the target was presented (Fig. 2d) and firing resumed, in the dark, towards the end of the overall multiple-step sequence. Fig. 2e shows the same trajectories now aligned on the end of the first plateau that followed the first gaze step. Surprisingly, if one refers to observations during single step saccades (Fig. 1b and Munoz and Wurtz, 1993a), the SCFN was silent during these plateaus, even though the visual axis was immobile and the cat was alert. In Fig. 2f, the movements are now aligned on the end of the multiple-step trajectories. The activity of the cell had fully resumed by then and in particular the cell was active during the last gaze saccade and the plateau that pre-

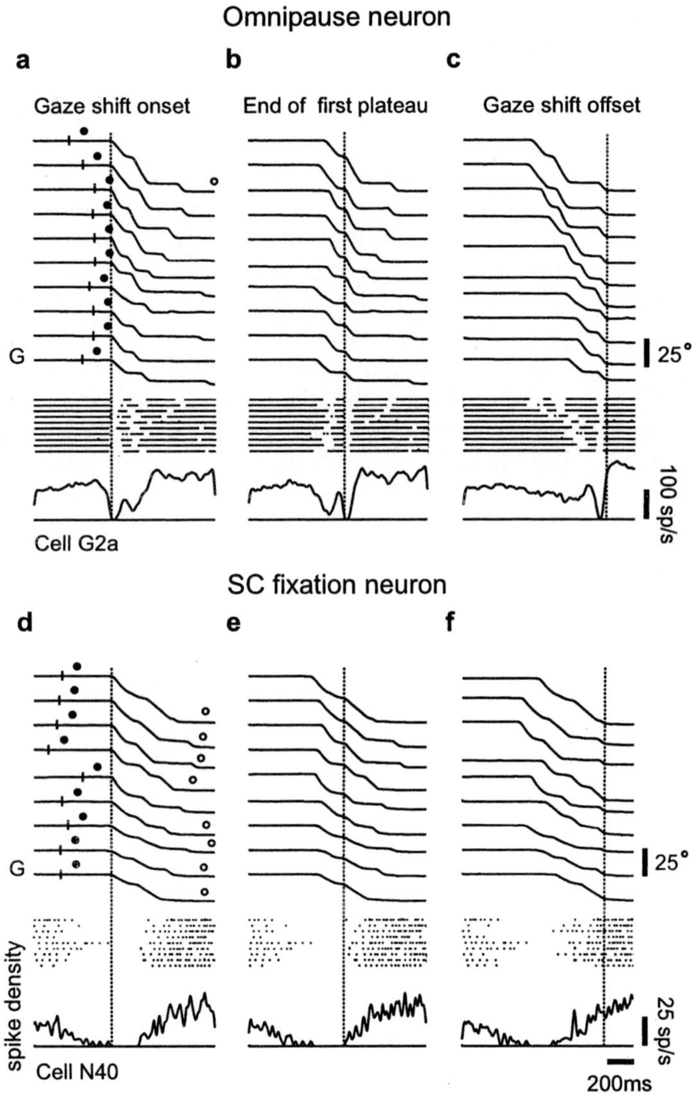

Fig. 2. Comparison of discharges of an OPN and a SCFN (cell N40 in right SC) during multiple-step gaze shifts. For each cell, same trials are shown in all panels except that in each panel traces are aligned on a specific feature of the gaze trajectory. (a,d) Movement-related discharges of cells when G traces are aligned on gaze shift onset (vertical dotted line). (b,e) Gaze traces aligned on end of the first fixation plateau. (c,f) Gaze traces aligned on end of gaze shifts. Same symbols and conventions as in Fig. 1.

ceded it. The firing rate continued to increase after the end of the gaze shift (also shown in Fig. 1c). This has been described previously for monkey SCFNs (Munoz and Wurtz, 1993a). Note that, like in the OPN, the discharge rate at the end of the multiple-step sequence, both in the light and dark, was greater than during the period preceding target presentation (as in Fig. 1c).

Why was a SCFN silent during the first plateau but often active during the last plateau? Put another way, what determined the end of the pause in SCFN activity? We have found that the activity of a particular SCFN resumed when the visual axis arrived at a specific angular distance from the remembered target location (Bergeron and Guitton, 2000). We have called this distance, a cell's preferred gaze-position

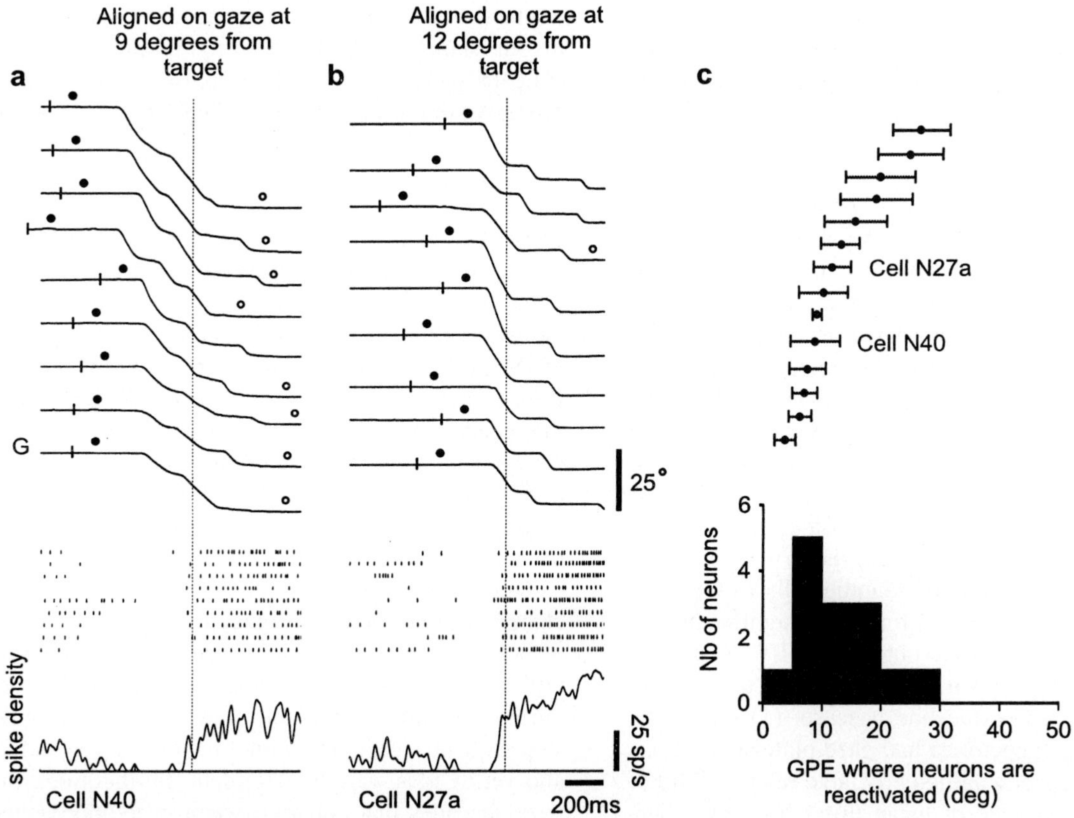

Fig. 3. Relationship of SCFN discharge to distance between G and target (GPE). (a,b) For cells N40 and N27a (in right SC) the pause in activity during multiple-step gaze shifts ended on average when the visual axis was at about 9 and 12°, respectively, from target. The example traces shown in panels a and b have been aligned on these values. (c) Mean values (closed circle) ± standard deviations of GPE (refer to lower graph's abscissa) at which activity in each SCFN in our sample reappeared. Each closed circle represents one cell. Bar graph shows distribution.

error (GPE). Fig. 3a shows the same trials as in Fig. 2, but now realigned to illustrate that the activity of cell N40 resumed when gaze was at 9 ± 4° from its goal; i.e. GPE = 9°. In another example (Fig. 3b) from a different cell (N27a) GPE = 12 ± 3°. For the other cells in our sample, the angular distance from the target at which the discharge resumed varied from 6 to 26° (Fig. 3c). The average for all cells was 13°.

The multiple-step sequences in Fig. 3a,b varied in overall amplitude from 25 to 50° because the cat initiated its orientation from different initial positions. It is important to note that a cell's 'preferred' GPE was independent of the size of the overall multiple-step sequence. Also, if the amplitude of the overall multiple-step gaze displacement was less than the cell's preferred GPE, the cell did not pause, but continued to discharge during the entire movement (not shown).

Note that a trajectory could reach the threshold GPE during a saccade (e.g. Fig. 3a, top trace) or at the start of a long plateau (Fig. 3a, 2nd trace from top). As a result, the reactivation time relative to the end of a gaze shift was highly variable and depended on plateau duration. For our 14 SCFNs combined, the mean standard deviation of the onset time of cell activity relative to the end (i.e. on goal) of the multiple-step sequences was 127 ms. By comparison for the population, the mean standard deviation of the onset time of cell activity relative to each cell's preferred GPE was 59 ms.

After the first spike, a cell's firing frequency did not necessarily immediately reach peak value

(Fig. 3a). This property is well illustrated for cell N27a, for which we were fortunate to have at least 10 multiple-step sequences in which the last gaze position plateau in each trace ended at about the same distance from the target (Fig. 4a). The spike density histogram shows that during the last plateau, where GPE is around 5°, the firing frequency was lower compared to when GPE = 0. A similar complementary result was found for cell N42a, recorded during multiple-step gaze shifts that had gaze-plateaus in many different positions relative to final gaze position (Fig. 4b). There are two segments to the relationship between firing frequency and GPE (Fig. 4b); one through the open circles where the cell did not discharge, the other through the black circles. Clearly, after the preferred GPE was reached at the black triangle on the abscissa (point through which regression line is forced) the firing frequency during plateaus increased monotonically as GPE approached zero. Regression lines with significant correlation coefficients were obtained in 10/18 SCFNs. In the remaining cells it was not possible to calculate a significant regression line because: (1) the multiple-step gaze trajectories had gaze-plateau positions that did not cover a sufficiently large range of GPEs; and (2) the estimate of mean firing frequency during plateaus that are close to the preferred GPE is inherently very 'noisy' due to the combination of low firing frequency and comparatively short plateau duration.

By comparison with SCFNs, the OPNs in our sample were active during all the plateaus of multiple-step gaze shifts (Fig. 2a–c). This constitutes a major difference between the discharge characteristics of these two cell types. However, we found that their discharges are not as totally decoupled as one might surmise from Fig. 2. Indeed, for many OPNs in our sample (8/16) the firing frequency during plateaus increased as GPE decreased (Fig. 4c,d), a property similar to that seen in SCFNs.

Discussion

These data lead to conclusions that are very different than those previously published based on observations of SCFN discharges during single saccades in monkey (Munoz and Wurtz, 1993a; Everling et al., 1998). In these, SCFN pause onset and offset times were linked, although less strongly than for OPNs, to saccade beginning and end, respectively. Saccades have a very stereotyped trajectory and a specific time relative to saccade-end tends to correspond to a specific GPE. Our results clearly distinguish between these two variables.

Our observations show that OPN and SCFN discharges can be totally decoupled. *Activity* in SCFNs is not a necessary condition either for activating OPNs or for assuring that gaze is immobile. Indeed, during the initial inter-step plateaus in a multiple-step sequence, gaze was immobile, OPNs were active and yet SCFNs were totally silent. Furthermore, the gaze saccades that occurred when gaze approached the salient target were generated when OPNs were silent but in spite of SCFN activity. By extension, our data also show that *silence* in SCFNs is neither necessary for silence in OPNs nor to permit gaze saccade generation. Thus, our OPN activity generally strongly reflected gaze motor behavior, whereas SCFN activity did not, but rather encoded that gaze was close to, or on, a cognitively significant target.

In spite of the obvious decoupling between SCFN and OPN discharges, our results also support some

Fig. 4. Relationship between firing frequency and gaze-position error at different gaze plateaus for SCFN (a,b) and OPN (c,d). (a) Multiple-step gaze shifts with amplitude of last saccade about 5°. Traces aligned on beginning of last saccade. SCFN, cell N27a, shows lower discharge when G is ~5° from goal compared to than when G is on goal at GPE = 0. (b) For cell N42a, mean firing frequency during plateau (black circle) increases as GPE of plateau decreases. Open circles on abscissa represent plateau positions for which cell did not discharge. The dark triangle on the zero of the abscissa indicates average GPE at which first spike occurred (18°) for this cell. Regression line was forced through this point. (c) Same as for SCFN in a. OPN, cell G4d, shows lower discharge when G is ~10° from goal compared to than when G is on goal at GPE = 0. Note that this typical cell's discharge pauses during gaze saccades. (d) For cell G4d, mean firing frequency during plateau (black circle) increases as GPE of plateau decreases. Horizontal line represents average firing frequency of neuron during 1st plateaus when gaze was more than about 10° from target. For these positions, cell discharge scatters about the line and was not modulated by GPE. This represents the postulated bias input to the OPN. We fit a regression line through all points lying more than two standard deviations above the horizontal line. Same symbols and conventions as in Figs. 1 and 2.

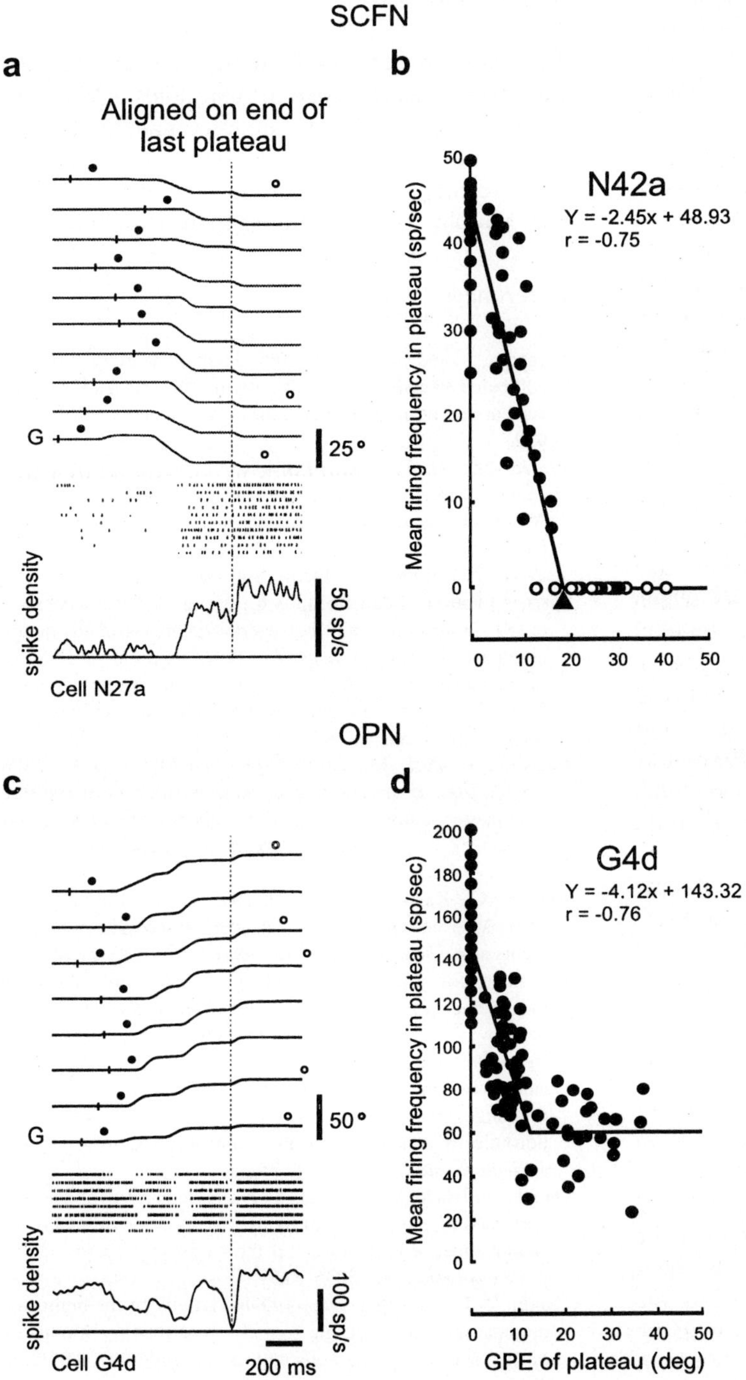
SCFN
a
b
Aligned on end of last plateau
G
25°
spike density
50 sp/s
Cell N27a
N42a
Y = -2.45x + 48.93
r = -0.75
Mean firing frequency in plateau (sp/sec)
0
10
20
30
40
50
OPN
c
d
G
50°
spike density
100 sp/s
Cell G4d
200 ms
G4d
Y = -4.12x + 143.32
r = -0.76
Mean firing frequency in plateau (sp/sec)
GPE of plateau (deg)

coupling between these cells. Thus, the firing frequency during gaze plateaus of both SCFNs and some OPNs increased as GPE approached zero. This suggests that SCFN activity did influence that of OPNs perhaps, in the context of Fig. 1, by superimposing on a simple bias input to OPNs — revealed by their discharge during the early plateaus when SCFNs are silent — that assures their steady firing (Fig. 4c,d). Such tonic firing would be useful, say, to suppress 'noise' in the gaze saccade generator, thereby preventing unwanted orienting gaze shifts. An increase in the tonic firing frequency of the OPN population at the end of a multiple-step sequence, when gaze is on target, would assure a period of steady fixation uninterrupted by intruding gaze shifts away from the target of interest.

Coupling between SCFNs and OPNs is suggested by other evidence. Some OPNs in the head-fixed cat have been described recently as having, like our SCFNs, target-related pauses in activity which continue during a sequence of saccades (Petit et al., 1999). This characteristic would make sense, in the context of Fig. 1a, if the proposed additional bias to some OPNs was weak, but so far in our present and another (Paré and Guitton, 1998) study in the head-unrestrained cat, we never saw total, SCFN-like, pauses in the discharge pattern of OPNs during plateaus.

It is noteworthy that multiple-step gaze shifts are commonly made by monkeys when they generate large gaze shifts (Crawford et al., 1999) and we anticipate that the present observations in cat can be generalized to include primates.

The present results bring up the interesting distinction between cognitive goals and motor goals. In our daily activities, a final goal can be the result of a series of motor acts that are quite distinct from each other. For example, if the reader of this article decides to go to the nearby bookshelf, this end-goal in itself implies a sequence of distinct intermediate motor sub-goals such as getting up from the chair, walking around the desk, etc. In this context, for the gaze control system, SCFNs are concerned with the achievement of the end goal, not the details of how it has been achieved. By comparison, OPNs seem better linked to the specific details of the motor output, but nevertheless maintain encoding of the important end-goal.

Acknowledgements

This research was Funded by the Medical Research Council of Canada (MRC). A.B. holds a MRC studentship. We thank and are very grateful to W.Y. Choi, D. Crawford, K. Cullen, and T. Herter for critically reading earlier versions of the manuscript and to J. Murphy for contributions to the experiments.

References

Bergeron, A. and Guitton, D. (2000) Fixation neurons in superior colliculus encode gaze-position-error, the distance between current and desired gaze positions. *Nat. Neurosci.*, 3(9): 932–939.

Büttner-Ennever, J.A. and Horn, A.K.E. (1995) Neuroanatomy of saccadic omnipause neurons in nucleus raphe interpositus. In: A.F. Fuchs, T. Brandt, U. Büttner and D.S. Zee (Eds.), *Contemporary Ocular Motor and Vestibular Research: a Tribute to David A. Robinson*. Thieme, Stuttgart, pp. 488–495.

Büttner-Ennever, J.A., Horn, A.K., Henn, V. and Cohen, B. (1999) Projections from the superior colliculus motor map to omnipause neurons in monkey. *J. Comp. Neurol.*, 413: 55–67.

Crawford, J.D., Ceylan, M.Z., Klier, E.M. and Guitton, D. (1999) Three-dimensional eye–head coordination during gaze saccades in the primate. *J. Neurophysiol.*, 81: 1760–1782.

Everling, S., Paré, M., Dorris, M.C. and Munoz, D.P. (1998) Comparison of the discharge characteristics of brain stem omnipause neurons and superior colliculus fixation neurons in monkey: implications for control of fixation and saccade behavior. *J. Neurophysiol.*, 79: 511–528.

Evinger, C., Kaneko, C.R. and Fuchs, A.F. (1982) Activity of omnipause neurons in alert cats during saccadic eye movements and visual stimuli. *J. Neurophysiol.*, 47: 827–844.

Freedman, E.G. and Sparks, D.L. (1997) Activity of cells in the deeper layers of the superior colliculus of the rhesus monkey — evidence for a gaze displacement command. *J. Neurophysiol.*, 78: 1669–1690.

Gandhi, N.J. and Keller, E.L. (1997) Spatial distribution and discharge characteristics of superior colliculus neurons antidromically activated from the omnipause region in monkey. *J. Neurophysiol.*, 78: 2221–2225.

Gandhi, N.J. and Keller, E.L. (1999a) Comparison of saccades perturbed by stimulation of the rostral superior colliculus, the caudal superior colliculus, and the omnipause neuron region. *J. Neurophysiol.*, 82: 3236–3253.

Gandhi, N.J. and Keller, E.L. (1999b) Activity of the brain stem omnipause neurons during saccades perturbed by stimulation of the primate superior colliculus. *J. Neurophysiol.*, 82: 3254–3267.

Grantyn, A. and Berthoz, A. (1985) Burst activity of identified tecto-reticulo-spinal neurons in the alert cat. *Exp. Brain Res.*, 57: 417–421.

Grantyn, A. and Grantyn, R. (1982) Axonal patterns and sites of termination of cat superior colliculus neurons projecting in the tecto-bulbo-spinal tract. *Exp. Brain Res.*, 46: 243–256.

Guitton, D. (1992) Control of eye–head coordination during orienting gaze shifts. *Trends Neurosci.*, 15: 174–179.

Guitton, D. and Munoz, D.P. (1991) Control of orienting gaze shifts by the tecto-reticulo-spinal system in the heat-free cat. I. Identification, localization and effects of behavior on sensory responses. *J. Neurophysiol.*, 66: 1605–1623.

Guitton, D., Buchtel, H.A. and Douglas, R.M. (1985) Frontal lobe lesions in man cause difficulties in suppressing reflexive glances and in generating goal-directed saccades. *Exp. Brain Res.*, 58: 455–472.

MacPherson, J.M. and Aldridge, J.W. (1979) A quantitative method of computer analysis of spike train data collected from behaving animals. *Brain Res.*, 175: 183–187.

Moschovakis, A.K., Scudder, C.A. and Highstein, S.M. (1996) The microscopic anatomy and physiology of the mammalian saccadic system. *Prog. Neurobiol.*, 50: 133–254.

Munoz, D.P. and Guitton, D. (1989) Fixation and orientation control by the tecto-reticulo-spinal system in the cat whose head is unrestrained. *Rev. Neurol. (Paris).*, 145: 567–579.

Munoz, D.P. and Guitton, D. (1991) Control of orienting gaze shifts by the tectoreticulospinal system in the head-free cat. II. Sustained discharges during motor preparation and fixation. *J. Neurophysiol.*, 66: 1624–1641.

Munoz, D.P. and Istvan, P.J. (1998) Lateral inhibitory interactions in the intermediate layers of the monkey superior colliculus. *J. Neurophysiol.*, 79: 1193–1209.

Munoz, D.P. and Wurtz, R.H. (1993a) Fixation cells in monkey superior colliculus. I. Characteristics of cell discharge. *J. Neurophysiol.*, 70: 559–575.

Munoz, D.P. and Wurtz, R.H. (1993b) Fixation cells in monkey superior colliculus. II. Reversible activation and deactivation. *J. Neurophysiol.*, 70: 576–589.

Munoz, D.P. and Wurtz, R.H. (1995) Saccade-related activity in monkey superior colliculus. II, Spread of activity during saccades. *J. Neurophysiol.*, 73: 2334–2348.

Munoz, D.P., Guitton, D. and Pelisson, D. (1991) Control of orienting gaze shifts by the tectoreticulospinal system in the head-free cat. III. Spatiotemporal characteristics of phasic motor discharges. *J. Neurophysiol.*, 66: 1642–1666.

Paré, M. and Guitton, D. (1994) The fixation area of the cat superior colliculus: effects of electrical stimulation and direct connection with brainstem omnipause neurons. *Exp. Brain Res.*, 101: 109–122.

Paré, M. and Guitton, D. (1998) Brain stem omnipause neurons and the control of combined eye–head gaze saccades in the alert cat. *J. Neurophysiol.*, 79: 3060–3076.

Paré, M., Crommelinck, M. and Guitton, D. (1994) Gaze shifts evoked by stimulation of the superior colliculus in the head-free cat conform to the motor map but also depend on stimulus strength and fixation activity. *Exp. Brain Res.*, 101: 123–139.

Peck, C.K. and Baro, J.A. (1997) Discharge patterns of neurons in the rostral superior colliculus of cat: activity related to fixation of visual and auditory targets. *Exp. Brain Res.*, 113: 291–302.

Petit, J., Klam, F., Grantyn, A. and Berthoz, A. (1999) Saccades and multisaccadic gaze shifts are gated by different pontine omnipause neurons in head-fixed cats. *Exp. Brain Res.*, 125: 287–301.

Richmond, B.J., Optican, L.M., Podell, M. and Spitzer, H. (1987) Temporal encoding of two-dimensional patterns by single units in primate inferior temporal cortex. I. Response characteristics. *J. Neurophysiol.*, 57: 132–146.

Robinson, D.A.A. (1963) Method of measuring eye movements using a scleral search coil in a magnetic field. *IEEE Trans. Biomed. Eng.*, 10: 137–145.

Sparks, D.L. and Hartwich-Young, R. (1989) The deep layers of the superior colliculus. *Rev. Oculomot. Res.*, 3: 213–255.

C. Casanova and M. Ptito (Eds.)
Progress in Brain Research, Vol. 134

CHAPTER 8

A possible role of the superior colliculus in eye–hand coordination

Lars Lünenburger [1], Raimund Kleiser [1], Veit Stuphorn [1], Lee E. Miller [2] and Klaus-Peter Hoffmann [1,*]

[1] *Lehrstuhl für Allgemeine Zoologie und Neurobiologie, Ruhr-Universität Bochum, Universitätsstr. 150, 44780 Bochum, Germany*
[2] *Department of Physiology, Northwestern University Medical School, Chicago, IL 60611, USA*

Abstract: Reaching with the arm to a newly appearing target is usually preceded by a saccadic eye movement. Neurons in the superior colliculus (SC) constitute one important brain structure controlling saccades. Yet, the SC also contains reach neurons activated during arm movements, whose location extends also deeper into the underlying mesencephalic reticular formation. Reach neurons can be divided into two classes based on their different modulation with respect to gaze position. For the first class, the gaze-independent reach neurons, the activity does not depend on which location is currently fixated, but solely on the position and movement of the (usually contralateral) arm. There is a correlation of the activity of these neurons with the activity of shoulder muscles. The second class, the gaze-related reach neurons, are active for reaches into a specific area relative to the current point of gaze. This means the target has to project on a certain part of the retina, while it is not important which arm is used or by which trajectory the target will be reached. Many fixation neurons in the rostral pole of the SC discharge tonically during fixation and pause during saccades. For some fixation neurons, the activity can be increased during simultaneous arm movements, for others decreased. Two psychophysical experiments with healthy human subjects show possible behavioral correlates of an interaction between these reach neurons and visuomotor neurons within the SC.

Introduction

The superior colliculus (SC) in the midbrain of mammals is a multilayered structure involved in an orienting response of eyes, ears, head or the whole body towards novel stimuli, termed 'visual grasp reflex' by Akert (1949). Within the different layers of the SC, topographical maps of the visual, acoustic and somatosensory 'worlds' of an animal are organized such that the spatial receptive fields in the different sensory modalities correspond (Updyke, 1977; Meredith and Stein, 1986). The coordinate frames of the different modalities, however, undergo dynamic changes according to the desired motor act, as has been demonstrated for visual and auditory stimuli in the awake monkey (Jay and Sparks, 1987a,b). In primates, motor reactions to targets of interest have been elaborated mostly with respect to gaze shifts and even more so for saccades, which has led to the misconception that the colliculus is merely triggering or inhibiting saccades. But the involvement of the superior colliculus in several other functions, such as fixation, accommodation and avoidance behavior, has also been described. We have been studying the role of neuronal activity in the superior colliculus during arm movements in primates and have identified at least three types of arm-movement-related neurons (Werner, 1993; Werner et al., 1997a,b; Stuphorn et

* Corresponding author: K.-P. Hoffmann, Lehrstuhl für Allgemeine Zoologie und Neurobiologie, Ruhr-Universität Bochum, Universitätsstr. 150, 44780 Bochum, Germany.

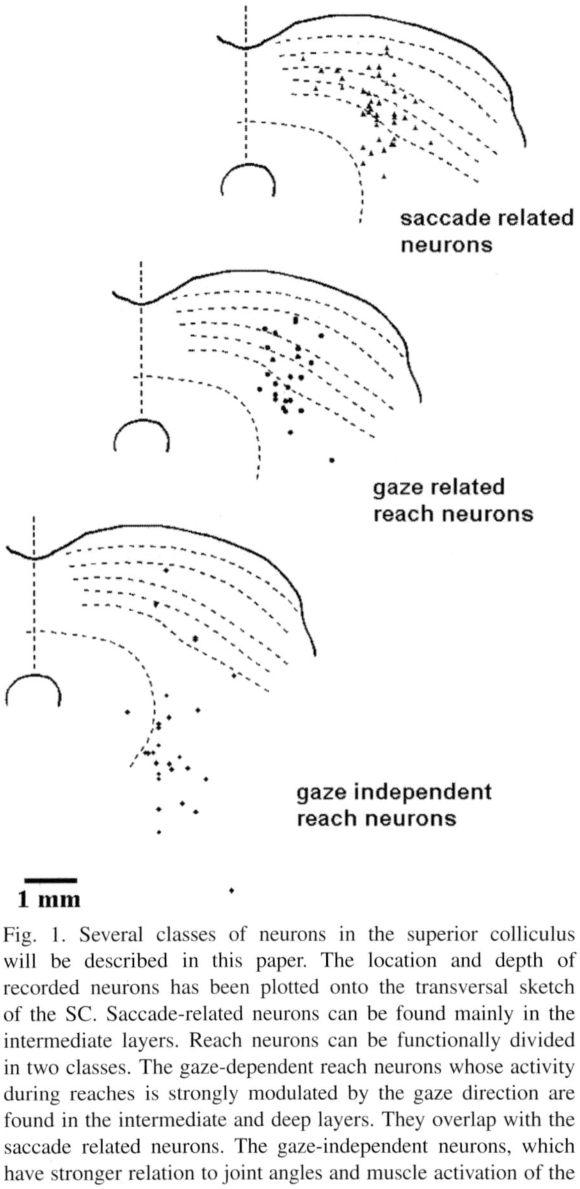

Fig. 1. Several classes of neurons in the superior colliculus will be described in this paper. The location and depth of recorded neurons has been plotted onto the transversal sketch of the SC. Saccade-related neurons can be found mainly in the intermediate layers. Reach neurons can be functionally divided in two classes. The gaze-dependent reach neurons whose activity during reaches is strongly modulated by the gaze direction are found in the intermediate and deep layers. They overlap with the saccade related neurons. The gaze-independent neurons, which have stronger relation to joint angles and muscle activation of the contralateral arm, are usually located deeper in the SC or lie in the underlying mesencephalic reticular formation.

al., 1999). See Fig. 1 for the location of these classes in the SC.

First, neurons in the deepest layers of the superior colliculus and in the underlying reticular formation are active mainly when the contralateral arm is being used; they fire independently of where gaze is being directed. Their firing rate correlates well with the EMG of one or several muscles. These neurons are organized most probably in a shoulder or body centered reference frame.

Second, neurons in the intermediate layers are active before and during arm movements to targets that are represented in a gaze-dependent reference frame. These neurons fire independently of the arm being used provided the target is presented in a particular sector of the retina.

Third, neurons in the rostral pole of the colliculus, which are known as fixation neurons in the oculomotor community, are strongly modulated by ongoing arm movements. So far, we have found examples where during the arm movement the firing rate is decreased or more interestingly increased.

In this article, we review our current knowledge along two lines: (1) Does the reach activity in the SC code the position of the target in retinal coordinates or is the modulation during reaching based on a spatial/body-centered reference frame? (2) In how far is the reach activity in the SC modulating eye–hand coordination or is the neuronal activity related to the EMG of muscles of the shoulder and arm?

Behavioral paradigms

Two different arm-movement tasks were used to probe the relationship of a cell to reach movements, a 'saccade-reach' (SR) task and a 'fixation-reach' (FR) task. The general outline of the two tasks is shown in Fig. 2. Both the SR and the FR tasks began in the same way. The monkey had to touch a metal bar located near its hip and to fixate a small light spot appearing on the screen. After a randomized interval (1–1.4 s), a target light was turned on. From here on the two tasks differed. In the saccade-reach task, the fixation LED was extinguished after a randomized delay (0.5–0.9 s). In response the monkey made a saccade to the illuminated target and fixated it (Fig. 2, left). After a second randomized delay (0.5–1.4 s), a tone ('go' signal) came on that instructed the monkey to reach towards the fixated target. In the fixation reach task, the starting cue for the arm movement (the acoustic 'go' signal) was given after a randomized delay (1–1.4 s), while the fixation light on the screen remained on. The monkey had to maintain fixation, while it reached to the peripheral target (Fig. 2, right). After touching the target for

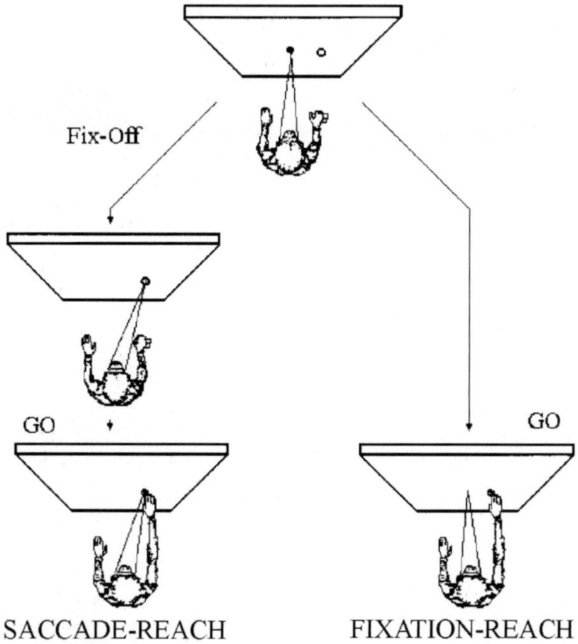

Fig. 2. The monkey performed two tasks that began in the same way, after it touched a metal knob near its hip. A visual target appeared on the screen that had to be fixated, while later a second visual target appeared peripherally. In the saccade-reach (SR) task (left part) the fixation point switched off and the monkey had to look to the peripheral target. An acoustic 'go' signal made the monkey to reach to the target. In the fixation-reach (FR) task the 'go' signal appeared while the fixation point was still on and had to be fixated. The monkey had to make a reach to the peripheral target, but had to keep fixating.

approximately 1 s, the monkey returned its arm to the initial starting position at hip level and received a liquid reward. A delayed saccade task and the two reach tasks were all performed in alternating blocks of at least five trials. The targets for the arm movements were an array of eight metal knobs, each containing an LED. The fixation light could appear at three different sites, i.e. either centrally (F1), or 19° lateral from the body midline (F2), or 19° below eye level (F3). The eight targets were arranged at a distance of 15° on the four corners of the three squares around the fixation points (compare Fig. 7). In that way, the monkey had to fixate at different locations, but make the very same arm movement.

For details on surgery and recording see Stuphorn et al. (1999, 2000). All procedures were approved by a local ethics committee and followed the European Communities Council Directive (86/609/EEC) and the National Institutes of Health Guidelines for Care and Use of Animals for Experimental Procedures.

Gaze-independent neurons

We describe here the activity of reach neurons recorded up to a depth of 6 mm below the collicular surface. Those up to 4 mm below the collicular surface are considered to be located in the SC for the following three reasons: (1) the overlap with saccadic neurons such as described e.g. by Sparks et al. (1976), and which are located mainly in the intermediate SC layers (sometimes reach and saccadic neurons in these layers could be recorded simultaneously); (2) the fact that the SC reaches approximately 1.5 mm deeper than the most ventrally located saccadic neurons described by Ma et al. (1991); (3) the location of small electrolytic lesions which were placed at recording sites of reach-related cells. Reach neurons deeper than 4 mm below the collicular surface are considered to be in the mesencephalic reticular formation. We found no differences in the properties of gaze-independent neurons related to recording depth.

Fig. 3 shows a cell exhibiting three types of neuronal modulation: Illumination of the peripheral target (T) located within the neuron's visual receptive field to the right of the fixation point (Fig. 3, upper panel) evoked a typical visual response with a latency of 42 ms. Upon extinction of the fixation light the monkey performed saccades (S) to the target which were accompanied by short bursts with high discharge rates. A third strong modulation component was visible with the beginning (M) of the arm movement. When located 15° to the left of the fixation point (Fig. 3, bottom), illumination of the target did not evoke any visual response, and the following saccade was not associated with an activity burst. Arm reaching movements to that target, however, were again accompanied by an activity increase. The activation during reaching was usually much stronger when the monkey used the arm contralateral to the recorded SC unit. The ratio calculated from the discharge rate during reaching with the contralateral relative to the ipsilateral arm was 3.19 (median value of 26 neurons). This test included midsagittal

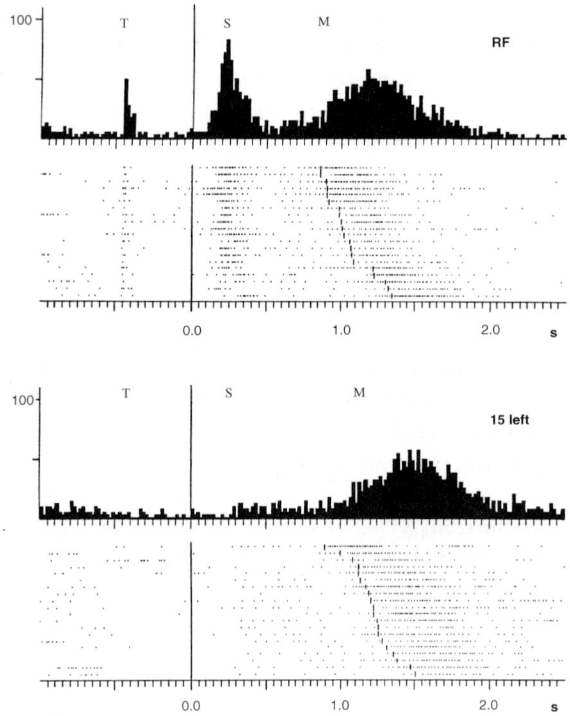

Fig. 3. Activity of a gaze-independent reach neuron in a saccade-reach task into the receptive field to the right (top) and in the opposite direction (bottom). For targets in the receptive field, the neuron shows increased activity in three time windows. The activity is higher after the appearance of the target (T), during the saccade (S) and during the arm movement (M). Targets 15° to the left did not fall into the visual receptive field and did not evoke any visual response (T). The saccade to this target did not lead to an activation during the saccade (S). The activation during the arm movement (M) is similar to the top panel. This indicates low spatial specificity for the reach activity of this neuron.

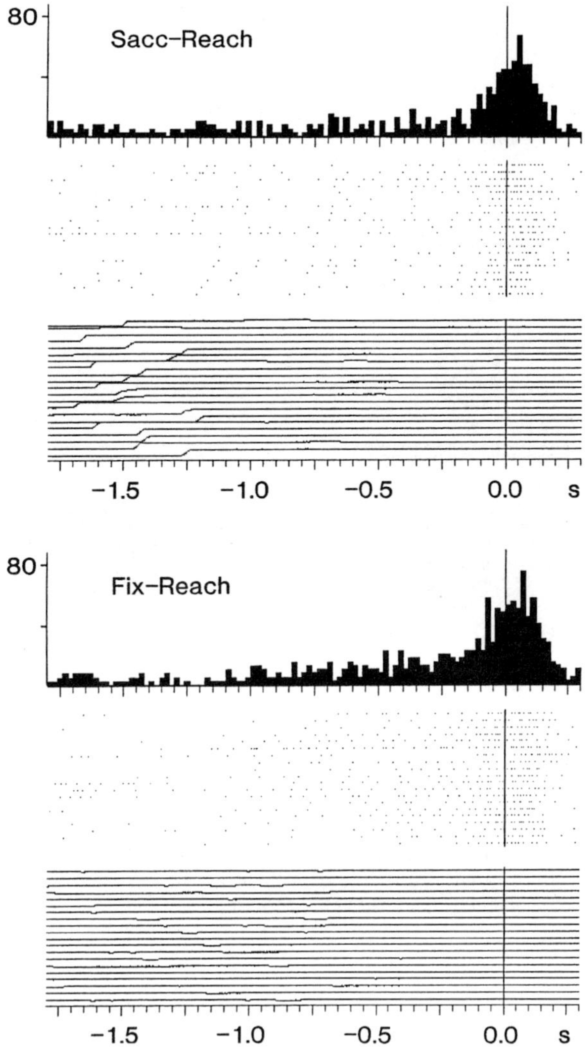

Fig. 4. The comparison of a reach activity for different fixation positions. In the SR task (top), the monkey made a saccade to the target and foveated it before starting with the arm (at 0 s). The activity before and during this arm movement is similar to the same time interval in a FR task (bottom) where the monkey was fixating a central target while reaching to the target projecting onto the peripheral retina.

or lateral targets with corresponding locations relative to the hand starting position, i.e. arm movements involving the same muscles of either side.

The possible independence of reach activity from oculomotor variables was further tested by investigating neuronal discharge during reaching to the same target, but with different eye positions. In the saccade-reach trials (Fig. 4, top) the monkey first performed saccades to the targets and then, while looking at them, started an arm movement in order to touch them. In the second condition, the monkey kept fixating the central LED while performing arm movements to the same targets, which in these trials were still on the peripheral retina (Fig. 4, bottom). Under both conditions, a comparable activity increase was found.

It was a general finding that the direction selectivity of visual and saccade responses was not strictly related to the tuning of the reach activity, which was broad and showed different preferred directions in different cells recorded at the same location. The ratio of discharge rates for preferred versus non-preferred reaching direction was 2.31 (median value of $n = 66$ neurons). To test whether there is a map-like arrangement of the preferred directions of gaze-independent neurons parallel to the collicular surface, the monkey had to reach to four to eight locations arranged on a circle on the tangent screen and the preferred reach direction was calculated as the vector sum. We then plotted these vectors of preferred direction on the simplified visual map of the SC (see Fig. 5)

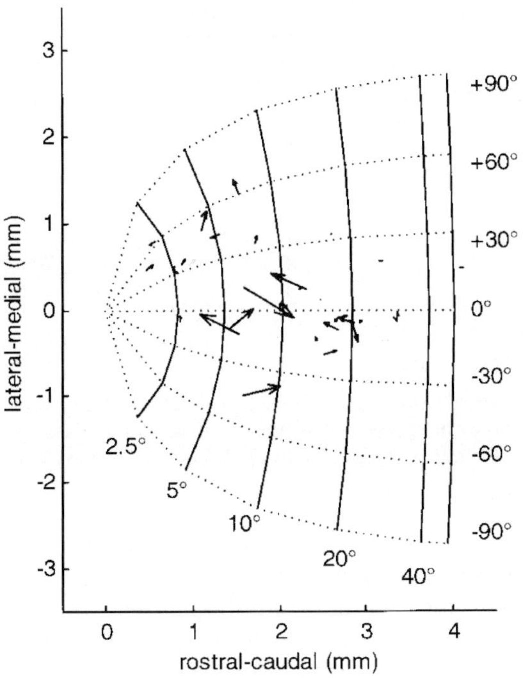

Fig. 5. Location of the preferred directions for the gaze-independent reach neurons with respect to their location in the SC. Location of the preferred direction was calculated by the vector sum of the discharge measured during arm movements in the fixation task to the four locations orthogonally arranged around the fixation point. The length of the vector indicates the directional selectivity determined by projecting the activity amplitudes of the four reaching movements on the calculated preferred direction vector. Although recordings were made from both SC, all calculated directions are plotted with respect to the left SC. Therefore vectors pointing to the right indicate preferred reach targets in the visual hemifield contralateral to the recorded SC. Vectors pointing to the left indicate preferred reach targets in the visual hemifield ipsilateral to the recorded SC. All vectors were plotted on a simplified oculomotor map of the SC (Ottes et al., 1986). Vector origin was placed at the coordinates of the visual receptive field measured in the same penetration while passing through the superficial layers.

using the equations of Ottes et al. (1986) to determine the anterior-posterior and medio-lateral position of a reach neuron in the SC from the visual receptive field measured in the same penetration during the passage of the superficial layers. The cell's location according to this visual map serves as the origin of the respective vector of preferred direction. The orientation of the resulting vector pointed in the direction of the reach, which yielded the strongest increase in discharge for that cell. The length of the vector increases with a sharper spatial selectivity of the cell. Most vectors are rather short and indicate that these neurons have a weak spatial tuning. The orientation of the preferred directions reveals no obvious topographic ordering. Adjacent vectors often have opposite directions. The gaze-independent neurons have a much weaker topographic organization than the gaze-related reach neurons, as we will see later (Fig. 10).

Correlation with EMGs of shoulder muscles

The contribution of a neuron in the SC to a reaching movement with the arm could be reflected either in the modulation of its discharge rate in relation to different reach directions or in the strength of the cross-correlation between its instantaneous discharge frequency and the EMGs of certain muscles involved in the reach. The contribution of discharge rate to the direction of the hand during the reach has been analyzed in a great number of papers for cortical neurons (Georgopoulos et al., 1986, 1988; Kettner et al., 1988; Schwartz et al., 1988) and for neurons in the superior colliculus by Kutz et al. (1997). Here we look at the number of significant correlations between the instantaneous discharge frequency of a collicular neuron and the EMGs of muscles in the shoulder and trunk during different reach directions. We do this to find out whether this correlation of a single SC neuron is more indicative of the direction of arm movement or of the muscles involved. In addition, discharge rate and correlation strength could be aligned. Therefore, we look at the tuning of correlation strength for different reach directions in comparison with the tuning of the discharge rate of the neuron. Recent results from Werner et al. (1997a,b) and Stuphorn et al. (1999) already suggested that there is a close relationship between the

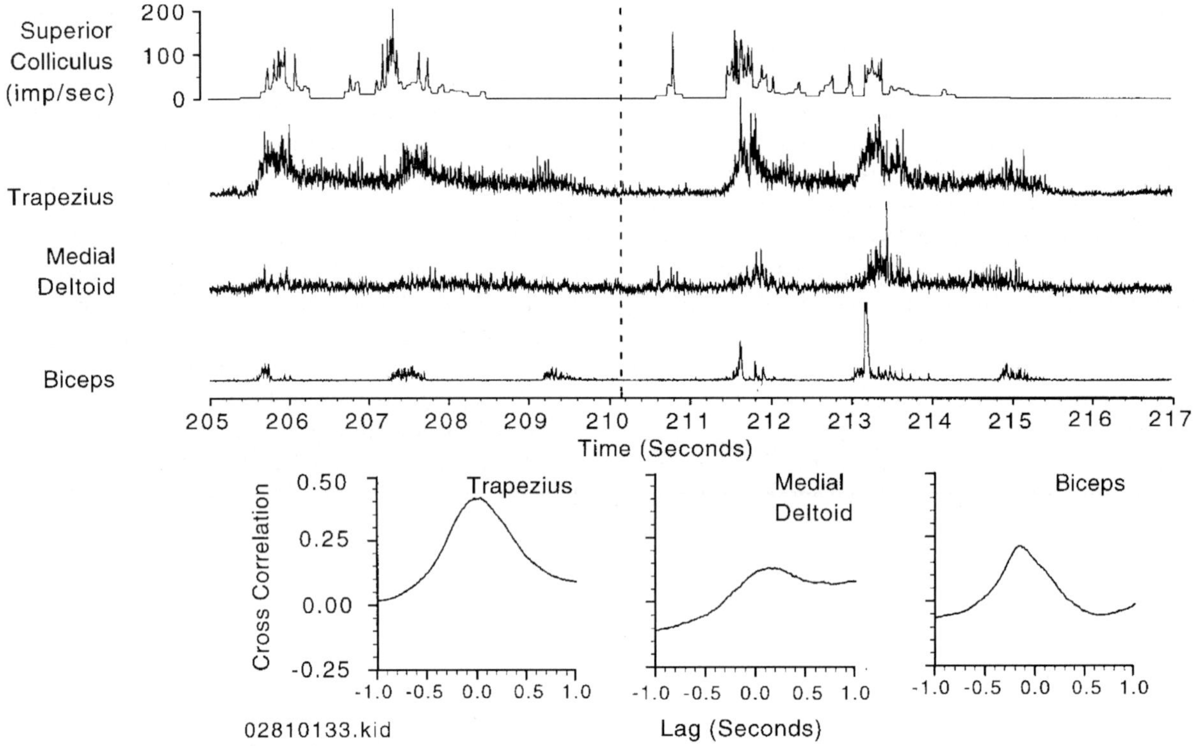

Fig. 6. Top: Firing rate of a collicular neuron (1.77 mm below the surface of the left SC) displayed with activity of several simultaneously recorded muscles. The trapezius electromyogram was very similar to the neuronal discharge during these two successive trials. The dotted line denotes the time where the recording was interrupted between the trials. Bottom: Cross-correlations between the neuronal and muscle activity for the entire file. The best correlation was found for the trapezius.

EMG activity pattern of shoulder muscles and neuronal activity of units in the deep layers of the SC as well as in the underlying reticular formation. In order to further quantify this functional relationship, the activity of single neurons in these structures was recorded in two monkeys while the animals reached to eight visual targets equally spaced along a circle on a tangent screen in a center-out-task. Thus, the monkey first moved its hand to the center of the target array and then moved it outwards to one of the targets. Simultaneously, the EMGs of 11 muscles of the arm and shoulder were recorded. To do this, bipolar 'patch' electrodes were chronically implanted in the M. deltoideus anterior (ADl), M. biceps brachii (Bic), M. flexor digitorum superficialis (FDS), M. infraspinatus (Inf), M. latissimus dorsi (Lat), M. deltoideus medialis (MD1), M. pectoralis major (Pec), M. rhomboideus major (Rhom), M. teres major (TMj), M. triceps brachii (Tri), and M. trapezius (Trp). We computed cross correlation functions between instantaneous discharge frequency of 126 neurons and the rectified EMGs of the 11 muscles separately for the eight different directions of arm movements. A shift predictor was always subtracted. Only peaks in the correlation function with lags between neural activity and EMGs of −200 ms (EMG leading) to +300 ms (neuron leading) were considered. We have found clear and highly specific correlations between the neuronal activity in the SC and the EMGs of muscles of the contralateral arm as well as shoulder (Fig. 6). These correlations of one neuron are present most often with one muscle in a narrow range of directions. About half of the neurons are correlated with several muscles. Again this correlation of one neuron is significant more often in one particular direction of arm movement than with particular muscles in different directions of arm movements. For a particular neuron, the vector sum of the movement directions with significant correlations has the tendency to point into the same spatial quadrant (up, left, down, right) as the vector sum of the neural activity, i.e. the preferred direction of a neuron and its strongest correlation with the EMG of shoulder and arm muscles coincide. This seems to suggest that the neurons in the colliculus we studied are more involved in the spatial parameters during the preparation of the arm movement than in a direct link to the motor output.

Gaze-dependent neurons

Characteristics of the gaze-related reach neurons

The typical activity pattern of a gaze-related reach neuron in the SR-task is shown in Fig. 7. The discharge of this sample neuron is presented in relation to onset of arm movements. The 12 histograms were compiled in sets of four according to the arrangement of four reach targets around each of the three fixation points (+). All movements were made with the contralateral (here the right) arm. They started with the hand approximately at waist level and were directed to one of the eight targets (1–8), positioned on a frontal screen as outlined in the sketch in the bottom right corner of Fig. 7. Activation was observed only when the arm was directed to a target at the lower right with respect to the fixation point. This occurred with targets 5, 6 and 8. But if the same arm movement (e.g. to target 5) was performed with eye positions, that shift the target location with respect to the gaze axis, i.e. to the upper right or lower left the neuron displayed no reach-related activity. The neuron was also not active during reaching when the same eight targets were fixated in the SR task (not shown).

Even for the same target location with respect to the gaze direction, the cell discharge is different for the three orbital positions of the eyes during the reach. It is very prominent in the histograms of Fig. 7 for reaches to the lower right, targets 5, 6 and 8 for the three fixation positions, respectively. This eye position effect occurred across the tested oculomotor range for all gaze-related reach cells.

All these experiments demonstrate that the reach-related activity of this neuron is locked to a gaze-related coordinate system and cannot be described in an allocentric or body-centered reference frame. Nevertheless, its activity is in close temporal relationship to the arm movement, preceding the onset of movement by approximately 200 ms. We call the area of target coordinates in a gaze-related frame of reference that is accompanied by neuronal activity the 'reach movement field' (RMF). It is important to note that both, the specific path of the arm movement and the muscle pattern that is necessary for its realization, are of no consequence for the neuron's discharge. Two neurons of the 25 gaze-related neurons also produced saccade-related bursts, but we found no relationship between these components and particular characteristics of the reach-related activity.

Activity of the gaze-related reach neurons during reaching with the ipsilateral arm

In order to see whether the reach neurons show a preference for the use of the arm contra- or ipsilateral to the recorded neuron in the SC we let the monkey perform the FR-task with either arm. A comparison of the neuronal discharge reveals that the neuron displays the same pattern of activity with an identical spatial tuning and almost the same amount of spikes irrespective of which arm is used, although anatomically different muscles execute the reach movements.

A quantitative comparison of the mean activity during the reach with the ipsilateral or contralateral arm is done for eight neurons for the eight targets accessible with both arms. The line of best fit shows that on average the cells are equally active irrespective of which arm is used (Fig. 8). All in all, a population of gaze-related reach neurons in the colliculus becomes activated during a goal-directed reach. The activation is independent of which muscles or arm are involved in the reach.

Reach movement fields (RMF)

We found that the RMFs of gaze-related reach neurons differed with respect to their peripheral borders. In six neurons, the RMFs were partially mapped by presenting reach targets further and further away from the preferred retinal target position. Fig. 9 shows three examples of these cells. Neuronal discharge of the cells is shown while the monkey fixated a certain position on the screen (the cross) and reached to a number of targets (indicated by position of the histograms). The amplitude of reach activity

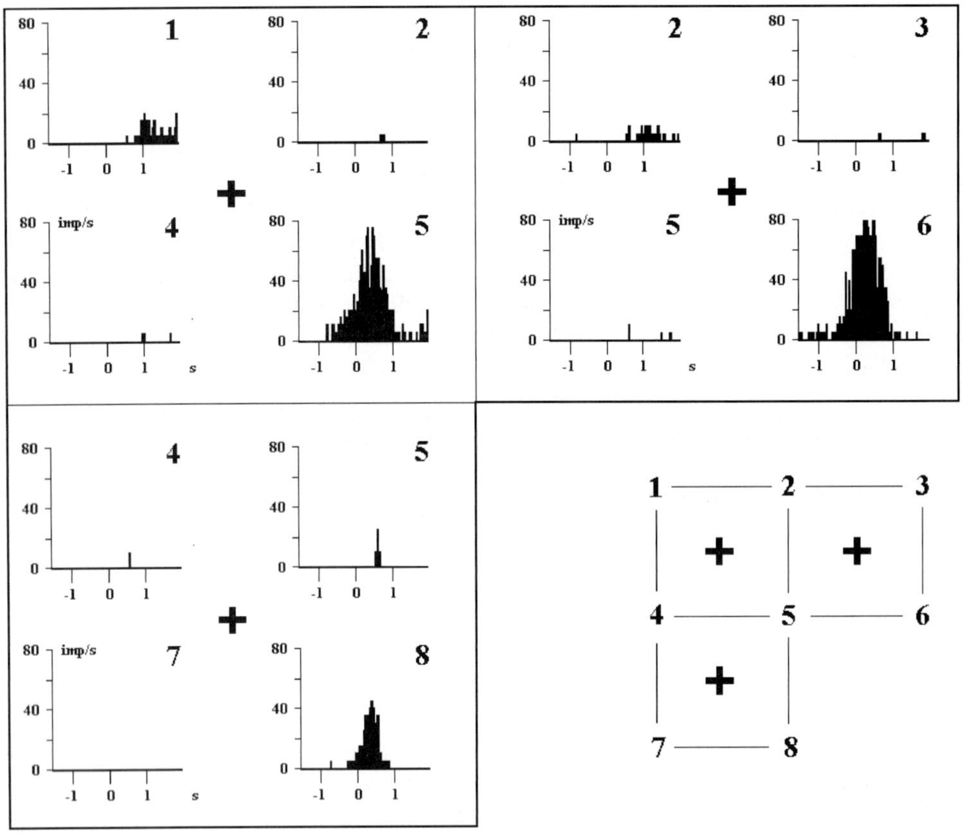

Fig. 7. Gaze-related reach neurons have different activity during reaches to the same target in space when the monkey fixates different points. This example neuron was recorded in the left colliculus 1.96 mm below the surface. The position of each histogram relative to the cross corresponds to the position of the reach target relative to the fixation point, the position of the block of histograms to the relative location of the fixation point. The numbers identify the eight reach targets, whose spatial positions are sketched in the inset. Although the movement of the arm is always the same for the histograms with the same target, i.e. the same number, the activity is different for different fixation positions.

increased when the monkey was reaching to more peripheral targets to the right in the cell presented in the top part of Fig. 9. This suggested that its RMF occupies a large area of the visual field and may possibly have no clear peripheral border at all. Such patterns of neuronal activation were seen in four of the six neurons tested. The other two cells allowed no clear conclusion due to the limited number of tested locations (see middle part of Fig. 9). In addition to these cells, we also recorded three neurons with a large difference in activity between saccade-reach and fixation-reach. The example in the lower part of Fig. 9 shows low activation for peripheral reaches (FR, left) and high activation for foveal reaches (SR, right). Another observation is the identical amplitude of the discharge for all spatial positions in the SR-task. Since the arm movements are the same in the two tasks, once again the difference in response must be due to the gaze-related target position. These neurons seem to have RMFs, which are positioned on the fovea and whose peripheral borders lie somewhere between the fovea and the targets with an eccentricity of 15°.

Distribution of RMF direction on the SC

Like for the gaze-independent neurons, we looked for a topographic map of the RMFs of the gaze-dependent neurons concerning their direction and spatial selectivity. Vectors characterizing the RMFs

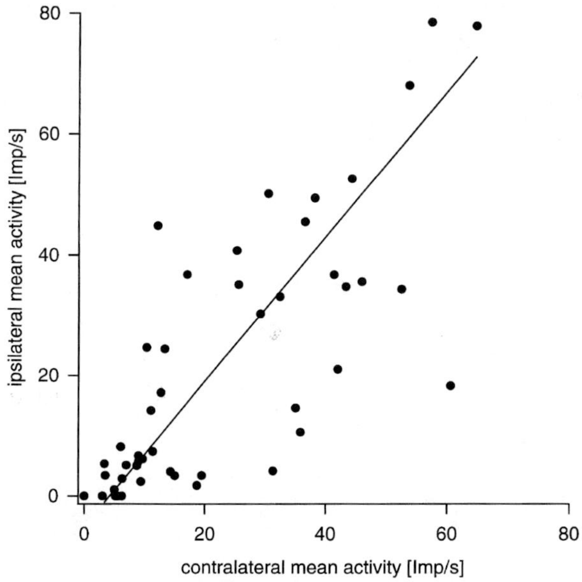

Fig. 8. The mean activity of gaze-related cells during use of the ipsi- and the contralateral arm to reach to the same target in space in the FR task. In the scatter plot, data from eight neurons are displayed. Each of the 64 dots shows the mean neuronal activity of one neuron while the monkey reached to one of the four targets surrounding each fixation point F1 and F2 (see Fig. 6). The many dots near the origin (not all are visible due to overlap) represent no or weak activity during reaches to non-preferred targets. Activity during the reach with the contralateral arm is presented on the *x*-axis and during the reach with the ipsilateral arm on the *y*-axis. Note that the neuronal activity of the gaze-related neurons is independent of the arm used to perform the movement (slope of line of best fit 1.2, $R^2 = 0.64$).

were constructed by the vector sum of the normalized neuronal activity during reaching to each of the four targets. Similarly to Fig. 5, we plotted the vectors of the RMFs onto the visual map of the SC (see Fig. 10). The RMFs of the gaze-related reach neurons could be directed either into the ipsi- or the contralateral hemifield, i.e. the preferred reach target location could be in the entire visual field and was not restricted to the contralateral hemifield, which is in sharp contrast to the organization of the visual map and saccadic movement fields. In addition, gaze-related reach cells recorded in a single penetration next to each other repeatedly showed clearly different RMF positions. Nevertheless, a closer inspection of Fig. 10 might reveal a weak organizing principle. The subpopulation that was recorded in the medial part of the colliculus corresponding to the upper visual field consisted mostly (8/13) of cells with RMFs also directed upwards. Correspondingly, the lateral part of the SC was dominated by gaze-related reach neurons with downward directed RMFs (8/12). All seven reach cells located in the rostral part of the SC (0–1 mm in Fig. 10) had RMFs directed into the ipsilateral hemifield whereas 13 of the 18 reach cells with more caudal locations in the SC (1–4 mm in Fig. 10) had RMFs directed into the contralateral hemifield. This organizational structure is much more pronounced for these gaze-dependent than for the gaze-independent reach neurons shown in Fig. 5.

Fixation neurons

The rostral pole of the superior colliculus contains neurons that are tonically active during fixation and are completely inhibited during saccades. The activity of these fixation neurons is thought to counterbalance the activity of saccadic build-up neurons (Munoz and Wurtz, 1993a,b, 1995a,b; Munoz and Istvan, 1998; Krauzlis et al., 2000).

Many recorded fixation neurons in our paradigm showed a modulation of their activity during arm movements. Fig. 11 shows a 'relative time histogram' of the activity of a fixation neuron during the SR task. To eliminate the trial-by-trial variation in the duration of different behavioral elements in the SR task, we divided these elements into a fixed number of bins that remained the same in each trial. The SR task was divided into eight successive behavioral elements. First, the 'waiting phase' (50 bins, before T) lasted from fixation onset until target onset. Second, the 'delay phase' (50 bins, T to O) lasted from target onset until the fixation point was switched off. Third, the 'saccadic reaction time' (12 bins, O to S) covered the time between fixation off and start of the saccade. Fourth, the 'saccade phase' (13 bins, S to F) extends from the start of the saccade to its end. Fifth, the 'fixation phase' (50 bins, F to G) starts at the end of the saccade and ends with the acoustic 'go' signal. Sixth, the 'reach reaction time' (20 bins, G to M) lasted from the 'go' signal to onset of the movement. Seventh, the 'movement phase' (10 bins, M to C) lasted from onset of the arm movement until the hand made contact with the target. Eighth, the 'target-hold phase' (35 bins, following C) finally

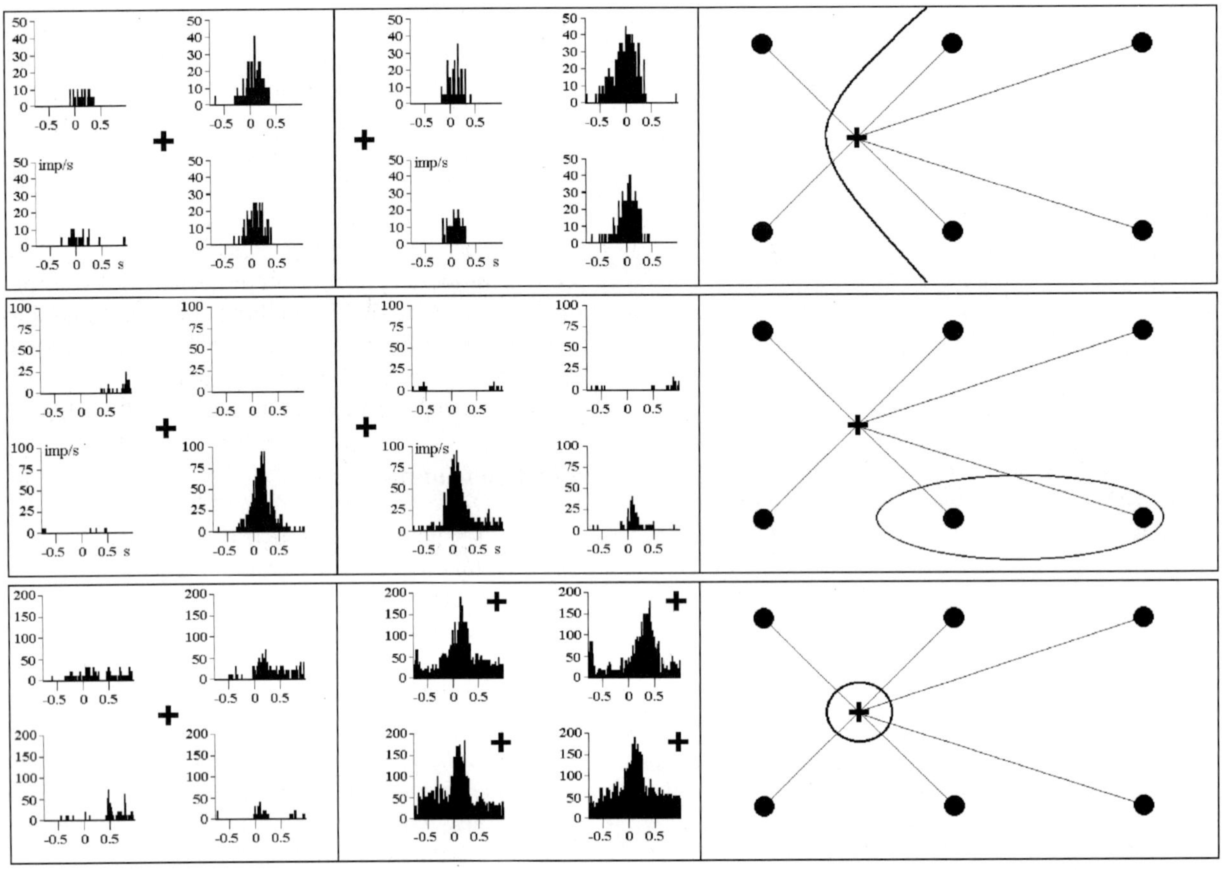

Fig. 9. If eye position effects play a small role, we were able to reconstruct reach movement fields (RMF) for some gaze-dependent reach neurons. The neuron in the top panel shows higher activity when the targets are further to the right of the fixation point. This may be depicted by an open RMF covering the right hemifield (right part). For the neurons in the middle panel, almost no activity was recorded for reaches above the fixation point. Because reaches with larger eccentricity elicited no response, the RMF seems closed and covers a part of the lower right quadrant. The neurons in the bottom panel show no activation in FR task, but high activation in SR task for all targets. The RMF covers an area around the fovea with eccentricities smaller than 15°.

lasted from contact with the target until its release at the beginning of the return movement. The number of bins for each phase was chosen in such a way that one bin accounted on average for about 20 ms. The actual time represented by such a bin could vary with the duration of the respective phase in the trials. Therefore the activity in a certain bin does not represent the mean activity in real time relative to a trigger point but rather the mean activity in a certain phase of the respective behavioral element. For example the first bin of the 'movement phase' shows the average discharge during the first 10% of the arm movement.

The fixation neuron in Fig. 11 is not active at all during the saccade to the target at S. After the saccade, it has again a steady-state rate higher than before (F–G). During the arm movement (M) after the 'go'-signal, the rate is even further increased.

The fixation neurons recorded so far show a diverse behavior. Some increase their discharge rate significantly during the arm movement, whereas others show a pause just like during saccades. Their role in eye hand coordination will be discussed later.

Eye–hand coordination

To examine the possible functional role of the reach-related neurons in the superior colliculus, we con-

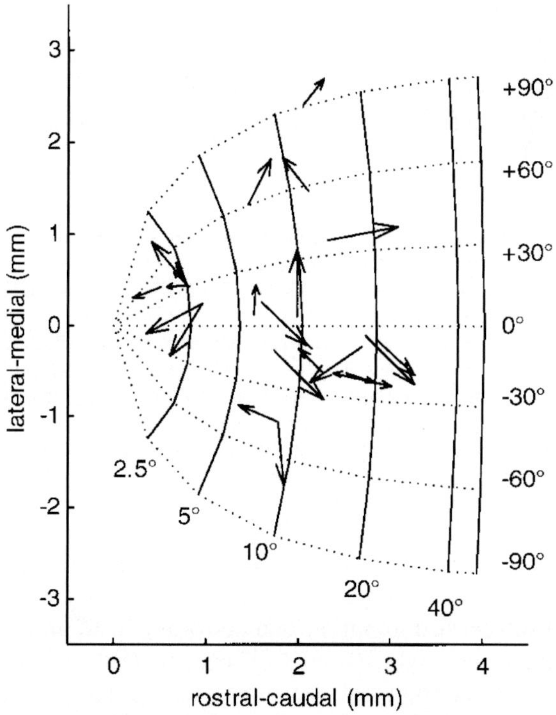

Fig. 10. Using the same construction methods as in Fig. 5 for gaze-related reach neurons ($n = 25$), we find a higher topographical organization than for gaze-independent neurons. However, it is not as strict as the visual or oculomotor map. Neurons in the medial half have preferentially upward RMFs; those in the lateral half have preferentially downward RMFs. Neurons in the rostral part have RMFs in the ipsilateral hemifield, a feature that is not present in the visual and oculomotor map in primates.

ducted psychophysical experiments in human subjects. The presence of information on arm movements in this structure leads one to expect an interaction between the control systems of eyes and arm. This interaction, i.e. influence of saccades on simultaneous arm movements or influence of the arm movement on the saccade, has been the subject of a large number of studies (Prablanc et al., 1979a,b; Biguer et al., 1982; Gielen et al., 1984; Rogal et al., 1985; Mather and Fisk, 1985).

In the present experiments, healthy human subjects had to look or look and point at a visual target. In the first experimental series, this target was displaced horizontally from a central to an eccentric position. With this single-step experiment, we explored how the initiation of eye and arm movements starting at the same point is coordinated. The second experiment involved double-step displaced targets, which required on-line correction of the ongoing movements. Here the different strategies for reacting to sudden target displacements were examined in both systems.

Single-step experiment

In the single-step experiment, the visual targets consisted of red LEDs. Buttons were mounted immediately below to record the manual responses (for more detailed description see Lünenburger et al., 2000). After extinction of the central LED, the target LED went on 29° eccentric, randomly to the left or the right. In half of the trials the eccentric LED went on only after 200 ms of darkness (gap-paradigm; Saslow, 1967; Boch et al., 1984; Fischer and Ramsperger, 1984). In saccade-reach tasks the subjects initially look at the central target while pressing the corresponding button with the (preferred) right hand (Fig. 12, left column). In the coupled saccade-reach task (cSRT), the computer moves the target after a random fixation period of 1500–1700 ms. When the target jumps, the subject has to look and reach as fast as possible to the lighted LED and press the corresponding button. In the saccade task, only eye movements were required and the hand rested on the table in front of the subject. Reaction times for the saccades were calculated from the eye traces recorded by the cornea-reflection system OBER2 (Permobil Meditech AB, Sweden) by a relative velocity threshold (10% of peak velocity) and visual inspection.

Subjects usually respond to such stimuli with a saccade in ST and a sequence of a saccade and a hand movement in SRT. Although this sequential response gives the possibility to visually guide the hand near the (already fixated) target, there might be a strong biomechanical constraint from the different inertia of the eyes and the arm.

In ST, the well-known gap-effect (Saslow, 1967; Fischer and Ramsperger, 1984) leads to reduced reaction times when the fixation point is off before target onset. In our case, the difference of the medians pooled over all 14 subjects and both directions is 27 ms (182 vs. 155 ms; cf. Fig. 12, right column). Simultaneous movement of the arm in cSRT leads to reduction in saccadic reaction time for movements

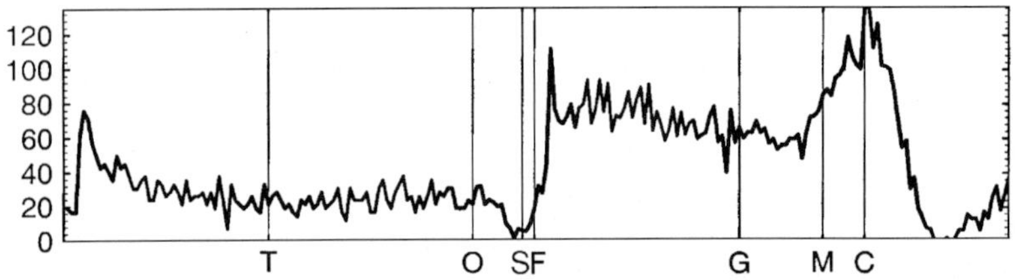

Fig. 11. Relative time histogram of a fixation neuron in the SR task. The time intervals between the behavioral events are normalized to the average values. The initial 'waiting phase' after fixating the central target and before the target appears (T) is divided into 50 bins. The monkey has to keep fixation further during the 'delay phase' (50 bins) until the fixation spot is switched off (O). The 'saccadic reaction time' (from O to S) is variable trial-by-trial, but partitioned into 12 bins. The 'saccade phase' (3 bins) from saccade start (S) to begin of fixation at the target position (F) is followed by the 'fixation phase', which comprises 50 bins until appearance of the acoustic 'go'-signal (G). The 'reach reaction time' from G to movement onset (M) is divided into 20 bins. The 'movement phase' from movement onset (M) until contact of the hand with the target button (C) contains 10 bins. The monkey had to hold this contact during the 'target holding phase' extending 35 bins after C. One bin accounted for 20 ms on average. The actual time represented by such a bin could vary with the duration of the respective phase in the trials. This fixation neuron shows decreased activity during saccades and transiently increased activity after saccades. This example shows a further increase during the reach movement.

to the right. This reduction is 11.5 ms without gap and 15 ms with gap. The contradiction to the reported increase in reaction time (Mather and Fisk, 1985; Bekkering et al., 1994, 1995) might be caused (apart from different pooling strategies) by the following difference in the paradigm. Given that the saccade is timed in a fixed temporal distance before the end of the hand movement (Helsen et al., 2000), the reduction of reaction time in our subjects results from the instruction to move as fast as possible.

When a saccade is not accurate enough to bring the target on the fovea, it is usually followed by a corrective saccade. Our subjects made at least one correction saccade in 62.1% of ST trials. When moving eyes and hand (cSRT trials) only 43.9% of the trials contained one or more correction saccades. Furthermore, the observed correction saccades in cSRT were smaller in median than those recorded in ST. In cSRT undershoot was −3.62% (median) of target amplitude in contrast to −4.15% in ST. However, the scatter of the endpoints of saccades that were followed by a correction saccade was larger in cSRT than in ST for most (9 of 13) subjects. This means that although the first saccade landed more often nearer (error rate and error size) to the target its endpoints were more scattered when a simultaneous arm movement was required.

The cSRT featured a common trigger and command to both — eye and hand — control systems, i.e. eye and hand moved from equal targets to equal targets after a common stimulus. This was changed in the uncoupled saccade-reach task (uSRT). Here the subject had to initiate and perform a hand movement to the right button (self-paced). Hand movement onset triggered the movement of the visual target, randomly to the right or the left. This means the subject had to produce a saccade to the same target the hand was is already moving to (compatible), or to the target contraversive to the on-going arm movement (incompatible). The saccadic reaction time is increased for incompatible movements compared to saccade alone (204 vs. 195 ms), it is decreased for compatible movements (195 vs. 200.5 ms).

Double-step experiment

For the double-step experiments, we built a virtual reality setup to allow arbitrary changes of position and timing of the targets. The subject views a downward-facing 20-inch computer screen via a half-silvered mirror tilted 45° with respect to vertical. The mirror image of the screen lies in a fronto-parallel plane 44 cm in front of the subject. The target — a red ball of 1.2 cm diameter — can be moved on a horizontal line in this plane. At the beginning of each trial, the target appeared on the midline. After 1500–1700 ms the target was displaced 10.2 cm (13.1°) to the right or the left. Afterwards the target was displaced either 5.1 cm back medially (6.5°) or further peripherally (6.0°) after a delay of 300 or

500 ms, or it stayed there. The target was visible for another 1500 ms before the next trial began after 100 ms of darkness. The subjects had to look at the target and make saccades to it in the ST. In cSRT, the subjects additionally had to point to the targets with the index finger of their (preferred) right hand (Fig. 13, top row). The ball had to be be touched with the tip of the index finger, which was visible through the mirror.

Example traces (Fig. 13) show that subjects respond with two distinct saccades and occasional correction saccades. The finger trajectory is much slower and usually does not allow discriminating two sub-movements. Especially for medial second steps one can see smooth redirection and online correction.

In ST, the median saccadic reaction times are 169 ms for the first saccade. For the second saccade, it is significantly higher, 196 ms with 300 ms delay and 171 ms with 500 ms delay (Fig. 13, bottom row). The reaction time for the first saccade is reduced to 161 ms in cSRT. However, it is increased for the second saccade for cSRT, 205.5 ms for 300 ms delay and 184 ms for 500 ms delay. This means that a simultaneous arm movement has a facilitating effect on the first saccade and a retarding effect on the second saccade.

Discussion

In this paper, we presented electrophysiological data from monkeys and psychophysical results from humans. Different classes of neurons in the SC have been described, differing in coding scheme and correlation to muscle activation. Gaze-independent reach neurons code in a shoulder or body centered reference frame, and their activity is often correlated with activity of individual shoulder and arm muscles. Gaze-dependent reach neurons are active independently of the motor implementation of the reach, as long as the reached target has a specific location relative to the current point of gaze. Some fixation neurons show modulation by a simultaneous arm movement. We will discuss the relation of the psychophysical finding with other recent psychophysical work, and will comment on the relevance of the reach neurons for the observed phenomena.

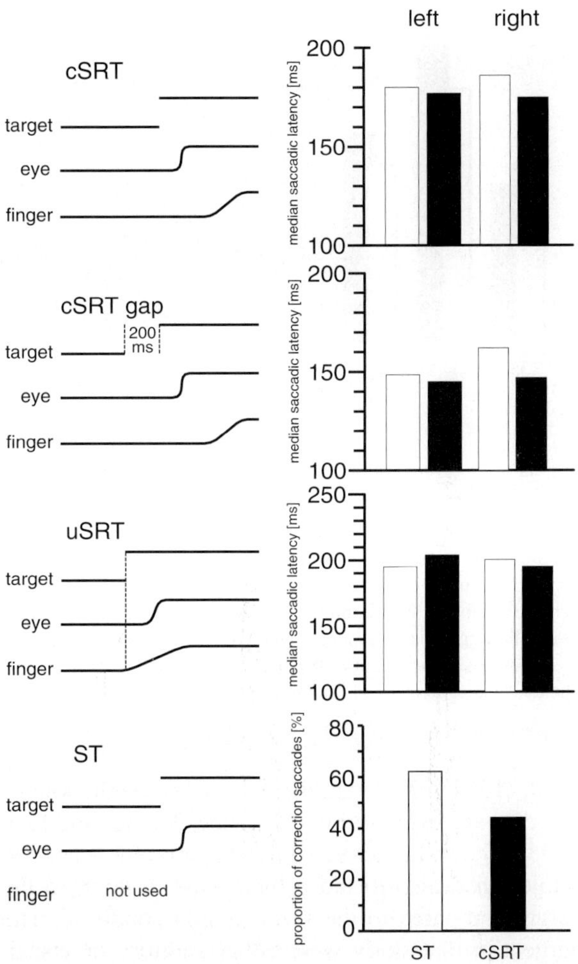

Fig. 12. The four different tasks used in this single-step experiment are depicted in the left column. Each row sketches the horizontal movements of target, eyes and fingertip. The medians of the resulting reaction times of all trials of all subjects are shown in the right column. White bars show the results in the saccade task (ST, only eye movements) in comparison to the saccade reach task in this row. Reaction times are reduced in the coupled saccade-reach task, both with and without gap (cSRT and cSRT gap), compared to ST. In the uncoupled saccade-reach task (uSRT, saccade-target displacement at onset of self-initiated hand movement to the right button), reaction times are shorter than in ST when the saccade was in the same direction as the ongoing hand movement (right). However, saccades in the opposite direction of the arm movement (left) had longer reaction times. The bottom figure in the right column shows that in cSRT trials fewer correction saccades occurred than in ST.

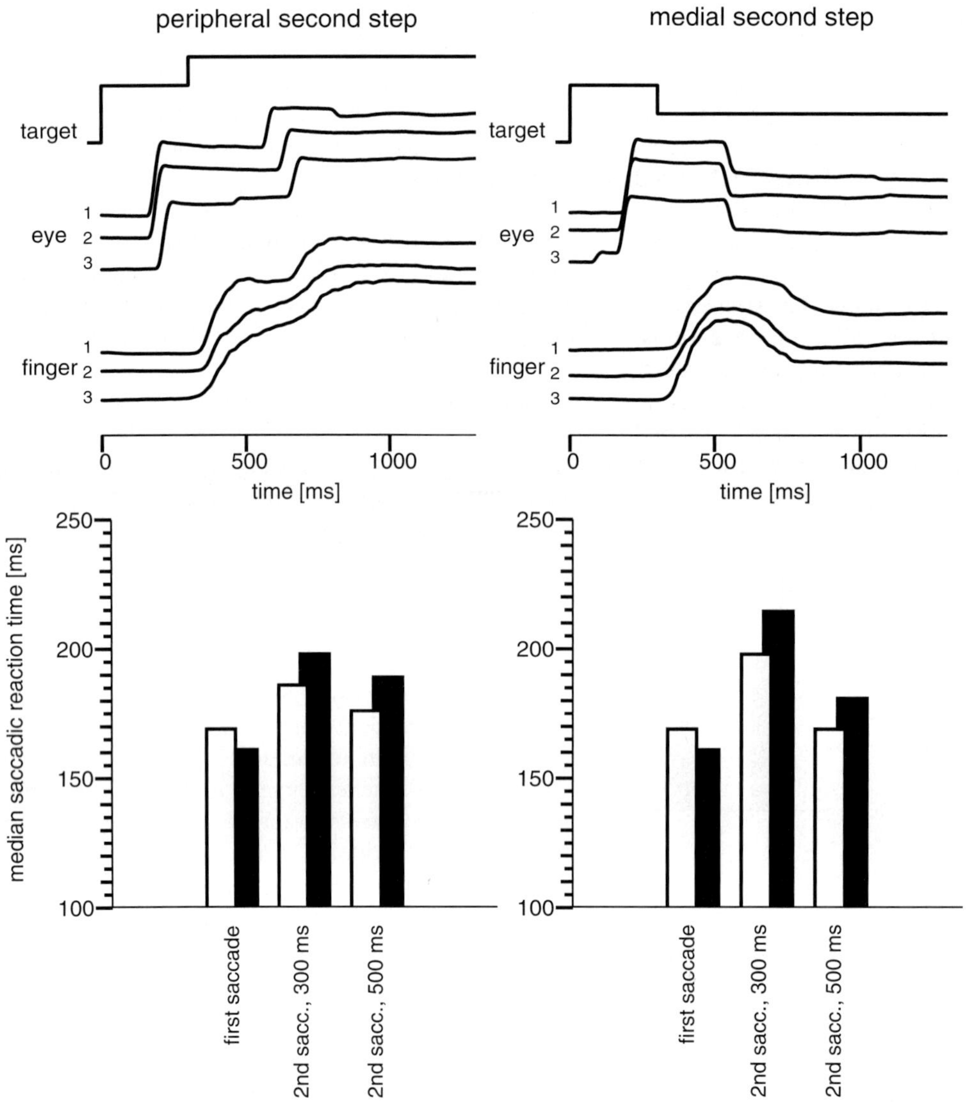

Fig. 13. Example trials (top row) and population medians of saccadic reaction time (bottom row) in double-step trials with a peripheral (left column) and medial second step (right column). The subject follows the target displacements quickly with two saccades and occasional correction saccades. In contrast, the hand movement starts later and is slower. Furthermore, in most trials, the hand trajectory does not show two distinct sub-movements like the eye, especially for the medial target displacement. Calculating the median of saccadic reaction times of all trials of all subjects for ST (white bars) and cSRT (black bars), we observe that the reaction time of the second saccade is higher than for the first. While the simultaneous use of the hand leads to a reduced reaction time for the first saccade, the second saccade is delayed.

Modulation of saccadic reaction times

As mentioned briefly above, the reduction of reaction time for the saccade in the single-step and the first saccade in the double-step task was not observed in the studies of Mather and Fisk (1985) and Bekkering et al. (1994, 1995). Yet there are some methodological clues to explain this difference. Mather and Fisk (1985) report higher saccadic reaction time when the subject had also to move their hand to point to the target compared to the saccade-only condition. The targets in that study were either auditory or visual.

It was reported that saccades to auditory targets had longer reaction times than to visual targets. Although the authors showed that coordination of eyes and arm depends on the modality of the targets (different correlation between saccadic and reach reaction times), they did not evaluate the effect of stimulus modality on the change of saccadic reaction time, when the subject is simultaneously pointing. Only the trials with visual targets would have been comparable to our results. Bekkering et al. (1994, 1995) asked the subjects to move a stylus over the surface of an x–y tablet when requiring simultaneous eye and arm movements. Drawing a line on that surface is reminiscent of a smooth pursuit eye movement, much less of a ballistic saccade. It might be that these two movements are already incompatible similar to the uSRT results.

If the eye movements in this task are used to improve the control of the arm movement (Prablanc et al., 1979a), it would be important to look at the end of the movements rather than on their start, because the movement times between both might vary. Helsen et al. (2000) approach that view by reporting that the end of the gaze movement coincided with the moment of peak hand velocity in a task where subjects made fast aiming movements with the arm. Furthermore, they report that the ratio between gaze and hand response time (reaction time + movement time) is 50%. Because saccadic movement duration is almost fixed, we might influence the saccadic reaction time by forcing the hand to arrive earlier or later. Subjects in our experiments were instructed to move as fast as possible.

Neggers and Bekkering (2000) recently reported a more pronounced increase of saccadic reaction time of 115 ms (from 255 ms for the first to 370 ms for the second saccade) in a comparable double-step experiment. This is an increase of about 45%. However, the crucial difference was that their subjects had to move the hand to the first target location, while a saccade to the second target location was required. This de-coupling of eyes and hand in the second sub-movement might have been solved by first completing the hand movement to target 1, which was still fixated, and initiate the second saccade afterwards. Then this is not on-line correction anymore.

Neuronal implementation

The presence of reach neurons in the SC supports the view that the SC of primates is more than a purely oculomotor structure. It is involved in the multisensory integration of signals to efficiently control and coordinate behavior. The two classes of coding schemes shown by the reach neurons reflect this sensorimotor integration. While the gaze-independent reach neurons code the arm movements similar to the motor signals of arm- and shoulder muscles, the code of gaze-dependent reach neurons resembles the retinotopic coding of the visual sensory input to the superficial collicular layers. However, this coding is also similar to the saccade-related neurons sending information to the brainstem saccade generator.

Combined use of one anatomical structure to code eye and arm movements should materialize in coordination or interference. The presented psychophysical experiments show both. The reaction time of the first saccade in a single-step or double-step experiment is reduced by a simultaneous arm movement to the same target. However, a saccade is delayed if it is the second in a double-step or has to go into the opposite direction of a simultaneously performed arm movement compared to the saccade alone. The obvious hypothesis would be that saccade triggering in the SC would be modulated for eye–hand coordination. For the facilitation of the first saccade, one could think of an excitatory input to the build-up neurons from the activated reach neurons. For the inhibition of the saccade to the second target we can think of three explanations:

(1) The reach neurons could excite the fixation neurons and by this elevate the saccadic trigger threshold and therefore increase the reaction time.
(2) The additional input of the reach neurons on the build-up cells leading to the quicker first saccade might also lead to a deeper inhibition in the saccadic initiation map (build-up neurons) thus increasing the reaction time of the next saccade.
(3) Although the target already moved to a new position, the internal target for the arm might still be at the first position, because it did not reach it so far and reprogramming takes some time. Then the reach neurons corresponding to that position could still be active and excite build-up neurons

at the corresponding position. The competition of this internal (wrong) input and the external (correct) visual input in the build-up layer would delay reaching the threshold for a saccade.

The main difference of these hypotheses is that the latter two predict a localized deficit for saccades with approximately the same size. The dynamic implementation of hypotheses 1 and 3 would also predict a dependence on the current arm movement instead of the previous one as hypothesis 2. The higher reaction time of the second saccade for a medial second step is likely to rule out hypothesis 2, because the ipsi- and contralateral SC are active successively for that task. Yet, the comparison of the hypotheses can only be resolved by further experiments.

The results of Bergeron and Guitton (also reported in these proceedings (Chapter 8), and Bergeron and Guitton, 2000) show that the role of some fixation neurons might be to signal the arrival of the eye near the target towards the end of a saccade. As described above, fixation neurons can be modulated — inhibited as well as excited — by arm movements. This modulation could have an influence on the neuron's reactivation at the end of a saccade, effectively changing the coded distance to the target. This might lead to a later or earlier end of the saccade and modify the end-point distribution around the target. The changes in error size and variance in the single-step experiment might reflect such a mechanism.

Conclusions

The superior colliculus in the midbrain of primates has information available on gaze and arm movements coded in compatible ways. The integration of this information might be important to control gaze and arm movements in a precise, effective and coordinated way. Thus the notion of the SC might be extended from a saccade trigger to a sensorimotor integrator.

Abbreviations

cSRT	coupled saccade-reach task
EMG	electromyogram
FR	fix reach
GD	gaze dependency index
RMF	reach movement field
SC	superior colliculus
SR	saccade reach
ST	saccade task
uSRT	uncoupled saccade-reach task

Acknowledgements

This study was supported by DFG Grants Ho 450 and a stipend to LL from the Boehringer Ingelheim Fonds.

References

Akert, K. (1949) Der visuelle Greifreflex. *Helv. Physiol. Acta*, 7: 112–134.

Bekkering, H., Adam, J.J., Kingma, H., Huson, A. and Whiting, H.T.A. (1994) Reaction time latencies of eye and hand movements in single- and dual-task conditions. *Exp. Brain Res.*, 97: 471–476.

Bekkering, H., Adam, J.J., Aarssen, A.v.d., Kingma, H. and Whiting, H.T.A. (1995) Interference between saccadic eye and goal-directed hand movements. *Exp. Brain Res.*, 106: 475–484.

Bergeron, A. and Guitton, D. (2001) The superior colliculus and its control of fixation behavior via projections to brainstem omnipause neurons. In: C. Casanova and M. Ptito (Eds.), *Vision: From Neurons to Cognition. Progress in Brain Research*, Vol. 134. Elsevier, Amsterdam, pp. 97–107.

Bergeron, A. and Guitton, D. (2000) Fixation neurons in the superior colliculus encode distance between current and desired gaze positions. *Nat. Neurosci.*, 3: 932–939.

Biguer, B., Jeannerod, M. and Prablanc, C. (1982) The coordination of eye, head, and arm movements during reaching at a single visual target. *Exp. Brain Res.*, 46: 301–304.

Boch, R., Fischer, B. and Ramsperger, E. (1984) Express-saccades of the monkey: reaction times versus intensity, site, duration, and eccentricity of their targets. *Exp. Brain Res.*, 55(2): 223–231.

Fischer, B. and Ramsperger, E. (1984) Human express saccades: extremely short reaction times of goal directed eye movements. *Exp. Brain Res.*, 57(1): 191–195.

Georgopoulos, A.P., Schwartz, A.B. and Kettner, R.E. (1986) Neuronal population coding of movement direction. *Science*, 233: 1416–1419.

Georgopoulos, A.P., Kettner, R.E. and Schwartz, A.B. (1988) Primate motor cortex and free arm movements to visual targets in three-dimensional space. II. Coding of the direction of movement by a neuronal population. *J. Neurosci.*, 8: 2928–2937.

Gielen, C.C.A.M., Heuvel, P.J.M.v.d. and Gisbergen, J.A.M.v. (1984) Coordination of fast eye and arm movements in a tracking task. *Exp. Brain Res.*, 56(1): 154–161.

Helsen, W.F., Elliott, D., Starkes, J.L. and Ricker, K.L. (2000) Coupling of eye, finger, elbow, and shoulder movements during manual aiming. *J. Mot. Behav.*, 32: 241–248.

Jay, M.F. and Sparks, D.L. (1987a) Sensorimotor integration in the primate superior colliculus. I. Motor convergence. *J. Neurophysiol.*, 57(1): 22.

Jay, M.F. and Sparks, D.L. (1987b) Sensorimotor integration in the primate sensory colliculus. II. Coordinates of auditory signals. *J. Neurophysiol.*, 57(1): 35–55.

Kettner, R.E., Schwartz, A.B. and Georgopoulos, A.P. (1988) Primate motor cortex and free arm movements to visual targets in three-dimensional space. III. Positional gradients and population coding of movement direction from various movement origins. *J. Neurosci.*, 8(8): 2938–2947.

Krauzlis, R.J., Basso, M.A. and Wurtz, R.H. (2000) Discharge properties of neurons in the rostral superior colliculus of the monkey during smooth-pursuit eye movements. *J. Neurophysiol.*, 84: 876–891.

Kutz, D.F., Dannenberg, S., Werner, W. and Hoffmann, K.-P. (1997) Population coding of arm movement related neurons in and below the superior colliculus of *Macaca mulatta*. *Biol. Cybern.*, 76: 331–337.

Lünenburger, L., Kutz, D.F. and Hoffmann, K.P. (2000) Influence of arm movements on saccades in humans. *Eur. J. Neurosci.*, 12: 4107–4116.

Ma, T.P., Graybiel, A.M. and Wurtz, R.H. (1991) Location of saccade-related neurons in the macaque superior colliculus. *Exp. Brain Res.*, 85: 21–35.

Mather, J.A. and Fisk, J.D. (1985) Orienting to targets by looking and pointing: parallels and interactions in ocular and manual performance. *Q. J. Exp. Physiol.*, 37A: 315–338.

Meredith, M.A. and Stein, B.E. (1986) Visual, auditory, and somatosensory convergence on cells in superior colliculus results in multisensory integration. *J. Neurophysiol.*, 56(3): 640–662.

Munoz, D.P. and Istvan, P.J. (1998) Lateral inhibitory interactions in the intermediate layers of the monkey superior colliculus. *J. Neurophysiol.*, 79: 1193–1209.

Munoz, D.P. and Wurtz, R.H. (1993a) Fixation cells in monkey superior colliculus. I. Characteristics of cell discharge. *J. Neurophysiol.*, 70: 559–575.

Munoz, D.P. and Wurtz, R.H. (1993b) Fixation cells in monkey superior colliculus. II. Reversible activation and deactivation. *J. Neurophysiol.*, 70: 576–589.

Munoz, D.P. and Wurtz, R.H. (1995a) Saccade-related activity in monkey superior colliculus. I. Characteristics of burst and buildup cells. *J. Neurophysiol.*, 73: 2313–2333.

Munoz, D.P. and Wurtz, R.H. (1995b) Saccade-related activity in monkey superior colliculus. II. Spread of activity during saccades. *J. Neurophysiol.*, 73: 2334–2348.

Neggers, S.F. and Bekkering, H. (2000) Ocular gaze is anchored to the target of an ongoing pointing movement. *J. Neurophysiol.*, 83: 639–651.

Ottes, F.P., Gisbergen, J.A.M.v. and Eggermont, J.J. (1986) Visuomotor fields of the superior colliculus: a quantitative model. *Vision Res.*, 26: 837–857.

Prablanc, C., Echallier, J.F., Komilis, E. and Jeannerod, M. (1979a) Optimal response of eye and hand motor systems in pointing at a visual target. I. Spatio-temporal characteristics of eye and hand movements and their relationships when varying the amount of visual information. *Biol. Cybern.*, 35: 113–124.

Prablanc, C., Echallier, J.E., Jeannerod, M. and Komilis, E. (1979b) Optimal response of eye and hand motor systems in pointing at a visual target. II. Static and dynamic visual cues in the control of hand movements. *Biol. Cybern.*, 35: 183–187.

Rogal, L., Reible, G. and Fischer, B. (1985) Reaction times of the eye and the hand of the monkey in a visual reach task. *Neurosci. Lett.*, 58: 127–132.

Saslow, M.G. (1967) Effects of components of displacement-step stimuli upon latency for saccadic eye movement. *J. Opt. Soc. Am.*, 57: 1024–1029.

Schwartz, A.B., Kettner, R.E. and Georgopoulos, A.P. (1988) Primate motor cortex and free arm movements to visual targets in three-dimensional space I.Relations between single cell discharge and direction of movement. *J. Neurosci.*, 8(8): 2913–2927.

Sparks, D.L., Holland, R. and Guthrie, B.L. (1976) Size and distribution of movement fields in the monkey superior colliculus. *Brain Res.*, 113: 21–34.

Stuphorn, V., Hoffmann, K.-P. and Miller, L.E. (1999) Correlation of primate superior colliculus and reticular formation discharge with proximal limb muscle activity. *J. Neurophysiol.*, 81: 1978–1982.

Stuphorn, V., Bauswein, E. and Hoffmann, K.P. (2000) Neurons in the primate superior colliculus coding for arm movements in gaze-related coordinates. *J. Neurophysiol.*, 83: 1283–1299.

Updyke, B.V. (1977) Topographic organization of the projections from cortical areas 17, 18 and 19 onto the thalamus, pretectum and superior colliculus in the cat. *J. Comp. Neurol.*, 173: 81–122.

Werner, W. (1993) Neurons in the primate superior colliculus are active before and during arm movements to visual targets. *Eur. J. Neurosci.*, 5: 335–340.

Werner, W., Dannenberg, S. and Hoffmann, K.P. (1997a) Arm-movement-related neurons in the primate superior colliculus and underlying reticular formation: comparison of neuronal activity with EMGs of muscles of the shoulder, arm and trunk during reaching. *Exp. Brain Res.*, 115: 191–205.

Werner, W., Hoffmann, K.P. and Dannenberg, S. (1997b) Anatomical distribution of arm-movement-related neurons in the primate superior colliculus and underlying reticular formation in comparison with visual and saccadic cells. *Exp. Brain Res.*, 115: 206–216.

C. Casanova and M. Ptito (Eds.)
Progress in Brain Research, Vol. 134

CHAPTER 9

Look and see: how the brain moves your eyes about

Peter H. Schiller * and Edward J. Tehovnik

Department of Brain and Cognitive Sciences, Massachusetts Institute of Technology, Cambridge, MA 02139, USA

Abstract: Two major cortical streams are involved in the generation of visually guided saccadic eye movements: the anterior and the posterior. The anterior stream from the frontal and medial eye fields has direct access to brainstem oculomotor centers. The posterior stream from the occipital cortices reaches brainstem oculomotor centers through the superior colliculus. The parietal cortex interconnects with both streams. Our findings suggest that the posterior stream plays an unique role in the execution of rapid, short-latency eye movements called 'express saccades'. Both the anterior and posterior streams play a role in the selection of targets to which saccades are to be generated, but do so in different ways. Areas V1, V2 and LIP contribute to decisions involved in where to look as well as where not to look. In addition, area LIP is involved in decisions about how long to maintain fixation prior to the execution of a saccade. Area V4 does not appear to be directly involved in eye-movement generation. In the anterior stream, the frontal eye fields, and to a lesser extent the medial eye fields, are involved in the correct execution of saccades subsequent to decisions made about where to look and where not to look.

Introduction

Our eyes are on the move most of the time during our waking hours. We make about three saccadic eye movements per second, some 170,000 a day, and about 5 billion in an average life time. With each shift in gaze, the numerous stimuli in the visual scene impinge on new retinal locations, to only one of which can the eye be shifted subsequently. This process of target selection necessitates the discrimination of objects, the assessment of temporal order and the determination of spatial location. In this presentation, some of the neural systems that are involved in the generation of visually guided saccadic eye movements are described. We have used several methods in our effort that include single-cell recordings, lesions and microstimulation. We have studied quite a number of brain areas that include V1, V2, V4, the lateral intraparietal sulcus (LIP), the frontal eye fields (FEF), the medial eye fields (MEF), and the superior colliculus (SC).

These experiments were carried out on trained rhesus monkeys because their eye movements are similar to those of humans. Fig. 1 shows records of eye movements made by one of our animals while he was restrained and looked at the displays shown on the left. The monkey received periodic juice reward. The eye movements are similar to those generated by humans as shown by Yarbus (1967).

Neural structures involved in the generation of saccadic eye movements

Fig. 2 shows schematically the central neural structures in the monkey from which saccadic eye movements can readily be elicited by electrical microstimulation. As indicated by the arrows in the circles, stimulation of regions of the occipital cortex, such as V1 and V2, elicits saccades whose vectors are

* Corresponding author: P.H. Schiller, Department of Brain and Cognitive Sciences, Massachusetts Institute of Technology, Cambridge, MA 02139, USA.
Tel.: +1-617-253-5754; Fax: +1-617-253-8943;
E-mail: phschill@mit.edu

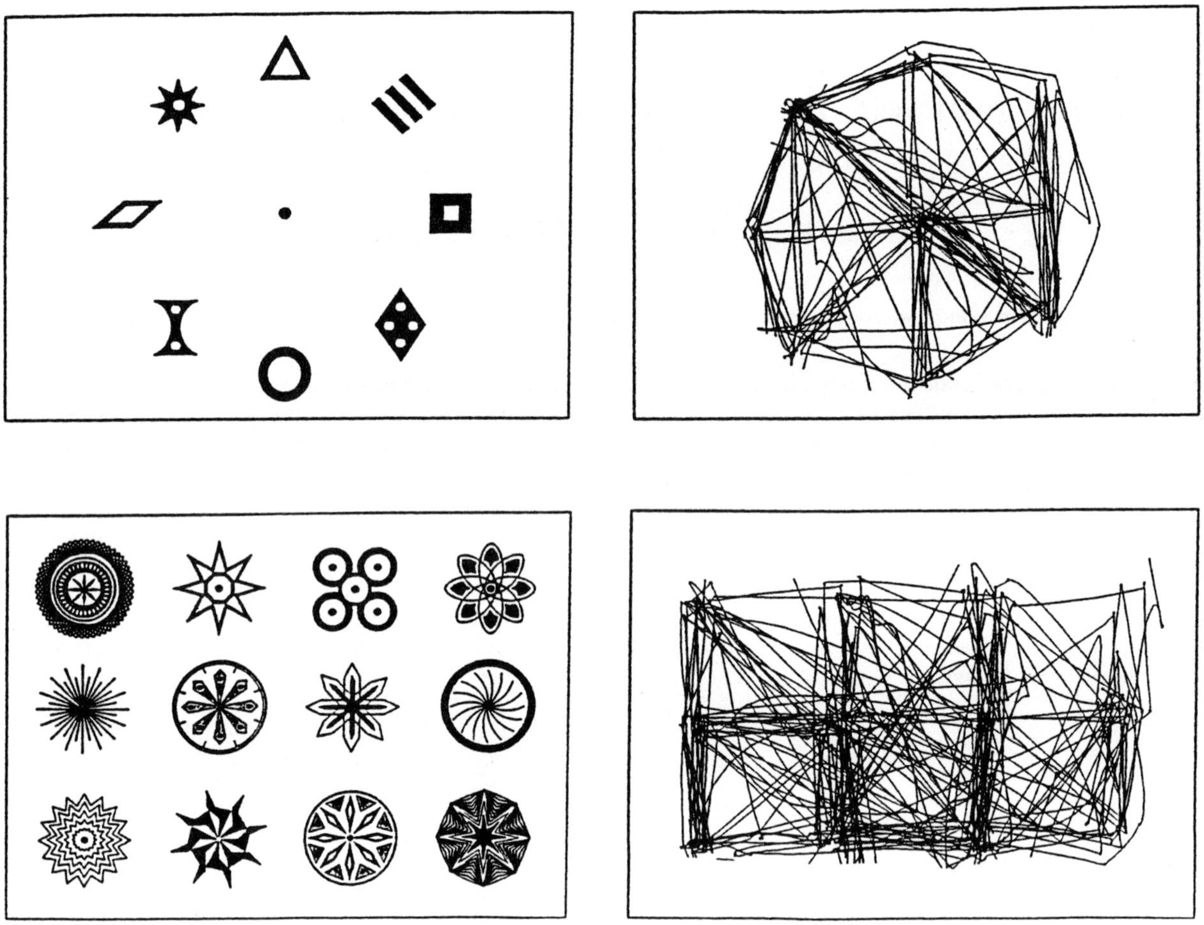

Fig. 1. Saccadic eye movements of a monkey, shown in the right panels, while the animal was viewing the stimulus displays shown on the left.

constant, and are independent of starting eye position (Schiller, 1972, 1977, 1998). The direction and amplitude of the saccades elicited depends on where one stimulates within the structure. When one records as well and finds the location of the receptive fields, stimulation takes the eye to the receptive field location prior to the eye movement. These areas therefore carry a vector code. What is computed is a retinal error signal between the center of gaze and the location of the receptive field activated by the target; the eye movement nulls this error. Like visual cortex, the superior colliculus and the frontal eye fields also carry a vector code (Robinson and Fuchs, 1969; Robinson, 1972; Schiller and Stryker, 1972). A different coding operation takes place in the medial eye fields where stimulation elicits a saccade that takes at the center of gaze to a particular location in craniotopic space (Schlag and Schlag-Rey, 1987; Tehovnik and Lee, 1993). Different subregions code for different spatial locations. In the different subregions of the parietal lobe, one can find either one or the other of these coding operations (Shibutani et al., 1984; Kurylo and Skavenski, 1991; Thier and Andersen, 1998).

Although it was thought that cortical signals for the generation of saccadic eye movements are conveyed entirely through the superior colliculus, more recent evidence indicates that this is not the case. When the colliculus is removed, monkeys still make

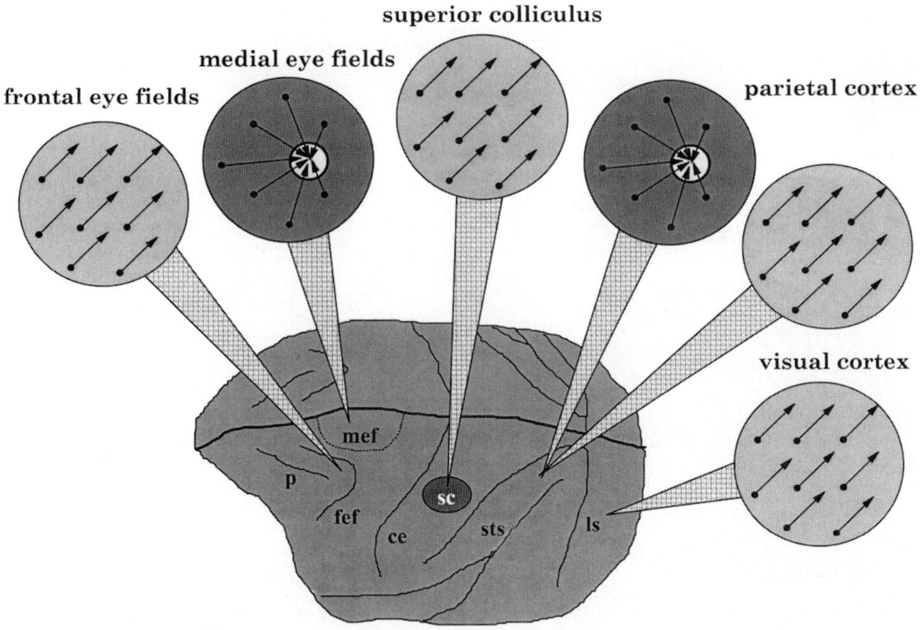

Fig. 2. Eye movements elicited by electrical stimulation of five areas. Stimulation of the superior colliculus, the visual cortex, regions of the parietal cortex, and the frontal eye fields produces saccades whose amplitude and direction depends on the subregion stimulated in each of these areas. Stimulation of the medial eye fields and some regions of the parietal cortex elicits saccades that take the eye to a particular orbital location.

pretty good visually guided eye movements (Schiller et al., 1980; Keating and Gooley, 1988a). Further work established that collicular removal has a selective effect on electrically triggered saccadic eye movements from the cortex. What happens is depicted in Fig. 3. After ablation of the superior colliculus, one can still elicit saccadic eye movements from the frontal and medial eye fields, but not from posterior cortex (Schiller, 1977; Keating et al., 1983; Keating and Gooley, 1988b; Tehovnik et al., 1994).

These findings have led to the formulation depicted in Fig. 4. According to this generalized scheme, there are two major streams for the generation of visually guided saccadic eye movements, the anterior and the posterior. The posterior stream gains access to the brainstem oculomotor centers through the superior colliculus whereas the anterior stream from the frontal and medial eye fields has direct connections to the brainstem. Although cortical areas are extensively interconnected, and the region of the parietal cortex that resides in the lateral intraparietal sulcus has connections both with the frontal cortex and the colliculus (Lynch et al., 1985; Huerta et al., 1987; Huerta and Kaas, 1990), there is one important additional piece of information in support of the two-stream hypothesis depicted in Fig. 4. This additional evidence is that ablation of both the superior colliculus and the frontal eye fields eliminates all visually guided saccadic eye movements (Schiller et al., 1980). This is a deficit from which there is virtually no recovery.

Given that there are quite a number of cortical areas involved in visually guided saccadic eye-movement control that appear to form two major streams to the brainstem oculomotor centers, the question arises as to what the functional contributions are of the cortical areas within each of these two streams. To address this question, in our recent work, we have concentrated on two methods. The first method examined the effects of selective lesions on the generation of visually guided saccadic eye movements. The second method examined the effects of subthreshold electrical microstimulation in various cortical areas on target selection and the execution of saccadic eye movements.

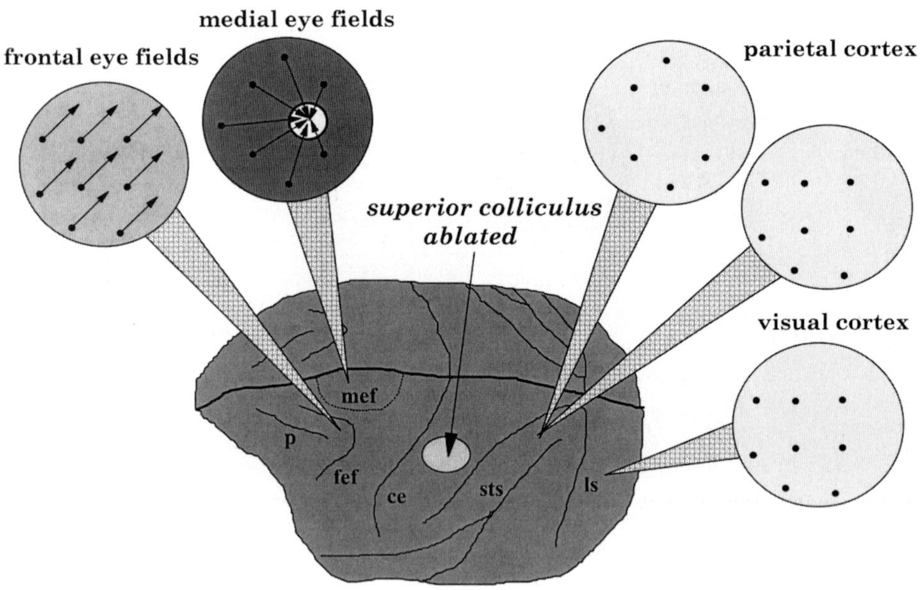

Fig. 3. After ablation of the superior colliculus, electrical stimulation no longer elicits saccadic eye movements from the occipital and parietal cortices, but continues to do so in the frontal lobe.

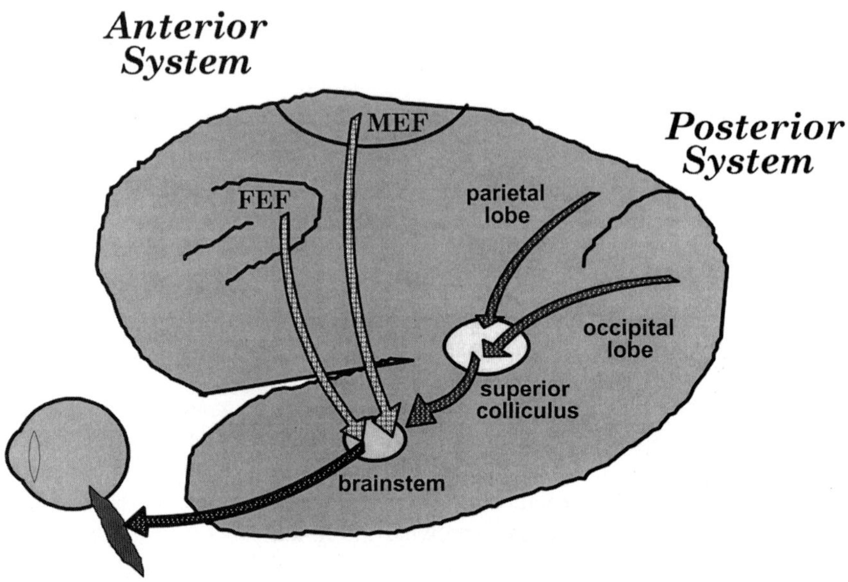

Fig. 4. Model of the hypothesized connections involved in visually guided eye-movement control. Two major streams control these eye movements: the anterior and the posterior. The anterior system has direct access to the brainstem oculomotor centers. The posterior stream reaches these centers through the superior colliculus.

Lesion studies

The aim of our lesion studies was to determine how the structures within the anterior and posterior streams contribute to different aspects of eye-movement generation. To block the posterior stream we removed the superior colliculus. We then compared that with lesions of the frontal and medial eye fields.

The first task to be discussed is depicted in Fig. 5. When a central fixation spot comes on, the monkey looks at it. Then a single target appears somewhere on the monitor and the monkey has to look at it to receive a drop of apple juice for reward. When a monkey performs this task repeatedly, the latency distribution becomes bimodal as first shown by Fischer and Boch (1983). An example of such a distribution appears in the top panel of Fig. 6. The first mode in this distribution that peaks at less than 100 ms is referred to as 'express saccades'. Those falling into the second mode are called 'regular saccades'. The heads of the animals were restrained during the experimental sessions.

So we can now ask what happens to the bimodal distribution of saccadic latencies when one makes lesions of either the superior colliculus or the frontal eye fields. After a frontal eye field lesion, there is very little effect (Schiller et al., 1987). The monkey still exhibits a bimodal distribution of saccadic latencies, although sometimes with a small overall shift towards slightly longer latencies. By contrast, a unilateral lesion of the superior colliculus abolishes all express saccades as depicted in the bottom panels in Fig. 6; after the left superior colliculus had been removed, the monkey never again makes express saccades to the right. On the other hand, saccades to the left retain their bimodal distribution. In addition, the regular saccades to the right have significantly longer latencies.

These findings suggest that the posterior stream is essential for the generation of express saccades.

Next we turn to a different task depicted in Fig. 7, which we refer to as the sequential task. In this case, we present two targets in succession and the monkey's task is to make a corresponding pair of saccades. The task is shown in Fig. 7. The duration of the targets and the interval between them is systematically varied. We studied performance on this task before and after unilateral frontal and medial eye field lesions. Fig. 8 shows eye-movement records obtained with this task for two sequence durations 18 and 60 weeks after a left frontal eye field lesion (Schiller and Chou, 2000a). The monkey does well toward the intact side, but does poorly, especially for the shorter sequence duration, for saccades to the right. More detailed data showing percent correct performance after frontal eye field and medial eye field lesions appear in Fig. 9. In this case, we ran the same four sets of sequences for several weeks. Recovery is quite rapid with the medial eye field lesions, but much slower after frontal eye field lesions. But even after the apparent recovery, when a new set of sequences is introduced, a large deficit is still evident. Fig. 8 in fact shows the eye movement records obtained with a sequence to which the monkey was only exposed a few times after 18 and 60 weeks.

A third task we used is shown in Fig. 10. We call this the paired target task. After the monkey centers his gaze on the fixation spot, two targets appear. He gets rewarded for looking at either target. In addition to presenting the two targets simultaneously, the temporal asynchrony with which

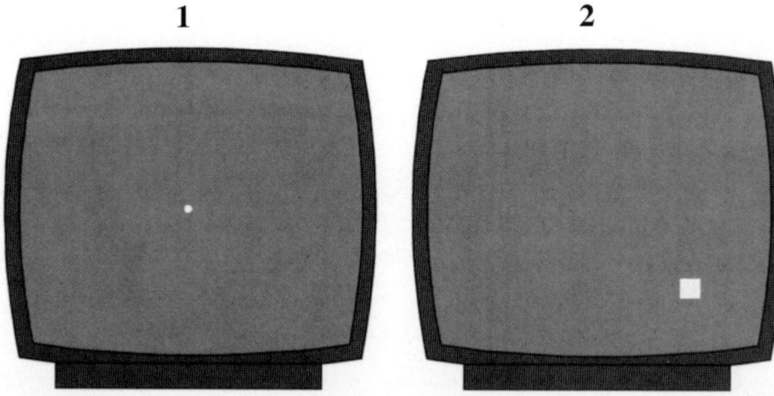

Fig. 5. Procedure to study eye movements made to single targets. First a fixation spot appears (1); when the monkey fixates it, a target appears in one of several locations (2). A saccade made to the target is rewarded with a drop of apple juice.

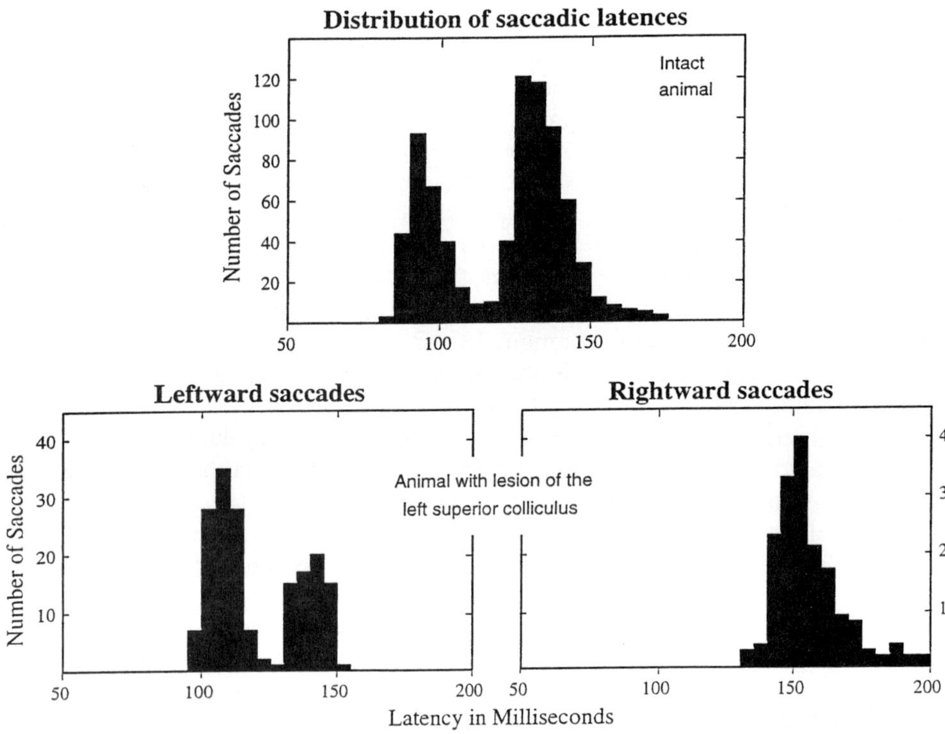

Fig. 6. The distribution of saccadic latencies before and after left superior colliculus lesion. Saccadic latencies made to single targets form a bimodal distribution the first mode of which has been called 'express saccades'. After a unilateral collicular lesion, monkeys no longer can make express saccades into the visual hemifield that had been represented by the removed colliculus. Regular saccades (the second peak in the distribution) have longer latencies after the collicular lesion.

they appear is also varied. This way we can determine what the probability is of selecting one target or the other as a function of the temporal asynchrony between them.

This task, using only simultaneous presentation conditions, has been extensively used in clinical studies showing that after unilateral cortical lesions the target presented in the hemifield contralateral to

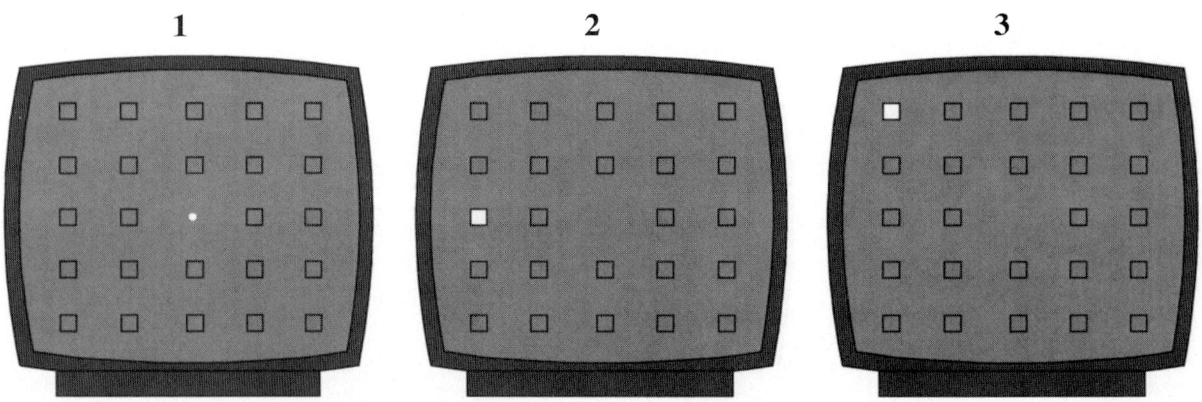

Fig. 7. Method for studying the execution of sequential saccades. After the animal fixates the fixation spot (1) two targets appear in succession (2 and 3). Target duration the interval between them is systematically varied.

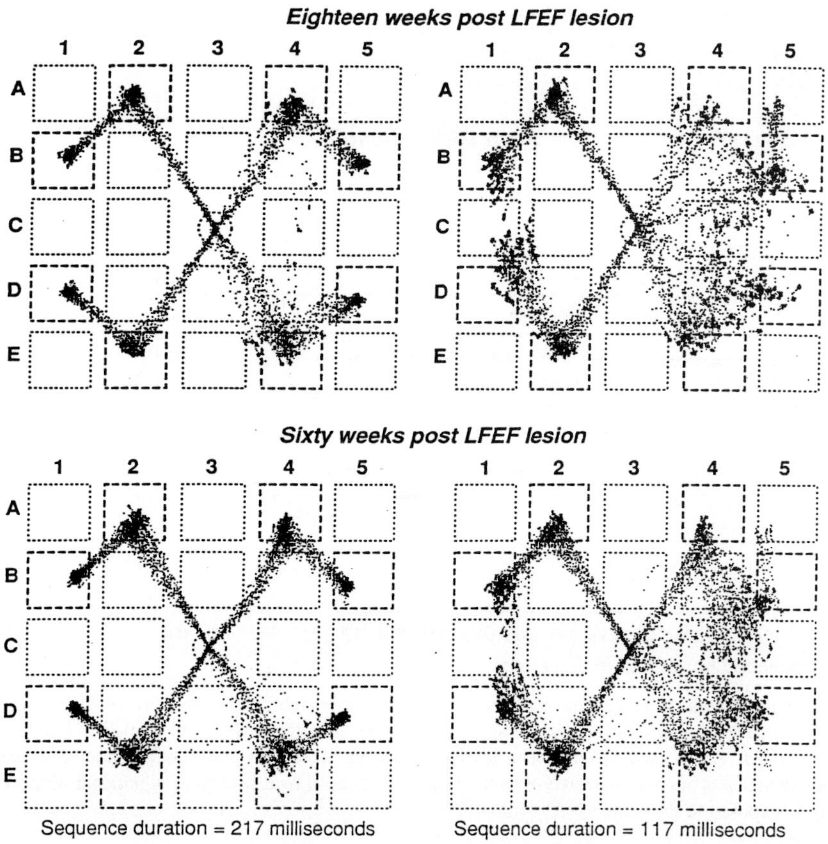

Fig. 8. Eye movements shown 18 and 60 weeks after a left frontal eye field lesion on a set of two target sequences presented for two sequence durations, 217 and 117 ms. The four sequences used were A2–B1, E2–D1, A4–B5 and E5–D5. Performance is much poorer to the right, especially for the shorter sequence duration. The monkey was exposed to the particular set of sequences shown here only occasionally.

the damaged area is ignored (Bisiach and Vallar, 1988). This has been termed the extinction phenomenon because the target presented in the hemifield ipsilateral to the damaged area 'extinguishes' the perception of the target in the intact hemifield; presented singly, a target is perceived at either location in many patients. This task with using just two targets is the simplest one we could devise to study target selection.

Fig. 11 shows data obtained on this paired target task after frontal and medial eye field lesions (Schiller and Chou, 1998, 2000b). Plotted here is the percent of time the left target is chosen as a function of the temporal asynchrony between the targets. Preoperative performance is shown by the solid lines and black squares; the probability with which the left and right targets are chosen is about the same when the two targets appear simultaneously. This equal probability choice shifts dramatically after a unilateral frontal eye field lesion. The target in the affected hemifield has to be presented much earlier than the target in the intact field to obtain equal probability choice for the left and right targets. This suggests that processing has been greatly slowed down as a result of the lesion. Recovery is slow and never complete. The effects are much smaller after medial eye field lesions (called dorsomedial frontal cortex, DMFC, by some investigators) and recovery is more rapid. The inset on the right shows actual eye-movement records obtained pre-operatively with the targets appearing either simultaneously or with 33 ms offsets. The paired targets on any given trial appeared either above or below fixation. In the simultaneous presentation case, the monkey makes about

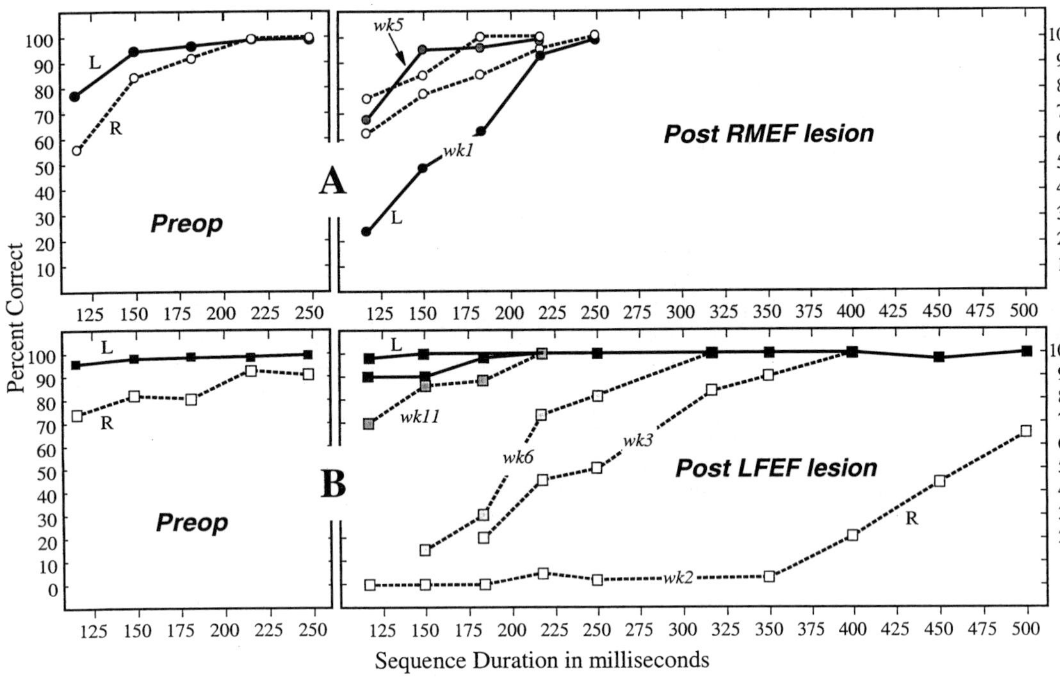

Fig. 9. Performance on another set of four sequences with varied sequence duration before and after right medial and left frontal eye field lesions. The same set of sequences were used repeatedly for 11 weeks starting 1 and 2 weeks after the RMEF and the LFEF had been ablated. The sequences used were C1–A1, C1–E1, C5–A5 and C5–E5. The RMEF lesion produced only mild deficits that recovered rapidly. The LFEF lesion produced a major deficit that recovered slowly over time. However, as shown in Fig. 8, significant recovery occurred only when the animal was repeatedly exposed to the same set of sequences.

the same number of saccades to the left and the right, whereas when the targets on the left appear first, most of the saccades are made to the left; the converse is the case when the targets appear first to the right of fixation.

Collectively, these lesion studies suggest then that the posterior stream plays an important role executing saccadic eye movements rapidly, and especially in generating express saccades. When it comes to more complex tasks, it appears that the frontal eye

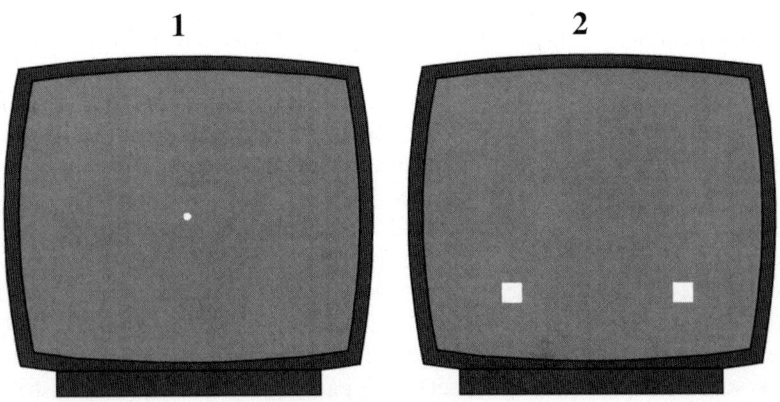

Fig. 10. The paired target task. After fixation, two targets appear. The monkey is rewarded for making a saccadic eye movement to either target. The targets are presented with various temporal asynchronies.

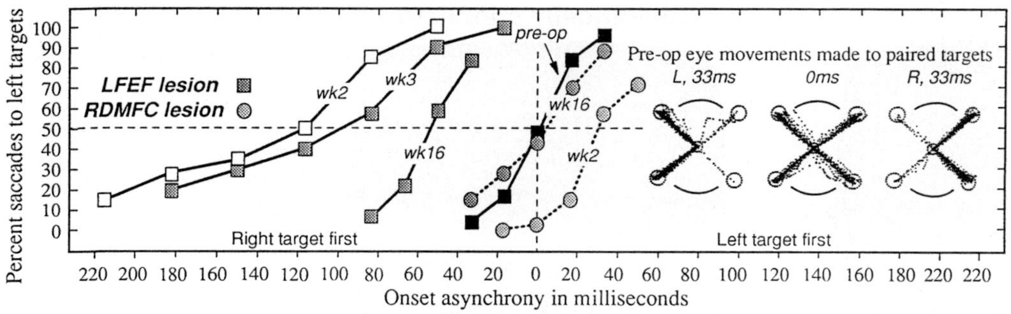

Fig. 11. Data obtained on the paired target task before and after LFEF and RMEF (labeled RDMFC) lesions. Percent of saccades made to the left targets is plotted as a function of the temporal asynchrony between the targets. In the intact monkey (pre-op), the left and right choices are made with equal probability when the two targets are simultaneous. After the LFEF lesion, the equal probability point shifts dramatically; the target in the affected hemifield has to be presented more than 100 ms before the target in the ipsilateral hemifield. There is gradual recovery over time. When tested over a year later, there is still a sizeable deficit after the LFEF lesion. The RMEF lesion produced much milder deficits that recovered fully by the 16th week. Pre-operative eye-movement traces are shown for targets presented simultaneously and with left and right target appearing first by 33 ms on the right side of figure.

fields in particular play an important role in temporal sequencing. The lesion data suggest that this structure also plays a significant role in target selection.

Microstimulation studies

To learn more about the role various brain structures play in target selection we have recently turned to microstimulation (Schiller and Tehovnik, 2000). The rationale of these experiments is that subthreshold electrical stimulation should be able to influence target selection in those cortical areas that are involved in this process. The nature of this influence should reveal how various areas contribute to the process.

The procedures we used are depicted in Fig. 12. We first record the activity of single neurons in the area under study. We then map the receptive or motor fields of the neurons from which we record, and we also examine their response characteristics. We then use the paired target task that are presented with various temporal asynchronies. One of the targets is placed into the receptive or the motor field of the cells. Next we electrically stimulate at low current levels to determine how target choice is altered. In addition, at each site we determine to what extent saccadic latencies to single targets are affected electrical stimulation.

We most commonly stimulated for 80 ms at 200 Hz. Stimulation was typically initiated 30 ms after the appearance of the first target. This delay time was chosen because we had found that in areas V1 and V2 single cells began discharging to the visual stimuli we used with that latency. The current levels we used are indicated for each curve generated in Figs. 14–15. Also indicated in these figures is the threshold level of the stimulation, expressed as the percent probability with which a saccade was elicited with electrical stimulation under our control condition in which the electrical stimulation was applied 120–140 ms after the termination at the fixation spot and no target was presented. These control conditions were randomly interspersed with the presentation of the paired targets. This procedure for establishing the lowest possible threshold was based on our earlier work in which we had found that the efficacy with which a saccade could be elicited with electrical stimulation was lowest when stimulation was applied well after the fixation spot was extinguished and no targets were presented. In the frontal eye fields, thresholds were three times lower, and in the medial eye fields they were 16 times lower when there were no targets and stimulation was delivered after the fixation spot had been terminated (Tehovnik et al., 1999).

Saccadic latencies elicited by above threshold electrical stimulation depended on the current levels used. This was true for all the brain sites we had studied. When the probability of eliciting saccades in the no target control condition was between 25 and 75%, latencies ranged between 75 and 150 ms. The majority of the effects reported on here were

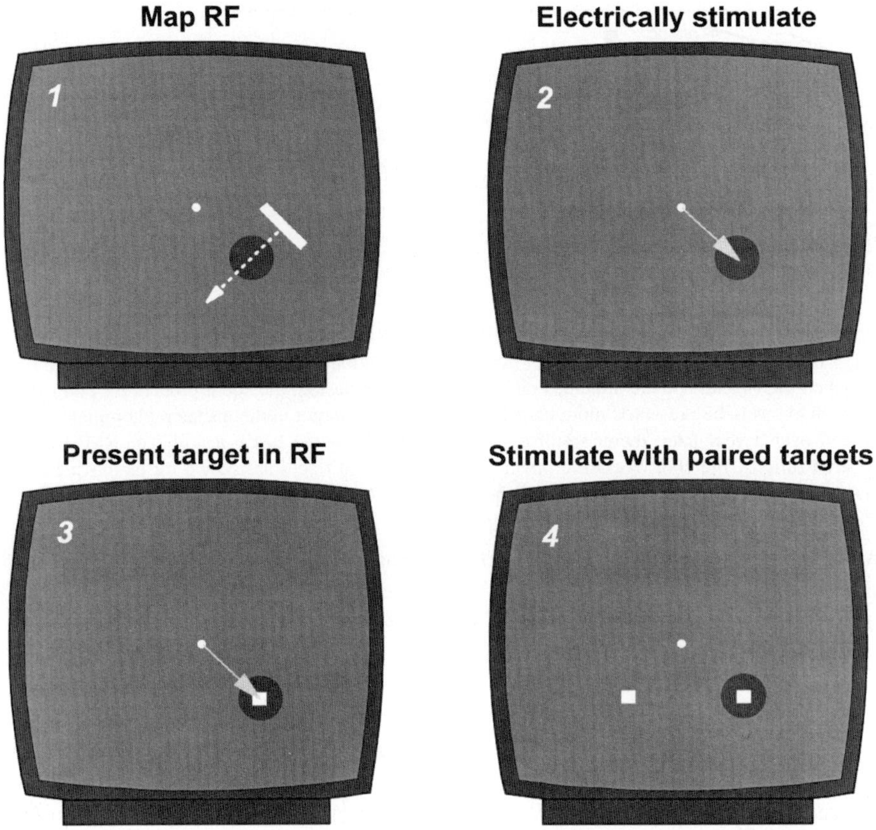

Fig. 12. Method used to study the effects of subthreshold electrical stimulation on target choice. After an electrode is lowered into a selected structure, the receptive field location of the neurons is plotted first. Then the area is stimulated at above threshold levels. The saccade elicited shifts the center of gaze to the receptive field. Thirdly, a target is placed into the receptive field to elicit the same direction and amplitude saccade that was elicited by electrical stimulation. Fourthly, two targets are presented with various asynchronies with one of them in the receptive field. We then proceed to determine to what extent subthreshold electrical stimulation alters they frequency with which the targets are selected.

obtained with current levels below which saccades were elicited under our control conditions.

Also interspersed with the presentation of the paired targets and the control condition were single targets that appeared at the same location as the paired targets. Stimulation was administered on a minority of trials with single targets as well which allowed us to determine the extent to which the latency of a visually triggered saccade could be influenced by subthreshold stimulation.

Fig. 13 depicts the cortical areas we had studied. They are areas V1, V2, V4, LIP, FEF and MEF.

In *area V1*, suprathreshold stimulation in the absence of any targets elicited saccades that shifted the center of gaze into the receptive field location of the stimulated neurons. Thresholds for eliciting such saccades were considerably higher in the upper layers than in the lower layers where saccades were often elicited with currents of less than 25 μA. Subthreshold stimulation administered with paired targets produced two effects. Unexpectedly, as shown in Fig. 14a, stimulation of the upper layers of V1 typically produced interference by *decreasing* the probability with which the target in the receptive field of the stimulated neurons was selected; the magnitude of the effect increased with increased subthreshold current. By contrast, stimulation in lower layers of V1 produced facilitation by increasing the probability with which the target in the receptive field was chosen. This is shown for one site in Fig. 14b.

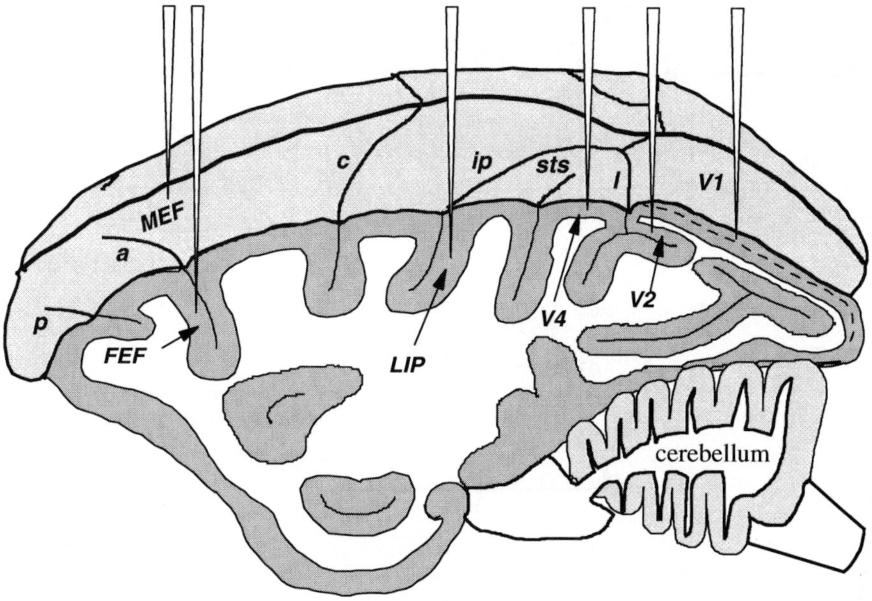

Fig. 13. A schematic showing the brain areas we had stimulated. They are V1, V2, V4, LIP, MEF and FEF.

At sites where stimulation produced an interference effect, stimulation administered in conjunction with single targets produced significant increases in saccadic latencies; on the other hand, stimulation at sites where facilitation was obtained had little effect on saccadic latencies to single targets. For the data shown in Fig. 14a and b, concurrently collected single target latency data are shown in Fig. 16, V1.

In *area V2*, similar results were obtained. Stimulation in the lower layers typically produced facilitation, whereas stimulation in the upper layers produced interference. In Fig. 14c, data are shown for conditions in which stimulation was delivered to two locations in the same electrode penetration using 50 μA. In the lower layers, this current was suprathreshold and resulted in driving eyes to the target in the receptive field. By contrast, the same current level in the upper layers decreased the probability of choosing the target in the receptive field.

Saccadic latencies to single targets appearing in the receptive field complemented these effects in V2. Differences in latencies for stimulated and unstimulated trials are shown in Fig. 16, V2, for the same data set that is graphed in Fig. 14c. For stimulation in the upper layers, which induced interference, saccadic latencies to single targets increased. By contrast, stimulation in the lower layers at the same current levels was above threshold and shortened saccadic latencies.

In *area V4*, electrical stimulation never produced saccades using currents levels up to 200 μA and failed to have any effect on target selection or saccadic latencies. Data are plotted in Figs. 14d and 16.

In *area LIP*, saccades could be elicited from a minority of sites (see Table 1). At such sites, subthreshold stimulation in the paired target case either produced facilitation or interference. In Fig. 15a, data are shown from a site where stimulation produced interference. Fig. 15b shows data for another site that yielded facilitation.

Saccadic latencies obtained in LIP to single targets appear in Fig. 16. Latency differences shown in Fig. 16, LIP, sections a and b, were obtained concurrently with the data collected for Fig. 15a and b. Single target latencies obtained at facilitatory sites were not significantly altered by stimulation. On the other hand, at sites that produced interference, higher subthreshold currents increased single-target latencies.

An additional effect in LIP was obtained at sites where neurons discharged with fixation (Lynch et

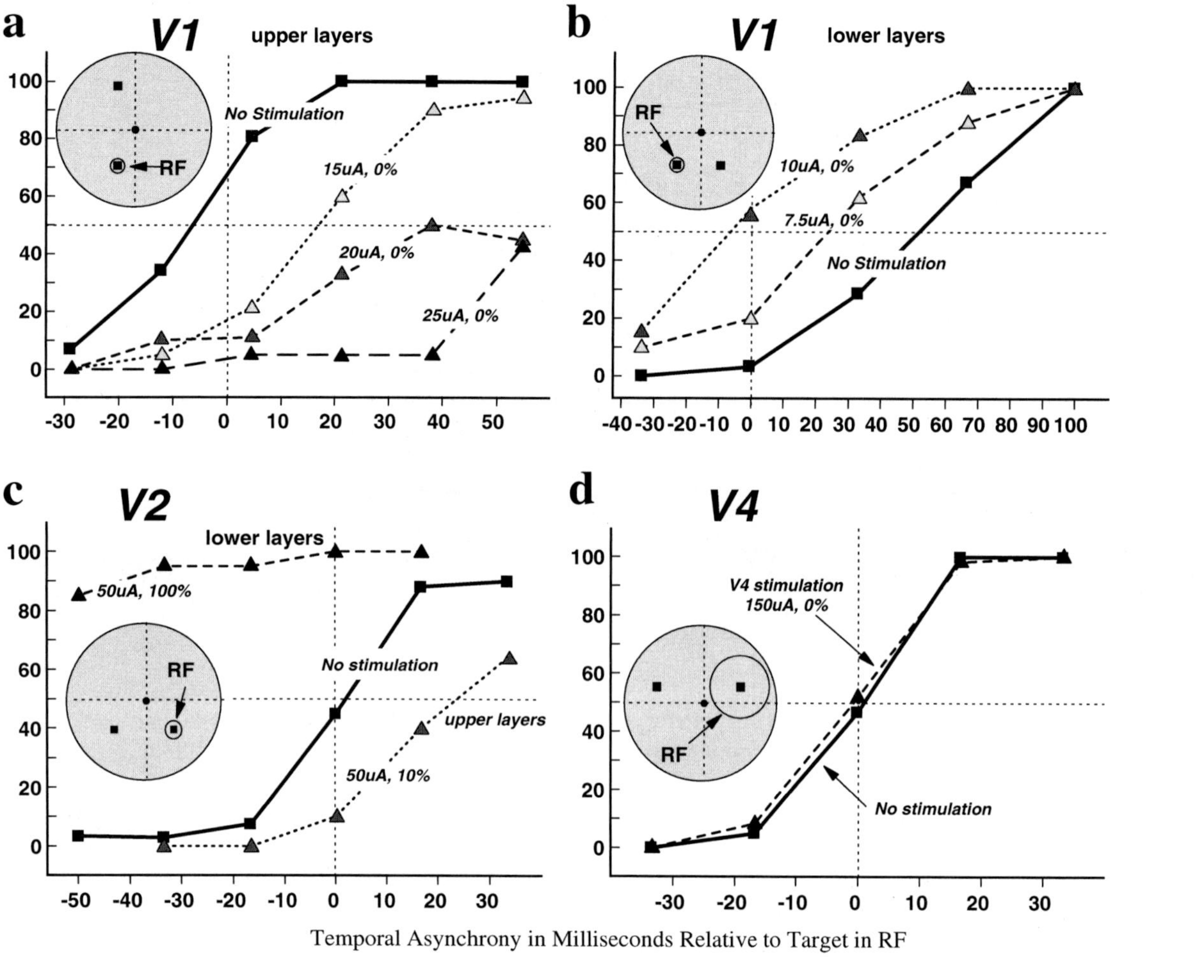

Fig. 14. The probability with which the target presented in the receptive field is chosen as a function of the temporal asynchrony between the two targets and the currents of electrical stimulation used. (a) Interference in V1. (b) Facilitation in V1. (c) Facilitation in the lower and interference in the upper layers of V2. (d) No effect in V4. The insets show arrangement of targets in the visual field. Currents and probability of eliciting a saccade when no target appeared (control condition) are shown for each line. The total number of trials from which the data are derived in this figure was 3480.

TABLE 1

Number of sites studied in each cortical area and their effects

	V1	V2	V4	LIP	DMFC	FEF
Sites electrically stimulated	47	11	21	156	63	92
Sites from which saccades were elicited	46	11	0	8	11	50
Sites tested with single and paired targets	44	11	12	33	9	24
Sites yielding increased choice of target in RF	12	6	0	10	9	24
Sites yielding decreased choice of target in RF	31	4	0	9	0	0
Sites yielding increased fixation times	0	0	0	14	0	0

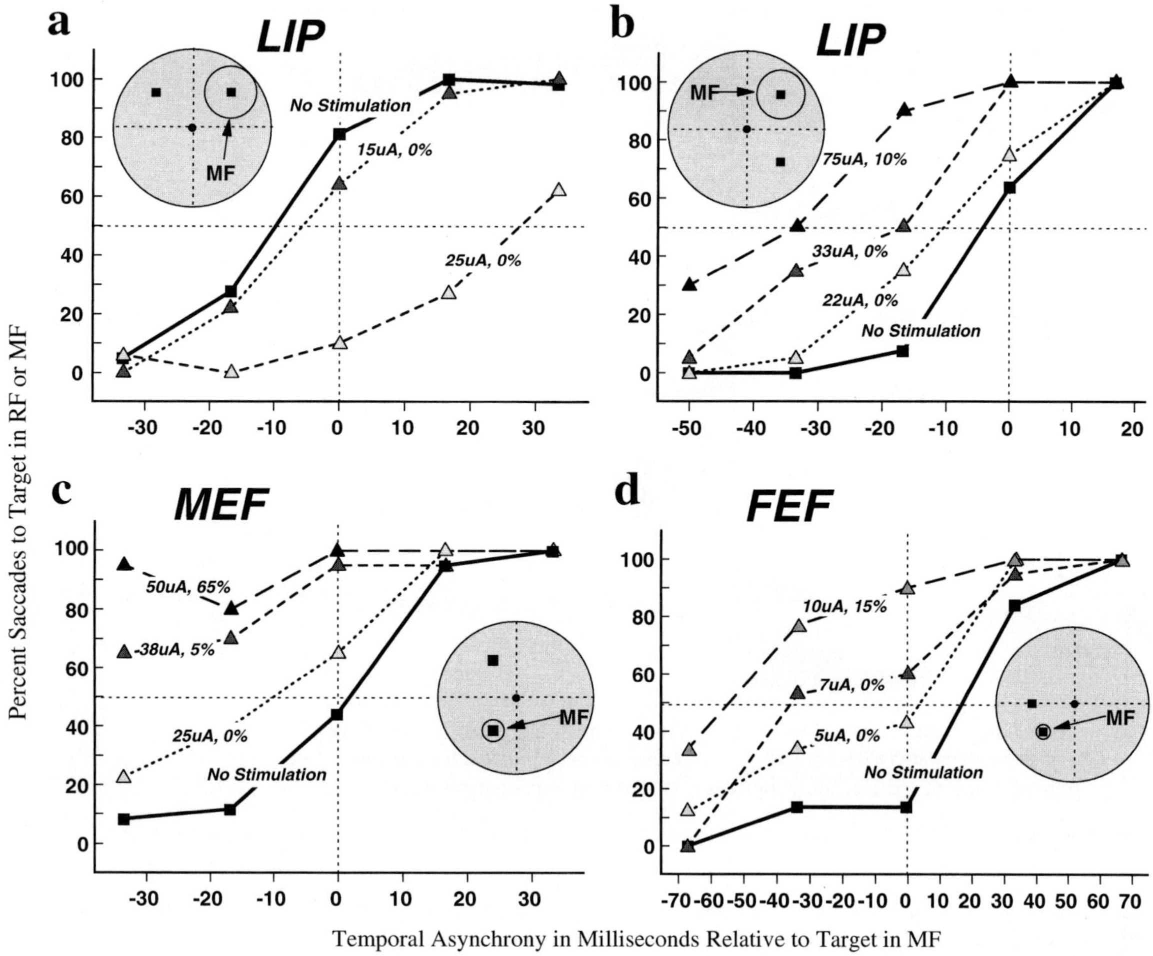

Fig. 15. The probability with which the target presented in the receptive field is chosen as a function of the temporal asynchrony between the two targets and the currents of electrical stimulation used. (a) Interference in LIP. (b) Facilitation in LIP. (c) Facilitation in MEF (d) Facilitation in FEF. The insets show the arrangement of targets in the visual field. Currents and probability of eliciting a saccade when no target appeared (control condition) are shown for each line. The total number of trials from which the data are derived in this figure was 4620.

al., 1977; Mountcastle et al., 1981); here currents of up to 200 μA failed to elicit saccades. The effect of stimulation at these sites was to prolong fixation. This effect differed from the already noted increases in saccadic latencies in V1, V2 and LIP by prolonging fixation duration no matter where targets appeared in the visual field. Data obtained from one such site are plotted in Fig. 16, LIP, section c. Similar increases in fixation time were obtained at 13 other sites in LIP (Table 1).

In area *MEF*, stimulation at 200 μA or lower elicited saccadic eye movements at the minority of the sites tested. At the effective sites, stimulation always produced facilitation. Data from one such site appear in Fig. 15c. Concurrently collected saccadic latencies to single targets were shortened moderately with stimulation as shown in Fig. 16, MEF.

In area *FEF* stimulation elicited saccades at the majority of sites. Subthreshold stimulation consistently produced facilitation. The effective currents were lowest in this area. Fig. 15d shows data from one site. Stimulation in the FEF also shortened saccadic latencies to single targets presented in the motor field. The mean decreases in saccadic latencies

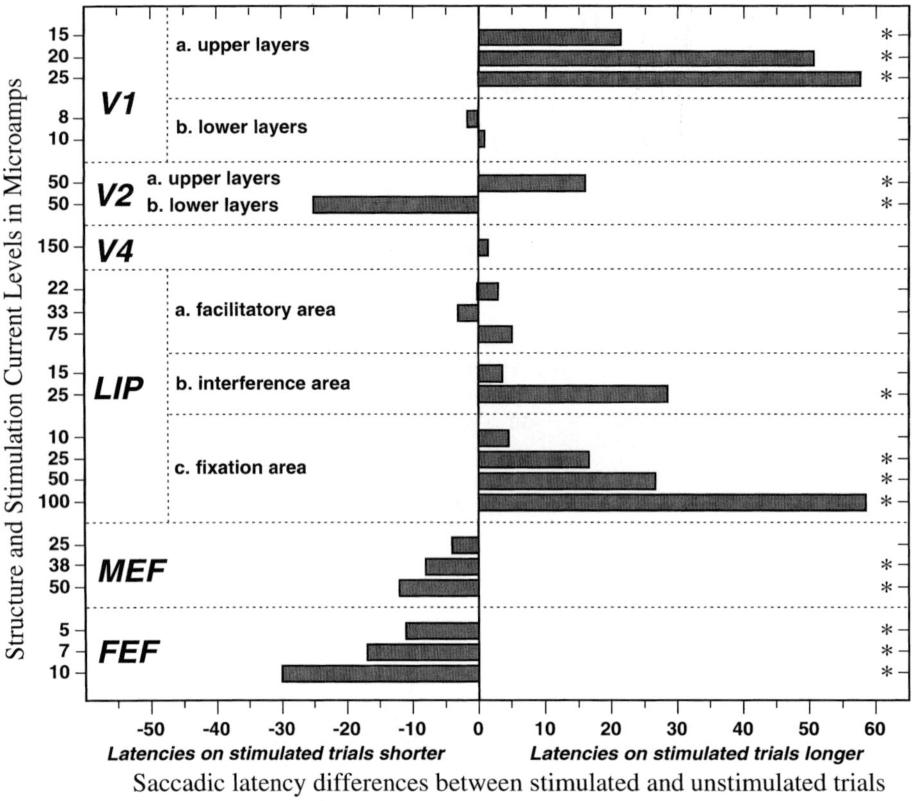

Fig. 16. Differences between the mean saccadic latencies made to single targets with and without electrical stimulation. The data shown were collected concurrently with those that appear in Figs. 14 and 15 with the exception of those for LIP in Fig. 15 subsections a and b, where the data shown were obtained from a site which contained cells that responded with fixation. No data were collected here with paired targets since the increases in saccadic reaction times were not target location specific. The stars next to the right tick marks in the figure indicate saccadic latency differences that were statistically significant ($P < 0.001$). The mean saccadic latencies without stimulation varied between 105 and 146 ms with standard deviations of 7–12 ms.

obtained with single targets in the motor field, collected concurrently with the data shown in Fig. 15d, are shown in Fig. 16, FEF.

Table 1 provides a tally of the number of sites at which the three effects on which we report had been found.

These microstimulation results suggest that both the anterior and the posterior system are involved in target selection. In the posterior system, it appears that decisions are made not only as to where to look, but also where not to look. This latter decision process, where not to look, seems to be a prominent feature of V1, V2 and LIP since, in these areas, stimulation at some of the sites decreased the probability of choosing the target that had been placed within the receptive field of the stimulated neurons.

Based on our lesion and microstimulation experiments we can now proceed to specify what goes on in the process of target selection with saccadic eye movements in the various cortical areas we had studied. Following each saccade to a new location, we see five computations being carried out for generating the next saccade as schematized in Fig. 17. The first under #1, is to determine *what* the objects are in the scene. This we know is carried out by many structures that include V1, V2, V4, inferotemporal cortex and LIP. Second, *one target needs to be chosen* to be looked at. This decision, based on the facilitatory effects we had found, appears to involve areas V1, V2, LIP, the FEF and the MEF. Our new finding showing that stimulation at some sites actually interfered with target selection suggests that a

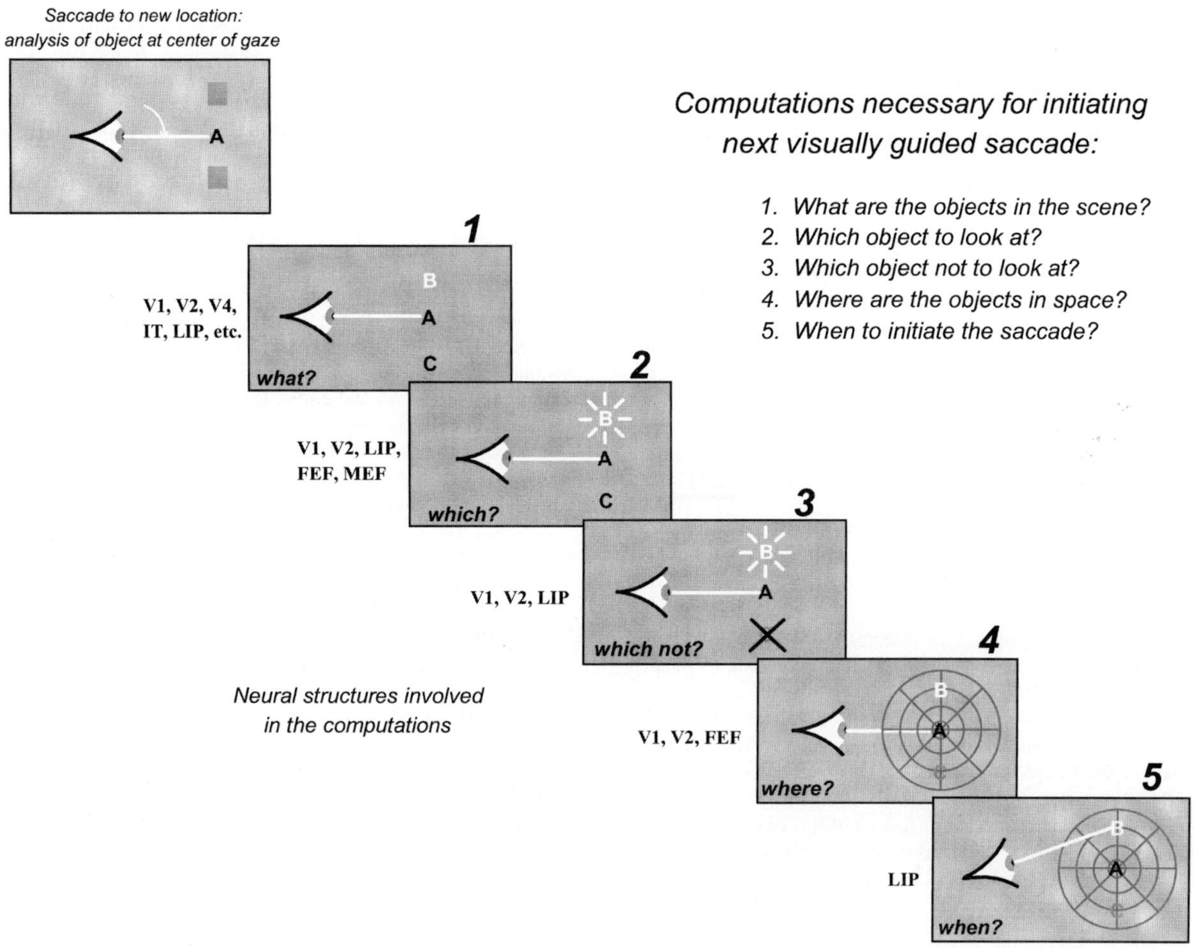

Fig. 17. Schematic representation of the computations involved in generating a saccadic eye movement to a selected target. After each saccade to a new location, the object to which the eye is directed is analyzed. At the same time, steps need to be taken for generating the next saccade. The five computations carried out are depicted as well as the structures involved.

decision also needs to be made as to which targets *not to look* at. This 'de-selection' process involves the upper layers of V1 and V2 and some regions of LIP since at these locations stimulation typically decreased the probability with which the targets in the receptive fields were chosen. This interference effect may well be a product of inhibitory feedback circuits activated by our electrical stimulation. Fourth, *the spatial location* of the targets needs to be computed to generate the correct saccade; in the cortex this probably involves V1, V2, and the FEF in each of which a nice topographic representation has been demonstrated. Lastly, #5, a decision needs to be made as to *when* to initiate the saccade which we believe lies largely in the domain of area LIP. These considerations suggest that both the anterior and the posterior streams are centrally involved in selecting targets with saccadic eye movements. One cannot help but be awed by the fact that this seemingly simple task of moving one's eyes about involves so many brain structures and so much computation.

Acknowledgements

Collaborators in the work described were I-han Chou, Andreas Tolias, John Maunsell, Julie Sandell, Michael Stryker, Janet Conway, and Sean True. We are also indebted to Warren Slocum and Christina Carvey for their contributions to this work.

References

Bisiach, E. and Vallar, G. (1988) Hemineglect in humans. In: E. Boller and J. Grafman (Eds.), *Handbook of Neuropsychology*, Vol. 1, Elsevier, Amsterdam, pp. 195–222.

Fischer, B. and Boch, R. (1983) Saccadic eye movements after extremely short fixation times in the monkey. *Brain Res.*, 260: 21–26.

Huerta, M.F. and Kaas, J.H. (1990) Supplementary eye field as defined by intracortical microstimulation: connections in macaques. *J. Comp. Neurol.*, 293: 299–437.

Huerta, M.F., Krubitzer, L.A. and Kaas, J.H. (1987) Frontal eye field as defined by intracortical microstimulation in squirrel monkeys, owl monkeys, and macaque monkeys. *J. Comp. Neurol.*, 265: 332–361.

Keating, E.G. and Gooley, S.G. (1988a) Saccadic disorders caused by cooling the superior colliculus or the frontal eye field, or from combined lesions of both structures. *Brain Res.*, 438: 247–255.

Keating, E.G. and Gooley, S.G. (1988b) Disconnection of parietal and occipital access to the saccadic oculomotor system. *Exp. Brain Res.*, 70: 385–398.

Keating, E.G., Gooley, S.G., Pratt, S.E. and Kelsey, J. (1983) Removing the superior colliculus silences eye movements normally evoked from stimulation of the parietal and occipital eye fields. *Brain Res.*, 269: 145–148.

Kurylo, D.D. and Skavenski, A.A. (1991) Eye movements elicited by electrical stimulation of area PG in the monkey. *J. Neurophysiol.*, 65: 1243–1253.

Lynch, J.C., Mountcastle, V.B., Talbot, W.H. and Yin, T.C.T. (1977) Parietal lobe mechanisms for directed visual attention. *J. Neurophysiol.*, 40: 362–389.

Lynch, J.C., Graybiel, A.M. and Lobeck, L.J. (1985) The differential projection of two subregions of the inferior parietal lobe of macaque upon deep layers of the superior colliculus. *J. Comp. Neurol.*, 235: 241–245.

Mountcastle, V.B., Andersen, R.A. and Motter, B.C. (1981) The influence of attentive fixation upon the excitability of the light-sensitive neurons of the posterior parietal cortex. *J. Neurosci.*, 11: 1218–1235.

Robinson, D.A. (1972) Eye movements evoked by collicular stimulation in the alert monkey. *Vision Res.*, 12: 1795–1808.

Robinson, D.A. and Fuchs, A.F. (1969) Eye movements evoked by stimulation of frontal eye fields. *J. Neurophysiol.*, 32: 637–648.

Schiller, P.H. (1972) The role of the monkey superior colliculus in eye movements and vision. *Invest. Ophthalmol.*, 11: 451–459.

Schiller, P.H. (1977) The effect of superior colliculus ablation on saccades elicited by cortical stimulation. *Brain Res.*, 122: 154–156.

Schiller, P.H. (1998) The neural control of visually guided eye movements. In: J. Richards (Ed.), *Cognitive Neuroscience of Attention*, Lawrence Erlbaum, London, Chapt. 1.

Schiller, P.H. and Chou, I. (1998) The effects of frontal eye field and dorsomedial frontal cortex lesions on visually guided eye movements. *Nat. Neurosci.*, 1: 248–253.

Schiller, P.H. and Chou, I. (2000a) The effects of anterior arcuate and dorsomedial frontal cortex lesions on visually guided eye movements in the rhesus monkey: I. Single and sequential targets. *Vision Res.*, 40: 1609–1626.

Schiller, P.H. and Chou, I. (2000b) The effects of anterior arcuate and dorsomedial frontal cortex lesions on visually guided eye movements in the rhesus monkey: II. Paired and multiple targets. *Vision Res.*, 40: 1626–1638.

Schiller, P.H. and Stryker, M. (1972) Single-unit recording and stimulation in superior colliculus of the alert rhesus monkey. *J. Neurophysiol.*, 3: 915–924.

Schiller, P.H. and Tehovnik, E.J. (2000) The role of cortical areas in target selection with saccadic eye movements. *Soc. Neurosci. Abstr.*, 26: 1075.

Schiller, P.H., True, S.D. and Conway, J.L. (1980) Deficits in eye movements following frontal eye field and superior colliculus ablations. *J. Neurophysiol.*, 44: 1175–1189.

Schiller, P.H., Sandell, J.H. and Maunsell, J.H.R. (1987) The effect of frontal eye field and superior colliculus lesions on saccadic latencies in the rhesus monkeys. *J. Neurophysiol.*, 57: 1033–1049.

Schlag, J. and Schlag-Rey, M. (1987) Evidence for a supplementary eye field. *J. Neurophysiol.*, 57: 179–200.

Shibutani, H., Sakata, H. and Hyvarinen, J. (1984) Saccade and blinking evoked by microstimulation of the posterior association cortex of the monkey. *Exp. Brain Res.*, 55: 1–8.

Tehovnik, E.J. and Lee, K.-M. (1993) The dorsomedial frontal cortex of the rhesus monkey. Topographic representation of saccades evoked by electrical stimulation. *Exp. Brain Res.*, 96: 430–442.

Tehovnik, E.J., Lee, K.-M. and Schiller, P.H. (1994) Stimulation-evoked saccades from the dorsomedial frontal cortex of the rhesus monkey following lesions of the frontal eye fields and superior colliculus. *Exp. Brain Res.*, 98: 179–190.

Tehovnik, E.J., Slocum, W.M. and Schiller, P.H. (1999) Behavioural conditions affecting saccadic eye movements elicited electrically from the frontal lobes of primates. *Eur. J. Neurosci.*, 11: 2431–2443.

Thier, P. and Andersen, R.A. (1998) Electrical microstimulation distinguishes distinct saccade-related areas in the posterior parietal cortex. *J. Neurophysiol.*, 80: 1713–1735.

Yarbus, A.L. (1967) *Eye Movements and Vision*. Plenum Press, New York.

C. Casanova and M. Ptito (Eds.)
Progress in Brain Research, Vol. 134

CHAPTER 10

Nonvisual influences on visual-information processing in the superior colliculus

Barry E. Stein *, Wan Jiang, Mark T. Wallace and Terrence R. Stanford

Department of Neurobiology and Anatomy, Wake Forest University School of Medicine, Winston-Salem, NC 27157-1010, USA

Abstract: Although visually responsive neurons predominate in the deep layers of the superior colliculus (SC), the majority of them also receive sensory inputs from nonvisual sources (i.e. auditory and/or somatosensory). Most of these 'multisensory' neurons are able to synthesize their cross-modal inputs and, as a consequence, their responses to visual stimuli can be profoundly enhanced or depressed in the presence of a nonvisual cue. Whether response enhancement or response depression is produced by this multisensory interaction is predictable based on several factors. These include: the organization of a neuron's visual and nonvisual receptive fields; the relative spatial relationships of the different stimuli (to their respective receptive fields and to one another); and whether or not the neuron is innervated by a select population of cortical neurons. The response enhancement or depression of SC neurons via multisensory integration has significant survival value via its profound impact on overt attentive/orientation behaviors. Nevertheless, these multisensory processes are not present at birth, and require an extensive period of postnatal maturation. It seems likely that the sensory experiences obtained during this period play an important role in crafting the processes underlying these multisensory interactions.

Nonvisual influences on vision

It is interesting to note that traditional scientific views are sometimes maintained despite the presence of compelling evidence that they are no longer tenable. For example, the neural bases for vision are generally studied as if they function independently of the influences of sensory cues from other modalities. Indeed, the history of the visual sciences has been one in which attempts to understand the brain's coding of visual stimuli have depended on experiments in which absolute control is exerted over the optical properties of stimuli, but little attention is paid to the influences of nonvisual cues. Yet, there is a long and rich history of perceptual studies in which the potent influences of nonvisual cues on visual judgements have been demonstrated. Until comparatively recently, however, the perceptual evidence had little impact on studies investigating the neural bases of vision.

Visual–nonvisual interactions represent one set of possible cross-modal interactions and there has been interest in such phenomena since at least the time of ancient Greece. Some investigators date the onset of discussions of cross-modal perceptual processes to Democritus (500 B.C., see Marks, 1978) and others to Aristotle (350 B.C., see Aristotle). But regardless of which of these scholars one prefers to use as the historical referent, they both appeared to have thought about how cues from different sensory modalities are used cooperatively in building a unified percept of the external world. Thus, there was early recognition of the influences of the different sensory modalities on one another, and especially of the influence of nonvisual cues on visual function. This has been demonstrated repeatedly by modern investigators. Some have shown that the vibration of the

* Corresponding author: B.E. Stein, Department of Neurobiology and Anatomy, Wake Forest University School of Medicine, Winston-Salem, NC 27157-1010, USA.
Tel.: +1-336-716-4368; Fax: +1-336-716-4534;
E-mail: bestein@wfubmc.edu

muscles on one side of the neck can make a stationary light in a darkened room appear to be displaced or to be moving toward the contralateral side (Biguer et al., 1988), others have shown that rotation of the body or a maintained tilt of the head and/or body can interfere with perceiving the orientation of a line (Clark and Graybiel, 1966; Wade and Day, 1968), and that changing gravitational forces can disrupt our visual judgements (Cohen, 1981). Even our simple judgements of visual intensity are influenced by the presence of a neutral auditory cue; it makes the light appear substantially brighter (Stein et al., 1996).

These cross-modal influences on visual perception reflect the fact that the senses have evolved to function in concert, in large part to serve a common purpose: detecting and interpreting changes in the external environment in order to guide and improve motor control. Not only can different senses substitute for one another for this purpose (hearing and touch can substitute for vision in the dark) and reduce the ambiguity of some events (e.g. events that look alike may be distinguished because they sound or feel different, and the correlations among the senses enhance predictions about events), but they can also enhance one another's effectiveness. For example, coupling a visual and an auditory cue can substantially enhance the likelihood that an event will be detected and that a response will be generated (Stein et al., 1989). Furthermore, the speed of one's reaction to either a visual or an auditory cue can be significantly enhanced by presenting them simultaneously (Zahn et al., 1978; Perrott et al., 1990; Lee et al., 1991; Hughes et al., 1994; Frens et al., 1995; Goldring et al., 1996; Harrington and Peck, 1998; Giard and Peronnet, 1999).

This synergy among sensory modalities is constructed in a way that facilitates the detection of events that have a common origin (e.g. the visual and auditory cues associated with an object hitting a surface, or a mouse rustling in the leaves). Presumably, this is effected via the enhancement of the individual neural signals initiated by the modality-specific stimuli derived from these events. As will be seen below, the spatial and temporal concordance of the visual–nonvisual cues that are generally associated with a single event can determine whether or not these multisensory cues will interact to produce enhanced neural signals.

Oddly enough, the importance of cross-modal synergy becomes most apparent when the cues normally associated with the same event are manipulated so that their normal spatial and/or temporal concordance is slightly disrupted. Under these conditions a cross-modal illusion may be produced, and there are many such illusions, which can significantly alter the apparent location of a sensory cue (e.g. see Howard and Templeton, 1966), or its meaning (e.g. see McGurk and MacDonald, 1976).

Although many perceptual and behavioral studies have demonstrated the potency of visual–nonvisual ('multisensory') integration, these laboratory demonstrations seem to involve situations that are uncommon in normal experience. Thus, it should be emphasized that because the environment is composed of stimuli that activate multiple sensory modalities and both the internal and external sensory environments are constantly in flux, the normal experience is one in which multisensory integrative processes are continuously in play. These processes are likely to have a more pervasive influence on perception and behavior than would be evident from even an extensive list of current laboratory demonstrations.

Multisensory convergence and cross-modal receptive field overlap

One of the most direct ways for nonvisual stimuli to affect the brain's 'visual' processes is via the convergence of nonvisual and visual signals onto the same neurons. This is far more common than one might think, and the convergence of multiple sensory afferents takes place at many levels of the neuraxis (see Stein and Meredith, 1993). One of the best known of these sites is the deep layers of the superior colliculus (SC). The SC is a midbrain structure that functions at the interface between sensory inputs and motor outputs. It receives inputs from the visual, auditory and somatosensory modalities and issues commands to control the orientation of the eyes, ears, head and limbs toward (or away from) these stimuli.

The visual and nonvisual sensory inputs to the SC are derived from numerous sources (see Edwards et al., 1979; Huerta and Harting, 1984), but most of these inputs are from structures that contain neurons only responsive to a single sensory modality. Thus, the SC, rather than reflecting a relay of the convergence patterns in its afferent structures, is a primary site of cross-modal convergence. This is particularly evident in the selective nature of the projections it receives from the anterior ectosylvian sulcus (AES), a region of association cortex that contains a mixture of modality-specific and multisensory neurons (Minciacchi et al., 1987; Kimura and Tamai, 1992; Wallace et al., 1992; Jiang et al., 1994a; Benedek et al., 1996; Kimura et al., 1996; Rauschecker, 1996). The AES sends a heavy direct projection to the deep SC (Stein et al., 1983) that consists of modality-specific neurons (Wallace et al., 1993); the region's multisensory neurons form a circuit independent of the SC. It is interesting to note, however, that many of the principles of multisensory integration that have been derived from work in the SC, and which will be described below, have proven to apply to the AES as well (see Jiang et al., 1994b; Wallace et al., 1992; Stein and Wallace, 1996).

Visual and nonvisual afferents to the SC are arranged to form topographic representations (see Stein and Meredith, 1993). In contrast to the topographies formed in primary sensory structures, experiments conducted in awake behaving animals suggest that sensory information in the SC has been transformed such that the visual, auditory, and somatosensory representations share a common 'motor' reference frame. Thus for example, rather than being referenced to the fovea (visual), head (auditory), and body surface (somatosensory), the 'sensory' topographies appear to represent the locations of stimuli with respect to the current position of gaze (Jay and Sparks, 1984; Hartline et al., 1995; Groh and Sparks, 1996; Peck et al., 1995). The consequence of this transformation for sensorimotor integration is that sensory maps, regardless of modality, are in register with the topographic representation of gaze metrics that is found within the same SC layers. Thus, for example, a stimulus 10° to the right of gaze will evoke activity in the same region of the SC for which motor-related activity produces a 10° rightward gaze shift. The topographies are such that rostral SC represents stimuli in near contralateral space (where motor activity produces small contralateral gaze shifts) and caudal SC represents stimuli in more eccentric regions of contralateral space (where motor activity produces larger contralateral gaze shifts). Stimuli in upper contralateral space (relative to gaze) would be represented medially and those in lower space represented laterally within the SC.

Referencing sensory representations to motor control is an important step in the process of transforming a sensory signal into an appropriate motor command. It also has important implications for multisensory integration, as it would ensure that the modality-specific receptive fields of multisensory neurons maintain their spatial congruence despite relative movements of the eyes, head, and body. As discussed below, the spatial register of modality-specific receptive fields is an important factor for multisensory integration. Cross-modal spatial register has been shown in recordings from anesthetized animals and is particularly evident in individual multisensory neurons (Drager and Hubel, 1975; Meredith and Stein, 1983; King and Palmer, 1985; Wallace et al., 1996). In these experiments, the eyes, ears, and head face forward such that the axes of visual, auditory, and somatosensory space are approximately aligned. Thus, a visual–auditory neuron whose visual receptive field is in central space will also have its auditory receptive field in central space (or its somatosensory receptive field on the face) (Fig. 1). The transformation of modality-specific sensory information into a common coordinate frame is likely to underlie the cross-modal receptive field register that characterizes multisensory neurons throughout the central nervous system (e.g. see Rizzolatti et al., 1981a,b; Gentilucci et al., 1983; Duhamel et al., 1991; Ramachandran et al., 1993; Graziano et al., 1994, 1997). Note however, that in other regions, the reference frame may differ from that found in the SC. For example, in premotor cortex, an area involved in the programming of reaching movements, sensory-receptive fields appear to be referenced to the body (e.g. hand) rather than the eye as in the SC (Gentilucci et al., 1983; Graziano et al., 1994, 1997).

Multisensory integration: response enhancement and response depression

A unique characteristic of multisensory SC neurons is their ability to synthesize their cross-modal inputs, resulting in a significantly enhanced or degraded neural response (Meredith and Stein, 1986; Wallace et al., 1996, 1998). The stimulus condi-

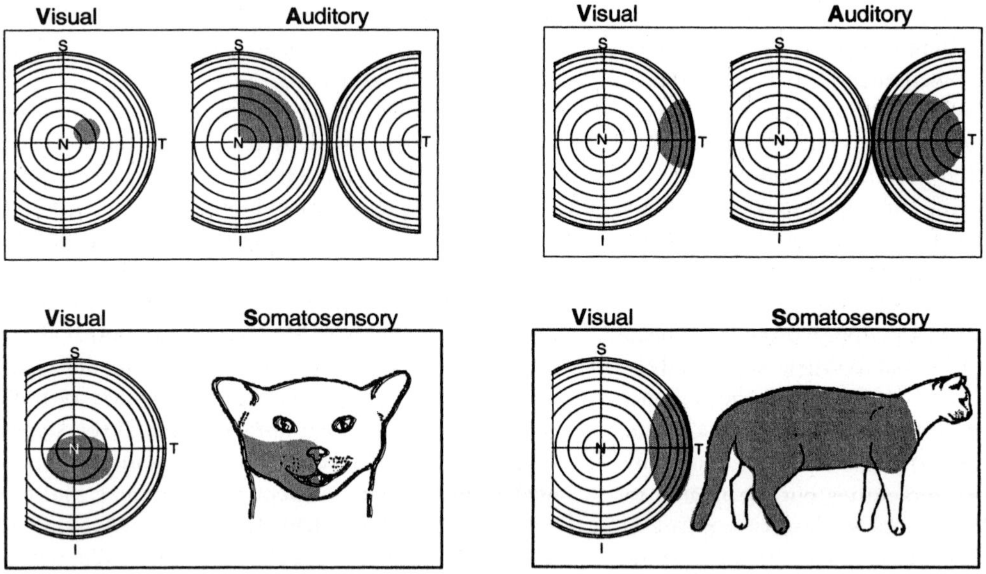

Fig. 1. Examples of cross-modal receptive field register, which characterizes multisensory neurons. Shown here are the receptive fields (shading) of four representative multisensory neurons studied in the cat SC. Visual and auditory space are represented from the animal's perspective in standardized conventions in which each concentric circle represents 10°. The caudal half of contralateral auditory space is shown as a the half circle on the right that has been folded forward (the caudal half of ipsilateral auditory space is not shown). Note the correspondence between the positions of the different receptive fields of the individual visual–auditory (top) and visual–somatosensory (bottom) SC neurons. N, nasal; T, temporal; S, superior; I, inferior.

tions that lead to an integrated multisensory response are also linked to an increase or decrease in the probability of an overt orientation response (Stein et al., 1989). The term 'multisensory integration' has been defined operationally as a statistically significant difference between the number of impulses evoked by a cross-modal combination of stimuli (e.g. a visual and an auditory stimulus) and the number evoked by the most effective of the modality-specific stimuli (Meredith and Stein, 1983). These integrated multisensory responses can be extremely potent. In some cases, response enhancement can exceed the arithmetic sum of the responses to the individual modality-specific stimuli that have been combined, and in others even a robust modality-specific response can be eliminated by the addition of a stimulus from another modality. Whether any given cross-modal stimulus combination produces a multisensory interaction in a given neuron, and whether this interaction results in response enhancement or response depression in that neuron, depends on the relationships among the stimuli and their respective receptive fields (Meredith and Stein, 1996; Kadunce et al., 1997). As will be shown below, for there to be any predictability in these integrated responses, a stable relationship must be maintained among a given neuron's cross-modal receptive fields.

When a given event gives rise to multiple sensory cues, these cues occur at the same time and are derived from the same location in space. Thus, they are all/both likely to fall within the multiple overlapping receptive fields of the same multisensory neurons. If they do so, it is likely that their combined excitatory influences will be dealt with in a synergistic fashion to produce an enhanced response (Fig. 2). The absolute magnitude of the enhancement depends on the effectiveness of the individual stimuli: modality-specific stimuli that are weak generally interact to produce the greatest response enhancement (Fig. 3). It is this observation that led to speculation that multisensory enhancement is of particular benefit when individual stimuli are weak and/or ambiguous. However, if these same cross-modal stimuli are derived from separate events, and are thus derived from different spatial locations such that, for example, the visual stimulus falls within its receptive field and the auditory stimulus falls outside its receptive field, there will be either no multisensory interaction or the auditory stimulus will inhibit visual excitation (Fig. 2). This cross-modal inhibition is produced when the extra-receptive-field stimulus activates the inhibitory region that borders some receptive fields.

Cortical influences on multisensory integration in the SC

It may seem reasonable to expect that any neuron that receives inputs from multiple sensory modalities is rendered capable of synthesizing these inputs. This is not correct. Approximately 20% of SC neurons in normal animals are able to respond to cues from different sensory modalities but are unable to integrate them to produce the response enhancement or depression described above. Furthermore, those SC neurons that are able to integrate their different sensory inputs are able to do so only in the presence of influences from two regions of association cortex: the anterior ectosylvian sulcus (AES) and the rostral aspect of the lateral suprasylvian sulcus (rLS) (Wallace and Stein, 1994; Jiang et al., 1999). This was determined from experiments in which the modality-specific and multisensory responses of SC neurons were examined before, during, and after reversible cryogenic deactivation of one or both of these cortical regions. During deactivation, the characteristic multisensory response enhancement of SC neurons (which was used as the index of multisensory integration) was eliminated (Fig. 5), and the responses of multisensory neurons to combinations of cross-modal cues became indistinguishable from those neurons that are normally incapable of multisensory integration. Yet, this capability was reinstated once the cortex was reactivated by warming.

The AES and rLS appear to function in cooperative fashion in mediating multisensory integration in SC neurons. In some cases SC neurons depend solely on inputs from the AES to express this capacity, and in rare cases they depend solely on the rLS. However, in many cases, SC neurons receive dual AES–rLS influences that function either in synergistic fashion (deactivation of either one compromises the multisensory integration capabilities of an SC neuron; Fig. 5) or redundant fashion (deactivation of either one alone has no effect, but their combined deactivation eliminates this SC capacity) (Jiang et al., 1999). These observations suggest that the primary difference between multisensory 'integrative' and 'nonintegrative' neurons is the presence or absence of a corticotectal projection from association cortex.

The importance of association cortex for the multisensory orientation/approach behaviors that are mediated by the SC is apparent from similar experiments in behaving cats (Wilkinson et al., 1996). Cats were trained in a perimetry device to orient to a light-emitting diode (LED) and approach its position in order to obtain a food reward. They were also trained to ignore a brief, broad-band, low-intensity sound that could occur at any location. Once trained, the intensity of each LED was lowered in order to evoke approximately 50% correct responses during normal modality-specific trials. When the visual and auditory stimuli were presented simultaneously at the same location, correct responding was enhanced to near 100%. On the other hand, when the visual and auditory stimuli were spatially disparate, correct responses to the visual stimuli were significantly degraded. These observations were consistent with the results of previous studies (Stein et al., 1989). However, when the AES was reversibly deactivated via injections of lidocaine through chronically implanted cannulae, the enhanced behavioral responding to spatially coincident visual–auditory cues was significantly degraded. The animals responded no better to the combination of cues than to the best of them alone. Similarly, the depression of the response to the visual cue induced by a spatially disparate auditory stimulus was also disrupted. These effects were specific to the AES (the rLS was not tested), and could not be induced by deactivation of other cortical areas that project to the SC (e.g. those from the posterior lateral suprasylvian sulcus, AI, or 17/18) or by saline injections into the AES. More recently, a more comprehensive evaluation of the effect of association cortex on these behaviors has found that deactivation of either the AES or the rLS could produce this behavioral effect (Jiang et al., 2000). That this inability to utilize multisensory cues behaviorally was likely due to the loss of multisensory integration in the SC, and not simply a consequence of eliminating the independent behavioral/perceptual contributions of the AES, is supported by the observation that ibotenic acid lesions of the SC produce a similar

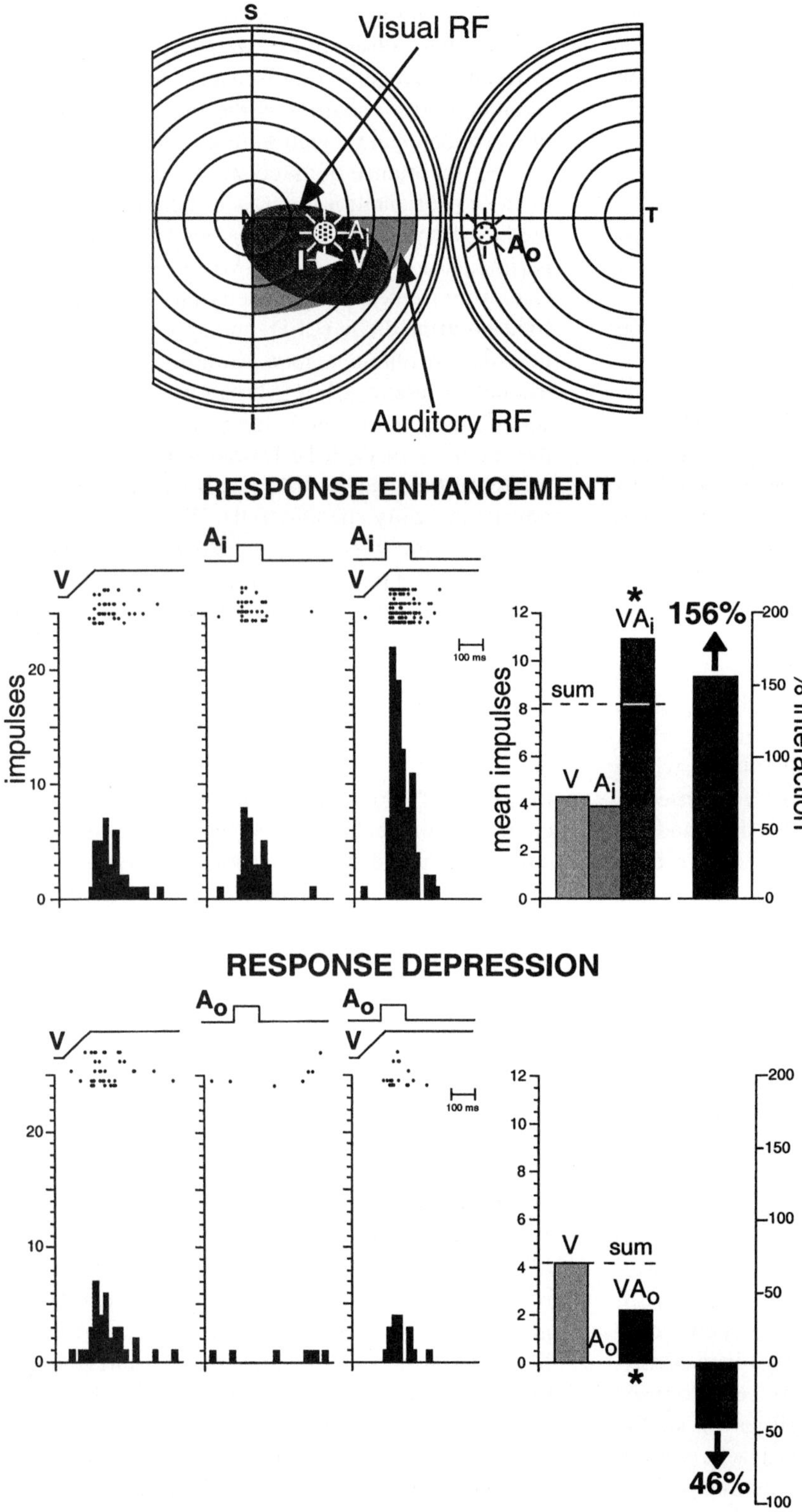
S
Visual RF
T
I
Auditory RF
V
A_i
A_o
RESPONSE ENHANCEMENT
impulses
mean impulses
sum
VA_i
156%
% interaction
100 ms
RESPONSE DEPRESSION
A_o
VA_o
46%

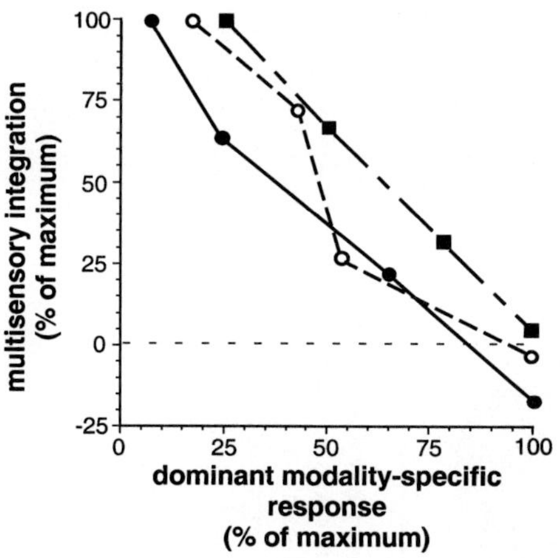

Fig. 3. Examples of inverse effectiveness. Multisensory neurons exhibit an inverse relationship between the effectiveness of the modality-specific stimuli and the magnitude of the multisensory interaction. Plotted here are data from three representative SC neurons. In each case, the maximal multisensory response enhancement was obtained at the lowest levels of effectiveness of the dominant modality-specific response (i.e. the sensory modality evoking the highest number of impulses). As the effectiveness of the dominant modality-specific stimulus increased, the relative magnitude of the integrated multisensory response decreased. Adapted from Stein et al. (2000b).

effect, despite the fact that the AES and rLS remaine functionally intact (Burnett et al., 2000).

In very rare cases, the normal cross-modal receptive field register does not develop (Wallace et al., 1996). Thus, even when all the sensory organs are properly aligned, their receptive fields are non-overlapping. In such instances, multisensory integration is seriously disrupted (Fig. 4).

Although the most straightforward way these influences can be exerted on SC neurons is via the direct corticotectal projections that originate from both areas (Stein et al., 1983), there are reciprocal rLS–AES connections (Miceli et al., 1985; Reinoso-Suarez and Roda, 1985; Scannell et al., 1995). Consequently, it is possible that, at least in the cases of synergy, these intracortical connections may also play a role. However these influences are mediated, it is important to note that, because these regions of association cortex are critical for SC multisensory integration, they perform some of their functions via connections to distant subcortical structures. Simultaneously, however, the multisensory neurons of the AES (we know very little about the neurons in rLS) are also capable of cross-modal synthesis. Interestingly, many of the same principles that govern multisensory integration in the SC also govern multisensory integration in the AES (Wallace et al., 1992, also see Minciacchi et al., 1987 and Jiang et al., 1994b).

What is most noteworthy about these corticotectal influences is, as noted earlier, their specificity for multisensory integration. The observation that during cortical deactivation, a visual–auditory neuron loses its ability to exhibit response enhancement to combinations of visual–auditory stimuli, but can still respond to individual visual and auditory stimuli, indicates that non AES–rLS inputs (e.g. ascending inputs) are capable of activating SC neurons independent of the AES or rLS. The SC receives a large number of such inputs, with the subcortical component alone numbering more than 40 (Edwards et al., 1979; Huerta and Harting, 1984). While there are many afferent convergence patterns in the SC, the data indicate that a common pattern is the convergence of cross-modal inputs from association cortex and from other, presumably ascending (or non-association cortical areas) (Wallace et al., 1993; Jiang et al., 1999).

Fig. 2. Multisensory response enhancement and multisensory response depression. Many multisensory SC neurons exhibit both response enhancement and response depression, depending on the spatial relationships of the stimuli relative to the locations of their receptive fields. The receptive fields of this visual–auditory neuron, and the locations of the visual and auditory stimuli, are shown at the top. The movement of the visual stimulus (a bar of light labelled V) is depicted by the arrow. The auditory stimulus (icon of speaker) was presented at two locations, one inside the auditory receptive field (Ai) and the other outside the receptive field (Ao). Rasters, histograms and summary bar graphs at the bottom show the responses of this neuron to the visual stimulus alone (movement is represented by a ramp), the auditory stimulus alone at each of the locations (represented by a square wave), and to the cross-modal stimulus combinations. Note that, whereas the stimulus combination in which both the stimuli are within their respective receptive fields resulted in a response enhancement that exceeded the sum of the individual modality-specific responses, the combination in which the auditory stimulus was outside its receptive field resulted in a significant depression of the response to the visual stimulus. $^{*}P < 0.05$. Adapted from Stein et al. (1999, 2000a).

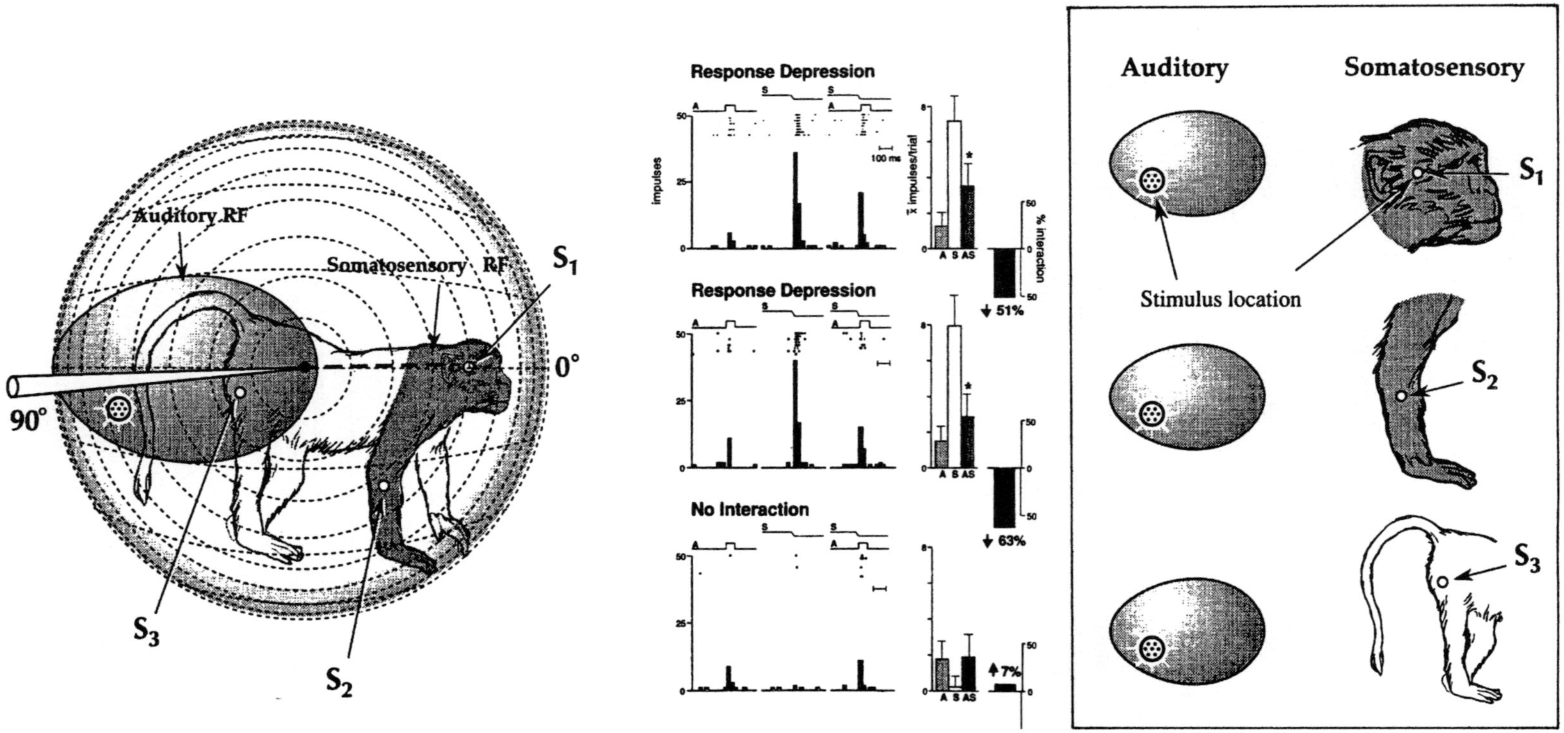

Fig. 4. Multisensory integration is abnormal with nonoverlapping receptive fields. The locations of the auditory and somatosensory receptive fields in this neuron in monkey SC were grossly mismatched. As a consequence, stimuli presented together in space could not fall within both receptive fields simultaneously. Rasters, peristimulus time histograms, and summary bar graphs illustrate that when both stimuli were presented within their respective receptive fields (AS_1, AS_2), response depression was generated, and that when the stimuli were presented in close spatial proximity (AS_3), no interaction was generated. Conventions are the same as in Fig. 2. For illustrative purposes, the monkey is shown within an imaginary bubble upon which the auditory receptive field is plotted. 0° represents the point directly in front of the animal, and 90° the point directly to the right in the interaural plane. Inset on right shows stimulus locations relative to receptive fields. From Wallace et al. (1996).

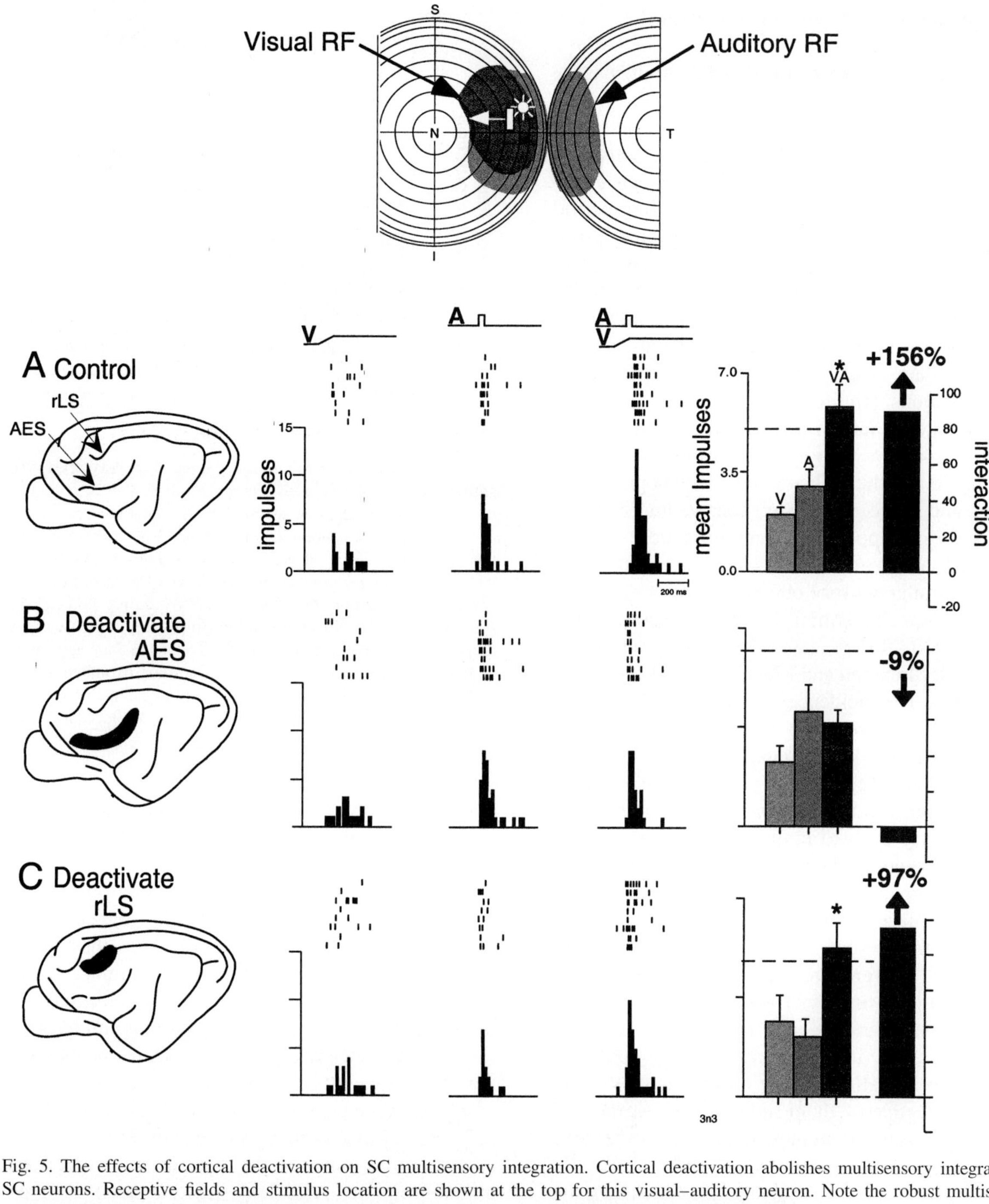

Fig. 5. The effects of cortical deactivation on SC multisensory integration. Cortical deactivation abolishes multisensory integration in SC neurons. Receptive fields and stimulus location are shown at the top for this visual–auditory neuron. Note the robust multisensory response enhancement to the stimulus combination in the control condition (prior to cortical deactivation). This multisensory response enhancement was eliminated during AES deactivation, yet there was no significant change in responses to either the visual or auditory stimuli. The multisensory integration of this neuron was unaffected by deactivation of rLS.

Development of multisensory integration

Earlier it was noted that not all adult multisensory SC neurons are capable of synthesizing cross-modal cues, and, thus, that multisensory integration is not an obligatory property of these neurons. This was particularly obvious in studies of neonatal cats (Wallace and Stein, 1997), which undergo a long period of maturation before their sensory response properties are adult-like. In very young kittens, there are no multisensory neurons in the SC: its neurons respond only to somatosensory cues. The first auditory-responsive neurons do not appear until 5 days postnatal (Stein et al., 1973a), and the first multisensory neurons (auditory–somatosensory) are not encountered until late in the second postnatal week. Visually responsive neurons in the multisensory (i.e. deep) layers of the SC are most developmentally delayed, and hence, visually responsive multisensory neurons do not appear until approximately 3 postnatal weeks (Kao et al., 1994; Wallace and Stein, 1997). A similar sensory chronology for orientation to modality-specific stimuli has been described (e.g. see Fox, 1970; Norton, 1974; Villablanca and Olmstead, 1979; Sireteanu and Maurer, 1982; Larson and Stein, 1984). The incidence of multisensory SC neurons increases progressively until reaching adult-like levels at 10–12 weeks postnatal.

As would be expected, the properties of neonatal sensory-responsive SC neurons are immature: they respond poorly even to high intensity stimuli, they have long response latencies, and their receptive fields are very large (Stein et al., 1973a,b; Kao et al., 1994; Wallace and Stein, 1997). Perhaps most interesting in the present context is that neonatal multisensory SC neurons are incapable of synthesizing their cross-modal inputs. They respond very much like the 'nonintegrative' multisensory SC neurons observed in adult animals, responding to combinations of two modality-specific stimuli as they do to the most effective of them individually. At the end of the first postnatal month, multisensory neurons begin to appear that are capable of synthesizing their cross-modal inputs by showing the characteristic response enhancements that were described above. Initially, there are very few such neurons, but their incidence gradually increases to adult-like levels by 3–4 months after birth (Fig. 6). What is surprising

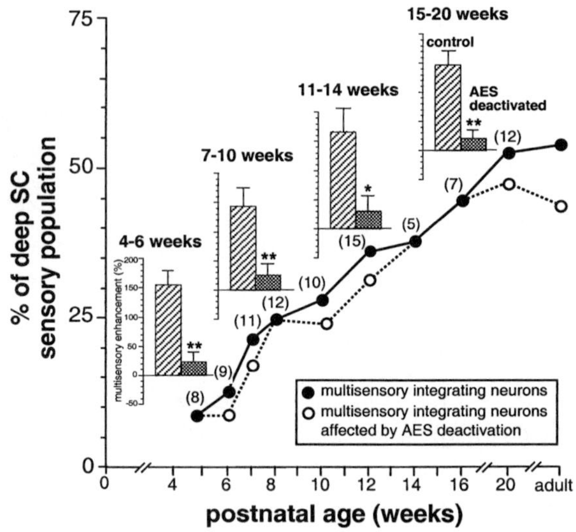

Fig. 6. The capacity for multisensory integration developed gradually for the population of SC neurons studied. This developmental change appeared to be a result of the functional maturation of corticotectal influences. The line graphs shown here plot the increasing prevalence of SC neurons capable of multisensory integration during postnatal maturation, and the increasing incidence of SC neurons that lost this ability during cortical (i.e. AES) deactivation. Note the striking similarities in the two functions. The bar graphs show that at each of the four age ranges represented, integrative multisensory neurons exhibited similar levels of response enhancement, and similar effects of AES deactivation. *$P < 0.05$, **$P < 0.01$. From Wallace and Stein (2000).

is that, with few exceptions, even the youngest neurons capable of synthesizing cross-modal cues do so in an adult-like manner. Although the time window during which multisensory integration can take place is shorter than it is in the adult, the same spatial and inverse effectiveness principles that govern multisensory integration in mature animals are already evident in the youngest SC neurons capable of multisensory integration. Even the magnitude of the response enhancements observed in neonates rivals that found in adults (Wallace and Stein, 1997).

As might be expected from the discussions above, the onset of multisensory integration in SC neurons appears to be linked to the maturation of functional inputs from the AES and rLS. As soon as a developing SC neuron is capable of synthesizing its cross-modal cues, this capacity is compromised by deactivation of association cortex (Fig. 6; Wallace and Stein, 2000). And, just as in the adult animal, deactivation of association cortex is selective: it eliminates the response enhancements produced by combinations of cross-modal cues, but does not preclude responses to these cues individually. However, now their combination produces a response that is comparable to the response to one of the modality-specific cues.

These data are consistent with the idea that when SC neurons mature from a stage where they can deal only with modality-specific cues to one at which they can deal with, but not integrate, inputs from more than a single sensory modality, there is a functional maturation of inputs from sources other than the AES and rLS. But, maturation from this condition to one in which multisensory integration takes place is linked to the functional maturation of corticotectal projections from association cortex. Presumably, then, the corticotectal projections from this region that have been shown to be present in newborn animals (McHaffie et al., 1988) are not yet functional.

Without conducting long-term recordings from the same neurons, it is not possible to determine whether each SC neuron that is capable of multisensory integration passes through sequential stages in which it is first modality-specific, then becomes multisensory and finally is rendered multisensory 'integrative.' But given that, from approximately 6 weeks of age to maturity there is no significant increase in the incidence of sensory neurons in the SC despite a substantial change in the incidence of multisensory integrative neurons, this is a plausible idea.

The abrupt developmental onset of multisensory integration in individual SC neurons, the adult-like capabilities of early integrating multisensory neurons, the correlation between the appearance of multisensory integration in a given neuron and the appearance of influences from association cortex, as well as the observation that the magnitude of the effect of cortical deactivation on multisensory integration does not change with age, all suggest that there is a 'gate-like' maturation of association cortex influences on individual SC neurons (Wallace and Stein, 1997, 2000). This sort of abrupt maturational change may be less unusual than it appears because it has also been noted in the development of corticotectal influences from the striate cortex over superficial layer SC visual responses (Stein and Gallagher, 1981).

The specific changes in the projections from association cortex neurons that must occur to render them capable of facilitating multisensory integration in SC neurons is unknown. Nevertheless, it has been shown that there are differences in the synaptic morphology that characterizes at least one set of ascending and descending tectopetal afferents: those in the somatosensory modality. Harting et al. (1997) showed that the somatosensory inputs to the SC derived from the trigeminal complex (i.e. ascending inputs) form small synapses in which there are round vesicles with dark mitochondria (i.e. RSD synapses). These synapses are on the distal dendrites of SC neurons. In contrast, somatosensory terminals from the AES are characterized by round vesicles, are large, and contain pale mitochondria (RLP synapses) and contact the proximal dendrites of SC neurons. These investigators raise the possibility that the synaptic differences between these two components of the somatosensory input to the SC distinguish between inputs that are capable only of activating SC neurons and those that are capable of facilitating multisensory integration. It remains to be seen whether this distinction holds for the visual and auditory modalities, and whether those corticotectal inputs that are uninvolved in multisensory integration (e.g. posterior lateral suprasylvian projections) lack RLP synaptic profiles.

But, whatever features are present that allow AES and rLS influences to facilitate SC multisensory integration give them control over these processes and the behavioral responses that depend on them. The question remains why such control is in place. One very real possibility is that this circuitry allows experiential influences to affect multisensory SC processes via corticotectal inputs. For it has been shown that while the response properties of SC neurons are changed through sensory experience, many of these changes are mediated via corticotectal influences (Wicklegren and Sterling, 1969).

Acknowledgements

We would like to thank Nancy London for her technical assistance. This work was supported by NIH Grants NS22543 and NS36916.

References

Aristotle. *De Anima*. Translated by R.D. Hicks, 1907. Reprint, Arno Press, New York, 1976.

Benedek, G., Fischer-Szatmari, L., Kovacs, G., Perenyi, J. and Katoh, Y.Y. (1996) Visual, somatosensory and auditory modality properties along the feline suprageniculate–anterior ectosylvian sulcus/insular pathway. *Prog. Brain Res.*, 112: 325–334.

Biguer, B., Donaldson, I.M.L., Hein, A. and Jeannerod, M. (1988) Neck muscle vibration modifies the representation of visual motion and direction in man. *Brain*, 111: 1405–1424.

Burnett, L.R., Stein, B.E. and Wallace, M.T. (2000) Ibotenic acid lesions of the superior colliculus (SC) alter multisensory orientation behaviors. *Soc. Neurosci. Abstr.*, in press.

Clark, B. and Graybiel, A. (1966) Contributing factors in the perception of the oculogravic illusion. *Am. J. Psychol.*, 79: 377–388.

Cohen, M.M. (1981) Visual-proprioceptive interactions. In: R.D. Walk and L.H. Pick, Jr. (Eds.), *Intersensory Perception and Sensory Integration*. Plenum, New York, pp. 175–314.

Drager, U.C. and Hubel, D.H. (1975) Responses to visual stimulation and relationship between visual, auditory and somatosensory inputs in mouse superior colliculus. *J. Neurophysiol.*, 38: 690–713.

Duhamel, J.-R., Colby, C.L. and Goldberg, M.E. (1991) Congruent representations of visual and somatosensory space in single neurons of monkey ventral intraparietal cortex (area VIP). In: J. Paillard (Ed.), *Brain and Space*. Oxford University Press, New York, pp. 223–236.

Edwards, S.B., Ginsburgh, C.L., Henkel, C.K. and Stein, B.E. (1979) Sources of subcortical projections to the superior colliculus in the cat. *J. Comp. Neurol.*, 184: 309–330.

Fox, M.W. (1970) Reflex development and behavioral organization. In: W.A. Himwich (Ed.), *Developmental Neurobiology*. Thomas, Springfield, IL, pp. 553–580.

Frens, M.A., Van Opstal, A.J. and Van der Willigen, R.F. (1995) Spatial and temporal factors determine auditory–visual interactions in human saccadic eye movements. *Percept. Psychophys.*, 57: 802–816.

Gentilucci, M., Scandolara, C., Pigarev, I.N. and Rizzolatti, G. (1983) Visual responses in the postarcuate cortex (area 6) of the monkey that are independent of eye position. *Exp. Brain Res.*, 50: 464–468.

Giard, M.H. and Peronnet, F. (1999) Auditory–visual integration during multimodal object recognition in humans: a behavioral and electrophysiological study. *J. Cogn. Neurosci.*, 11: 473–490.

Goldring, J.E., Dorris, M.C., Corneil, B.D., Ballantyne, P.A. and Munoz, D.P. (1996) Combined eye–head gaze shifts to visual and auditory targets in humans. *Exp. Brain Res.*, 111: 68–78.

Graziano, M.S., Yap, G.S. and Gross, C.G. (1994) Coding of visual space by premotor neurons. *Science*, 266: 1054–1057.

Graziano, M.S., Hu, T. and Gross, C.G. (1997) Visuospatial properties of ventral premotor cortex. *J. Neurophysiol.*, 77: 2268–2292.

Groh, J.M. and Sparks, D.L. (1996) Saccades to somatosensory targets. III. Eye-position-dependent somatosensory activity in primate superior colliculus. *J. Neurophysiol.*, 75: 439–453.

Harrington, L.K. and Peck, C.K. (1998) Spatial disparity affects visual–auditory interactions in human sensorimotor processing. *Exp. Brain Res.*, 122: 247–252.

Harting, J.K., Feig, S. and Van Lieshout, D.P. (1997) Cortical somatosensory and trigeminal inputs to the cat superior colliculus: light and electron microscopic analyses. *J. Comp. Neurol.*, 388: 313–326.

Hartline, P.H., Pandey Vimal, R.L., King, A.J., Kurylo, D.D. and Northmore, D.P.M. (1995) Effects of eye position on auditory localization and neural representation of space in superior colliculus of cats. *Exp. Brain Res.*, 104: 402–408.

Howard, I.P. and Templeton, W.B. (1966) *Human Spatial Orientation*. Wiley, London.

Huerta, M.F. and Harting, J.K. (1984) The mammalian superior colliculus. Studies of its morphology and connections. In: H. Vanegas (Ed.), *Comparative Neurology of the Optic Tectum*. Plenum, New York, pp. 687–773.

Hughes, H.C., Reuter-Lorenz, P.A., Nozawa, G. and Fendrich, R. (1994) Visual–auditory interactions in sensorimotor processing: saccades versus manual responses. *J. Exp. Psychol.: Human Percept. Perf.*, 20: 131–153.

Jay, M.F. and Sparks, D.L. (1984) Auditory receptive fields in primate superior colliculus shift with changes in eye position. *Nature*, 309: 345–347.

Jiang, H., Lepore, F., Ptito, M. and Guillemot, J.-P. (1994a) Sensory modality distribution in the anterior ectosylvian cortex (AEC). *Exp. Brain Res.*, 97: 404–414.

Jiang, H., Lepore, F., Ptito, M. and Guillemot, J.-P. (1994b) Sensory interactions in the anterior ectosylvian cortex of cats. *Exp. Brain Res.*, 101: 385–396.

Jiang, W., Wallace, M.T., Jiang, H., Vaughan, J.W. and Stein, B.E. (1999) Two cortical areas contribute to the multisensory integration in superior colliculus neurons. *Soc. Neurosci. Abstr.*, 25: 1413.

Jiang, W., Jiang, H. and Stein, B.E. (2000) Influences from the anterior ectosylvian sulcus (AES) and rostral lateral suprasylvian sulcus (rLS) are critical for multisensory orientation behavior. *Soc. Neurosci. Abstr.*, 26: in press.

Kadunce, D.C., Vaughan, J.W., Wallace, M.T., Benedek, G. and Stein, B.E. (1997) Mechanisms of within- and cross-modality suppression in the superior colliculus. *J. Neurophysiol.*, 78: 2834–2847.

Kao, C.-Q., McHaffie, J.G., Meredith, M.A. and Stein, B.E. (1994) Functional development of a central visual map in cat. *J. Neurophysiol.*, 72: 266–272.

Kimura, A. and Tamai, Y. (1992) Sensory response of cortical neurons in the anterior ectosylvian sulcus, including the area evoking eye movement. *Brain Res.*, 575: 181–186.

Kimura, A., Hamada, Y., Kawai, Y. and Tamai, Y. (1996) Sensory response properties of cortical neurons in the anterior ectosylvian sulcus of cats: intracellular recording and labeling. *Neurosci. Res.*, 26: 357–367.

King, A.J. and Palmer, A.R. (1985) Integration of visual and auditory information in bimodal neurones in the guinea-pig superior colliculus. *Exp. Brain Res.*, 60: 492–500.

Larson, M. and Stein, B.E. (1984) The use of tactile and olfactory cues in neonatal orientation and localization of the nipple. *Dev. Psychobiol.*, 17: 423–436.

Lee, C., Chung, S., Kim, J. and Park, J. (1991) Auditory facilitation of visually guided saccades. *Soc. Neurosci. Abstr.*, 17: 862.

Marks, L.E. (1978) *The Unity of the Senses*. Academic Press, New York.

McGurk, H. and MacDonald, J. (1976) Hearing lips and seeing voices. *Nature*, 264: 746–748.

McHaffie, J.G., Kruger, L., Clemo, H.R. and Stein, B.E. (1988) Corticothalamic and corticotectal somatosensory projections from the anterior ectosylvian sulcus (SIV cortex) in neonatal cats: an anatomical demonstration with HRP and 3H-leucine. *J. Comp. Neurol.*, 274: 115–126.

Meredith, M.A. and Stein, B.E. (1983) Interactions among converging sensory inputs in the superior colliculus. *Science*, 221: 389–391.

Meredith, M.A. and Stein, B.E. (1986) Visual, auditory, and somatosensory convergence on cells in superior colliculus results in multisensory integration. *J. Neurophysiol.*, 56: 640–662.

Meredith, M.A. and Stein, B.E. (1996) Spatial determinants of multisensory integration in cat superior colliculus. *J. Neurophysiol.*, 75: 1843–1857.

Miceli, D., Reperant, J. and Ptito, M. (1985) Intracortical connections of the anterior ectosylvian and lateral suprasylvian visual areas in the cat. *Brain Res.*, 347: 291–298.

Minciacchi, D., Tassinari, G. and Antonini, A. (1987) Visual and somatosensory integration in the anterior ectosylvian cortex of the cat. *Brain Res.*, 410: 21–31.

Norton, T.T. (1974) Receptive-field properties of superior colliculus cells and development of visual behavior in kittens. *J. Neurophysiol.*, 37: 674–690.

Peck, C.K., Baro, J.A. and Warder, S.M. (1995) Effects of eye position on saccadic eye movements and on the neuronal responses to auditory and visual stimuli in cat superior colliculus. *Exp. Brain Res.*, 103: 227–242.

Perrott, D.R., Saberi, K., Brown, K. and Strybel, T.Z. (1990) Auditory psychomotor coordination and visual search performance. *Percept. Psychophys.*, 48: 214–226.

Ramachandran, R., Wallace, M.T. and Stein, B.E. (1993) Distribution and properties of multisensory neurons in rat cerebral cortex. *Soc. Neurosci. Abstr.*, 19: 1447.

Rauschecker, J.P. (1996) Substitution of visual by auditory inputs in the cat's anterior ectosylvian cortex. *Prog. Brain Res.*, 112: 313–323.

Reinoso-Suarez, F. and Roda, J.M. (1985) Topographical organization of the cortical afferent connections to the cortex of the anterior ectosylvian sulcus in the cat. *Exp. Brain Res.*, 59: 313–324.

Rizzolatti, G., Scandolara, C., Matelli, M. and Gentilucci, M. (1981a) Afferent properties of periarcuate neurons in macaque monkeys. I. Somatosensory responses. *Behav. Brain Res.*, 2: 125–146.

Rizzolatti, G., Scandolara, C., Matelli, M. and Gentilucci, M. (1981b) Afferent properties of periarcuate neurons in macaque monkeys. II. Visual responses. *Behav. Brain Res.*, 2: 147–163.

Scannell, J.W., Blakemore, C. and Young, M.P. (1995) Analysis of connectivity in the cat cerebral cortex. *J. Neurosci.*, 15: 1463–1483.

Sireteanu, R. and Maurer, D. (1982) The development of the kitten's visual field. *Vision Res.*, 22: 1105–1111.

Stein, B.E. and Gallagher, H. (1981) Maturation of cortical control over superior colliculus cells in cat. *Brain Res.*, 223: 429–435.

Stein, B.E. and Meredith, M.A. (1993) *The Merging of the Senses*. MIT Press, Cambridge, MA.

Stein, B.E. and Wallace, M.T. (1996) Comparisons of cross-modality integration in midbrain and cortex. *Prog. Brain Res.*, 112: 89–299.

Stein, B.E., Labos, E. and Kruger, L. (1973a) Sequence of changes in properties of neurons of superior colliculus of the kitten during maturation. *J. Neurophysiol.*, 36: 667–679.

Stein, B.E., Labos, E. and Kruger, L. (1973b) Determinants of response latency in neurons of superior colliculus in kittens. *J. Neurophysiol.*, 36: 680–689.

Stein, B.E., Spencer, R.F. and Edwards, S.B. (1983) Corticotectal and corticothalamic efferent projections of SIV somatosensory cortex in cat. *J. Neurophysiol.*, 50: 896–909.

Stein, B.E., Meredith, M.A., Honeycutt, W.S. and McDade, L. (1989) Behavioral indices of multisensory integration: orientation of visual cues is affected by auditory stimuli. *J. Cogn. Neurosci.*, 1: 12–24.

Stein, B.E., London, N., Wilkinson, L.K. and Price, D.D. (1996) Enhancement of perceived visual intensity by auditory stimuli: a psychophysical analysis. *J. Cogn. Neurosci.*, 8: 497–506.

Stein, B.E., Wallace, M.T. and Stanford, T.R. (1999) Development of multisensory integration: transforming sensory inputs into motor output. *Mental Retard. Dev. Disab. Res. Rev.*, 5: 72–85.

Stein, B.E., Wallace, M.T., Stanford, T.R. and McHaffie, J.G. (2000a). Integrating information from different senses in the superior colliculus. In: J.J. Bohuis (Ed.), *Brain Mechanisms of Perception, Learning and Memory*. Oxford University Press, Oxford, in press.

Stein, B.E., Stanford, T.R. and Wallace, M.T. (2000b). Neural mechanisms of cross-modal synthesis. In: E.B. Goldstein (Ed.), *Blackwell's Handbook of Perception*. Oxford University Press, Oxford, in press.

Villablanca, J.R. and Olmstead, C.E. (1979) Neurological development of kittens. *Dev. Psychobiol.*, 12: 101–127.

Wade, N.J. and Day, R.H. (1968) Apparent head position as a basis for a visual aftereffect of prolonged head tilt. *Percept. Psychophys.*, 3: 324–326.

Wallace, M.T. and Stein, B.E. (1994) Cross-modal synthesis in the midbrain depends on input from cortex. *J. Neurophysiol.*, 71: 429–432.

Wallace, M.T. and Stein, B.E. (1997) Development of multisensory neurons and multisensory integration in cat superior colliculus. *J. Neurosci.*, 17: 2429–2444.

Wallace, M.T. and Stein, B.E. (2000) The onset of cross-modal synthesis in the neonatal superior colliculus is gated by the development of cortical influences. *J. Neurophysiol.*, 83: 3579–3582.

Wallace, M.T., Meredith, M.A. and Stein, B.E. (1992) Integration of multiple sensory modalities in cat cortex. *Exp. Brain Res.*, 91: 484–488.

Wallace, M.T., Meredith, M.A. and Stein, B.E. (1993) Converging influences from visual, auditory, and somatosensory cortices onto output neurons of the superior colliculus. *J. Neurophysiol.*, 69: 1797–1809.

Wallace, M.T., Wilkinson, L.K. and Stein, B.E. (1996) Representation and integration of multiple sensory inputs in primate superior colliculus. *J. Neurophysiol.*, 76: 1246–1266.

Wallace, M.T., Meredith, M.A. and Stein, B.E. (1998) Multisensory integration in the superior colliculus of the alert cat. *J. Neurophysiol.*, 80: 1006–1010.

Wicklegren, B.G. and Sterling, P. (1969) Effect on the superior colliculus of cortical removal in visually deprived cats. *Nature*, 224: 1032–1033.

Wilkinson, L.K., Meredith, M.A. and Stein, B.E. (1996) The role of anterior ectosylvian cortex in cross-modality orientation and approach behavior. *Exp. Brain Res.*, 112: 1–10.

Zahn, J.R., Abel, L.A. and Dell'Osso, L.F. (1978) Audio-ocular response characteristics. *Sensory Proc.*, 2: 32–37.

C. Casanova and M. Ptito (Eds.)
Progress in Brain Research, Vol. 134

CHAPTER 11

Beyond the classical receptive field in the visual cortex

Ralph D. Freeman *, Izumi Ohzawa and Gary Walker

Group in Vision Science, School of Optometry, University of California, Berkeley, CA 94720-2020, USA

Abstract: We have investigated the organization of regions outside the classical receptive field (CRF) for neurons in the visual cortex. First, we have determined the incidence and nature of interactions from outside the CRF. We find interaction from regions outside the CRF for a majority of cortical cells and it is almost always of a suppressive nature. Second, we have determined that most interaction is from specific well-defined regions outside the CRF. These regions are generally as effective as what is found for a complete annulus. Third, it is possible to reverse the inhibition from outside the CRF by the addition of a second grating that is orthogonal to the preferred orientation. This disinhibition may completely offset the suppressive influence of the surround. Additional experiments suggest that this process is not necessarily involved in figure/ground analysis.

Introduction

The classical receptive field (CRF) of cells in central visual pathways is a crucial concept. It is the neural transducer by which we are able to describe the transformation between an optically created image on the retina and the conscious perception of the imaged scene. The definition of the CRF specifies clearly that it refers to the region within which it is possible to activate or suppress a cell or fiber. However, the region outside the CRF may also be relevant to the activity of the cell or fiber. Specifically, even though, by definition, a stimulus in the outer zone cannot activate the cell directly, it can influence the response. The influence of the effect of stimulation in the region beyond the CRF has been discussed in previous reviews (e.g. Allman et al., 1985). Unfortunately, published accounts of this area contain considerable discrepancies. Nearly every parameter of study has been reported to have widely varying values. This applies to the incidence of influence from areas outside the CRF, the size and distribution of the areas, and the nature of the effects i.e. excitatory or inhibitory. In addition, there is a study in which it is reported that cortical cells may be activated by a stimulus presented in the CRF at an orientation orthogonal to the preferred, when it is accompanied by a grating at the preferred orientation presented to a region outside the CRF (Sillito et al., 1995).

The wide discrepancies in nearly all the parameters of interest make it difficult to assess the mechanisms that may be at play in the regions outside the CRF. We therefore undertook a series of studies in order to first establish in a rigorous manner the variables of importance. We then investigated the possibility that the effective interactive region outside the CRF may be limited to a specific zone instead of the entire surround. Finally, we addressed the possibility that the surround of the CRF may be part of a mechanism by which figure/ground analysis may be accomplished. Our main results are as follows. First, the incidence of effects from outside the CRF is relatively high. The majority of cortical cells show it. Second, we find that nearly all the influence from outside the CRF is of a suppressive

* Corresponding author: R. Freeman, Group in Vision Science, School of Optometry, University of California, Berkeley, CA 94720-2020, USA. Tel.: +1-510-642-6341; Fax: +1-510-642-3323;
E-mail: freeman@neurovision.berkeley.edu

nature. If care is taken in centering visual stimuli so that the CRF is accurately defined, there is almost no evidence of facilitation from outside the CRF. Third, it is generally assumed that the influence from outside the CRF is derived uniformly from the entire region. In fact, we find that for nearly all cortical cells, the effective area is localized to a region above, below, or to the side of the CRF. Finally, our tests of a possible figure/ground role for the surround area suggest that all effects may be accounted for by local processes. Some findings are consistent with a disinhibition process by which the suppressive influence of the surround may be offset by an orthogonal superimposed stimulus.

Methods

Our experiments were performed with anesthetized paralyzed cats. The apparatus and procedures have been described previously (Walker et al., 1999, 2000). The following description covers the main information. Prior to anesthetic induction, animals are tranquilized and given a secretion blocking drug. Anesthesia is induced with isoflurane and cannulas are positioned for intravenous infusions. A tracheal tube and rectal thermometer are inserted, ECG and EEG leads are connected, and a craniotomy and durotomy are performed over area 17. Once anesthesia level is stabilized with thiopental sodium, the animal is paralyzed with a bolus of gallamine triethiodide. The cat is then ventilated with a mixture of N_2O and O_2 and anesthesia is maintained with an infusion of thiopental sodium. Dextrose and lactated Ringer's solution are also infused. The animal is hydrated with a drip system and core body temperature is maintained at around 38°C. The following physiological parameters are monitored continuously throughout each experiment. End-tidal CO_2 (maintained at 4–4.5%), ECG, EEG, heart rate, and core body temperature. Pupils are dilated, nictitating membranes are retracted, and contact lenses with artificial pupils (3.5 mm diameter) are positioned. Chloromycetin is given prophylactically.

The apparatus used for the experiments includes all the standard equipment required for physiological procedures. The visual stimulation techniques are accomplished with a computer based system. A visual stimulator generates images on CRT displays. Custom software is used to create the visual patterns required for the experiments described here. Custom software is also used to discriminate and process individual action potentials. Microelectrodes are used to isolate and monitor spike waveforms from individual neurons. A search program is used to estimate the main parameters of a small patch of a drifting sinusoidal grating that activates optimally the cell under study. Quantitative tests are then run in order to determine firm values for a series of parameters. For the grating runs, we define response amplitude in terms of mean firing rate or amplitude of the first harmonic for complex and simple cells, respectively.

Once specific preferred parameters for a given cell are determined, we use a small grating patch to obtain center coordinates of the CRF. A quantitative evaluation is then made of spatial summation, size, and surround suppression for each cell. Size–tuning responses are quantified by fitting data with a difference of integrals of two Gaussian functions. The first integral describes spatial summation of excitation within the CRF. The second integral represents summation of inhibitory inputs from the surround. In addition to the variable size grating stimuli, we also use reverse correlation and m-sequence procedures with sparse and dense noise stimuli for some cells in order to get detailed two- or three-dimensional spatio-temporal RF maps. These methods provide an independent means to assess RF boundaries for center and surround regions.

Results

At the outset, we must establish clear definitions of the CRF and the region beyond it that has an influence on the cell's response. We use the classical definition of a CRF as the area in space within which stimuli can elicit an excitatory response. The 'surround' is defined as a region outside the CRF within which stimuli do not elicit an excitatory response. However, stimuli within the surround may modulate a response in a facilitatory or suppressive manner. We begin with these definitions in order to proceed from a broad perspective. The results described below allow for more specific statements to be made.

The first task is to obtain size–tuning characteristics of cortical cells. To do this, a series of drifting grating patches of variable sizes is used. The resulting size–tuning curves provide estimates of the size and nature of the CRF. These data are not unique, of course, since many similar estimates have been made previously. However, in the present case, we have taken extreme care to obtain proper centering of the stimulus. It turns out that this is of prime importance in obtaining accurate maps of both the CRF and the surrounding regions.

Examples of these size–tuning curves are shown in Fig. 1. Responses for four cells are given, two simple (A and B) and two complex (C and D) types. There are two basic response patterns exhibited here. In one (A and C), responses reach a peak and then level off. This is more obvious in A. There is a minimal increase in response level in C following the initial peak. Responses in B and D are clearly different in that they demonstrate specific tuning for a given grating size. These response types are akin to the 'standard' and 'special' categories of previous studies (see Hubel and Wiesel, 1962; Palmer and Rosenquist, 1974).

What is the nature of surround effects? We studied a relatively large population of cortical cells (271 neurons) and find that nearly all surround effects are of a suppressive nature. In nearly all cases where it appeared that surround facilitation was present, careful examination of the CRF revealed that we had initially misjudged the borders. When this was corrected, the initially apparent facilitation was no longer valid. There were, however, some instances of what appeared to be genuine facilitation, such as the example shown in Fig. 1C. But even in this case, it is possible that the RF was elongated and all our stimuli were contained within the CRF.

Given that the type of interaction is nearly always suppressive, the next question concerns the degree

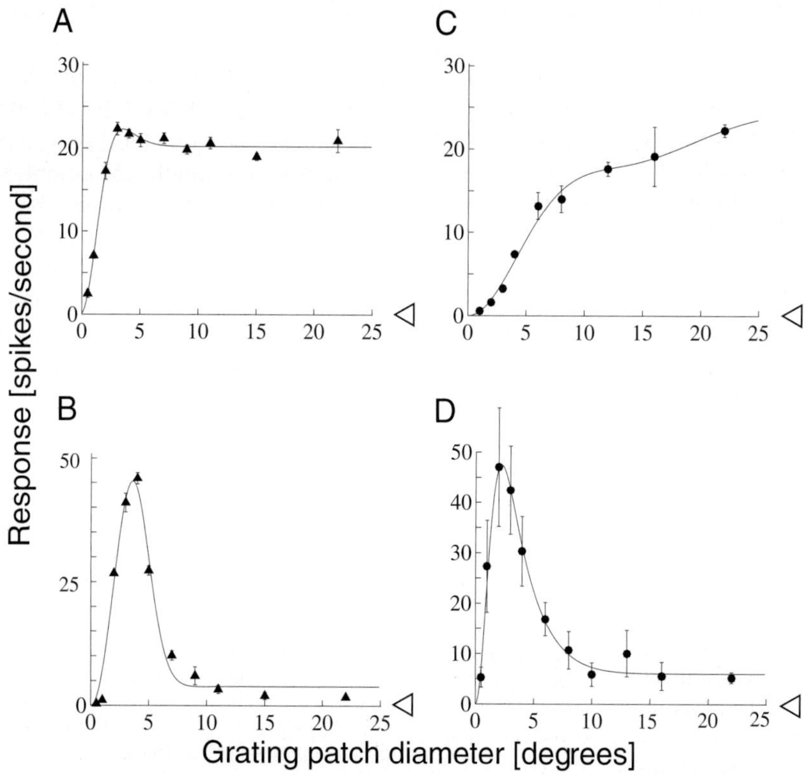

Fig. 1. Monocular size–tuning functions are shown for two simple cells (A and B) and two complex cells (C and D). Response in this and all subsequent figures is given in impulses per second. Spontaneous activity in this and subsequent figures is indicated by open triangles on the right of each graph. Small grating patches are carefully centered in each RF. They are gradually increased in size, as indicated by abscissa values, and responses are obtained for each. Each set of data is fit with suitable functions to obtain the smooth curves (see Methods). Error bars represent ±1 standard error of the mean.

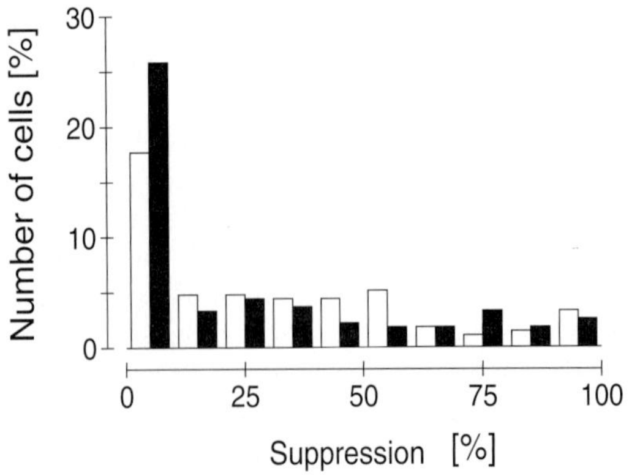

Fig. 2. This histogram gives the distribution of the degree of suppression exhibited by enlarging the grating stimulus beyond the CRF. Values of suppression are relative, given in percent, as determined through the dominant eye in a population of 271 cortical neurons. Filled and unfilled bars represent complex and simple cells, respectively. In total, 44% of the cells in the sample exhibited a suppression of less than 10%. The other cells in the sample, 56%, had suppression values ranging uniformly from 10 to 100%.

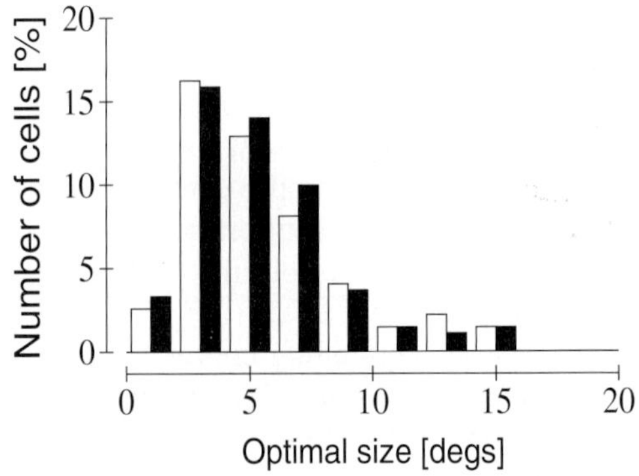

Fig. 3. Optimal RF size is given here for our sample of 271 cells. As before, these values are derived from monocular measurements through the dominant eye for each cell. These measurements were made with circular grating patches and each value is optimal for a given cell. Once again, complex and simple cells are represented by filled and unfilled bars, respectively.

of suppression. We classed the extent of suppression for the population of cells using as an arbitrary criterion a value of 10% as a minimal value. The majority of the cells in our sample (56%) exhibited values greater than 10%. Therefore, a majority of cortical cells exhibit surround suppression. The distribution in our sample is shown in Fig. 2. Unfilled and filled bars represent simple and complex cells, respectively. For both cell types, the most likely degree of suppression is in the lowest range shown. Simple cells exhibit suppression slightly more often and to a greater extent than that for complex cells. But the differences are not significant.

Since we have carefully determined response characteristics for different grating patch sizes, data on optimal sizes of CRFs are available. The distribution of optimal CRF sizes for our population of cortical cells is shown in Fig. 3. Optimal size is determined from the peak of each size–tuning curve. If suppression is less than 10%, size is estimated by a fitting procedure using the difference of integrals of two Gaussian functions, as mentioned above. As seen in Fig. 3, most of the CRF sizes are from 2° to 8° in diameter. Median values for simple and complex cells are 4.6° and 4.8°, respectively. Therefore, simple and complex cells do not differ significantly in size. This is contrary to the original subjective impression that complex cell RFs are generally larger (Hubel and Wiesel, 1962).

For around one-third of the cell population, we obtained size–tuning data through both right and left eyes. Typical results, in the same format as Fig. 1, are shown in Fig. 4. The data are for simple and complex cells in A and B, respectively. In general, the size–tuning functions are similar in shape in both cases with ordinate differences that reflect variations in response strength. Stimuli through the more responsive eye yields suppressive values of around 50% in

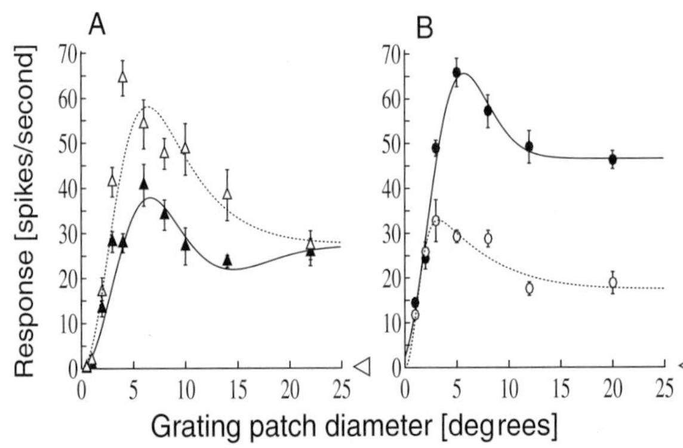

Fig. 4. Binocular size–tuning functions such as those of Fig. 1, are given here. One simple cell and one complex cell (A and B, respectively), are presented here. Dashed and solid curves represent left and right eye responses, respectively. All other symbols are as represented in Fig. 1.

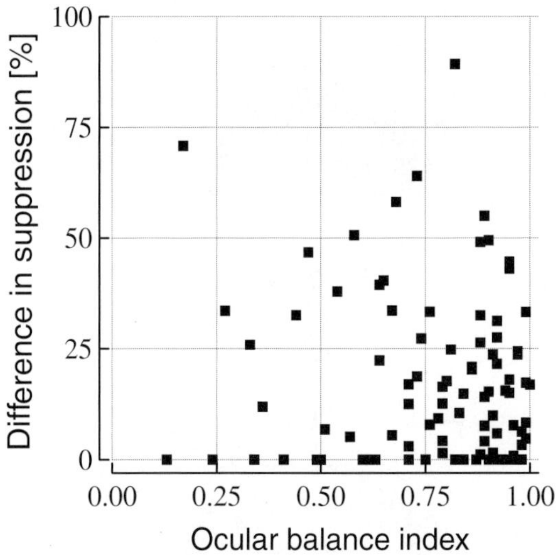

Fig. 5. The difference in suppression between left and right eyes is given here as a function of the degree to which one eye dominates a cortical cell. For this test, 99 cells were studied. The ocular balance index, (OBI) is: $\mathrm{OBI} = 1 - 2\left[R_\mathrm{I}/(R_\mathrm{I} + R_\mathrm{C})\right]$, where R_I and R_C represent responses from ipsilateral and contralateral eyes, respectively.

each case. The difference in degree of suppression between the two eyes is plotted as a function of ocular balance index in Fig. 5. The ocular balance index (OBI) is a quantitative designation of ocular dominance as follows:

$$\mathrm{OBI} = 1 - 2\left[\frac{R_\mathrm{I}}{(R_\mathrm{I} + R_\mathrm{C})}\right]$$

where R_I and R_C represent ipsilateral and contralateral responses to an optimal stimulus, respectively. The data of Fig. 5 are skewed to the right and this shows that most of the cells we have studied are nearly binocularly balanced. Filled symbols represent percent suppression. The scale on the ordinate is for percent suppression. A scale for absolute values is not given. Most of the data points of Fig. 5 are in the lower part of the graph indicating that suppression is similar for the two eyes.

In summary, the results presented so far show that the majority of cells (56%) exhibit surround suppression. There is a wide range of suppression but most cells display modest levels. Simple and complex cells do not differ in the RF size or incidence or strength of surround suppression. The amount of surround suppression is similar for left and right eyes. This is consistent with the notion that surround suppression originates in pathways after the combination of monocular inputs.

We next examine the specific spatial organization of surround suppression. In previous work, assumptions were made about the nature of surround effects that biased the experimental protocols. In early studies, attention was paid to end zones in connection with end-stopped or length-tuned properties. (Hubel and Wiesel, 1959, 1962, 1965, 1968). Side zones were investigated later both alone (e.g. Maffei and Fiorentini, 1976; Born and Tootle, 1991; Von der Heydt et al., 1992) and in relation to end zones (Born and Tootle, 1991; DeAngelis et al., 1994). In other work, stimuli that encircled the CRF were used (Lamme et al., 1997; Levitt and Lund, 1997). However, there has not been a previous attempt to explore systematically the organization of the regions surrounding the CRF. To do that, we used the stimulus configuration depicted in Fig. 6A. A grating framed by the rectangle in Fig. 6A was presented to the CRF. A second grating, as depicted in the figure, was presented simultaneously at one of a number of positions outside the CRF.

Generally, eight positions were used. Cells of the original sample of 271 were chosen for further study if they exhibited strong surround suppression. In addition, several cells were studied that had not shown suppressive behavior. In total, the sample for this part of the study was 101 cells.

The purpose of using relatively small patches of grating to study surround effects was to localize interactions as much as possible. It is possible, for example, that facilitation and suppression could originate from separate discrete locations surrounding the CRF. In this case, effects from both locations could be cancelled if very large stimuli are used in the surround of the CRF. With the relatively small patches of gratings used in the surrounds, it should be possible to identify antagonistic pockets of inhibition and excitation. This should apply even if a cell exhibits no apparent suppression in its size–tuning function. For most of the tests we conducted, grating parameters for the CRF stimulus and the second grating presented to the surround region, were of optimal values for the CRF.

Typical results are depicted in Fig. 6. In A, the stimulus configuration is illustrated for the CRF

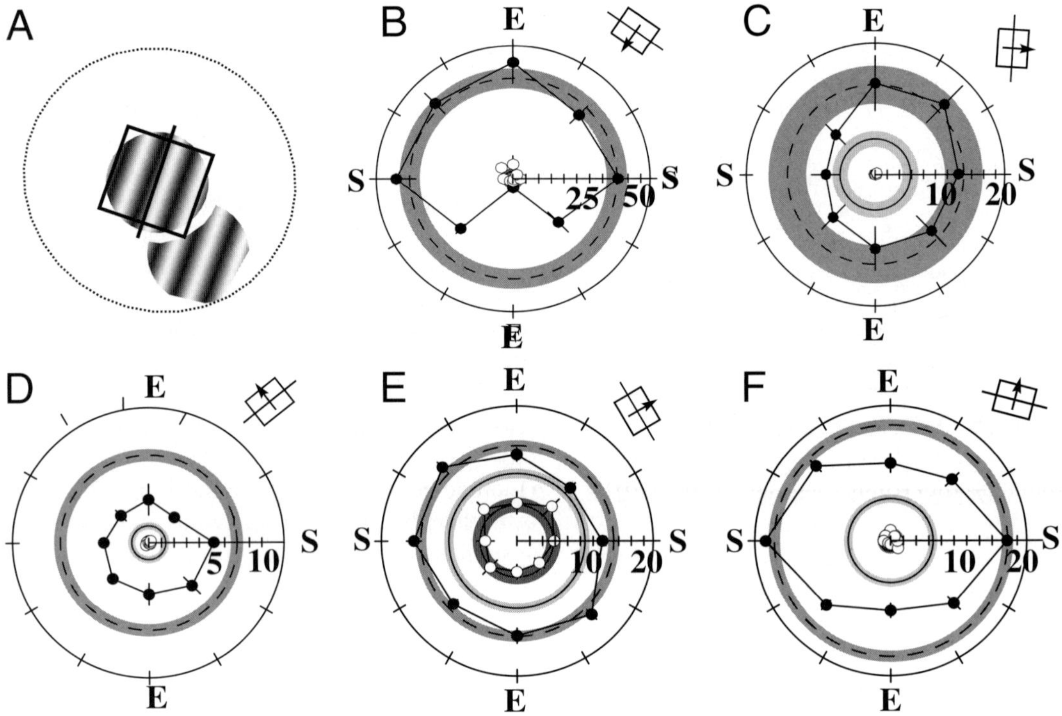

Fig. 6. To determine regional effects of stimuli outside the CRF, small satellite patches were positioned as illustrated in A. They could be placed anywhere outside the CRF at end, side, or oblique positions. Typical results are shown for cortical cells in B–F. In all cases, responses are for optimal values of gratings in the central and satellite positions. Numbers on each radial axis represent response values in impulses per second. Outer dashed circles represent baseline responses to stimulation of the CRF. Dark gray regions surrounding each dashed line circle represents ±1 standard error of the mean (SEM). Inner solid circles represent responses to stimulation of the CRF plus the entire annular surround. Light gray regions surrounding each solid circle represent SEM. Note inner solid circles may not be visible (as in B) if responses are suppressed nearly completely. Spontaneous activity is indicated by a solid circle and dark shaded area (as in E). Plots of cells are rotated so that preferred orientation is vertical. Actual orientation preferences are indicated by icons above and to the right of each cell's representation. E and S for each plot represent end and side, respectively. Filled data points are responses to the CRF plus one of the satellite surround grating patches at the positions indicated. Error bars here represent ±1 SEM. Unfilled data points represent control tests in which satellite grating patches are presented alone. Data shown in B are for a complex cell which exhibits asymmetrical suppression at the bottom end of the RF. Similar asymmetry is evident for the simple cell in C only in this case, suppression is from the left side. The example in D shows relatively symmetrical suppression from the satellite grating patches. The entire annulus causes much more suppression than any of the surround patches. The complex cell in E exhibits asymmetrical suppression from an oblique, and to a lesser extent, right side and upper end areas. Note the relatively high spontaneous level. In F, results for a complex cell are shown which has axial surround symmetry in which both ends are strongly suppressed. Even stronger suppression is observed with an annulus covering the entire surround.

grating and the second grating patch used to probe various positions adjacent to the center. To get a general idea of the response pattern, we used four positions of the satellite grating. For a more detailed response, we used eight positions. An example in which the major suppressive influence was nearly all from the bottom end of the RF is shown in B. In this and the other examples of this figure, the radial axis represents the response rate in impulses per second. Angular position of the data points indicates location of the satellite patch. The outer dashed circle represents the baseline response to stimulation of the CRF. This value is measured in separate trials interleaved with those in which the satellite is also presented simultaneously. The dark gray zone around the dashed circle is ± the standard error of the mean. The solid circle and light gray region surrounding it represents stimulation to the center and annular surround together. This circle is not visible, as in B, when the response of the cell is suppressed to near spontaneous levels. Spontaneous activity is indicated by a circle with a dark shaded region as in E. All plots are rotated so that preferred orientation and direction are vertical and to the right, respectively. Ends and sides of the CRF are denoted by E and S, respectively. Rectangles next to each plot represent actual orientations and direction preferences of the cells. Filled data points connected by solid lines represent mean responses to stimulation of the CRF plus the satellite grating patch. Error bars denote ±1 SEM. Unfilled data points represent responses to the satellite gratings alone. These runs are also interleaved with the other test stimuli and they verify that the surround grating patches are outside the CRF and do not drive the cell.

The complex cell whose data are shown in Fig. 6B was suppressed almost entirely by the annular surround (unfilled data points). The satellite grating patch was also highly effective in suppressing the cell's response when it was positioned at the lower end of the CRF. Intermediate levels of suppression are seen when the satellite patch is positioned obliquely on either side of the end. The main suppressive region is around 3.5°. The cell in Fig. 6C is suppressed mainly by satellite patches to the left side. The maximum suppression is around 61%. Grating patches above and below also cause suppression to a slightly lesser degree. The amount of suppression from the satellite patch is only slightly less than that from the annular surround (solid circle and light gray background). Although there are clear asymmetries in the suppression patterns of most cells, some neurons exhibit relatively uniform profiles. An example is shown in Fig. 6D. In this case, all satellite positions produce similar patterns of suppression. None of the grating patches cause as much suppression as the annular surround stimulus. Other cells exhibit symmetrical patterns of suppression as in the case of the example of Fig. 6E. In this case, suppression arises from the oblique regions outside the CRF. This complex cell also exhibits some suppression from adjacent end (E) and side (S) regions. Note that the surround-only control condition response is equivalent to that of the spontaneous activity (unfilled symbols and inner solid circle, respectively). Finally, an example is shown (Fig. 6F) in which suppression is also symmetrical only in this case, it arises from upper and lower end positions. For this neuron, a complex cell, strong suppression is observed with the complete annulus. With the satellite patches, intermediate but still strong levels of suppression are observed which are roughly equal from either end (E). Oblique regions yield weaker suppression. Side areas (S) of the CRF have no influence on the cell's response.

For some cells, we obtained detailed maps of the CRF and surround suppression as illustrated in Fig. 7. A standard map obtained as in the examples of Fig. 6, is shown in A. In this case, there is a clear asymmetry in which the lower oblique region outside the CRF is the source of substantial suppression. There is also suppression from the lower end zone. In addition to the satellite probe, we used a modified reverse correlation procedure (Jones and Palmer, 1987a,b; Freeman and Ohzawa, 1990) to obtain detailed maps of the CRF and surround. The procedure, depicted in Fig. 7B, utilizes an optimal grating as a conditioning stimulus presented on one monitor. At the same time, a second grating is presented as a probe on another monitor. The two gratings are optically superimposed. The probe grating is presented at various locations within a two-dimensional array so that the entire CRT and surround regions are covered. By using repeated sequences of presentations, it is possible to obtain detailed CRF and surround maps such as that shown in Fig. 7C. The dots represent the 144 grid locations that were studied. Dark shading represents cell response levels higher than maintained discharge and lighter regions depict suppressed conditions while the probe stimulus was used. Since the reverse correlation procedure can be used to analyze different time delays between spike occurrence and stimulus presentation, a temporal response pattern may be derived. The data in Fig. 7D represent averaged temporal response patterns derived from the contour map in C. The trace at the top is the response pattern from the CRF. The middle trace is that from the suppressive region. Values for this curve are smaller than that for the excitatory CRF and the curve is normalized to facilitate comparisons. In the bottom traces, a direct comparison is made between the CRF response pattern and an inverted version of that from the surround zone. In this example, surround suppression peaks around 15 ms

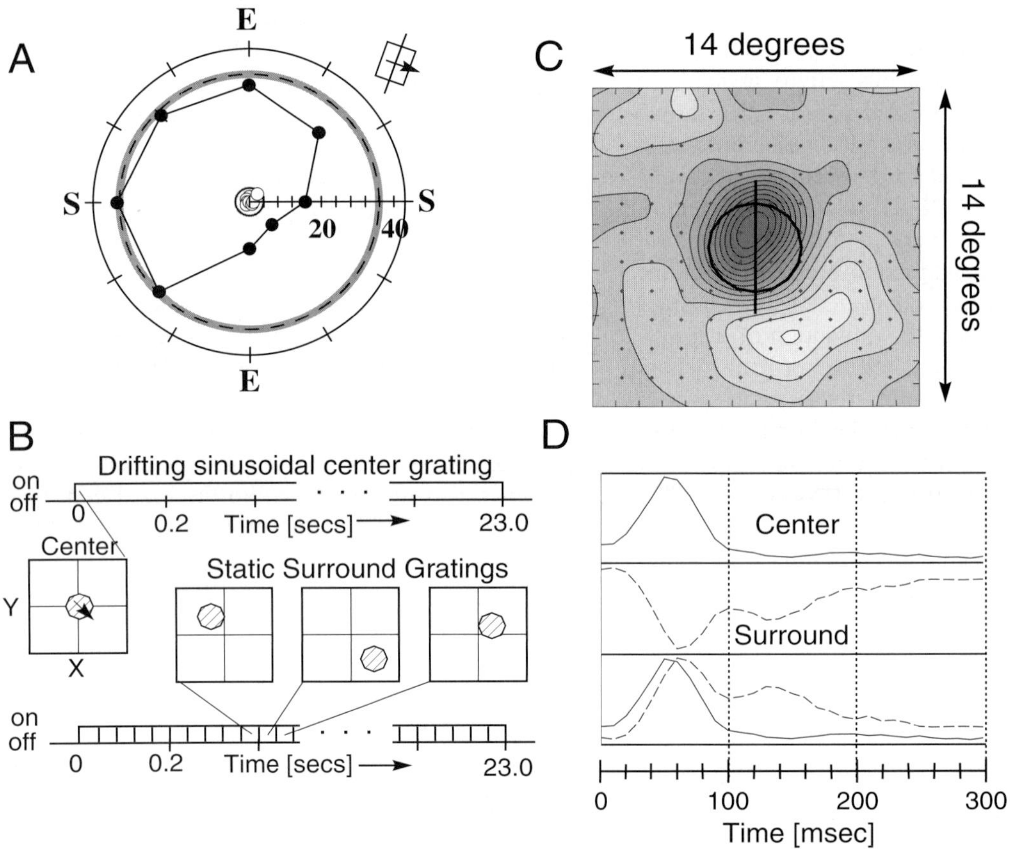

Fig. 7. An asymmetrical suppression profile, similar to those shown in Fig. 6, is illustrated here in A. In addition to the standard method of grating patch presentation to the CRF and to satellite positions in the surround, we used a modified reverse correlation technique as illustrated in B (Walker et al., 1999). The resulting two dimensional spatial map of excitation (dark shading) and relative suppression (light shading) is shown in C. The CRF is represented by the thick circle. The 144 grid locations are represented by dots in the field. In D, an average temporal response pattern is shown as derived from the contour map in C, taken at different spatial locations. The top trace (solid line) is from the CRF. The middle trace (dashed line) is from the suppressive surround. These two curves are normalized to facilitate comparison. In the bottom trace, the surround curve is inverted to allow direct comparison.

after the excitatory center. In addition, it has a flatter decay slope and a possible second peak around 70 ms after the first.

A summary of the spatial regions causing suppression outside the CRF is shown in Fig. 8. The polar plot in A gives the distribution of suppressive regions from the sample of cells (40) that exhibited 30% or more suppression with an annulus. Each point represents a vector from a given cell. To visualize differences between end, side, and oblique locations, we folded the axes so that all data fall into the first quadrant and this is shown in Fig. 8B. Note that nearly twice as many cells fall in the end zone area compared to the other two areas. So although the data points are scattered within all three zones, there is a clear bias for maximal suppression to arise from the end zones. This may help explain why earlier studies were focused on end-stopped behavior (Dreher, 1972; Sillito, 1977; Kato et al., 1978; Nelson and Frost, 1978; Albus and Fries, 1980). Finally, in Fig. 8C, the distribution is shown for magnitude of suppression for each of the eight positions of the satellite grating patch. Note that in all cases, the histograms are skewed to the left indicating that lower levels of suppression are encountered most frequently.

In summary, a relatively small satellite grating presented at a particular location outside the CRF

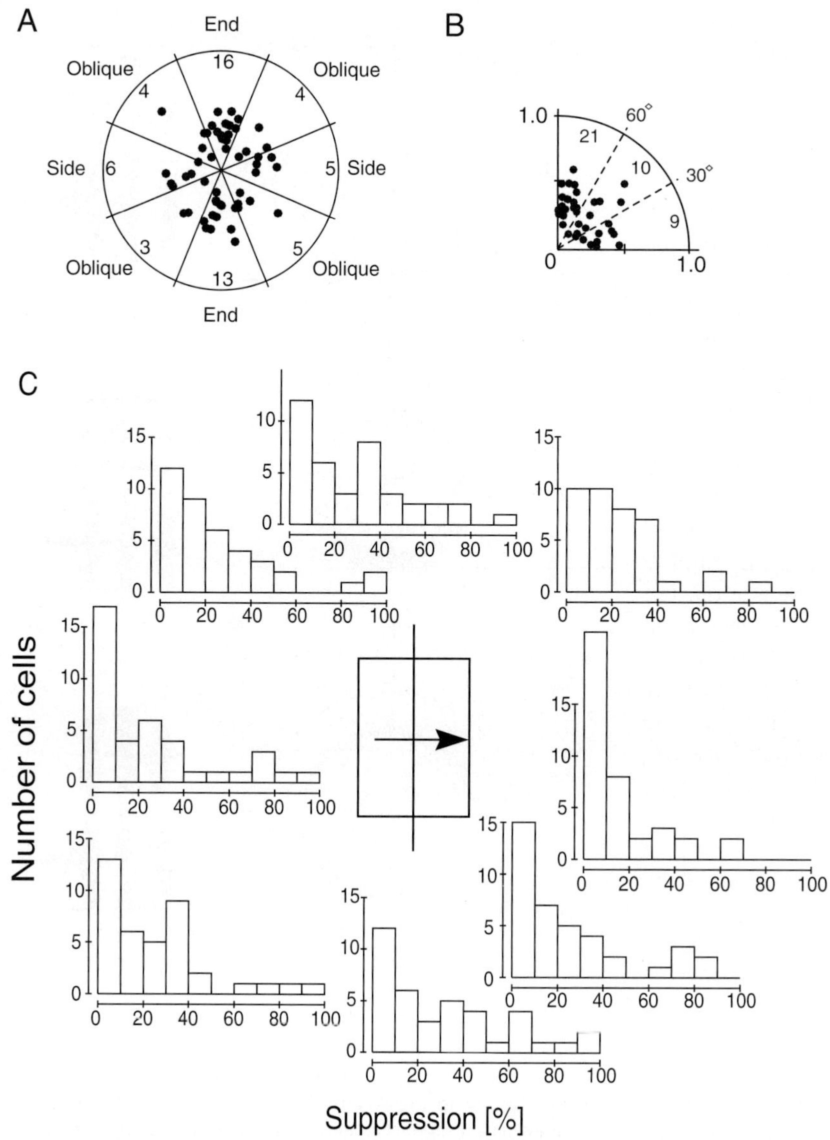

Fig. 8. A summary is shown here of the distribution of suppressive regions from our cell sample. We restricted this analysis to cells that exhibited 30% or more of suppression with a full annular surround. In A, each point represents a specific analysis vector from a given cell (see Walker et al., 1999 for details of the vector analysis). The angular position of each point represents the location of the suppressive region. Numbers in the sectors refer to the number of cells with strongest suppression in a given location. The pie-shaped distribution in A is folded twice and presented in B. The resulting 30° bins give relative distributions of cell locations in end, side, and oblique locations. About twice as many cells fall in the end zone compared to the other locations. In C, histograms are given of the distribution of degrees of suppression for the cell population shown in A.

can have a substantial inhibitory effect. This occurs when the satellite is presented with a second grating patch located within the CRF. In general, the extent of inhibition elicited by a small satellite grating patch in the correct position is nearly equivalent to that caused by an annulus that covers the entire surround.

So far, all tests that have been described were conducted with grating patches of optimal parameters. We used that procedure because it reduced the number of testing variables and we knew from previous work, that surround suppression is generally strongest for matched CRF and surround grating orientations. (DeAngelis et al., 1994) However, the asymmetric suppression patterns that we have determined here raise questions about suppressive mechanisms. One obvious question is whether grating orientation in the surround is relevant. Specifically, for a given satellite region, does orientation of the grating determine the degree of suppression? Data relevant to this question are given for a complex cell in Fig. 9. In A, the basic pattern for four satellite positions shows substantial suppression at the lower end of the region outside the CRF. In B, the orientation of the satellite grating is rotated 90° so that it is orthogonal to the preferred orientation. Note that in this configuration, overall suppression is reduced and the spatial pattern is changed. In C, the satellite grating is once again at the optimal orientation, but it is drifted in the opposite direction to that of the CRF grating. In this case, the suppression pattern is very similar to that of A. In general, for most of the cells we tested using different orientations for the satellite gratings, suppression was strongest for optimally oriented surround stimuli. There were some rare cases (about 14% of the 42 cells tested with nonoptimal surround gratings) in which the strongest suppression was found for nonoptimal stimuli in the satellite position.

Our main results of the satellite experiments are as follows. We confirm, using careful probe satellite stimuli that nearly all surround effects from outside the CRF are of a suppressive nature. The spatial organization of the surround is typically asymmetrical. A relatively small satellite area provides most or all of the inhibitory signal. The location of the inhibitory patch can be anywhere surrounding the CRF but end zone suppression is the most commonly encountered.

The last topic of interest in this series of experiments concerns the functional nature of surround effects from outside the CRF. One possibility that has been proposed concerns figure/ground segregation (Lamme, 1995; Zipser et al., 1996; Lamme et al., 1997). The surround of the CRF could be the background component of a visual image with the main object contained within the CRF (Lamme, 1995). Another possibility is that surround effects

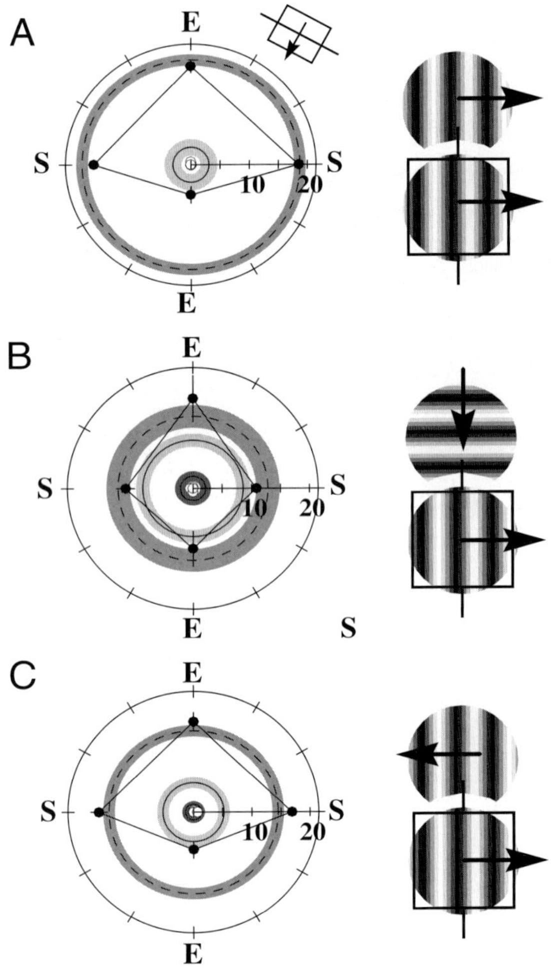

Fig. 9. For this complex cell, a comparison is made between results for optimal stimuli in the satellite surround and nonoptimal parameters. The CRF grating is always of optimal parameters. The satellite is optimal, as in A, orthogonal, as in B, or optimal but opposite to the preferred direction, as in C. With optimal parameters in both the center and the surround, there is strong suppression from the lower end (A). With a complete annulus, this cell exhibits 100% suppression. With an orthogonal orientation of the satellite, suppression is weaker and not as symmetrical (B). With a complete annulus at an orthogonal orientation, the suppression level is 36%. For optimal orientation of the satellite but opposite direction of drift, the suppression pattern is nearly identical to that for the optimal direction (C). Suppression for the complete annulus with opposite directional drift is 84%.

are an intrinsic property of RF organization and are not necessarily involved in figure/ground segregation. In either case, it should be possible to design tests that would allow predictions consistent with one but not necessarily the other explanation. That is the goal of some of the experiments that we have performed. In the basic tests, a grating of optimal parameters was presented to the CRF and a maximum response level was determined. The grating was then expanded to cover both the CRF and the surround. Next, an orthogonal grating of the same spatial frequency and contrast was added to the surround. Initially, the contrast of the orthogonal grating was set to a very low value. In this condition, the surround orthogonal grating had minimal effect. Generally, the surround grating suppressed the overall response of the cell so that when the orthogonal surround grating was added at a higher contrast level, it had the effect of reversing the suppression to some degree. In some cases, this disinhibition process was complete.

An example of this procedure is illustrated in Fig. 10. In A, results are shown for a complex cell which exhibits strong suppression in the center plus surround condition (dashed line). There is no effect when a low contrast orthogonal grating is added. But at contrasts above 30%, the orthogonal grating has the clear effect of neutralizing the suppression. At the highest contrast level, suppression is completely offset and response magnitude is equivalent to that from stimulation of the CRF alone. Another example is shown in Fig. 10B. In this case, the cell's response is completely suppressed in the condition in which the CRF and surround are both stimulated. As for the previous cell, addition of an orthogonal grating of low contrast has no effect. But as the contrast is increased, the suppression is diminished. At the highest contrast level of the orthogonal grating, the cell's response recovers to about half that of the optimal response to the CRF grating.

Most of the cells we tested using this protocol responded in similar ways to the examples described above. Varying amounts of disinhibition are expressed. To test directly the notion of figure/ground analysis, we conducted additional tests. An example, given in Fig. 11, illustrates disinhibition for two different surround conditions. The first is like the ones described above in which the orthogonal grating covers the entire surround annulus. The result, shown in Fig. 11A, is nearly complete initial suppression with low contrast orthogonal grating stimulation. As contrast levels are increased, disinhibition occurs and

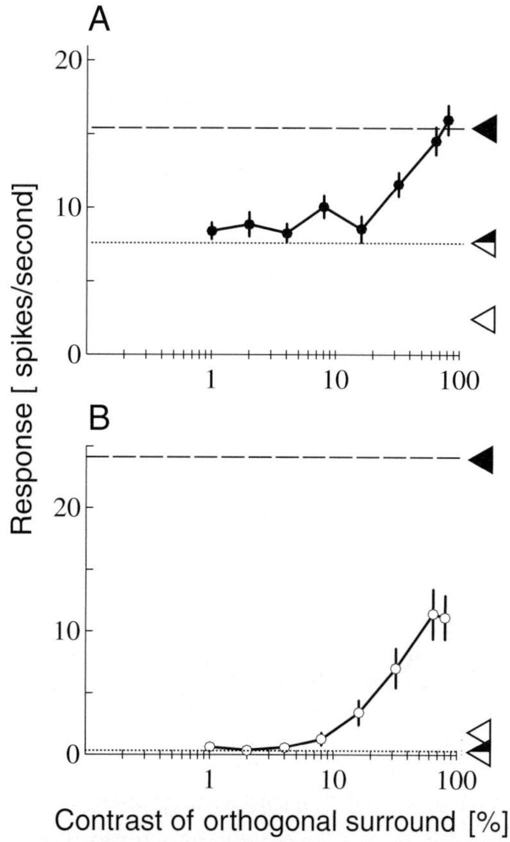

Fig. 10. Examples are shown here of two cells that are disinhibited by orthogonal gratings that overlap optimal patterns in the surround. In each case, dashed lines and filled triangles indicate responses to the optimal grating presented to the CRF alone. Dotted lines and half filled triangles refer to responses to the CRF stimulus plus the annular surround stimulus. Unfilled triangles represent spontaneous levels of activity. The complex cell in A responds well to a high contrast grating in the CRF and is suppressed when the grating is expanded to fill the surround area. With the addition of an orthogonal grating in the surround, there is a gradual disinhibition that increases with the contrast of the added grating. When contrast is high enough, there is a complete disinhibition. A similar pattern is seen for the simple cell in B. In this case, the response is completely suppressed by the optimal surround. With addition of the orthogonal grating in the surround, the cell's response is disinhibited and at the highest contrast of the orthogonal grating, it recovers around half of the response to an optimal grating presented to the CRF.

it is complete at 60% so that the cell's response is equal to that for the optimal stimulus to the CRF. A control condition is included as follows. The CRF is stimulated with an optimal grating. In addition, an

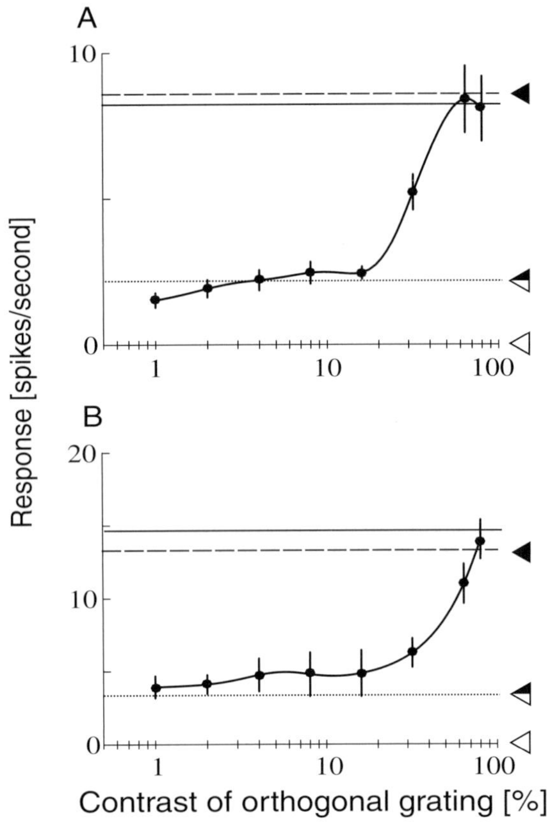

Fig. 11. To explore the figure/ground notion of CRF and surround function, two different stimulus configurations are used for a neuron that exhibits full disinhibition with a high contrast orthogonal grating. Symbols and patterns are as in Fig. 10. In addition, there are solid horizontal lines in A and B that represent responses in a control condition in which the CRF is stimulated with an optimal grating and an orthogonal grating is presented to the surround. In this case, responses are nearly identical to those of the CRF alone. The pattern obtained in A is for a stimulus configuration in which the entire annulus is disinhibited. The pattern in B is for responses when only one end is stimulated with an orthogonal grating patch. In previous measurements, this end was shown to be the main source of suppression of the cell. The similar patterns of disinhibition for these two stimulus conditions suggest that figure/ground analysis may not occur at this level of the visual cortex.

orthogonal grating of high contrast is presented to the surround. The result is that the cell's response is nearly identical to that for CRF stimulation alone. In other words, the orthogonal grating had no direct effect on the cell's response. However, it clearly modulates the suppressive influence of the optimally oriented grating.

The other condition tested for this cell is concerned with the possible functional purpose for the suppression. A possibility that has been proposed in previous publications is that the surround suppression serves as background for figure/ground analysis (Lamme, 1995; Zipser et al., 1996; Lamme et al., 1997). We have found that a small patch of grating at a critical satellite location just outside the CRF can be as effective in causing suppression as a surround stimulus that covers the entire annulus (Walker et al., 1999). It is therefore possible that the disinhibition described above can be generated in the same position as that within which there is a suppressive effect. This may be tested by the addition of a second grating which is orthogonal to and overlays the surround grating. The response to this condition, for the same cell as shown in Fig. 11A, is presented in Fig. 11B. Note first that the response curves for the two panels of the figure are closely similar. The main finding here is that complete disinhibition is achieved in a very similar manner in both cases. The isolated patch of orthogonal grating is essentially as effective as the full surround grating in reversing the suppression. Note that in both cases, complete disinhibition is attained when the orthogonal grating is of sufficiently high contrast. The same control run as described above for the full annular surround was also conducted for the satellite grating patch test of Fig. 11B. A similar result was attained demonstrating once again that the orthogonal grating patch outside the CRF had no direct effect on the response of the cell.

Discussion

The work described here is concerned with organization of the cortical RF in area 17. We are interested in the relationship between the CRF and the surrounding region that has been shown to have an influence on a cell's response (Blakemore and Tobin, 1972; Allman et al., 1985; Knierim and Van Essen, 1992). Specifically, we wish to establish the incidence of surround effects, the nature of the effects, the spatial configuration of the surround interactions, and the possible functional significance of the surround.

This review covers three studies. In the first, we have determined the incidence and nature of surround effects. Specifically, we find that the majority of cells in striate cortex (56%) are affected by stimulation outside the CRF. Furthermore, the nature of the interaction is almost always one of suppression. We arbitrarily classified cells as having surround effects if the change of a cell's response was at least 10% compared to the response of optimal stimulation of the CRF. Very few cells exhibited facilitation. We conducted size–tuning tests to determine the spatial extent over which the CRF is sensitive to visual stimuli. As size increases, responses increase monotonically and reach a plateau or decrease. When responses change, we assume that the surround mechanisms are invoked. These tests enable estimates of CRF size for the population of cells we have studied. Interestingly, there is no apparent size difference between simple and complex cells in contradiction to the traditional assumption (Hubel and Wiesel, 1962). There is also no difference between these two cell types in incidence or strength of surround suppression. Furthermore, the amount of surround suppression is well correlated between the two eyes. This indicates that surround effects may occur after the combination of monocular inputs.

The second study concerns the general characteristics of surrounding regions of the CRF. Specifically, we are interested in the spatial organization of the surround. It has generally been assumed that surrounds are uniform regions that encircle the entire CRF. The original work on RF organization in the visual cortex suggested that the ends of CRFs are of prime importance. We have determined here that for most cells that exhibit suppression, the region of interest outside the CRF is generally limited to a specific area. Within this area, which can be located anywhere outside the CRF, a grating of appropriate parameters can cause substantial suppression of the cell's response. Suppressive regions are located most often at the end zones of the CRF. Finally, we have explored the tuning characteristics of the surround region. There appears to be a wide range of parameters of the surround grating patch that are effective in causing suppression. However, the suppressive effect is generally strongest when the surround grating parameters are matched to those of the CRF.

The third study addresses the possible utility of surround suppression. One notion that has been proposed in previous work is that the zone outside the CRF could serve as background for a particular portion of a scene that is imaged within the CRF (Lamme, 1995). In this way, the scene could generate a perceptual pop-out or figure/ground image. We have carried out studies in order to determine if there is an alternative explanation for the interactions that occur between the CRF and surround regions. By using a grating that overlays the satellite surround grating, it is possible to block the suppressive influence of the surround stimulus. Although we cannot rule out feedback from another cortical region that could be generated via the satellite surround stimulus, it is possible to account for the results we have obtained by local interactions of specific areas within and beyond the CRF. These interactions are not necessarily involved in figure/ground analysis.

Acknowledgements

The work reported here was done was supported by research and CORE grants from the National Eye Institute (EY 01175 and EY 03176).

References

Allman, J., Miezin, F. and McGuinness, E. (1985) Stimulus specific responses from beyond the classical receptive field: neurophysiological mechanisms for local–global comparisons in visual neurons. *Annu. Rev. Neurosci.*, 8: 407–430.

Albus, K. and Fries, W. (1980) Inhibitory sidebands of complex receptive fields in the cat's striate cortex. *Vision Res.*, 20: 369–372.

Blakemore, C.B. and Tobin, E.A. (1972) Lateral inhibition between orientation detectors in the cat's visual cortex. *Exp. Brain Res.*, 15: 439–440.

Born, R.T. and Tootle, R.B.H. (1991) Single-unit and 2-deoxyglucose studies of side inhibition in macaque striate cortex. *Proc. Natl. Acad. Sci. USA*, 88: 7071–7075.

DeAngelis, G.C., Freeman, R.D. and Ohzawa, I. (1994) Length and width tuning of neurons in the cat's primary visual cortex. *J. Neurophysiol.*, 71: 347–374.

Dreher, B. (1972) Hypercomplex cells in the cat's striate cortex. *Invest. Ophthalmol. Vis. Sci.*, 11: 355–356.

Freeman, R.D. and Ohzawa, I. (1990) On the neurophysiological organization of binocular vision. *Vision Res.*, 30: 1661–1676.

Hubel, D.H. and Wiesel, T.N. (1959) Receptive fields of single neurones in the cat's striate cortex. *J. Physiol. (Lond.)*, 148: 574–591.

Hubel, D.H. and Wiesel, T.N. (1962) Receptive fields, binocular interaction, and functional architecture in the cat's visual cortex. *J. Physiol. (Lond.)*, 160: 106–154.

Hubel, D.H. and Wiesel, T.N. (1965) Receptive fields and functional architecture in two non-striate visual areas (18 and 19) of the cat. *J. Neurophysiol.*, 41: 229–289.

Hubel, D.H. and Wiesel, T.N. (1968) Receptive fields and functional architecture of monkey striate cortex. *J. Physiol. (Lond.)*, 195: 215–243.

Jones, J.P. and Palmer, L.A. (1987a) The two-dimensional spatial structure of simple receptive fields in the cat striate cortex. *J. Neurophysiol.*, 58: 1187–1211.

Jones, J.P. and Palmer, L.A. (1987b) An evaluation of the two-dimensional Gabor filter model of simple receptive fields in cat striate cortex. *J. Neurophysiol.*, 58: 1233–1258.

Kato, H., Bishop, P.O. and Orban, G.A. (1978) Hypercomplex and simple/complex cell classifications in cat striate cortex. *J. Neurophysiol.*, 41: 1071–1095.

Knierim, J.J. and Van Essen, D.C. (1992) Neuronal responses to static texture patterns in area V1 of the alert macaque monkey. *J. Neurophysiol.*, 67: 961–980.

Lamme, V.A.F. (1995) The neurophysiology of figure-ground segregation in primary visual cortex. *J. Neurosci.*, 15: 1605–1615.

Lamme, V.A.F., Zipser, K. and Spekreijse, H. (1997) Figure-ground signals in V1 depend on extrastriate feedback. *Invest. Ophthalmol. Vis. Sci. (Suppl.)*, 38: 969.

Levitt, J.B. and Lund, J.S. (1997) Contrast dependence of contextual effects in primate visual cortex. *Nature*, 387: 73–76.

Maffei, L. and Fiorentini, A. (1976) The unresponsive regions of visual cortical receptive fields. *Vision Res.*, 16: 1131–1139.

Nelson, J.I. and Frost, B.J. (1978) Orientation-selective inhibition from beyond the classic visual receptive field. *Brain Res.*, 139: 359–365.

Palmer, L.A. and Rosenquist, A.C. (1974) Visual receptive fields of single striate cortical units projecting to the superior colliculus in the cat. *Brain Res.*, 67: 27–42.

Sillito, A.M. (1977) The spatial extent of excitatory and inhibitory zones in the receptive field of superficial layer hypercomplex cells. *J. Physiol. (Lond.)*, 273: 791–803.

Sillito, A.M., Grieve, K.L., Jones, H.E., Cudeiro, J. and Davis, J. (1995) Visual cortical mechanisms detecting focal orientation discontinuities. *Nature*, 378: 492–496.

Von der Heydt, R., Peterhans, E. and Dursteler, M.R. (1992) Periodic-pattern-selective cells in monkey visual cortex. *J. Neurosci.*, 12: 1416–1434.

Walker, G.A., Ohzawa, I. and Freeman, R.D. (1999) Asymmetric suppression outside the classical receptive field of the visual cortex. *J. Neurosci.*, 19: 10536–10553.

Walker, G.A., Ohzawa, I. and Freeman, R.D. (2000) Suppression outside the classical cortical receptive field. *Vis. Neurosci.*, 17: 1–11.

Zipser, K., Lamme, V.A.F. and Schiller, P.H. (1996) Contextual modulation in primary visual cortex. *J. Neurosci.*, 16: 7376–7389.

C. Casanova and M. Ptito (Eds.)
Progress in Brain Research, Vol. 134

CHAPTER 12

Processing of second-order stimuli in the visual cortex

Curtis L. Baker, Jr. [1,*] and Isabelle Mareschal [2]

[1] *Department of Ophthalmology, McGill University, 687 Pine Ave. W. H4-14, Montreal, PQ H3A 1A1, Canada*
[2] *Center for Neural Science, Room 809, New York University, New York, NY 10003, USA*

Abstract: Naturally occurring visual stimuli are rich in examples of objects delineated from their backgrounds simply by differences in luminance, so-called first-order stimuli, as well as those defined by differences of contrast or texture, referred to as second-order stimuli. Here we provide a brief overview of visual cortical processing of second-order stimuli, as well as some comparative background on first-order processing, concentrating on single-unit neurophysiology, but also discussing relationships to human psychophysics and to neuroimaging. The selectivity of visual cortical neurons to orientation, spatial frequency, and direction of movement of first-order, luminance-defined stimuli is conventionally understood in terms of simple linear filter models, albeit with some minor nonlinearities such as thresholding and gain control. However, these kinds of models fail entirely to account for responses of neurons to second-order stimuli such as contrast envelopes, illusory contours, or texture borders. Second-order stimuli constructed from sinusoidal components have been used to analyze the neurophysiological mechanisms of such responses; these experiments demonstrate that the same neuron can exhibit three distinct kinds of tuning to spatial frequency, and also to orientation. These results can be understood in terms of a type of nonlinear 'filter → rectify → filter' model, which has been widely used in human psychophysics. Finally, several general issues will be discussed, including potential artifacts in experiments with second-order stimuli, and strategies for avoiding or controlling for them; caveats about definitions of first- vs. second-order mechanisms and stimuli; the concept of form–cue invariance; and the functional significance of second-order processing.

Introduction

Our visual world is most simply thought of in terms of local variations in luminance, and thus it is not surprising that until recently most theoretical conceptions of visual processing, as well as stimuli used to characterize it, were cast in terms of responses to local luminance differences. Nevertheless, we readily detect objects which differ from their background in other aspects than luminance. In the natural image in Fig. 1A, the up-turned fishing boats are clearly delineated from their background by luminance differences, but the fine texture of the foreground vegetation is distinguished from the coarse stripes of the boat ramp much less by luminance differences than by changes in texture and contrast.

Simple visual stimuli whose principal attributes can be characterized as variations in local luminance are referred to as *first-order* stimuli. A first-order stimulus which has proven particularly useful for visual science experiments is a sinewave grating (Fig. 1B): note it is spatially one-dimensional, and in a static image is entirely specified by parameters of orientation, spatial frequency, spatial phase, and contrast. A smoothly moving grating is additionally characterized by its temporal frequency, in Hertz (cycles/s); thus the speed or velocity of its motion is the ratio of its temporal frequency to its spatial frequency, with dimensions of degrees per second. Notice that attributes of this stimulus, such as its orientation and spatial frequency, are entirely specified by changes in luminance across space.

Visual stimuli which portray variations in stimulus properties other than luminance, such as contrast

* Corresponding author: C.L. Baker Jr., Department of Ophthalmology, McGill University, 687 Pine Ave. W. H4-14, Montreal, PQ H3A 1A1, Canada. Tel.: +1-514-842-1231, ext. 4819; Fax: +1-514-843-1691;
E-mail curtis@astra.vision.mcgill.ca

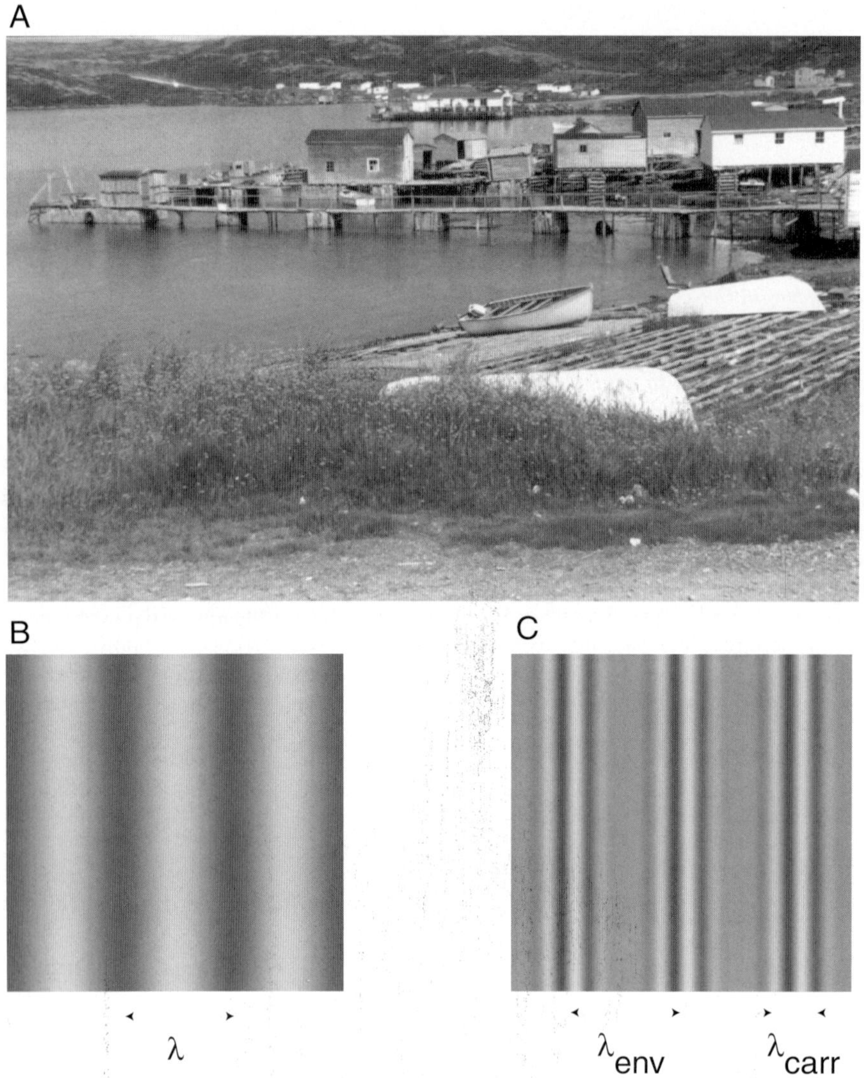

Fig. 1. From natural scenes to analytical stimuli. (A) Objects are delineated from one another as much by changes of texture and contrast as by luminance differences, as in this photograph of Goose Cove, an outport fishing village in Newfoundland, Canada. (B) Sinewave grating, a first-order stimulus whose orientation and spatial frequency ($1/\lambda$) are defined by variations in luminance. (C) Contrast envelope stimulus, consisting of a fine-grain 'carrier' pattern (grating of high spatial frequency, $1/\lambda_{carr}$) whose contrast is modulated by a coarse-grain 'envelope' pattern (grating of low spatial frequency, $1/\lambda_{env}$). Orientation and spatial frequency of the envelope are second-order stimulus attributes, defined by variations of contrast rather than luminance.

or texture, are referred to as *second-order* stimuli — also sometimes called 'non-Fourier' stimuli (Chubb and Sperling, 1988; Cavanagh and Mather, 1989). An example of such a stimulus which has proven experimentally useful is the contrast envelope stimulus (Fig. 1C), consisting of a finely detailed pattern (carrier — here a sinewave grating at a high spatial frequency), whose contrast varies on a coarse spatial scale (envelope — here a sinewave grating of low spatial frequency). In this example, the carrier and envelope waveforms have the same orientation, though this does not necessarily have to be the case. Note that the envelope of this stimulus is not defined by a variation in luminance across space, but rather by a variation in the change of luminance across space, i.e. a second-order statistic — the rate of change of the rate of change of luminance.

In this review, we introduce some theoretical background regarding filtering models of cortical receptive fields, building a foundation with conventional first-order processing concepts before delving into experimental data and models for second-order responses. Second-order processing will be introduced with a variety of examples from the literature, followed by a summary of our analysis of its nature at the single neuron level using contrast envelope stimuli. A type of model will be discussed, which not only provides a framework for understanding these results, but also suggests a linkage to a wide variety of other kinds of visual processing. While our principal emphasis will be on single unit neurophysiology, relationships to human psychophysics and brain imaging experiments will also be pointed out.

First-order processing

Spatial selectivity

Early visual cortex neurons are selective for a remarkable variety of stimulus attributes. Like neurons earlier in the visual pathway, they respond only to stimuli presented within a small region of visual space, the neuron's receptive field. The seminal experiments of Hubel and Wiesel (1962) additionally demonstrated a narrow selectivity for orientation of simple luminance-defined stimuli such as bars or edges. Later studies demonstrated a similarly impressive selectivity for the orientation and also the spatial frequency of sinewave gratings (Campbell et al., 1969). These and other kinds of stimulus selectivity are easily understood for at least one kind of cortical neuron, termed 'simple cells' by Hubel and Wiesel (1962): the receptive fields of these neurons have spatially segregated sub-regions, alternating in excitatory and inhibitory effect (Fig. 2A). A light bar presented in an excitatory region will elicit a transient discharge at its onset, an 'On-response'; it will also elicit a transient discharge when removed from an inhibitory region (presumably due to a rebound from inhibition), termed an 'Off-response'. Dark bars have the opposite effects, eliciting On-responses from inhibitory zones and Off-responses from excitatory zones (Ferster, 1988; Hirsch et al., 1998). In visual cortex receptive fields, these excitatory and inhibitory regions are elongated and occur in alternation. The stimulus orientation selectivity of such a neuron can be understood in terms of the competing influences of these regions, if it is assumed that they are linearly additive (Hubel and Wiesel, 1962), prior to a simple threshold. Thus if a light bar or a grating (Fig. 2B) is presented at an orientation different from that of the elongated sub-regions, their excitatory and inhibitory influences will cancel one another out. But an oriented bar or grating at the same orientation (Fig. 2C) will cause consistent stimulation of these sub-regions, which will synergistically sum to a strong response. Hubel and Wiesel (1962) first demonstrated this correspondence between the orientation of the simple cell sub-regions and the neurons' preferred stimulus orientation.

Selectivity for spatial frequency of sinewave gratings can be understood similarly. A maximal response is obtained only if the spacing of light and dark regions of a grating correspond well with the spacing of excitatory and inhibitory regions (Fig. 2C), otherwise there will be a failure of effective summation, even if the orientation is optimal (Fig. 2D). But the sinewave grating which maximally activates a simple type cell will be one whose light and dark bars are in register with the alternating excitatory and inhibitory sub-regions (Fig. 2C). Such a correspondence between spacing of sub-regions and optimal grating spatial frequency has been demonstrated quantitatively (Movshon et al., 1978; Andrews and Pollen, 1979; DeAngelis et al., 1993; McLean et al., 1994).

Velocity tuning

These neurons are also selective for the speed, and often the direction of motion, of moving bars or gratings: it turns out that this spatiotemporal selectivity can also be understood in an analogous manner. Since the stimuli are spatially elongated, and presented at the neuron's preferred orientation, they have only one spatial dimension which is relevant: the luminance profile along the orthogonal direction (i.e. the direction of motion). Therefore these spatiotemporal stimuli can be represented as two-dimen-

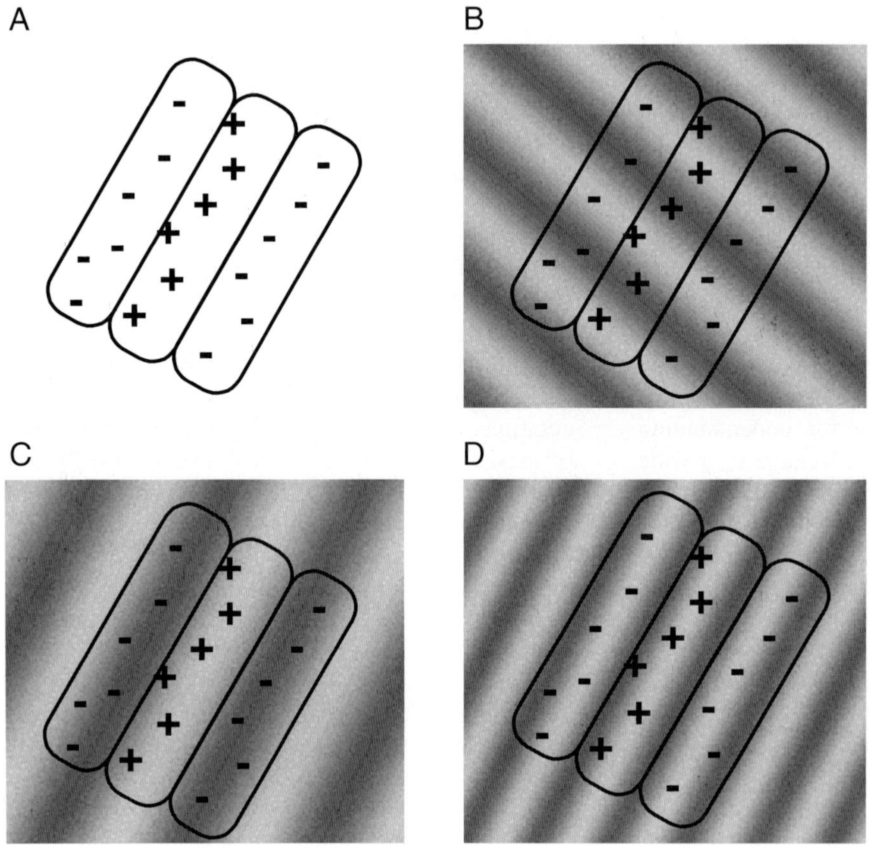

Fig. 2. Spatial selectivity of cortical neurons for sinewave gratings understood in terms of linear summation. (A) Cartoon model of oriented, excitatory and inhibitory sub-regions of simple-type receptive field in visual cortex. (B) Sinewave grating at differing orientation elicits poor summation of sub-regions, and no response. (C) An optimal grating is one whose dark and light bars have orientation and spacing corresponding to the neuron's sub-regions, eliciting maximally effective summation. (D) Grating of correct orientation, but nonoptimal spatial frequency gives poor response because bars are not matched in size with neuron's sub-regions.

sional images, as functions of time and of one spatial dimension. Such 'space–time diagrams' are shown in Fig. 3, for drifting bars (top row) and gratings (bottom row), which are drifting rightwards (left column) or leftwards (right column). Thus considered in this way, motion becomes a kind of orientation, but in space–time rather than space–space; higher speeds correspond to orientations closer to horizontal (note that a stationary stimulus would have a vertical orientation). Then it is easy to see by analogy that selectivity for velocity (speed and direction) can be obtained with a spatiotemporal filter which is oriented, as indicated with overlaid cartoons of excitation and inhibition in Fig. 3.

What does it mean to have a receptive field which is 'space–time oriented'? It means that the temporal response of the neuron varies systematically with position in the receptive field. Start by considering only the excitation (+) in Fig. 3A (with time running downwards, the latency of the neuron's response is the distance from the top of the diagram) and in this case as we proceed from left to right, the peak response is at progressively greater latencies. The inhibitory responses are constructed similarly, but in an alternating spatial relationship. As illustrated in Fig. 3, such a space–time oriented filter would have a net cancellation of excitation and inhibition in response to stimuli moving in the opposite direction to its space–time orientation (right panels), and a good summation of response for those moving at its preferred velocity (left panels). Such a linear spatiotemporal

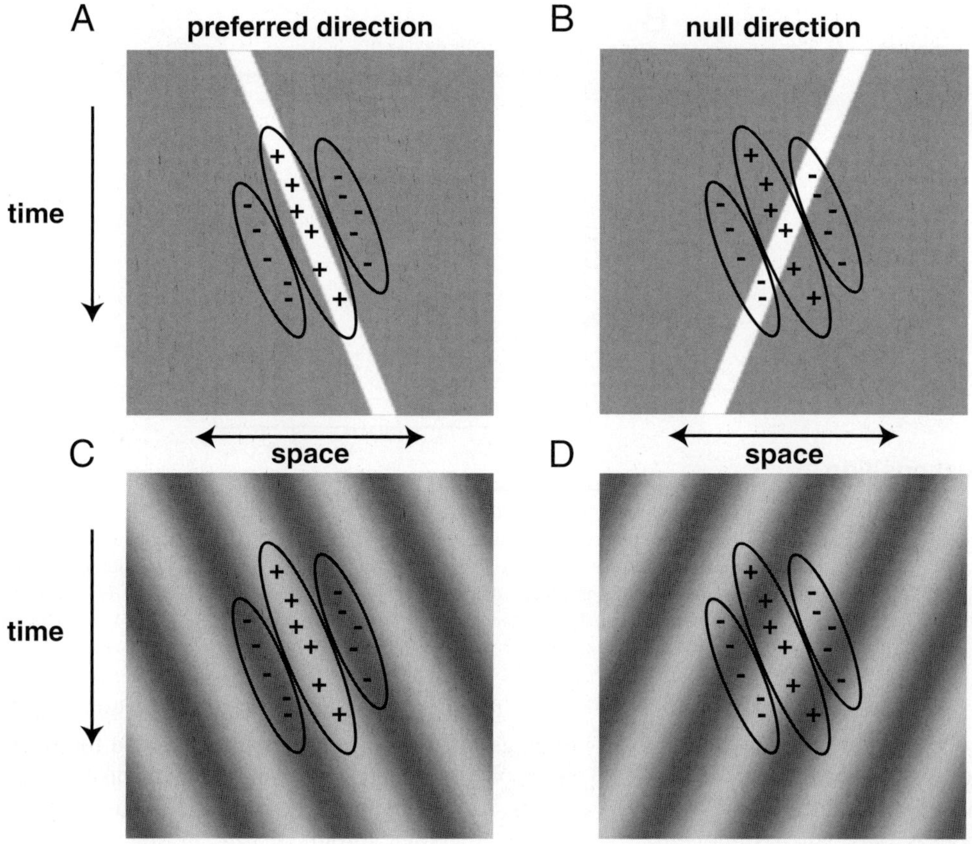

Fig. 3. Conventional model of how linear summation might explain direction selectivity. In each panel, cartoon spatiotemporal receptive field is superimposed on stimulus, depicted as spatial luminance profile along direction of motion (abscissa), with time progressing downwards. (A) Rightwards-moving luminance bar gives synergistic summation to neuron receptive field, and therefore strong response. (B) Leftwards-moving bar fails to match receptive field regions, giving cancellation and poor response. (C) Rightwards-moving sinewave grating gives good match-up to receptive field, and good response. (D) Leftwards-moving grating causes cancellation of responses from neuron receptive field.

filtering account of visual motion processing has been proposed as an integral part of computational models of biological motion detection (Adelson and Bergen, 1985). The temporally delayed responses may arise from a population of lateral geniculate neurons, 'lagged cells' (Saul and Humphrey, 1990, 1992).

Neuronal properties understood in terms of the linear filter model

The linear filter model has provided a basis on which to understand important relationships between a neuron's responses to different stimuli, including bars, gratings, and random noise. The space–time filter function can be experimentally measured with 'reverse-correlation', which entails taking the average space–time stimulus history preceding each neuronal spike, using a white noise stimulus — an example (Baker and Boulton, 1990; Baker, 2001) is shown in Fig. 4A. McLean et al. (1994) demonstrated that the space–time orientation of such plots could quantitatively predict a neuron's preferred velocity to moving bars. The ratio of a neuron's optimal temporal frequency to its optimal spatial frequency, in response to drifting sinewave gratings, can also be a good predictor of its optimal velocity for a moving bar (Baker, 1990) (Fig. 4B).

Of course cortical neurons do not behave linearly in every respect (Bonds, 1992), but some of the best-

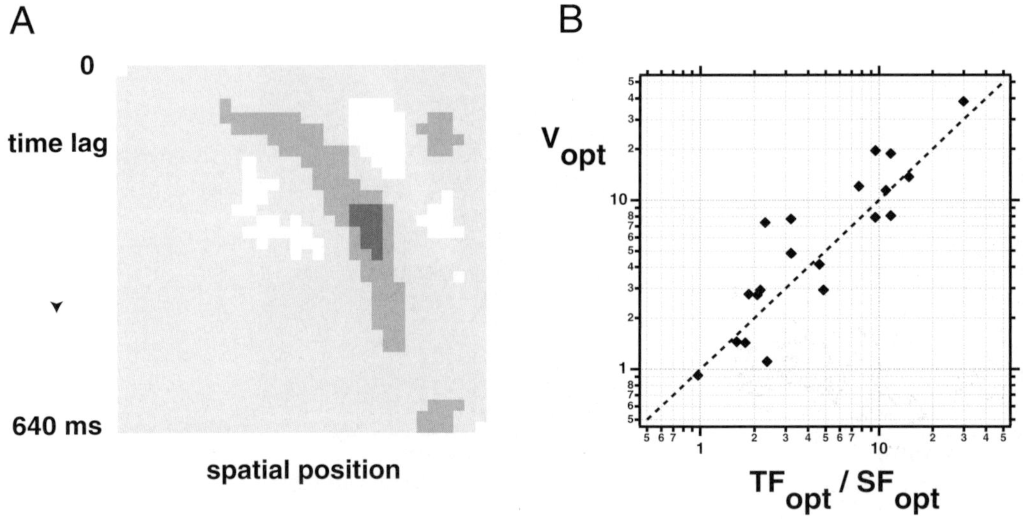

Fig. 4. Examples of evidence for linear model of neuronal direction selectivity. (A) First-order reverse correlation analysis of a direction-selective visual cortex neuron, which provides an estimate of the cell's linear spatiotemporal filtering operation. Note the spatiotemporally oriented correlation, corresponding to the neuron's preferred direction of motion. (B) Optimal velocity of a moving bar (V_{opt}) correlates with predictions from optimal temporal and spatial frequencies for sinewave gratings (TF_{opt}/SF_{opt}). Each point represents data from one neuron; dashed line shows unity ratio. Data replotted from Baker (1990).

known nonlinearities can be accommodated with simple modifications to the linear filter model. The most obvious nonlinearity is a threshold — cortical neurons usually have relatively little spontaneous activity, and give responses only when sufficiently excited — this can be modeled as a simple threshold operation following the linear spatiotemporal filter.

Many cortical neurons, termed 'complex cells', differ from simple-type cells in having On- and Off-responses which are not spatially segregated; nevertheless they also show a strong selectivity for orientation, spatial frequency, and velocity. However their selectivity can be understood in similar terms, if they add up the responses of a small pool of nearby simple-type cells, having the same selectivity but slightly differing receptive field positions (Hubel and Wiesel, 1962).

A number of other nonlinear behaviors of early cortical neurons could be accounted for with simple modifications to the linear filter model. For example, a cortical neuron maintains its selectivity to a given stimulus parameter across a range of contrasts (Albrecht et al., 1984; Skottun et al., 1987), and its response to an optimal stimulus is inhibited by superimposing a nonoptimal stimulus (Morrone et al., 1982; Bonds, 1989; DeAngelis et al., 1993). Such findings have been interpreted to indicate the operation of a nonlinear gain control mechanism which serves to 'normalize' the response to a stimulus, relative to other stimuli nearby in space or time. An example of a simple model which might account for such results is one (Heeger, 1992) in which the cell's response gain is scaled by the pooled responses of nearby neurons, having different stimulus selectivities but the same receptive field location (Fig. 5A).

Physiological basis of linear filter model

It is easy to imagine that the excitatory and inhibitory sub-regions of a simple cell arise from linear summation of aligned sets of lateral geniculate nucleus (LGN) afferents (Hubel and Wiesel, 1962). This idea has been extended with evidence that excitatory sub-regions may receive both excitation for LGN On-cells and inhibition from LGN Off-cells (and conversely for inhibitory sub-regions), a 'push–pull' model which gives more truly linear behavior (Ferster, 1988; Carandini et al., 1999). This idea has been extended to direction selectivity, with lagged-type LGN cells providing space–

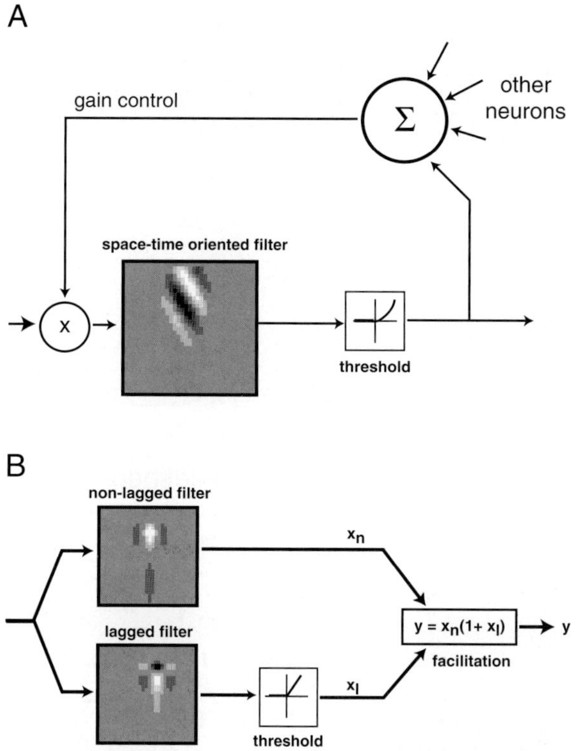

Fig. 5. Quasi-linear models of first-order direction selectivity. (A) Conventional linear space–time oriented filter model, with subsequent half-squaring, and gain control from pooled responses of similar neurons selective for other orientations and spatial frequencies. (B) Alternative model, suggested by experiments on two-flash motion at large SOAs and white noise analysis, in which signals from quadrature-phase linear filters are combined nonlinearly.

time orientation (Saul and Humphrey, 1992). The model is supported by superposition experiments in intracellular recordings (Jagadeesh et al., 1977), and by cross-correlation analysis of simultaneously recorded cells in LGN and area 17 (Reid and Alonso, 1995).

However, a simple linear filter model has been challenged by evidence for a crucial role of lateral inhibitory interactions in shaping orientation selectivity (Ringach et al., 1997). Another kind of challenge has been evidence for nonlinear summation (e.g. shunting inhibition, facilitation), based on intracellular recording (Borg-Graham et al., 1998), integrative properties of NMDA receptors (Rivadulla et al., 1999), direction-selectivity for apparent motion at very large onset asynchronies (Baker and Cynader, 1994), and nonlinear white noise analysis (Baker, 2001) (see Fig. 5B).

In spite of these and other caveats, the linear filter model has proven to be a useful metaphor for understanding a variety of spatial and temporal integrative behaviors of many early visual cortex neurons. The best characterized nonlinearities can be modeled as part of an adaptive gain control which affects the overall response gain of the neuron, but with its fundamental stimulus selectivity being controlled by the linear filter (Carandini et al., 1999).

Human psychophysics

A very large body of human psychophysics has supported the idea that the visual system can be considered an ensemble of such linear spatial filters, selective for orientation and spatial frequency. In such a 'bank of filters' scheme, threshold for stimulus detection is determined by the most sensitive filter (e.g. Campbell and Robson, 1968; Blakemore and Campbell, 1969); for review see Graham (1980). The contrast sensitivity function of the visual system is interpreted as representing the envelope of sensitivities of these filters.

Motion detection thresholds can be understood similarly (Levinson and Sekuler, 1975). For suprathreshold stimuli, the theory successfully predicts that the spatial limits of apparent motion ('D_{max}') scale inversely with spatial frequency content of the displaced stimulus (Bischof and DiLollo, 1990; Cleary and Braddick, 1990; Boulton and Baker, 1993b).

Contrast gain control has also proven a useful concept in models of first-order motion psychophysics, for example in how apparent motion is affected by unequal durations (Bischof and DiLollo, 1996) or differing contrasts (Georgeson and Scott-Samuel, 1999) on successive exposures.

Second-order processing: detection of borders defined by contrast or texture

Form–cue invariance

The earliest report of neuronal responses to second-order motion was by Albright (1992), who showed that neurons in primate area MT/V5 responded to

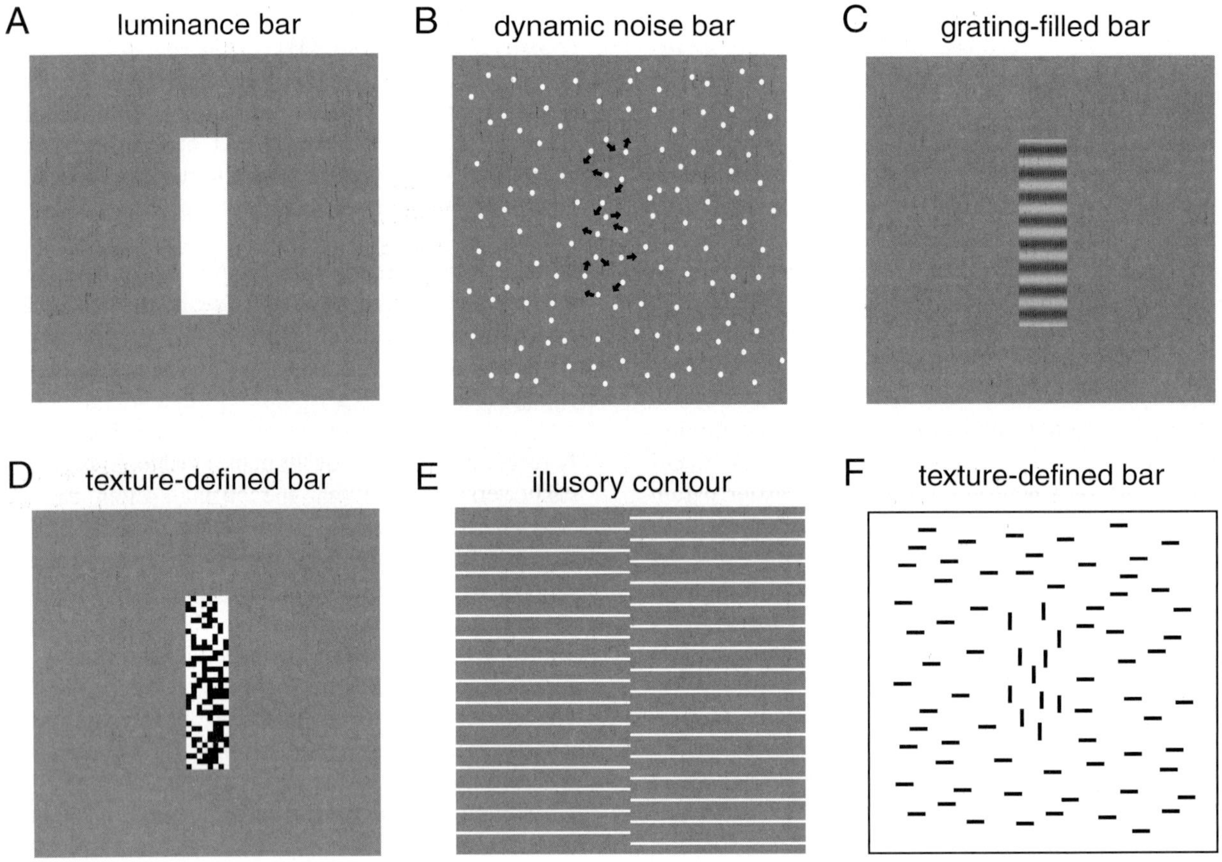

Fig. 6. Examples of vertically oriented second-order stimuli, defined by various carriers. (A) Luminance-defined bar (first-order), for comparison. (B) Bar defined by dynamic noise, on background of static noise. (C) Oriented grating patch, on background of same average luminance. (D) Oriented patch of noise, on background of same average luminance. (E) Illusory contour stimulus, defined by phase-shifted abutting gratings or bars. (F) Bar of vertical micro-elements, on background of horizontal elements.

moving regions of dynamic noise, on a static noise background (Fig. 6B). The same neurons also responded to luminance-defined stimuli, with the same preferred direction of motion, leading to the notion of 'form–cue invariance' — the property of a neuron being selective to a stimulus attribute (e.g. direction of motion) regardless of the 'cue' defining it (here, either temporal contrast, or luminance contrast). Presumably neurons displaying such form–cue invariance would be functionally useful in mediating responses to overall objects regardless of the cue (or, in our terms, carrier) by which they are segregated from the background.

Similar findings of form cue invariance for bar-shaped stimuli have been reported in other brain areas, for different stimuli and stimulus attributes. Geesaman and Andersen (1996) demonstrated a similar invariance for complex motion attributes in MT/V5 neurons, using stimuli defined by a variety of carrier types. Chaudhuri and Albright (1997) described responses to dynamic noise bars in primate V1 — rarely direction selective (for either kind of stimulus), but having the same selectivity to orientation of the bar, whether defined by luminance or by dynamic noise. In area 18 neurons of the cat, Leventhal et al. (1998) found single neurons with consistent direction selectivity to bars defined either by luminance, or by gratings or texture on a gray background of the same luminance (Fig. 6C,D).

Using drifting periodic contrast modulation stimuli (Fig. 1C), Zhou and Baker (1993, 1996) also found single neurons in cat areas 17 and 18, which responded both to luminance and contrast-defined stimuli with a consistent preferred direction of motion. For a given neuron, the preferred contrast envelope spatial frequency was similar to, but often significantly lower than, the optimal spatial frequency for luminance gratings (Zhou and Baker, 1996; Mareschal and Baker, 1998b). Area 18 neurons were shown to have consistent optimal orientations for envelopes and luminance gratings (Mareschal and Baker, 1998a, 1999). Unlike the above studies, however, the use of narrowband carrier waveforms led to finding surprisingly narrow tuning to both carrier spatial frequency and orientation (Zhou and Baker, 1996; Mareschal and Baker, 1999); these findings will be described much more extensively below. This specificity of a neuron's response to carrier parameters may provide an important qualification to the notion of form–cue invariance, though it does not preclude the possibility that other neurons might exist whose envelope responses are invariant to the nature of the carrier.

Illusory contours, texture borders

A rather differently motivated line of research involved searching for neural correlates of human perception of 'illusory contours', formed for example by abutting gratings which have an abrupt discontinuity at their juncture (Fig. 6E); these stimuli have no luminance-defined edge along the illusory contour, and so they might be considered as 'second-order' (see below). Neurons have been reported in cat area 18 (Peterhans and von der Heydt, 1991) and in primate area V2 (Grosof et al., 1993), to respond to motion of such illusory contours with a similar selectivity to orientation and direction of motion as for luminance edges.

Yet another line of research has investigated possible mechanisms of texture segregation, using stimuli having a central region differing from its background in local texture properties (Fig. 6F) — again, with the same net luminances in the figure and ground, these could be considered second-order stimuli. For example, Olavarria et al. (1992) demonstrated responses in primate MT/V5 neurons using textures of small lines, differing in orientation, and responses to texture borders were also found in primate area V1 (Nothdurft et al., 1999).

Human psychophysics

Henning et al. (1975) introduced contrast envelope stimuli, like that shown in Fig. 1C, arguing that their detection could not be accounted for in terms of linear filter schemes. Several subsequent studies (e.g. Derrington and Badcock, 1985; Ledgeway and Smith, 1994b) indicated that contrast envelopes were detected by a different mechanism.

Chubb and Sperling (1988) introduced 'drift-balanced' motion stimuli which were constructed such that their motion would be invisible to any motion detector based on linear filtering: this was achieved by using a dynamic noise carrier which has no coherent motion signals. These authors also introduced early versions of 'filter → rectify → filter' models (see below), and proposed an analogous kind of processing for spatial vision. This work inspired many subsequent studies of such 'non-Fourier' processing, in spatial vision tasks (Sutter et al., 1989; Graham and Sutter, 1998) as well as motion perception (see Smith, 1994).

A continuing question has been whether second-order stimulus attributes are processed by a distinct mechanism from that which handles first-order ones. Numerous studies have provided evidence for such separate processing, but the question has remained controversial (Taub et al., 1997) (see below). Particularly compelling psychophysical evidence has emerged from recent work showing that adaptation to first- or second-order stimuli selectively affects thresholds only for target stimuli of the same type, but that cross-adaptation is absent (Nishida et al., 1997), and that subthreshold facilitation is similarly specific to the type of stimulus (Schofield and Georgeson, 1999).

Analysis of the mechanism of second-order processing

Use of contrast envelope stimuli to characterize second-order responses in single neurons

To demonstrate and characterize second-order responses from early visual cortex neurons, we employed contrast envelope stimuli (Fig. 1C) consisting of a high spatial frequency sinewave carrier whose contrast is modulated by a lower spatial frequency,

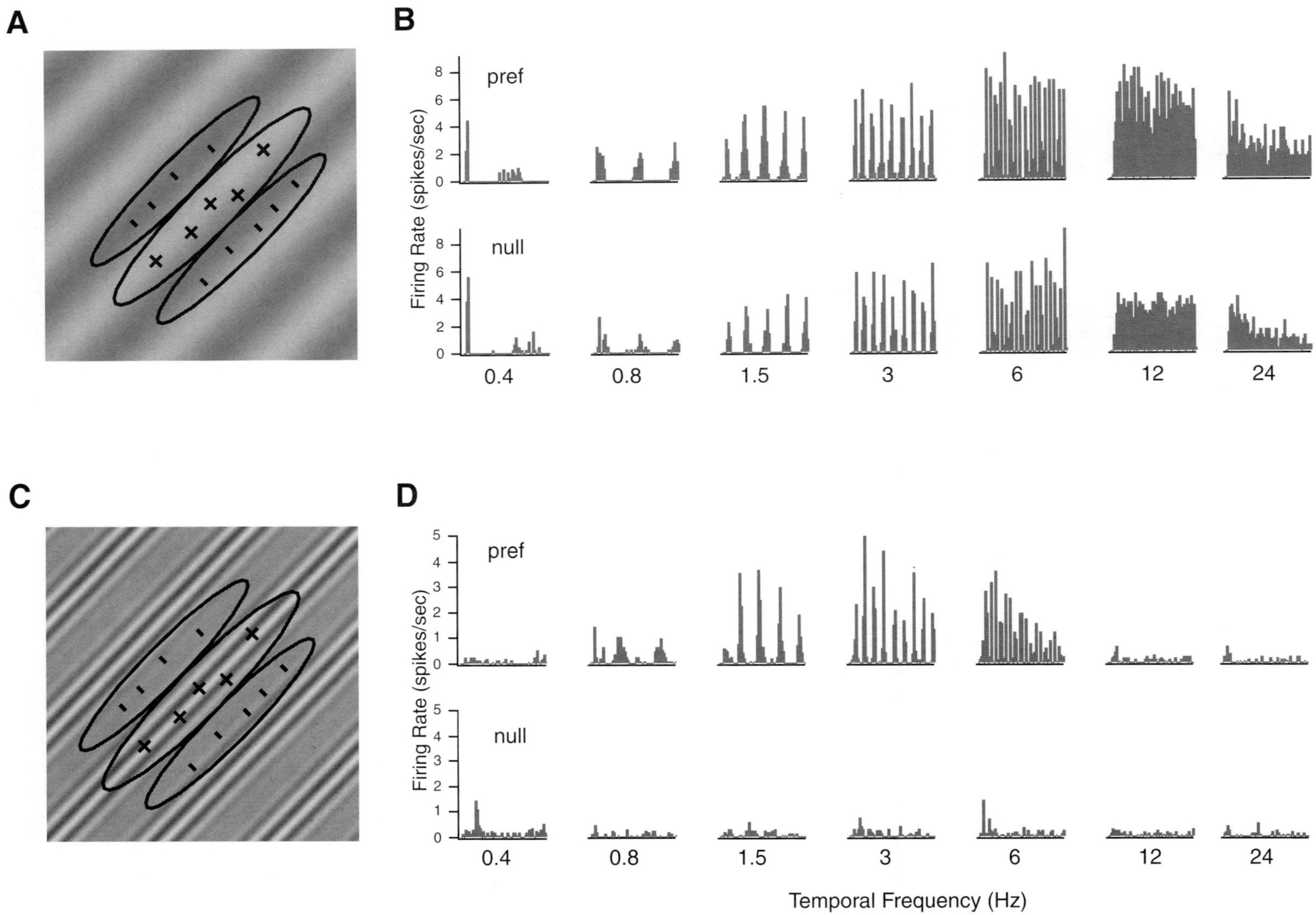

Fig. 7. Responses of linear model and cortical neuron to first- and second-order stimuli. (A) Sinewave grating stimulus which is optimal for a linear model (superimposed cartoon receptive field). (B) Post-stimulus time histograms of cortical simple cell's response to drifting grating, at a series of temporal frequencies in both preferred and nonpreferred directions. Note modulated discharge, indicative of a simple type cell, preference for temporal frequencies of 3–12 Hz, and very little direction selectivity. (C) Contrast envelope stimulus, which would fail to activate a linear receptive field. (D) Response of same neuron as in A, to contrast envelope drifting at a series of temporal frequencies. Note that response is again modulated, but with a greater degree of direction selectivity and tuning to lower temporal frequencies of about 1.5–6 Hz. Post-stimulus time histograms (B and D) from Mareschal and Baker (1998b).

drifting sinewave envelope (e.g. Zhou and Baker, 1993; Mareschal and Baker, 1998a). In most of these experiments the carrier was stationary, and the carrier and envelope were of the same orientation (i.e. the stimuli were spatially one-dimensional). Fig. 7 shows images of a luminance grating (A) and contrast envelope (C), each with a cartoon spatially linear receptive field overlaid on the stimuli, to illustrate how such a neuron should respond well to the luminance grating, but not the contrast envelope: in the latter case, the effects of the fine-grain light and dark regions of the carrier would cancel out within the much larger summation sub-regions of the linear receptive field. To put this another (equivalent) way, the carrier spatial frequency is so high as to be outside the passband of the luminance-responsive linear receptive field.

Each neuron's receptive field was first characterized conventionally using sinewave gratings, establishing its preferred orientation, spatial frequency, temporal frequency and direction selectivity. Then contrast envelope stimuli were tested, setting the envelope parameters in accordance with those found optimal for the luminance gratings, and testing a series of high carrier spatial frequencies. At least half the neurons in area 18 of the cat, and a minority of those in area 17, were found to respond significantly to contrast envelopes (Zhou and Baker, 1993). In most cases, a neuron's response to the envelope stimulus was weaker than to luminance gratings, but both kinds of stimuli elicited consistent preferred directions of motion, though with differing degrees of direction selectivity (Mareschal and Baker, 1998b; Zhou and Baker, 1996). Both simple and complex type cells were envelope responsive, though more frequently for complex cells. Simple cells showed modulated discharges to drifting stimuli of either type (Fig. 7B,D), demonstrating that the nonlinearity underlying second-order responses is not related to that which distinguishes complex from simple type cells.

Three kinds of spatial frequency tuning in the same neuron

A theoretically important early result was that envelope responses were highly dependent on carrier spatial frequency, typically being tuned to frequencies 5–30 times greater than for luminance gratings (Zhou and Baker, 1996; Mareschal and Baker, 1999) (see Fig. 8A,B). Bandpass tuning was also found for envelope spatial frequency (Fig. 8C), for frequencies similar to (though often somewhat lower than) those for luminance gratings (Mareschal and Baker, 1998b). Bandwidths of all three types of spatial tuning were similarly narrow (Mareschal and Baker, 1999), such that the carrier bandwidth was unambiguously well outside the luminance passband of the neuron (e.g. in Fig. 8, the tuning curves in A and B are nonoverlapping).

Optimal carrier spatial frequencies for these neurons were typically 1–3 cycles per degree (cpd), sometimes as high as 4 cpd, which is very high relative to the cat's spatial acuity of 5–10 cpd (Cleland et al., 1979; Ulrich et al., 1981). In this respect, the cat is a highly advantageous choice of species for studies of second-order responses, since practical use of spatial frequencies which are comparably high for the monkey would be awkward.

Across the population of sampled neurons, the optimal carrier spatial frequency was not in any characteristic fixed ratio to either the optimal luminance or envelope spatial frequencies (Zhou and Baker, 1996; Mareschal and Baker, 1999). A given individual neuron's optimal carrier spatial frequency was not dependent on the envelope spatial frequency at which it was measured. The independence of these tunings to luminance, carrier, and envelope spatial frequencies suggest that they are mediated by separate mechanisms.

Three kinds of orientation tuning in the same neuron

While our earlier studies employed spatially one-dimensional stimuli produced by lookup table animation, our later use of digital movies (Brainard, 1997) allowed us to vary independently the orientations of carrier and envelope in our second-order stimuli (Mareschal and Baker, 1998a, 1999). Fig. 9 shows orientation tuning curves as polar plots, with distance from the origin indicating strength of response. Luminance gratings always elicited narrow orientation tuning (Fig. 9A) as expected; second-order stimuli also showed similarly narrow tuning to the envelope waveform (the carrier orientation was held constant). Most interesting was that many neurons also showed a bandpass tuning to the carrier (with envelope orientation held constant (Fig. 9C)),

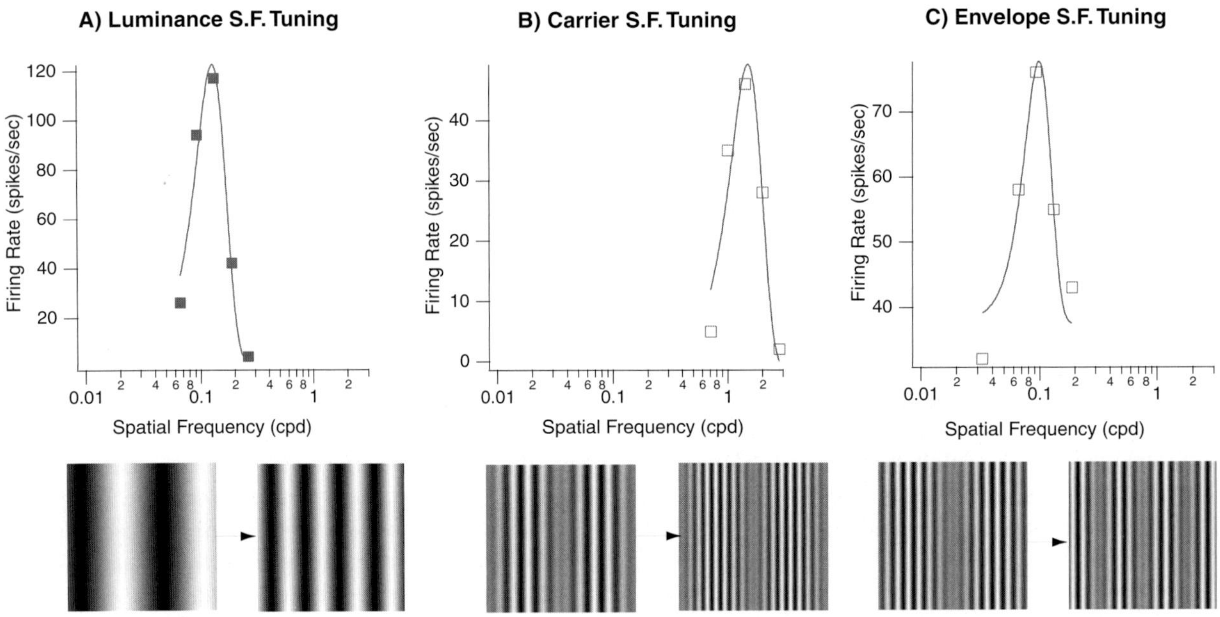

Fig. 8. Three kinds of spatial frequency tuning in a single A18 neuron. In each case, average response of the neuron is plotted against spatial frequency, with examples of stimuli shown below the graphs. (A) Response to luminance grating is sharply tuned, peaking about 0.15 cpd. (B) Response to contrast envelope, with fixed envelope spatial frequency and varying carrier frequency; response is again very sharp, tuned to much higher frequency of about 1.5 cpd. (C) Response to contrast envelope, with fixed carrier frequency and varying envelope frequency. Optimum is about 0.09 cpd similar to, but slightly lower than for luminance grating in A. Reprinted with the permission of Cambridge University Press, from Mareschal and Baker (1999).

though often with a much broader bandwidth. This result suggests that the mechanism of carrier selectivity is almost certainly cortical (Mareschal and Baker, 1998a, 1999).

Fig. 10 shows scatterplots of the measured optimal orientations, across the population of sampled neurons. Neurons' optimal orientation for the envelope was very similar to that for luminance gratings (Fig. 10A), consistent with a 'form–cue invariance' (Albright, 1992); but a given neuron's preferred carrier orientation was totally unpredicatable from its optimal envelope or luminance orientation (Fig. 10B). The independence of carrier orientation tuning again suggests that the carrier is processed by a different set of neurons than those which determine selectivity for the envelope component, or for luminance gratings.

Temporal properties

A large proportion of neurons in cat area 17 and 18 are at least partially direction-selective to luminance gratings, and this was seen also in the same neurons' responses to contrast envelopes. A given neuron always showed a consistent preferred direction for luminance and envelope motion, though the quantitative degree of directionality could differ considerably (Zhou and Baker, 1996; Mareschal and Baker, 1998b; Fig. 7B,D). Envelope responses were temporally bandpass, with optimal temporal frequencies of typically 2–6 Hz; the bandwidths of tuning for envelope and luminance motion were quantitatively similar. A given neuron's optimal temporal frequency for envelope motion was similar to, but often quantitatively somewhat less, than that for luminance grating motion; in addition, simple type cells also exhibited much greater temporal phase lags to contrast envelope responses than to luminance gratings (Mareschal and Baker, 1998b).

These findings of slower temporal properties for second-order than for first-order motion are consistent with the majority of human psychophysical evidence — for example, a lower temporal acuity for contrast envelopes than for luminance grat-

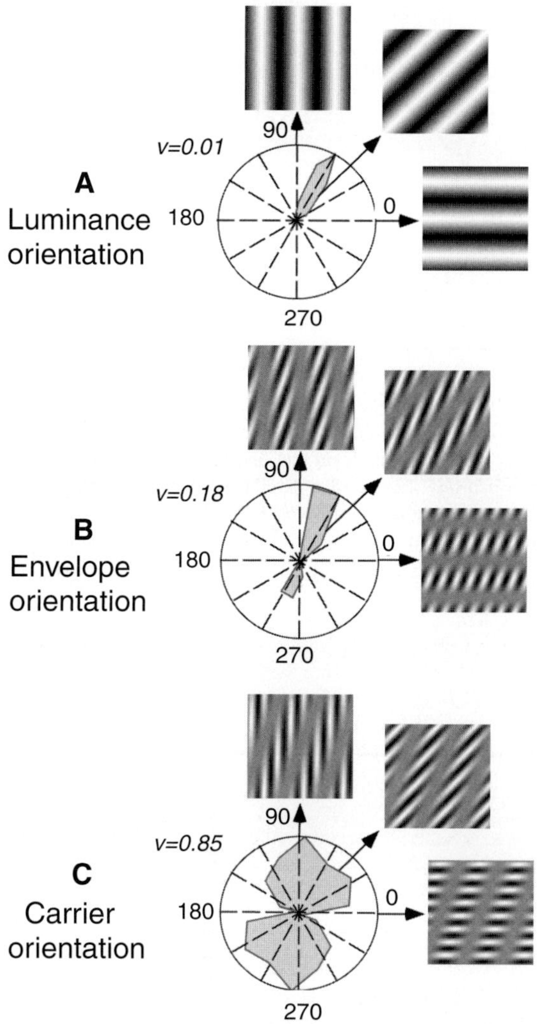

Fig. 9. Three kinds of orientation and directional tuning of an A18 neuron. Data are shown as polar plots: distance from origin represents magnitude of neuron's response, angle represents stimulus orientation. In each case, three examples of the stimulus are shown alongside the polar plot. (A) Response to luminance-defined sinewave grating. (B) Response to contrast envelope stimulus, varying envelope orientation while holding carrier orientation fixed. (C) Same as B, but varying carrier orientation, with envelope orientation fixed. Reprinted with the permission of Cambridge University Press, from Mareschal and Baker (1999).

ings (Derrington et al., 1993), a larger optimal onset asynchrony for nonlinear (second-order) than for quasi-linear (first-order) apparent motion (Boulton and Baker, 1993a), and better performance for second-order motion at lower temporal frequencies (Smith and Ledgeway, 1998). However recent work using double-pulse summation suggests that the temporal properties of the two kinds of processing might be less different if tested with stimuli of comparable bandwidth (Schofield and Georgeson, 2000).

A model of envelope-responsive neurons

That a neuron can show different preferred spatial and temporal frequency preferences, and differing degrees of direction selectivity, to luminance and envelope stimuli suggests that its firing reflects a combination of inputs from two distinct pathways or 'streams', one mediating first-order and the other second-order responses. An adequate model for the one handling luminance grating responses could be a conventional linear filter model like that discussed above, but such a model would be entirely incapable of producing envelope responses for reasons outlined earlier.

Contrast envelopes can be thought of as analogous to AM ('amplitude modulation') radio signals, in which the amplitude of a radio frequency carrier has been modulated by a much lower frequency audio signal; in an AM radio, the audio signal is 'demodulated' by rectification followed by low-pass filtering to smooth out the irregularities introduced by the high frequency carrier. While a signal-processing scheme of this kind might mediate neuronal responses to contrast envelopes, some important modifications are needed to account for the physiological data. Firstly, the spatial and temporal tuning characteristics for envelope responses require that the filter following the rectifier be band-pass rather than low-pass. Secondly, to achieve the tuning to carrier spatial frequency and orientation, we need a front-end filter prior to the rectification (analogous to the radio frequency tuner which selects which station we receive). The intervening rectification ensures that the fine-grain positive and negative portions of the carrier-frequency signal do not cancel one another when smoothed by the later filter. Thus we are led to a 'filter → rectify → filter' (F→R→F) model, for the second-order stream mediating a cortical neuron's response to contrast envelopes (Fig. 11).

This is a very attractive idea because the results of our neurophysiological data map on to it so straightforwardly. The very different tunings for orientation

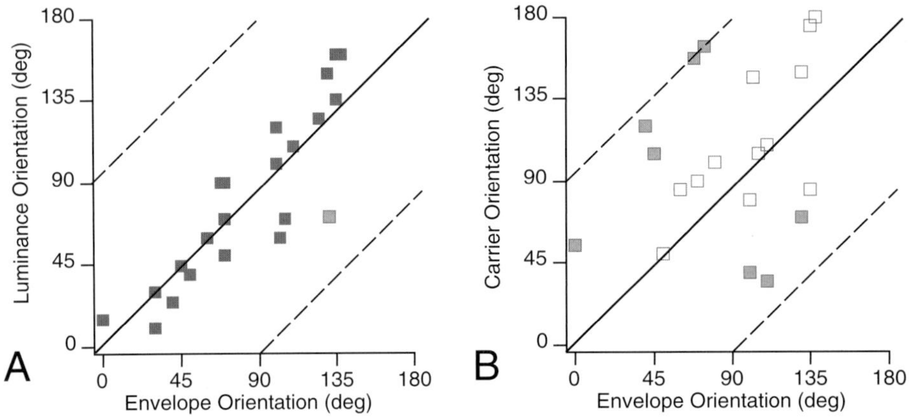

Fig. 10. Relationships of different kinds of orientation tuning. (A) Optimal orientation to luminance grating, compared to optimal orientation of envelope of a contrast modulation stimulus. Each point represents measurements from one neuron; solid line shows unity ratio, dashed lines represent orthogonal preferred orientations. Note that most neurons showed very similar orientation preference for luminance gratings and envelopes. (B) Similar plot, for orientation of carrier of contrast modulation. Note the lack of correlation between the two kinds of tuning, with many neurons preferring carrier orientations close to orthogonal to the envelope (darkened symbols). From Mareschal and Baker (1998a).

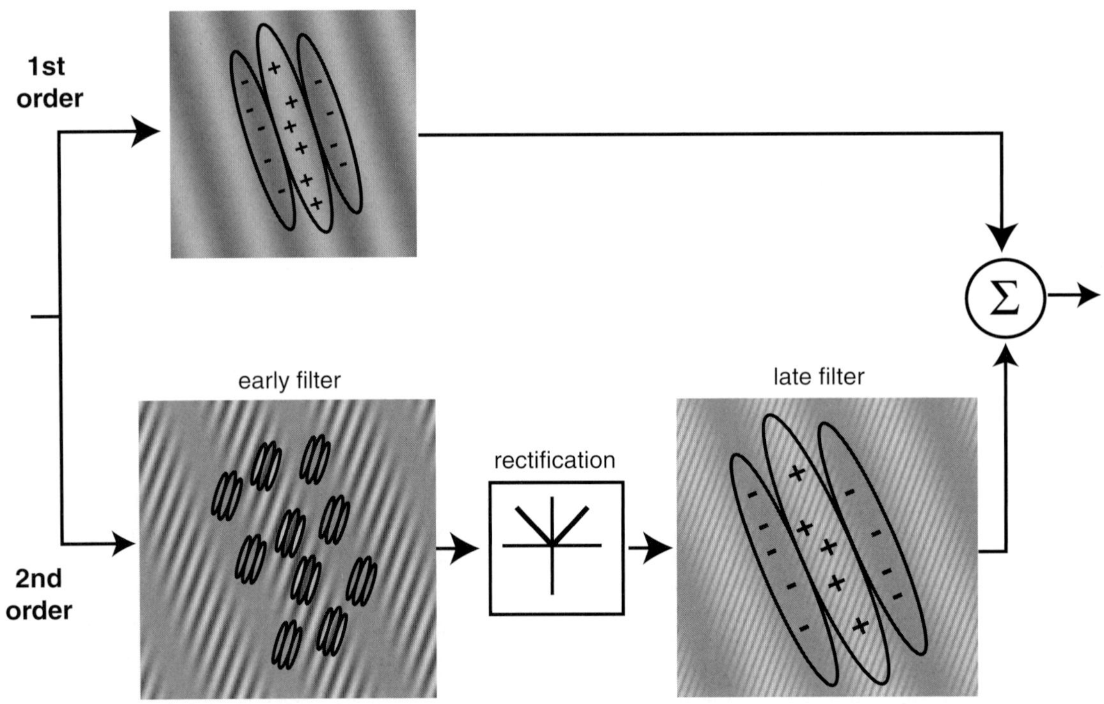

Fig. 11. Model of cortical neuron response, having separate parallel signal-processing pathways for first- and second-order stimuli. In the top path, luminance-defined stimuli are processed conventionally with a linear spatiotemporal filter. The bottom path processes second-order stimuli, and has a 'filter → rectify → filter' cascade consisting of early linear filtering subunits, a nonlinearity (e.g. rectification), and a late linear filter. The early filters are shown superimposed on a contrast envelope stimulus, to illustrate how they could mediate selectivity for carrier properties, while the late filter is shown on the full-wave rectified stimulus to illustrate its selectivitiy for properties of the envelope. The neuron's response reflects a combination of both pathways.

and spatial frequency of the carrier and envelope are easily understood: the selectivity for stimulus parameters of the carrier reflect the properties of the first filter, while the selectivity for envelope attributes reflects the tuning of the second filter.

Fig. 11 illustrates the complete model with separate streams or paths for processing first- and second-order stimuli. A simple luminance grating can elicit a response only via the first-order pathway: regardless of its spatial frequency, it can never satisfy the conflicting demands of the highly discrepant spatial frequency tunings of the early and late filters of the F→R→F stream. Similarly, a contrast envelope stimulus will exert an effect on the final output only via the F→R→F stream, for the reasons discussed already.

Many findings from human psychophysics can be similarly understood in terms of a F→R→F scheme. For example, second-order operations which are selective for carrier spatial frequency and orientation (Green, 1986; Ledgeway and Smith, 1994b; Dakin and Mareschal, 2000) may indicate characteristics of the early filter, while specificity to attributes of the envelope could reflect properties of the late filter (Nishida et al., 1997). But in addition to second-order processing, F→R→F models have also been used in various forms to understand spatial vision tasks such as detection of texture borders (Landy, 1991; Graham and Sutter, 1998), illusory contours (Wilson, 1999), terminators (Loffler and Orbach, 1999), and non-Cartesian stimuli (Gallant et al., 1993; Gallant et al., 1996; Wilson, 1999). By making either the early or late filters selective for other attributes, this kind of model might conceivably handle an even wider variety of stimuli, such as 'theta motion' (Zanker, 1993) if the early filters are selective to direction or speed of motion, or second-order stereopsis (Hess and Wilcox, 1994) if the late filters are disparity-selective. Appropriately arranged early and late filters could be designed for specific responses to optic flow invariants (expansion–contraction, rotation, etc.), or for contour integration (Field et al., 1993).

Possible physiological substrates of second-order processing

In the model of Fig. 11, the upper branch which handles first-order processing could be any of the quasi-linear neurons of early visual cortical areas, though the low preferred spatial frequencies in our data suggest a greater contribution from second-tier areas (A18, V2). Our findings of selectivity for carrier spatial frequency and orientation suggest that the early filters of the F→R→F branch must be cortical, and the quite high optimal carrier frequencies suggest quasi-linear neurons in first-tier areas (A17, V1) as very likely candidates.

The more interesting question is the neural substrate of the later filters of the F→R→F branch: neurons corresponding to this stage, if they exist, would in this scheme be exclusively responsive to second-order stimuli. They would not respond to full-field sinewave gratings, of any spatial frequency or orientation, but would respond to contrast envelope stimuli, with the same selectivities already described for spatial frequency and orientation of both carrier and envelope, and in many cases also to direction of envelope motion. Neurons having all these properties have never been reported, though this might well be a consequence of not having used appropriate 'search stimuli', and use of protocols (such as ours) in which neurons are always first characterized with sinewave gratings.

The possible existence of neurons exclusively responsive to second-order stimuli in humans is supported by psychophysics showing separable adaptation and masking subthreshold facilitation of first- and second-order stimuli (Nishida et al., 1997; Schofield and Georgeson, 1999). A possible extrastriate locus is suggested by brain imaging experiments (Smith et al., 1998) and by descriptions of brain-damaged patients having selective deficits for either first- or second-order motion (Vaina et al., 1999). A higher order site would also be consistent with the slower temporal processing characteristic of second-order processing.

Utility of stimuli composed of sinusoidal components

While it might seem counterintuitive to use stimuli comprised of sinusoidal components to analyze nonlinear mechanisms of second-order processing, this strategy has actually proven invaluable. The use of a band-limited carrier, at a spatial frequency well above the neuron's measured spatial frequency response to simple gratings, provides a way to ensure definitively that a neuron's response is genuinely second-order, and not simply mediated by the same linear filtering assumed to mediate conventional grating responses. Using narrowband carriers also led to the finding of surprisingly narrow carrier spatial frequency tuning (Zhou and Baker, 1993; Zhou and Baker, 1996), and later to demonstration of independent orientation tuning for carrier and envelope (Mareschal and Baker, 1998a, 1999). Similarly, sinusoidal envelope waveforms allow measurement of narrow tunings to envelope spatial and temporal frequency. For both carrier and envelope, sinusoidal signals permit useful quantitative comparisons of bandwidths as well as optimal values to luminance responses in the same and in other neurons. Finally, the close relationship of sinusoidal signals to linear filtering theory facilitates interpretation of the data in terms of a nonlinear model composed of linear elements.

Is it really second order?

Perceived change-of-position

The ability to perceive a visual stimulus, or for a neuron to respond to it, might not necessarily require a separate specialized, low-level mechanism. For example, human perception of second-order motion might be mediated by a high-level appreciation of the change-of-position of salient stimulus attributes, sometimes called 'feature-tracking' (e.g. Lu and Sperling, 1995; Derrington and Ukkonen, 1999; Seiffert and Cavanagh, 1999). However, much evidence argues otherwise: motion after-effects to second-order motion (Ledgeway, 1994; Ledgeway and Smith, 1994a; Nishida et al., 1994; Nishida and Sato, 1995), a very different vulnerability to added noise (Bex and Baker, 1999), and direction-selective single neuron responses as discussed above.

Early nonlinearity

A more serious and frequently touted possibility is that a subtle nonlinearity prior to the linear filtering of first-order processing might accomplish the necessary demodulation (i.e. by giving a slightly different gain to light and dark regions of the carrier, preventing cancellation) (e.g. Burton, 1973; Taub et al., 1997). To plausibly accommodate the body of psychophysical and neurophysiological findings which led to the notion of linear summation, such an 'early nonlinearity' would have to be slight. Using a luminance-nulling technique to psychophysically measure the contribution of such early nonlinear demodulation in human vision, Scott-Samuel and Georgeson (1999) demonstrated that second-order motion could be mediated this way only at quite high stimulus contrasts, and at temporal frequencies above about 8 Hz. Their findings are consistent with those of Holliday and Anderson (1994) using a different method, who reported genuine second-order motion at low temporal frequencies but operation of a different mechanism at higher rates. (Note that our single neuron responses to contrast envelopes showed optimal temporal frequencies of 2–6 Hz.)

Such a simple early nonlinearity could not account for most neurophysiological reports of second-order responses. The necessity of only a slight nonlinearity implies that responses would be extremely weak to second-order stimuli, whereas at least some neurons can give responses roughly equal in magnitude to those from comparable first-order stimuli (e.g. Leventhal et al. (1998); see Fig. 7B,D). Such an early nonlinearity scheme would predict the same tuning to envelope spatial frequency as to luminance spatial frequency, and would fail to predict the selectivity to carrier spatial frequency and orientation which we observe.

First-order intrusion

Another potential pitfall is that responses to second-order stimuli might be mediated by their first-order attributes, i.e. responses mediated by the carrier rather than by the envelope. A very simple and instructive example is that of a conventional complex type cell (or, an 'energy model' (Adelson and Bergen, 1985) of first-order motion), which would give a strong response to an envelope stimulus whose *carrier* is its optimal grating: literally a response to a second-order stimulus, but critically lacking in selectivity for attributes of the *envelope* such as its direction of motion, spatial frequency or orientation. In general, one must ask whether a second-order stimulus is actually being detected by a first-order mechanism.

For A17/18 neurons, we could cleanly avoid this problem by constraining ourselves to carrier spatial frequencies well outside a given neuron's measured spatial frequency pass-band (Zhou and Baker, 1994; Mareschal and Baker, 1998b). Effective strategies for human psychophysics include use of stochastic carriers (Chubb and Sperling, 1988; Smith and Ledgeway, 1997), tasks requiring judgments of envelope-specific attributes, and inference from the pattern of the data that only envelope attributes could have mediated performance (Boulton and Baker, 1993b; Baker and Hess, 1998). This remains a particularly challenging problem for the design of brain imaging experiments on second-order processing.

The serious potential for confusion to be generated by use of the same terminology (first- and second-order), for both stimuli and mechanisms, is quite comparable to the analogous unfortunate situation for luminance vs. color. Just as we must beware that a chromatic stimulus might inadvertently activate a luminance mechanism (e.g. via optical chromatic aberrations), so also the response to a second-order stimulus can sometimes be due to 'cross-activation' of a first-order mechanism (e.g. Smith and Ledgeway, 1997).

When used with reference to stimuli, the terms first- and second-order best refer to stimulus attributes (e.g. orientation or direction of motion), rather than to stimuli themselves. Indeed, many stimuli may have both first- and second-order attributes, for example in the carrier and envelope of a contrast modulation.

Caveats about the definition of 'second-order'

Contemporary vision researchers would typically use the term 'second-order' to denote stimuli whose principal attributes, such as direction of motion, are not defined by first-order statistics of luminance or color (Cavanagh and Mather, 1989) — this image statistical definition has its origins in work on texture segregation (Julesz, 1981). In view of recent human psychophysics demonstrating that quasi-linear apparent motion appears to use only luminance and not chromatic mechanisms, whereas nonlinear (second-order) motion does use chromatic information (Baker et al., 1998; Yoshizawa et al., 2000), it seems unwise to exclude color as one of the defining properties of second-order stimuli.

A related approach might be to define second-order stimuli in terms of nonlinear processing, with first-order corresponding to linear filtering. However, it then becomes a 'trash-can category' which is overly inclusive. For example, cross-orientation inhibition (Morrone et al., 1982; Bonds, 1989) is certainly highly nonlinear (and, literally, a 'second-order' interaction), but it is thought to reflect the operation of a contrast gain control, of linear (first-order) filtering mechanisms. One way around this is to tie the definition to F→R→F processing (Wilson, 1999); however, while the F→R→F model has proven an extremely useful metaphor for understanding second-order processing, it seems undesirable to have a rigidly model-dependent definition.

Many of these semantic problems are complicated by the now prevailing usage of the terms 'first- and second-order' to refer both to visual *stimuli* and to *mechanisms* which are specific to their processing. This usage is in retrospect undesirable, but now seems too entrenched to attempt prescriptive reform. As noted already, this situation and its problems are reminiscent of those with using 'luminance' and 'chromatic' to refer both to stimuli and to mechanisms.

Our interim (working) definition of second-order stimuli would be those whose principal attributes are defined by variations in contrast or texture. This definition leaves ill-defined a number of stimuli whose status seems presently uncertain, for example spatial differentials of local motion (e.g. rotation, expansion–contraction), 'theta motion' (Zanker, 1993), cyclopean motion (Smith and Scott-Samuel, 1998), plaid coherence, contour integration (Field et al., 1993), non-Cartesian stimuli (Gallant et al., 1996; Wilson, 1999), and 'salience-defined' (also termed 'third-order') stimuli (Lu and Sperling, 1995). In future, when we have learned much more about the neuronal processing of these stimuli, it may be feasible to construct more mature definitions which are biologically rather than mathematically motivated.

Function of second-order processing

One could argue that second-order processing is of very limited functional significance, since 'pure' second-order stimuli are ecologically rare — most natural contours contain luminance as well as textural differences. In this view, second-order processing might be a marginally useful evolutionary accident which merely supplements abundant luminance-defined information, and might be critically useful for only a few special situations. Such a limited role seems unlikely, however, in view of the lack of difficulty in finding neurons which respond to such stimuli, and the impressive specificity of those neurons to characteristics of second-order stimuli (particularly, to carrier spatial frequency). But there are computationally motivated reasons why second-order information might be important.

While first-order luminance information is ecologically abundant, it is often highly unreliable in defining objects due to the vagaries of illumination — indeed the ambiguities introduced by shadows and by gradients of shading are an important part of what makes vision a difficult problem (Marr, 1982). False edges provided by shadows can be disambiguated by differences of texture, color, motion, or disparity — all second-order cues, or their close relatives [1]. Indeed, we might turn the above argument on its head, and propose that a good computational strategy for image understanding might be to ignore first-order information entirely, and only use second-order cues! Perhaps it should not be surprising that many neurons in extrastriate cortical areas respond relatively poorly to sinewave gratings (e.g. Gallant et al., 1996).

Natural images have first-order statistics like those of fractals, with an amplitude that falls with the reciprocal of spatial frequency (Field, 1987). But random fractal images which satisfy this relationship look very unnatural, because they lack the rich spatial 'structure' of natural images (Field, 1994), from edges, terminations, occlusions, etc. Natural images also differ from random fractals in being 'sparse' (i.e. high kurtosis in the luminance distribution), having a differentiation of local regions varying in contrast (Field, 1994). Thus it seems a possibility that second-order processing mechanisms might play an important role in representing the higher-order statistical structure in natural images. For example, a F→R→F model responds best to images that are sparse within a (carrier) spatial frequency/orientation passband.

Thus asking, "What is second-order analysis good for?", might be akin to earlier, similar questions about orientation-selective and spatial frequency-selective neurons or psychophysical channels: the answer might not simply be to encode one particular class of stimulus or solve one specific problem, but rather to provide a general-purpose, low-level representation, which serves as a 'basis set' for representing higher-order structural features occurring in natural images; for example F→R→F operators could play an important role in detection of the pattern motion of plaids (Wilson et al., 1992), and contribute to higher order form recognition (Wilkinson et al., 1998; Wilson, 1999).

Natural images contain visual information at a wide range of spatial scales, from small striations of the bark on a tree, to a forest of trees. While the visual system can represent this information with neurons spanning a large range of receptive field sizes or spatial frequencies, it must also be able to encode attributes of large-scale structures defined by finely scaled, textured surfaces, as well as sparse images containing objects which are largely devoid of texture. Second-order processing may provide a common basis for this kind of representation.

[1] While color has often been considered first-order, as noted previously, our findings suggest its processing is more closely related to second-order operations (Baker et al., 1998; Yoshizawa et al., 2000).

Acknowledgements

We wish to thank David Field, Fred Kingdom, Stacey Maher, and Nick Scott-Samuel for useful comments on the manuscript. This research was supported by Canadian CIHR (MA 9685) and NSERC (OPG0001978) grants to C.B., an FCAR fellowship to I.M., and supplementary funds from FRSQ.

References

Adelson, E.H. and Bergen, J.R. (1985) Spatiotemporal energy models for the perception of motion. *J. Opt. Soc. Am. A*, 2: 284–299.

Albrecht, D.G., Farrar, S.B. and Hamilton, D.B. (1984) Spatial contrast adaptation characteristics of neurones recorded in the cat's visual cortex. *J. Physiol.*, 347: 713–739.

Albright, T.D. (1992) Form–cue invariant motion processing in primate visual cortex. *Science*, 255: 1141–1143.

Andrews, B.W. and Pollen, D.A. (1979) Relationship between spatial frequency selectivity and receptive field profile of simple cells. *J. Physiol.*, 287: 163–176.

Baker Jr., C.L. (1990) Spatial and temporal frequency selectivity as a basis for velocity preference in cat striate cortex neurons. *Vis. Neurosci.*, 4: 101–113.

Baker Jr., C.L. (2001) Linear filtering and nonlinear interactions in direction-selective visual cortex neurons: a noise correlation analysis. *Visual Neurosci.*, in press.

Baker, C.L., Jr. and Boulton, J.C. (1990) Neurobiological mechanisms of cortical direction selectivity. In: T.B. Lawton (Ed.), *Computational Vision Based on Neurobiology*, Vol. 2054.

Baker Jr., C.L. and Hess, R.F. (1998) Two mechanisms underlie processing of stochastic motion stimuli. *Vision Res.*, 38: 1211–1222.

Baker Jr., C.L., Boulton, J.C. and Mullen, K.T. (1998) A nonlinear chromatic motion mechanism. *Vision Res.*, 38: 291–302.

Baker, C.L.J. and Cynader, M.S. (1994) A sustained input to the direction selective mechanism in cat striate cortex neurons. *Vis. Neurosci.*, 11: 1083–1092.

Bex, P. and Baker Jr., C.L. (1999) Motion perception over long interstimulus intervals. *Percept. Psychophys.*, 61: 1066–1074.

Bischof, W.F. and DiLollo, V. (1990) Perception of directional sampled motion in relation to displacement and spatial frequency: evidence for a unitary system. *Vision Res.*, 30.

Bischof, W.F. and DiLollo, V. (1996) Psychophysical evidence of a sustained input to directionally selective motion mechanisms. *Perception*, 25: 65–76.

Blakemore, C. and Campbell, F.W. (1969) On the existence of neurones in the human visual system selectively sensitive to the orientation and size of retinal images. *J. Physiol.*, 203: 237–261.

Bonds, A.B. (1989) Role of inhibition in the specification of orientation selectivity of cells in the cat striate cortex. *Vis. Neurosci.*, 2: 41–55.

Bonds, A.B. (1992) Spatial and temporal nonlinearities in receptive fields of the cat striate cortex. In: R.B. Pinter and B. Nabet (Eds.), *Nonlinear Vision*. CRC Press, Boca Raton, FL, pp. 329–352.

Borg-Graham, L.J., Monier, C. and Fregnac, Y. (1998) Visual input evokes transient and strong shunting inhibition in visual cortex neurons. *Nature*, 393: 369–373.

Boulton, J.C. and Baker Jr., C.L. (1993a) Dependence on stimulus onset asynchrony in apparent motion: evidence for two mechanisms. *Vision Res.*, 33: 2013–2019.

Boulton, J.C. and Baker, C.L.J. (1993b) Different parameters control motion perception above and below a critical density. *Vision Res.*, 33: 1803–1811.

Brainard, D.H. (1997) The psychophysics toolbox. *Spat. Vis.*, 10: 443–446.

Burton, G.J. (1973) Evidence for non-linear response processes in the human visual system from measurements on the thresholds of spatial beat frequencies. *Vision Res.*, 13: 1211–1225.

Campbell, F.W. and Robson, J.G. (1968) Application of Fourier analysis to the visibility of gratings. *J. Physiol.*, 197: 551–566.

Campbell, F.W., Cooper, G.F. and Enroth-Cugell, C. (1969) The spatial selectivity of the visual cells of the cat. *J. Physiol.*, 203: 223–235.

Carandini, M., Heeger, D.J. and Movshon, J.A. (1999) Linearity and gain control in V1 simple cells. In: E.G. Jones and P.S. Ulinski (Eds.), *Cerebral Cortex*, Vol. 13, *Cortical Models*. Kluwer Academic/Plenum, New York, pp. 401–443.

Cavanagh, P. and Mather, G. (1989) Motion: The long and short of it. *Spat. Vis.*, 4: 103–129.

Chaudhuri, A. and Albright, T.D. (1997) Neuronal responses to edges defined by luminance vs. temporal texture in macaque area V1. *Vis. Neurosci.*, 14: 949–962.

Chubb, C. and Sperling, G. (1988) Drift-balanced random stimuli: a general basis for studying non-Fourier motion perception. *J. Opt. Soc. Am.*, 5: 1986–2007.

Cleary, R. and Braddick, O.J. (1990) Direction discrimination for bandpass filtered random dot kinematograms. *Vision Res.*, 30: 303–316.

Cleland, B.G., Harding, T.H. and Tulanay-Keesey, U. (1979) Visual resolution and receptive field size: Examination of two kinds of cat retinal ganglion cell. *Science*, 205: 1015–1017.

Dakin, S.C. and Mareschal, I. (2000) Sensitivity to contrast modulation depends on carrier spatial frequency and orientation. *Vision Res.*, 40: 311–329.

DeAngelis, G.C., Ohzawa, I. and Freeman, R.D. (1993) Spatiotemporal organization of simple-cell receptive fields in the cat's striate cortex. II. Linearity of temporal and spatial summation. *J. Neurophysiol.*, 69: 1118–1135.

Derrington, A.M. and Badcock, D.R. (1985) Separate detectors for simple and complex grating patterns? *Vision Res.*, 25.

Derrington, A.M. and Ukkonen, O.I. (1999) Second-order motion discrimination by feature-tracking. *Vision Res.*, 39: 1465–1475.

Derrington, A.M., Badcock, D.R. and Henning, G.B. (1993) Discriminating the direction of second-order motion at short stimulus durations. *Vision Res.*, 33: 1785–1794.

Ferster, D. (1988) Spatially opponent excitation and inhibition in simple cells of the cat visual cortex. *J. Neuroscience*, 8: 1172–1180.

Field, D.J. (1987) Relations between the statistics of natural images and the response properties of cortical cells. *J. Opt. Soc. Am.*, 4: 2379–2394.

Field, D.J. (1994) What is the goal of sensory coding? *Neural Comput.*, 6: 559–601.

Field, D.J., Hayes, A. and Hess, R.F. (1993) Contour integration by the human visual system: evidence for a local association field. *Vision Res.*, 33: 173–193.

Gallant, J.L., Braun, J. and Van Essen, D.C. (1993) Selectivity for polar, hyperbolic, and Cartesian gratings in macaque visual cortex. *Science*, 259: 100–103.

Gallant, J.L., Connor, C.E., Rakshit, S., Lewis, J.W. and Van Essen, D.C. (1996) Neural responses to polar, hyperbolic, and Cartesian gratings in area V4 of the macaque monkey. *J. Neurophysiol.*, 76: 2718–2739.

Geesaman, B.J. and Andersen, R.A. (1996) The analysis of complex motion patterns by form/cue invariant MSTd neurons. *J. Neurosci.*, 16: 4716–4732.

Georgeson, M.A. and Scott-Samuel, N.E. (1999) Motion contrast: a new metric for direction discrimination. *Vision Res.*, 39: 4393–4402.

Graham, N. (1980) Spatial-frequency channels in the human visual system: detecting edges without edge-detectors. In: C.S. Harris (Ed.), *Visual Coding and Adaptability*. Erlbaum, Hillsdale, NJ, pp. 215–262.

Graham, N. and Sutter, A. (1998) Spatial summation in simple (Fourier) and complex (non-Fourier) texture channels. *Vision Res.*, 38: 231–257.

Green, M. (1986) What determines correspondence strength in apparent motion? *Vision Res.*, 26: 599–607.

Grosof, D.H., Shapley, R.M. and Hawken, M.J. (1993) Macaque V1 neurons can signal 'illusory' contours. *Nature*, 365: 550–552.

Heeger, D.J. (1992) Normalization of cell responses in cat striate cortex. *Vis. Neurosci.*, 9.

Henning, G.B., Hertz, B.G. and Broadbent, D.E. (1975) Some experiments bearing on the hypothesis that the visual system analyses spatial patterns in independent bands of spatial frequency. *Vision Res.*, 1975: 887–897.

Hess, R.F. and Wilcox, L.M. (1994) Linear and nonlinear filtering in stereopsis. *Vision Res.*, 18.

Hirsch, J.A., Alonso, J.M., Reid, R.C. and Martinez, L.M. (1998) Synaptic integration in striate cortical simple cells. *J. Neurosci.*, 18: 9517–9528.

Holliday, I.E. and Anderson, S.J. (1994) Different processes underlie the detection of second-order motion at low and high temporal frequencies. *Proc. R. Soc. Lond. B*, 257: 165-173.

Hubel, D.H. and Wiesel, T.N. (1962) Receptive fields, binocular interaction and functional architecture in the cat's visual cortex. *J. Physiol.*, 1962: 106–154.

Jagadeesh, B., Wheat, H.S., Kontsevich, L.L., Tyler, C.W. and Ferster, D. (1977) Direction selectivity of synaptic potentials in simple cells of the cat visual cortex. *J. Neurophysiol.*, 78: 2772–2789.

Julesz, B. (1981) Textons, the elements of texture perception, and their interactions. *Nature*, 290: 91–97.

Landy, M.S. (1991) Texture segregation and orientation gradient. *Vision Res.*, 31: 679–691.

Ledgeway, T. (1994) Adaptation to second-order motion results in a motion aftereffect for directionally-ambiguous test stimuli. *Vision Res.*, 34: 2879–2889.

Ledgeway, T. and Smith, A.T. (1994a) The duration of the motion aftereffect following adaptation to first-order and second-order motion. *Perception*, 23: 1211–1219.

Ledgeway, T. and Smith, A.T. (1994b) Evidence for separate motion-detecting mechanisms for first- and second-order motion in human vision. *Vision Res.*, 34: 2727–2740.

Leventhal, A.G., Wang, Y., Schmolesky, M.T. and Zhou, Y. (1998) Neural correlates of boundary perception. *Vis. Neurosci.*, 15: 1107–1118.

Levinson, E. and Sekuler, R. (1975) The independence of channels in human vision selective for direction of movement. *J. Physiol.*, 250: 347–366.

Loffler, G. and Orbach, H.S. (1999) Computing feature motion without feature detectors: a model for terminator motion without end-stopped cells. *Vision Res.*, 39: 859–871.

Lu, Z.L. and Sperling, G. (1995) The functional architecture of human visual motion perception. *Vision Res.*, 35: 2697–2722.

Mareschal, I. and Baker Jr., C.L. (1998a) A cortical locus for the processing of contrast-defined contours [see comments]. *Nat. Neurosci.*, 1: 150–154.

Mareschal, I. and Baker Jr., C.L. (1998b) Temporal and spatial response to second-order stimuli in cat area 18. *J. Neurophysiol.*, 80: 2811–2823.

Mareschal, I. and Baker Jr., C.L. (1999) Cortical processing of second-order motion. *Vis. Neurosci.*, 16: 1–14.

Marr, D. (1982) *Vision*. Freeman, San Francisco.

McLean, J., Raab, S. and Palmer, L.A. (1994) Contribution of linear mechanisms to the specification of local motion by simple cells in areas 17 and 18 of the cat. *Vis. Neurosci.*, 11: 271–294.

Morrone, M.C., Burr, D.C. and Maffei, L. (1982) Functional implications of cross-orientation inhibition of cortical visual cells. I. Neurophysiological evidence. *Proc. R. Soc. Lond. B*, 216: 335–354.

Movshon, J.A., Thompson, I.D. and Tolhurst, D.J. (1978) Spatial summation in the receptive fields of simple cells in the cat's striate cortex. *J. Physiol.*, 283: 53–77.

Nishida, S., Ashida, H. and Sato, T. (1994) Complete interocular transfer of motion aftereffect with flickering test. *Vision Res.*, 34: 2707–2716.

Nishida, S., Ledgeway, T. and Edwards, M. (1997) Dual multiple-scale processing for motion in the human visual system. *Vision Res.*, 37: 2685–2698.

Nishida, S. and Sato, T. (1995) Motion aftereffect with flickering test patterns reveals higher stages of motion processing. *Vision Res.*, 35: 477–490.

Nothdurft, H.-C., Gallant, J.L. and Van Essen, D.C. (1999) Response modulation by texture surround in primate area V1: Correlates of 'popout' under anesthesia. *Vis. Neurosci.*, 16: 15–34.

Olavarria, J.F., DeYoe, E.A., Knierim, J.J., Fox, J.M. and van Essen, D.C. (1992) Neural responses to visual texture patterns in middle temporal area of the macaque monkey. *J. Neurophysiol.*, 68: 164–181.

Peterhans, E. and von der Heydt, R. (1991) Subjective contours-bridging the gap between psychophysics and physiology. *Trends Neurosci.*, 14: 112–119.

Reid, R.C. and Alonso, J.M. (1995) Specificity of monosynaptic connections from thalamus to visual cortex. *Nature*, 378: 281–284.

Ringach, D.L., Hawkin, M.J. and Shapley, R. (1997) Dynamics of orientation tuning in primary visual cortex. *Nature*, 387: 281–284.

Rivadulla, C., Sharma, J. and Sur, M. (1999) Role of NMDA and AMPA glutamate receptors in orientation and direction selectivity of V1 neurons. *Soc. Neurosci. Abstr.*, 25: 270.11.

Saul, A.B. and Humphrey, A.L. (1990) Spatial and temporal response properties of lagged and nonlagged cells in cat lateral geniculate nucleus. *J. Neurophysiol.*, 64: 206–224.

Saul, A.B. and Humphrey, A.L. (1992) Evidence of input from lagged cells in the lateral geniculate nucleus to simple cells in cortical area 17 of the cat. *J. Neurophysiol.*, 68: 1190–1208.

Schofield, A.J. and Georgeson, M.A. (1999) Sensitivity to modulations of luminance and contrast in visual white noise: separate mechanisms with similar behaviour. *Vision Res.*, 39: 2697–2716.

Schofield, A.J. and Georgeson, M.A. (2000) The temporal properties of first- and second-order vision. *Vision Res.*, 40: 2475–2487.

Scott-Samuel, N.E. and Georgeson, M.A. (1999) Does early non-linearity account for second-order motion? *Vision Res.*, 39: 2853–2865.

Seiffert, A.E. and Cavanagh, P. (1999) Position-based motion perception for color and texture stimuli: effects of contrast and speed. *Vision Res.*, 39: 4172–4185.

Skottun, B.C., Bradley, A., Sclar, G., Ohzawa, I. and Freeman, R.D. (1987) The effects of contrast on visual orientation and spatial frequency discrimination: a comparison of single cells and behavior. *J. Neurophysiol.*, 57: 773–786.

Smith, A.T. (1994) The detection of second-order motion. In: A.T. Smith and R.J. Snowden (Eds.), *Visual Detection of Motion*. Academic Press, London, pp. 145–176.

Smith, A.T., Greenlee, M.W., Singh, K.D., Kraemer, F.M. and Hennig, J. (1998) The processing of first- and second-order motion in human visual cortex assessed by functional magnetic resonance imaging (fMRI). *J. Neurosci.*, 18: 3816–3830.

Smith, A.T. and Ledgeway, T. (1997) Separate detection of moving luminance and contrast modulations: fact or artifact? *Vision Res.*, 37: 45–62.

Smith, A.T. and Ledgeway, T. (1998) Sensitivity to second-order motion as a function of temporal frequency and eccentricity. *Vision Res.*, 38: 403–410.

Smith, A.T. and Scott-Samuel, N.E. (1998) Stereoscopic and contrast-defined motion in human vision. *Proc. R. Soc. Lond. B*, 265: 1573-1581.

Sutter, A., Beck, J. and Graham, N. (1989) Contrast and spatial variables in texture segregation: testing a simple spatial-frequency channels model. *Percept. Psychophys.*, 46: 312–332.

Taub, E., Victor, J.D. and Conte, M.M. (1997) Nonlinear preprocessing in short-range motion. *Vision Res.*, 37: 1459–1477.

Ulrich, D.J., Essock, E.A. and Lemkuhle, S. (1981) Cross-species correspondence of spatial contrast sensitivity functions. *Behav. Brain Res.*, 2: 291–299.

Vaina, L.M., Cowey, A. and Kennedy, D. (1999) Perception of first- and second-order motion: separable neurological mechanisms? *Hum. Brain Mapp.*, 7: 67–77.

Wilkinson, F., Wilson, H.R. and Habak, C. (1998) Detection and recognition of radial frequency patterns. *Vision Res.*, 38: 3555–3568.

Wilson, H. (1999) Non-Fourier cortical processes in texture, form, and motion perception. In: P.S. Ulinski and E.G. Jones (Eds.), *Cerebral Cortex*, Vol. 13., *Cortical Models*. Kluwer Academic/Plenum, New York, pp. 445–477.

Wilson, H.R., Ferrera, V.P. and Yo, C. (1992) A psychophysically motivated model for two-dimensional motion perception. *Vis. Neurosci.*, 9: 79–97.

Yoshizawa, T., Mullen, K.T. and Baker, C.L.J. (2000) Quasi-linear and nonlinear motion mechanisms for chromatic and luminance stimuli in foveal vision. *Vision Res.*, 40: 1993–2010.

Zanker, M.J. (1993) Theta motion: a paradoxical stimulus to explore higher-order motion extraction. *Vision Res.*, 33: 553–569.

Zhou, Y.X. and Baker Jr., C.L. (1993) A processing stream in mammalian visual cortex neurons for non-Fourier responses. *Science*, 261: 98–101.

Zhou, Y.X. and Baker Jr., C.L. (1994) Envelope-responsive neurons in areas 17 and 18 of cat. *J. Neurophysiol.*, 72: 2134–2150.

Zhou, Y.X. and Baker Jr., C.L. (1996) Spatial properties of envelope-responsive cells in area 17 and 18 neurons of the cat. *J. Neurophysiol.*, 75: 1038–1050.

C. Casanova and M. Ptito (Eds.)
Progress in Brain Research, Vol. 134

CHAPTER 13

The role of feedback connections in shaping the responses of visual cortical neurons

Jean Bullier *,[1], Jean-Michel Hupé [2], Andrew C. James [1] and Pascal Girard [1]

Cerveau et Vision INSERM 371, 18 avenue du Doyen Lépine, 69675 Bron Cedex, France

Abstract: The results of a previous study [Hupé et al. (1998) *Nature*, 394: 784–787] led us to conclude that feedback connections are important for differentiating a figure from the background, particularly in the case of low salience stimuli. This conclusion was principally based on the observation in area V3 neurons that inactivating MT by cooling led to a severe weakening of the center response and of the center–surround interactions, and that these effects were particularly strong for low salience stimuli. In the present paper, we first show that the results extend to areas V1 and V2. In particular, the inhibitory center–surround interactions in areas V1, V2 and V3 disappear almost completely in the absence of feedback input from MT for low salience stimuli, whereas the effects are much more limited for stimuli of middle and high salience. We then compare the results obtained in studies of feedback connections from MT to those obtained in a study of the feedback action of area V2 onto V1 neurons [Hupé et al. (2001) *J. Neurophysiol.*, 85: 146–163], in which the same effects were observed on the center mechanism (decrease in response), but no effects were seen on the center–surround interactions. We conclude that feedback connections act in a non-linear fashion to boost the gain of the center mechanism and that they combine with horizontal connections to generate the center–surround interactions.

Introduction

Despite the large number of feedback connections between visual cortical areas of the mammalian brain, very few studies have been devoted to elucidating the role of these connections in cortical processing. These studies generally demonstrated that lesion or inactivation of a higher order area leads to a decrease of the neuron response in the lower order area to a stimulus activating the RF center (Mignard and Malpeli, 1991; Sandell and Schiller, 1982; Vanduffel et al., 1997; Wang et al., 2000). Thus, feedback connections appear to potentiate the RF center response of neurons in lower order areas.

In a series of publications in the 1990s, we studied the visuotopic organizations of feedforward and feedback connections and concluded that feedback connections are not visuotopically organized in the same manner as feedforward connections (Salin et al., 1992; Salin and Bullier, 1995). Recipient neurons of feedforward connections have RF centers that include those of their inputs. This corresponds to the strategy employed at numerous levels of the visual system that consists in increasing the specificity of the receptive field properties of neurons in higher-order areas by convergence of appropriate feedforward inputs. Feedback connections, on the other hand, link neurons in such a way that the RF centers of neurons providing the feedback connections cover a much wider part of the visual field than

* Corresponding author: J. Bullier, Centre de Recherche Cerveau et Cognition, CNRS-UPS UMR 5549, Université Paul Sabatier, 133, route de Narbonne, 31062 Toulouse Cedex, France. Tel.: +33-5-6217-2800; Fax: +33-5-6217-2809; E-mail: bullier@cerco.ups-tlse.fr
[1] Present address: Centre de Recherche Cerveau et Cognition, CNRS-UPS UMR 5549, Université Paul Sabatier, 133, route de Narbonne, 31062 Toulouse Cedex, France.
[2] Present address: Center for Neural Science, New York University, 4 Washington Place, New York NY 10003, USA.

that represented in the RF center of the recipient neuron. For this reason, we concluded that the feedback connections are organized in a non-retinotopic or a loose retinotopic fashion.

The loose retinotopic character of the feedback connections suggested that these connections may be involved in controlling the modulatory influences of the RF surround on the response elicited by stimulating the RF center. This was tested in a first series of studies in the monkey in which we inactivated the superior temporal sulcus at the location of visual cortical area MT, and observed the responses of neurons in areas V1, V2 and V3. The stimuli were similar to those illustrated in the bottom part of Fig. 1. A central bar of variable luminance moved back and forth across the cell RF center. This bar was superimposed on a background composed of gray rectangles of same width and orientation. The contrast of the background checks was too low to activate the RF center of the neuron when it was moving (see responses corresponding to bkg alone in Fig. 1). The contrast was nonetheless sufficient to activate the surround mechanism, as seen in Fig. 1 by comparing the responses to the bar moving on a stationary background (BS histograms) with the responses to the bar moving together with the background (BM histograms). The response decrease for stimulus BM compared to BS is due to the suppressive effect of the moving background on the response of the neuron to the bar alone. This suppressive effect is principally due to activation of the inhibitory surround of the receptive field.

Area MT neurons show vigorous responses at low contrast (Sclar et al., 1990) and we were therefore particularly interested in studying the responses of neurons in lower order areas to activation by a moving bar of low contrast. Because the structured background stimulus acted as a mask, such a low contrast bar was hardly seen when stationary and became visible when it started to move. To quantify the visibility of the bar, we defined the salience of the stimulus by the ratio of the contrast of the central bar divided by that of the background. We subdivided the scale of salience in three categories: low salience (from 1 to 7), middle salience (from 7 to 15) and high salience (above 15; see Hupé et al., 1998) for further details).

From the results of these studies, we concluded that the role of feedback connections is to help differentiate the figure from the background, particularly in the case of stimuli of low salience. This conclusion was principally based on the observation in area V3 that inactivating MT by cooling led to a severe weakening of the center response and of the center–surround interactions, and that these effects were particularly strong for low salience stimuli (Hupé et al., 1998). In the present paper, we report the results concerning areas V1, V2 and V3, as we wished to determine to what extent the findings observed in V3 were also observed in the other two areas. The first two sections of this paper are devoted to this question of the generality of our original findings in area V3. We then draw some general conclusions concerning the role of the feedback connections from MT in differentiating figures from the background in lower order areas.

In the final two sections, we compare the results obtained in studies of feedback connections from MT to those obtained in a study of the feedback action of area V2 onto V1 neurons, and we discuss the possible role of feedback connections in controlling the gain of center–surround interactions in lower order areas.

All experiments were conducted on anesthetized and paralyzed macaque monkeys. Details of experimental methods can be found in the figure legends of the present paper or in the methods sections of our earlier publications (Hupé et al., 1998, 2001a,b).

Effect of stimulus salience on feedback action

Fig. 1 illustrates the effects of inactivating MT on the responses of selected neurons in areas V1, V2 and V3 to the central bar moving across the RF center with the background stationary (BS), and to the bar moving together with the background (BM). Mean responses per stimulus presentation of these different stimuli are shown for both the control runs and the runs when MT was inactivated by cooling. Two groups of examples are presented: on the left, responses to high salience stimuli (Fig. 1A–C); and on the right, responses to low salience stimuli (Fig. 1D–F).

Fig. 1A illustrates a case with no statistically significant change during MT inactivation. Fig. 1B and C present cases for which decreases in response are observed during MT cooling for the central moving

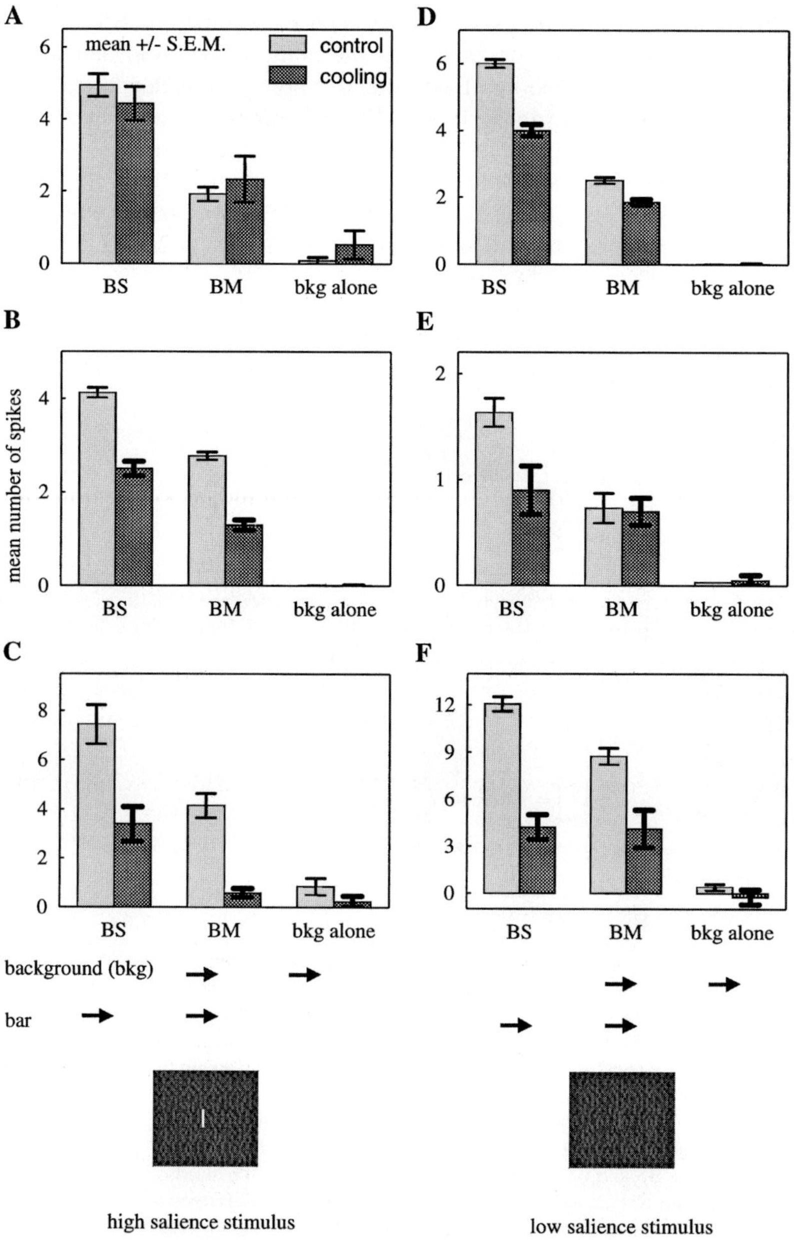

Fig. 1. Examples of neurons for which the response to the moving bar is decreased by a moving background. (A–C) Neurons tested with a high salience stimulus. There is no significant change of the background suppression index (BM − BS)/BS) when MT is inactivated. (D–F) Neurons tested with a low salience stimulus. There is a decrease of the background suppression index or even a disappearance of background suppression during the cooling of MT. (A) Layer 2 V1 neuron, single unit, case lba14. (B) Layer 2/3 V1 neuron, single unit, case lca24. (C) Layer 2/3 V2 neuron, single unit, case kal21. (D) Layer 2/3 V1 neuron, single unit, case lcb14. (E) Layer 2/3 V1 neuron, single unit (but not isolated), case lcb15. (F) Layer 2/3 V2 neuron, single unit, case kbt24.

bar (BS) and for the bar moving together with the background (BM). During inactivation, the amount of suppression of the response to the central bar induced by the moving background is maintained or only slightly changed relative to the control situation.

In contrast, for low salience stimuli (Fig. 1D–F), the response suppression induced by the moving background is strongly diminished by MT inactivation. This can be seen by comparing BS and BM responses during the control condition and during cooling. Background suppression is decreased in the example in Fig. 1D and completely abolished in the examples shown in Fig. 1E and F (responses to BS and BM stimuli become equal during MT cooling).

The population data are illustrated in Fig. 2 for neurons recorded in areas V1, V2 and V3 with

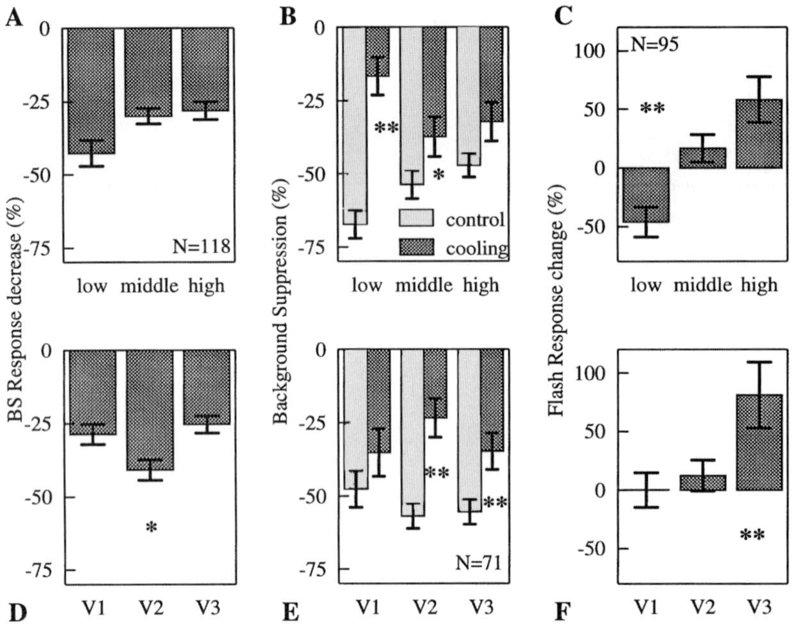

Fig. 2. (A,D) Mean (± SEM) decrease (neurons showing increases are excluded) of the response to the stimulus BS during the inactivation of MT for neurons tested at low, middle and high salience stimulus (A) in areas V1, V2, V3 (D). We carried out a two-way ANOVA with the independent variables 'area' and 'salience' (the variances are homogenous, and the distribution of the residuals is not different from a Normal distribution). There is a significant effect of the salience of the stimulus ($P = 0.046$, A) and of the area of recording ($P = 0.002$, D). The interaction between these two factors is not significant ($P = 0.21$). The asterisks on this graph and all the others (unless specified) correspond to the results of 2 × 2 post-hoc comparisons (Tukey test): $^{*}P < 0.05$; $^{**}P < 0.01$; and $^{***}P < 0.001$. (B,E) Mean (± SEM) change of the background suppression index during the inactivation of MT for neurons tested at low, middle and high salience stimulus (B) in areas V1, V2, V3 (E). The background suppression index (also called bsup in Table 1) is defined as 100 × (BM − BS)/BS_c where BS and BM are the responses to the BS and BM stimuli during control or during MT inactivation and BS_c is the response to BS during control. Normalization was done with respect to BS_c to limit the influence of large changes in the BS responses during inactivation which produced many outliers. All these 71 neurons were significantly suppressed by the moving background before the cooling of MT. A three-way ANOVA was done (Table 1). There is a significant dependence on the salience of the stimulus for the effect of cooling on the background suppression (salience × treatment: $P < 10^{-3}$, B): the effect is stronger at low salience. The effect on the background suppression does not significantly depend on the area of recording (area × treatment: $P = 0.064$, E): the background suppression decreased during cooling in areas V1, V2 and V3. (C,F) Mean (± SEM) change of the ON response to the flash stimulus during the inactivation of MT for all the neurons ($n = 95$) tested at low, middle and high salience stimulus (C) in areas V1, V2, V3 (F). A two-way ANOVA could not be performed as the distributions were far away from the Normal distribution. Two one-way non-parametric ANOVA were done instead. There is a significant effect of the salience of the stimulus (Kruskal–Wallis test, $P = 0.003$, C): the mean response decreased for neurons tested at low salience, whereas it increased for the neurons tested at high salience. The area where the neurons were recorded has also a significant effect (Kruskal–Wallis test, $P = 0.006$, F): there is a strong increase of the responses in V3. Here (C and F), the two asterisks mean that the group was significantly different ($P < 0.01$, Mann–Whitney) from the two other groups.

stimuli at different levels of salience. Fig. 2A illustrates how the mean decrease in BS response during MT inactivation varies as a function of stimulus salience ($P = 0.046$, see legend of Fig. 2) for the neurons in V1/V2/V3 showing BS response decreases (118/154 neurons). The response decrease is more pronounced for low salience stimuli (Tukey, $P = 0.08$). This suggests that the potentiating effect of the feedback connections on the center response is stronger for poorly visible stimuli than for highly salient stimuli.

A similar but stronger effect of stimulus salience on the suppression of the center response by the moving background ($P < 10^{-3}$; see Table 1) is illustrated in Fig. 2B for all the neurons showing statistically significant background-induced suppression (71 neurons/135 neurons tested for background suppression). For low salience stimuli, the background suppression changes from about 70% to 15%. In other words, under MT inactivation, the background suppression is almost totally abolished for low salience stimuli. For middle and high salience stimuli, the background suppression also decreases but to a much smaller extent (significant at the 0.05 level for middle salience; $P = 0.058$ for high salience)

Fig. 2C illustrates the observation that stimulus salience is also an important factor governing the cooling-induced changes in response to a small bar flashed in the RF center (Hupé et al., 2001b). During MT inactivation at low stimulus salience, the response decreases by almost 50%, whereas it increases by the same amount for high salience stimuli.

The scattergram presented in Fig. 3 shows how the background suppression (bsup) varies between the control and the cooling condition for different levels of salience of the stimulus (same data as shown in Fig. 2B). For middle and high salience, there are a few neurons for which the background suppression increases (below the 45° line) and some for which there is little change or some decrease during MT inactivation. For low salience on the other hand, all the neurons show a decrease of the background suppression (above the 45° line). For a few cases, background suppression is converted to facilitation during MT inactivation (points above the horizontal line at zero bsup).

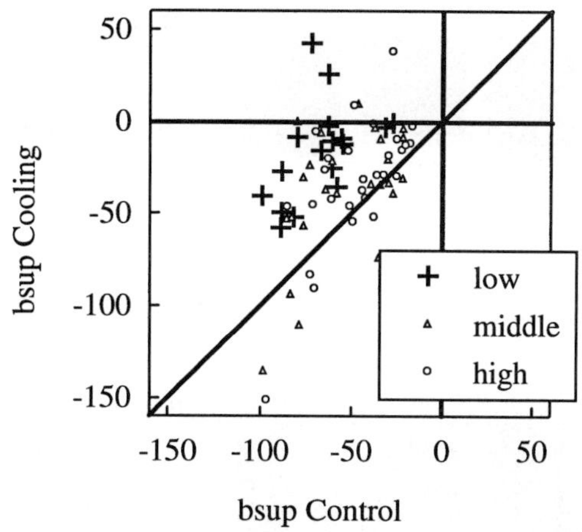

Fig. 3. Scattergram of the values of background suppression (bsup) during control and cooling runs for different categories of stimulus salience: +, low salience; triangle, middle salience; circles, high salience. Note that bsup increases for all neurons tested at low salience, whereas variable effects are observed for the middle and high salience cases.

Effect of MT inactivation in different cortical areas at different saliences

Recordings were done in areas V1, V2 and V3 and we were interested in determining whether similar results are found in these different areas. The bottom histograms in Fig. 2 show the influence of the area in which the neurons were recorded. Response decreases to the central bar (BS) are stronger in V2 than in V1 or V3 (Fig. 2D). Although the background suppression varied in the same direction (decrease) for neurons in all three areas (no significant interaction, $P = 0.064$, see Table 1), there was also a tendency for the decrease to be more marked in area V2 (Fig. 2E). Finally, for flashed stimuli, increases are principally observed in V3 whereas variable effects (increases and decreases) are recorded in areas V1 and V2 (Fig. 2F).

Next, we wished to determine whether similar effects of salience were observed in all three visual areas. Interactions between salience and area are presented in Fig. 4. The interaction for the response decreases to the central bar (BS) is not significant (two-way ANOVA, $P = 0.21$); however, we can see that in areas V2 and V3, the decrease is more pronounced for low salience than for medium or high salience stimuli (Fig. 4B,C),

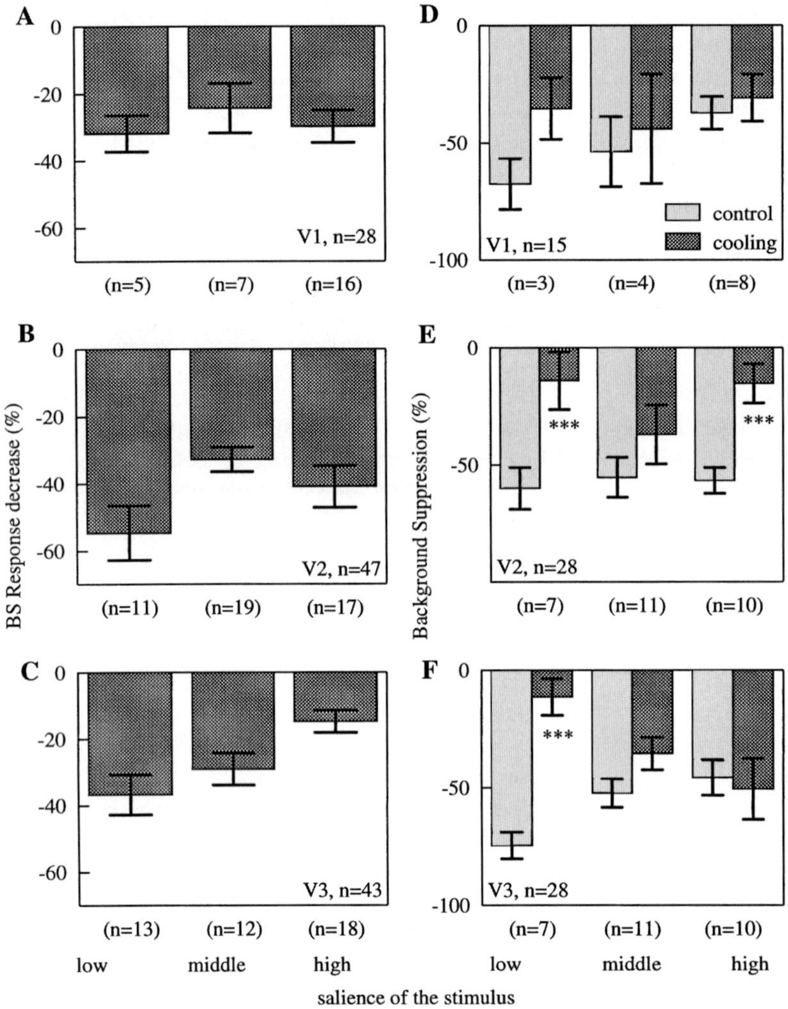

Fig. 4. (A–C) Interactions between area and stimulus salience for the BS response in the 118 neurons with decreased responses during MT inactivation. The post-hoc 2 × 2 comparisons (Tukey test) are not significant. (D–F) Interactions between area and stimulus salience for the background suppression in the 71 neurons for which the moving background decreased significantly the response to the center stimulus. In all three areas, the background suppression is decreased strongly at low salience, and this decrease is significant in V2 and V3 (Tukey post-hoc 2 × 2 comparison, $P < 10^{-3}$). In addition, in V2 some decreases of background suppression at high salience were also observed (E, right columns). These effects are responsible for the significant three-way interaction (see Table 1).

whereas the salience effect is not apparent in V1 (Fig. 4A).

Table 1 summarizes the results obtained by a three-way ANOVA on the bsup values (background suppression values in per cent; see legend of Fig. 2 for definition) with the independent variables ‘area’ and ‘salience’ and the repeated measured variable ‘treatment’ (cooling or control). The ANOVA was made on the bsup values of the 71 neurons showing statistically significant background suppression. The results indicate that treatment (cooling/control) had a highly significant effect. Interaction between area and treatment is not significant (Fig. 2E). Interaction between salience and treatment is highly significant (Fig. 2B), which supports our claim that the effect on background suppression is much stronger at low salience. The three-way interaction between salience, area and treatment is also highly significant.

The dependence of the background suppression on stimulus salience is particularly strong in area

TABLE 1

Summary of the results of the three-way ANOVA done on background suppression values for the 71 neurons showing significant background suppression with the three factors: area, salience and treatment

Area (1)	$F(2, 62) = 0.35$	0.707
Salience (2)	$F(2, 62) = 0.47$	0.626
Treatment (3)	$F(1, 62) = 64.18$	0.000
1 × 2	$F(4, 62) = 0.51$	0.726
1 × 3	$F(2, 62) = 2.88$	0.064
2 × 3	$F(2, 62) = 9.99$	0.000
1 × 2 × 3	$F(2, 62) = 4.12$	0.005

V3 (Fig. 4F), as reported earlier. The background suppression at low salience changes from 75% to less than 10% when MT is inactivated, whereas no significant change is observed for medium and high salience stimuli. In V3, the decrease in background suppression at low salience is due to a decrease in BS response and to an increase in BM response (Hupé et al., 1998). This was not the case in V2 and V1 in which the BS response decreases, but the BM remains unchanged (Hupé, 1999). In V2 also, the decrease in background suppression is marked at low salience, not significant at medium salience, but is strong and highly significant for high salience stimuli (Fig. 4E). This effect is mainly responsible for the three-way significant interaction. It should be noted that among the 10 neurons tested at high salience in V2, three had an almost complete response suppression to the BS stimulus and two had color-selective responses. In V1, the trend is also observed of stronger effects on background suppression for low salience stimuli (Fig. 4D), despite the lack of statistical significance due to the small sample at low salience.

Thus, the effects of salience on the response changes to BS and BM stimuli during MT cooling tend to be observed in all three areas but are particularly strong in areas V2 and V3: during MT inactivation, the BS response and the background suppression both show a stronger decrease at low salience.

What does this effect on center and surround mechanisms mean for the role of feedback connections in information processing in the visual system? Fig. 5 summarizes in a schematic fashion the effects of inactivating area MT on the cortical responses of neurons in a lower order area such as V1, V2 or V3. The cortex is seen from above and the white or gray rectangles represent the neuronal activity evoked by a low salience bar moving across the stationary background (BS stimulus, left) or together with the background (BM stimulus, right). The white area in the cortex for the BS stimulus (Fig. 5A) represents the robust responses of neurons with RF centers crossed by the moving bar. In normal conditions, because of the strong inhibitory influences of surround stimulation for most neurons (Hupé et al., 2001a; Knierim and Van Essen, 1992; Li and Li, 1994; Nothdurft et al., 1999), the cortical activation by the BM stimulus is much weaker, as illustrated by the dark gray color of the activated cortical region (Fig. 5B).

When area MT is inactivated, the response to the central bar is decreased by 40% on average, which corresponds to the light gray color of the activated cortical region (Fig. 5C). Because of the almost complete disappearance of the background-induced suppression when MT is blocked, the response to the BM stimulus differs only slightly from that of the BS stimulus, as illustrated by the gray color of the activated cortical region (Fig. 5D).

The consequence of inactivating the feedback is therefore that the cortical response to the BS stimulus is strongly reduced and that it is no longer substantially different from that to the BM stimulus. In other words, in the absence of feedback connections, the cortical area loses the ability to differentiate the BS and BM stimuli, particularly at low salience. This led us to conclude that feedback connections act to differentiate figure from background in low visibility conditions (Hupé et al., 1998).

Effects of V2 inactivation on responses in area V1

In another series of experiments published elsewhere (Hupé et al., 2001a), we studied the effects of inactivating with GABA a small region (around 2–3 mm in diameter) of V2 on the responses of neurons in the retinotopically corresponding region in V1. The stimuli used were similar to those used by Knierim and Van Essen (1992): the RF center was activated by a small flashed bar of optimal orientation and the surround was stimulated by an array of flashed bars with different positions and orientations (optimal or orthogonal to the optimal orientation).

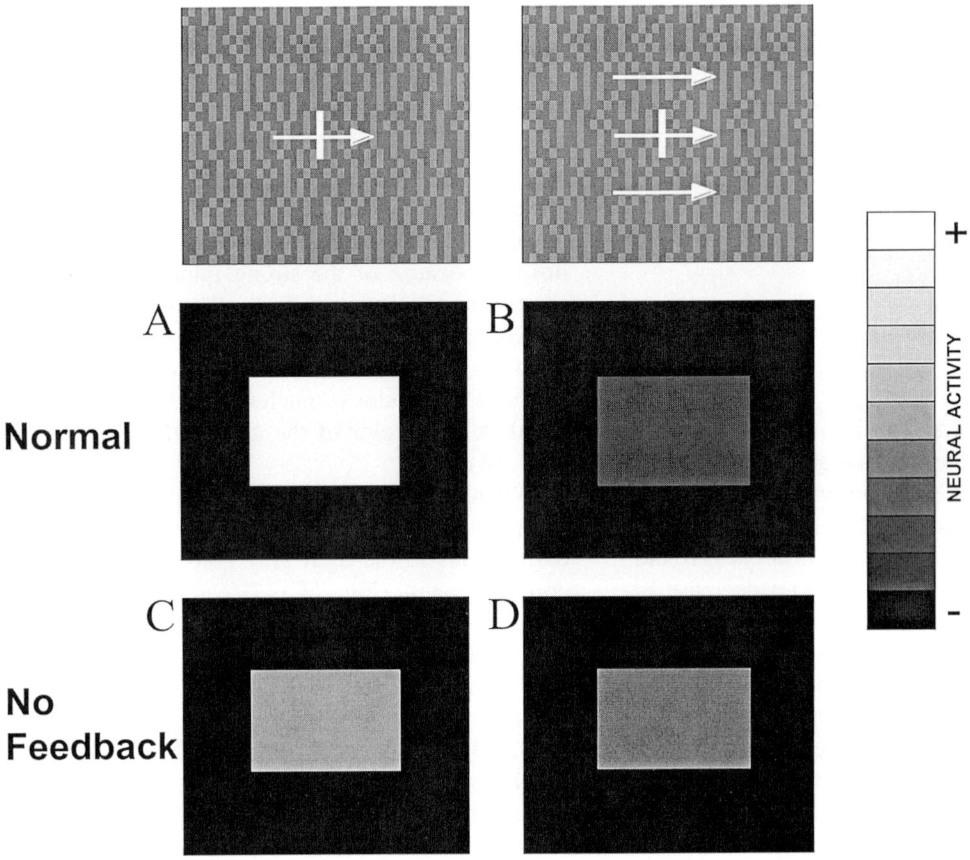

Fig. 5. Schematic representation of the effects of feedback removal on the ability of cortical neurons to differentiate between the BS and BM stimuli at low salience. The rectangular white or gray squares in A–D represent the average neural activity of neurons activated by the stimulus. A single bar moving on a stationary background (BS stimulus) strongly activates the neurons whose RF centers are on the trajectory of the stimulus. (B) Because of the strong background suppression, the response to the BM stimulus is much weaker (dark gray). When the feedback is removed, the response to the BS stimulus is decreased by 40% on average (C) and the background suppression is strongly decreased (D). As a result, the cortical area responds more weakly to the BS stimulus and does not properly differentiate between the BS and BM stimuli.

In keeping with an earlier preliminary report (Bullier et al., 1996), we observed statistically significant changes in the responses to the bar flashed in the RF center for 10% of the sampled neurons. In all cases, the response was a decrease of the V1 response when V2 was inactivated. The average response decrease was around 30%. Thus, the feedback connections from V2 to V1 appear to play a similar role in boosting the response to a central stimulus as observed in the feedback from MT to V1, V2 and V3.

Using sets of oriented bars flashed in the RF surround we also studied the center–surround interactions in V1 neurons during V2 inactivation. Contrary to what we had observed in the study of MT feedback, we could not find any change in surround suppression in V1 neurons during V2 inactivation (Hupé et al., 2001a). We also failed to replicate an earlier observation of general response increases to surround stimulation during V2 inactivation (Bullier et al., 1996). We interpreted the differences between these two studies as due to the strict monitoring of the EEG traces during control and V2 inactivation in the second set of experiments. Indeed, it has recently been shown (Worgotter et al., 1998) that during phases of power increases of low frequency components of the EEG, RF centers of cortical neurons tend to increase in such a way that could have produced the effects we observed in our earlier study.

Conclusion: feedback influences on center responses and center–surround interactions

Center responses

In both systems of feedback connections that we studied, the effect of inactivation of a higher order area led to a decrease of the center response: this was observed for 85% of the neurons that were affected by MT inactivation and for 100% of the V1 neurons that were affected by V2 inactivation. This is in keeping with earlier results concluding that feedback connections tend to boost the responses in lower order areas (Mignard and Malpeli, 1991; Sandell and Schiller, 1982; Vanduffel et al., 1997). The higher proportions of response decreases versus increases during inactivation in our results compared to those of Sandell and Schiller (1982) may be due to different inactivation techniques and to a more rigorous statistical treatment of the data that allowed us to eliminate many false-positive results.

The fact that we observed effects on a smaller proportion of neurons in V1 after inactivation of V2 than in areas V1, V2, V3 after MT inactivation may be due to the fact that the inactivation of V2 by GABA was less extensive than that of MT by cooling. Another possibility is related to the fact that the central stimulus in the V1/V2 experiment was highly salient. If feedback connections from V2 to V1 are particularly important for differentiating figure from background in the case of low salience stimuli as it is for the MT feedback (Figs. 3–5), we may have missed the major effects that could be seen with other types of low salience or ambiguous stimuli such as Kanisza-type stimuli. Responses to such stimuli have been reported for neurons in areas V1 and V2 (Peterhans and von der Heydt, 1989; Von der Heydt and Peterhans, 1989; Grosof et al., 1993; Leventhal et al., 1998) and in imaging studies (Hirsch et al., 1995; Sheth et al., 1996; Seghier et al., 2000).

The effects of feedback connections can be surprisingly strong: during MT inactivation, the responses of some neurons appear to be almost completely abolished (Hupé et al., 1998). Despite this strong influence, it appears that the feedback connections do not drive their target neurons as feedforward connections do. This conclusion is based on two observations.

(1) When V1 is reversibly blocked, practically all neurons in V2 loose their visual responses (Girard and Bullier, 1989), despite the presence of a strong residual activity in area MT (Girard et al., 1992) that should be able to drive V2 neurons if feedforward and feedback connections were combined in a linear fashion.

(2) If feedback connections acted in a linear fashion, we should have observed activity changes outside the RF center of V1/V2/V3 neurons during MT inactivation. This results from the fact that the moving stimulus activates the RFs of several feedback neurons before entering the RF center of the recorded neuron, because of the loose visuotopic nature of feedback connections. However, the changes in responses of neurons in areas V1, V2 and V3 during MT inactivation are observed only during the period of response to the central bar (BS) in the RF center. No significant changes of activity are observed when the bar crosses the surround region. This restriction of changes to the RF center was observed both for response increases and for response decreases during MT inactivation (Hupé et al., 2001b).

Thus, feedback connections appear to interact in a non-linear fashion with feedforward and horizontal connections to boost the center response by controlling the gain of the center mechanism. Although we lack experimental evidence, it is likely that the effect of feedback connections on center–surround mechanisms also corresponds to a non-linear mechanism such as gain control.

These differences in mechanisms between feedforward and feedback connections are in keeping with differences in anatomy (for example laminar distributions of terminals) and synaptic mechanisms (Felleman and Van Essen, 1991; Salin and Bullier, 1995; Shao and Burkhalter, 1996).

Center–surround interactions

As suggested by many authors, horizontal connections are the most likely basis for center–surround interactions. This possibility is supported by measurements of timing of responses. With the exception of fibers in layer 4B, horizontal connections in primate area V1 are non-myelinated and very fine in diameter, and are therefore likely to be slow conducting. From electrical stimulation experiments in monkey V1 we concluded that their median conduction velocity is 0.3 m/s (Girard et al., 2001). This value is consistent with those found for center–surround interactions using optical imaging (Grinvald et al., 1994) and for long distance interactions in the receptive field demonstrated by intracellular recordings in the cat (Bringuier et al., 1999). Thus, at least in terms of conduction speed, horizontal connections could be the main basis of center–surround interactions.

On the other hand, there are reasons to think that horizontal connections cannot be the sole substrate of center–surround interactions in cortical neurons and that feedback connections are involved in these effects. Horizontal connections have a limited spread and therefore cannot be the substrate of long-range lateral interactions in the visual field, at least monosynaptically. For example, in area V1 at 2.5° eccentricity (corresponding to our recording position), an axonal length of 3 mm corresponds to approximately 0.5° in the visual field (Dow et al., 1981). This is much smaller than the maximal extent of the modulatory surround region of neurons in this area (Levitt and Lund, 1997). Indeed the extent of cortex spanned by horizontal connections in macaque V1 appears to correspond to the RF center and the most proximal part of the surround (Angelucci et al., 2000). Reaching out to several degrees in visual field would require multisynaptic connections. On the other hand, because of their loose visuotopic organization, feedback connections could transfer information from distant regions of the visual field and could therefore be the substrate of distant influences in the RF surround.

In that case, one could expect that these distant influences should be delayed, because of the supposedly slow nature of feedback connections and the delayed activation of higher order areas. The orientation-selective component of the surround effect in V1 is indeed delayed by 15–20 ms with respect to the onset of the population response (Knierim and Van Essen, 1992; Nothdurft et al., 1999), and by about 40 ms at the single cell level (Hupé et al., 2001a). But, in fact, we showed that feedback connections have a very rapid action (Hupé et al., 2001b), and there appears to be no participation of feedback connections from V2 in center–surround interactions tested with such stimuli in V1 (Hupé et al., 2001a). The delay for the observed surround modulations agrees therefore better with the horizontal connection hypothesis.

The results obtained at high salience in the study of MT feedback point to the same conclusion: at middle and high salience, there is on average a minimal change in the suppression of the center response by activating the surround with a moving background. This suggests that our failure to observe strong effects of feedback inactivation on center–surround interactions in V1 was not simply due to an incomplete inactivation of V2.

The most likely explanation of our failure to demonstrate strong feedback influences on center–surround interactions at middle and high salience is that the different sets of feedback connections from different cortical areas and the horizontal connections combine with an OR-gate mechanism to control the gain of the inhibitory surround. Thus, for high salience stimuli, all feedback and local inputs are active, and removal of one has a minimal effect on center surround interactions. If feedback and horizontal connections combine their effects in this way, one should be able to demonstrate effects on center–surround mechanisms by activating neurons in a single area by chemical means or by inactivating most cortical areas providing feedback connections. Another way to address specifically the role of feedback connections from one area on center–surround interactions would be to work near the threshold limits for responses in that area, by adjusting parameters such as speed differences, spatial or temporal frequencies, or chromatic differences. This is probably what we did by using low contrast moving stimuli that activated mostly area MT.

For reasons explained above, it appears difficult for horizontal connections to mediate the longest range interactions measured physiologically in V1 (Levitt and Lund, 1997; Angelucci et al., 2000). It is therefore likely that feedback connections are involved in these long-range center–surround interactions. In our study of feedback from MT we used a large background stimulus that did not enable us to study specifically some parts of the surround. The stimuli used in the V1–V2 study were mostly confined to the proximal part of the surround as we wished to activate the most sensitive part of the surround. Thus we have not specifically tested the role of feedback connections in providing surround effects for large distances in the visual field and this remains to be done.

Another way to interpret our failure to identify strong feedback effects on center surround interactions for high salience stimuli is to consider the possibility that this is simply not the main role of feedback connections. Center–surround interactions are present from the earliest stages of processing in the retina and orientation-specific surround effects could be provided by horizontal connections at least for proximal interactions. Feedback connections may be important for providing an 'intelligent' input to different sets of neurons in lower order areas depending on interpretations reached at higher levels of the hierarchy (Gilbert et al., 2000). In a recent publication, we showed that feedback connections act on the early part of the visual responses of neurons in lower order areas (Hupé et al., 2001b). Information can be rapidly transferred to higher order areas through the population of magnocellular neurons that are activated early (Nowak and Bullier, 1997) and a first-pass analysis can be performed in higher order areas. According to this first-pass analysis, the gains of the center mechanism and the center–surround interactions could be adjusted in lower order areas to perform an optimal processing of the second wave of information carried by the parvocellular neurons. Recent results of feedback inactivation on neural activity evoked by plaid patterns in cat area 18 are in keeping with such an interpretation of the role of feedback connections in providing a global-to-local interface to neurons in low order areas (Schmidt et al., 2000).

Acknowledgements

We thank Alessandra Angelucci for helpful discussions and for reading the text and suggesting changes. We are also grateful to Frédéric Sarrato for help with the iconography.

References

Angelucci, A., Levitt, J.B., Hupé, J.M., Walton, E.J.S., Bullier, J. and Lund, J.S. (2000) Anatomical circuits for local and global integration of visual information: intrinsic and feedback connections in macaque visual cortical area V1. *Eur. J. Neurosci.*, 12: 285.

Bringuier, V., Chavane, F., Glaeser, L. and Frégnac, Y. (1999) Horizontal propagation of visual activity in the synaptic integration field of area 17 neurons. *Science*, 283: 695–699.

Bullier, J., Hupé, J.-M., James, A.C. and Girard, P. (1996) Functional interactions between areas V1 and V2 in the monkey. *J. Physiol. (Paris)*, 90: 112–119.

Dow, B.M., Snyder, A.Z., Vautin, R.G. and Bauer, R. (1981) Magnification factor and receptive field size in foveal striate cortex of the monkey. *Exp. Brain Res.*, 44: 213–228.

Felleman, D.J. and Van Essen, D.C. (1991) Distributed hierarchical processing in the primate cerebral cortex. *Cereb. Cortex*, 1: 1–47.

Gilbert, C., Ito, M., Kapadia, M. and Westheimer, G. (2000) Interactions between attention, context and learning in primary visual cortex. *Vision Res.*, 40: 1217–1226.

Girard, P. and Bullier, J. (1989) Visual activity in area V2 during reversible inactivation of area 17 in the macaque monkey. *J. Neurophysiol.*, 62: 1287–1302.

Girard, P., Salin, P.A. and Bullier, J. (1992) Response selectivity of neurons in area MT of the macaque monkey during reversible inactivation of area V1. *J. Neurophysiol.*, 67: 1–10.

Girard, P., Hupé, J.M. and Bullier, J. (2001) Feedforward and feedback connections between areas V1 and V2 of the monkey have similar rapid conduction velocities. *J. Neurophysiol.*, 85: 1328–1331.

Grinvald, A., Lieke, E.E., Frostig, R.D. and Hildesheim, R. (1994) Cortical point-spread function and long-range lateral interactions revealed by real-time optical imaging of macaque monkey primary visual cortex. *J. Neurosci.*, 14: 2545–2568.

Grosof, D.H., Shapley, R.M. and Hawken, M.J. (1993) Macaque V1 neurons can signal 'illusory' contours. *Nature*, 365: 550–552.

Hirsch, J., DeLaPaz, R.L., Relkin, N.R., Victor, J., Kim, K., Li, T., Borden, P., Rubin, N. and Shapley, R. (1995) Illusory contours activate specific regions in human visual cortex: evidence from functional magnetic resonance imaging. *Proc. Natl. Acad. Sci. USA*, 92: 6469–6473.

Hupé, J.M. (1999) Rôle des connexions corticales feedback dans la perception visuelle, Université Claude Bernard, Lyon, 183 pp.

Hupé, J.M., James, A.C., Payne, B.R., Lomber, S.G., Girard, P. and Bullier, J. (1998) Cortical feedback improves discrimination between figure and background by V1, V2 and V3 neurons. *Nature*, 394: 784–787.

Hupé, J.M., James, A.C., Girard, P. and Bullier, J. (2001a) Response modulation by static texture surround in area V1 of the macaque monkey do not depend on feedback connections from V2. *J. Neurophysiol.*, 85: 146–163.

Hupé, J.M., James, A.C., Girard, P.S.L., Payne, B. and Bullier, J. (2001b) Feedback connections act on the early part of the responses in monkey visual cortex. *J. Neurophysiol.*, 85: 134–145.

Knierim, J.J. and Van Essen, D.C. (1992) Neuronal responses to static texture patterns in area V1 of the alert macaque monkey. *J. Neurophysiol.*, 67: 961–980.

Leventhal, A.G., Wang, Y., Schmolesky, M.T. and Zhou, Y. (1998) Neural correlates of boundary perception. *Vis. Neurosci.*, 15: 1107–1118.

Levitt, J.B. and Lund, J.S. (1997) Spatial summation properties of macaque striate neurons. *Soc. Neurosci. Abstr.*, 23: 455.

Li, C.-Y. and Li, W. (1994) Extensive integration of field beyond the classical receptive field of cat's striate cortical neurons-classification and tuning properties. *Vision Res.*, 34: 2337–2355.

Mignard, M. and Malpeli, J.G. (1991) Paths of information flow through visual cortex. *Science*, 251: 1249–1251.

Nothdurft, H.C., Gallant, J.L. and Van Essen, D.C. (1999) Response modulation by texture surround in primate area V1: correlates of 'popout' under anesthesia. *Vis. Neurosci.*, 16: 15–34.

Nowak, L.G. and Bullier, J. (1997) The timing of information transfer in the visual system. In: J.H. Kaas, K.L. Rockland and A.L. Peters (Eds.), *Extrastriate Visual Cortex in Primates*, Vol. 12. Plenum, New York, pp. 205–241.

Peterhans, E. and von der Heydt, R. (1989) Mechanisms of contour perception in monkey visual cortex. II. Contours bridging gaps. *J. Neurosci.*, 9: 1749–1763.

Salin, P.-A. and Bullier, J. (1995) Corticocortical connections in the visual system: structure and function. *Physiol. Rev.*, 75: 107–154.

Salin, P.A., Girard, P., Kennedy, H. and Bullier, J. (1992) The visuotopic organization of corticocortical connections in the visual system of the cat. *J. Comp. Neurol.*, 320: 415–434.

Sandell, J.H. and Schiller, P.H. (1982) Effect of cooling area 18 on striate cortex cells in the squirrel monkey. *J. Neurophysiol.*, 48: 38–48.

Schmidt, K.E., Goebel, R., Castelo-Branco, M., Lomber, S., Payne, B.R. and Galuske, R.A.W. (2000) Global motion representation in primary visual cortex of the cat and the influence of feedback. *Eur. J. Neurosci.*, 12: 75.

Sclar, G., Maunsell, J.H.R. and Lennie, P. (1990) Coding of contrast in central visual pathways of the macaque monkey. *Vision Res.*, 30: 1–10.

Seghier, M., Dojat, M., Delon-Martin, C., Rubin, C., Warnking, J., Segebarth, C. and Bullier, J. (2000) Moving illusory contours activate primary visual cortex: an FRMI study. *Cereb. Cortex*, 10: 663–670.

Shao, Z.W. and Burkhalter, A. (1996) Different balance of excitation and inhibition in forward and feedback circuits of rat visual cortex. *J. Neurosci.*, 16: 7353–7365.

Sheth, B.R., Sharma, J., Rao, S.C. and Sur, M. (1996) Orientation maps of subjective contours in visual cortex. *Science*, 274: 2110–2115.

Vanduffel, W., Payne, B.R., Lomber, S.G. and Orban, G.A. (1997) Functional impact of cerebral connections. *Proc. Natl. Acad. Sci. USA*, 94: 7617–7620.

Von der Heydt, R. and Peterhans, E. (1989) Mechanisms of contour perception in monkey visual cortex. I. Lines of pattern discontinuity. *J. Neurosci.*, 9: 1731–1748.

Wang, C., Waleszczyk, W.J., Burke, W. and Dreher, B. (2000) Modulatory influence of feedback projections from area 21a on neuronal activities in striate cortex of the cat. *Cereb. Cortex*, 10: 1217–1232.

Worgotter, F., Suder, K., Zhao, Y., Kerscher, N., Eysel, U.T. and Funke, K. (1998) State-dependent receptive-field restructuring in the visual cortex. *Nature*, 396: 165–168.

C. Casanova and M. Ptito (Eds.)
Progress in Brain Research, Vol. 134

CHAPTER 14

Cortical mechanisms of binocular stereoscopic vision

A.J. Parker * and B.G. Cumming

University Laboratory of Physiology, Parks Road, Oxford, OX1 3PT, UK

Abstract: The early neurophysiology of binocular vision is largely dominated by measurements of disparity selectivity in cortical neurons in various visual areas. Incisive progress has been made by the intensive study of the mechanism of disparity selectivity of V1 in cortical neurons and the development of a number of tests for the involvement of single neurons in the perception of stereoscopic depth. The picture that now emerges is that cortical area V1 must be a preliminary processing stage for the analysis of stereoscopic depth, whereas some of the extrastriate areas may actually be responsible for the generation of neuronal signals that underlie the perception of binocular depth.

Introduction

This article is concerned with the way in which the visual areas of the cerebral cortex process information arising from the two eyes. It has long been established by psychophysical experiments that small differences in the images on the left and right retinae are sufficient to generate a sensation of depth. The basic geometric relationships are outlined in Fig. 1. When the eyes are binocularly fixating a single target in the three-dimensional world, any object that is closer to or further from the depth plane of the fixation target falls on non-corresponding retinal points. Wheatstone (1838, 1852) demonstrated that binocular stimulation of this form is sufficient to provide observers with the impression that objects are at different distances. Julesz (1964, 1971) showed that this process is driven automatically by luminance edges or other low-level image features, in that no explicit recognition of form is required at the monocular level in order for the observer to experience binocular depth.

* Corresponding author: A.J. Parker, University Laboratory of Physiology, Parks Road, Oxford, OX1 3PT, UK. Tel.: +44-1865-272504; Fax: +44-1865-272469; E-mail: andrew.parker@physiol.ox.ac.uk

The intention here is to review recent progress towards understanding the neuronal basis of binocular depth perception and related phenomena. Much of the relevant evidence comes from studies of V1, the primary visual cortex. However, these experiments highlight some significant limitations of stereoscopic processing in area V1, a conclusion that points the way to a fresh look at the contributions of extrastriate cortex. Although many studies have measured the tuning characteristics for binocular disparity in extrastriate visual areas, it is argued here that a new range of tests needs to be applied to reveal more precisely the role of neurons in the various extrastriate areas.

Before embarking on these issues, we should address briefly the most significant issue of all, namely the functional role of stereoscopic vision and how it fits together with other important sensory and motor functions.

Functions of stereoscopic vision

There can be no doubt that the fact that our species possesses two eyes bears no simple relationship to a single visual function. The bilaterality of eyes and ears clearly owes more to the midline symmetry of vertebrate development, than any specific selective advantage reinforced by evolutionary mechanisms.

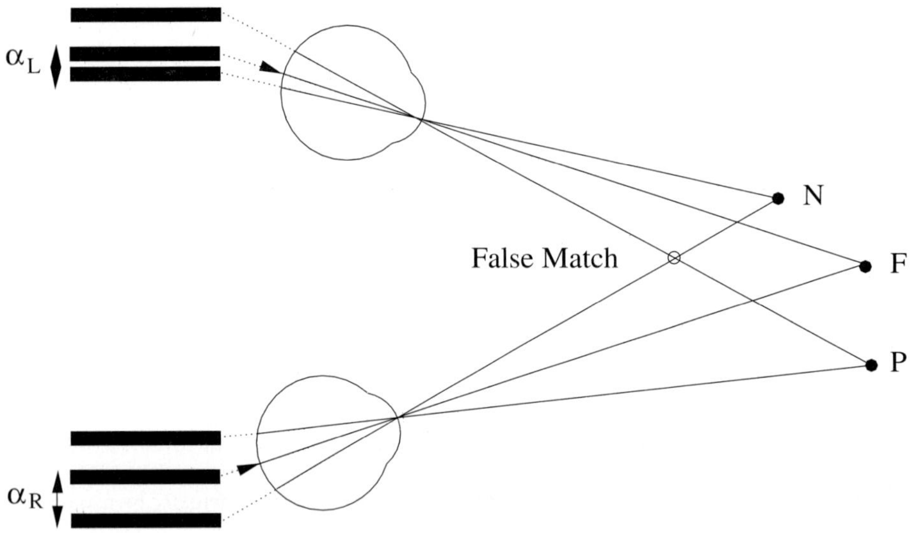

Fig. 1. Diagram to illustrate stereoscopic viewing geometry for horizontal disparities. The eyes are fixating point F. Point N has a non-zero disparity with respect to point F because its distance is less than F. Point P is at zero disparity because it is at the same distance as the fixation point. The angles subtended at the left and right eyes (α_L and α_R, respectively) by the gap between features N and F are different, whereas the angles between F and P are the same. The open circle marked 'False Match' shows that if N and P give rise to similar image features then there is the possibility of confusion about how to pair up the image features between the left and right eyes. The brain is remarkably adept at eliminating these potential confusions.

The different ways in which this symmetry has been exploited by lateral-eyed and frontal-eyed animals illustrates the opportunistic effect of biological selection. In lateral-eyed animals, such as the rabbit, the two eyes are used primarily to provide a panoramic view of the world with only a small region of binocular overlap. In frontal-eyed animals, such as primates, the basic sensory input from the two eyes is coordinated and exploited in a variety of ways.

Bifoveation and vergence control

First, it is used for bifoveation, to ensure that the foveas of the two eyes remain locked on a single target, for example during a pursuit eye movement. Related to this function is the control of vergence position, which allows the system to acquire new targets at different depths or even to track the movement of a target in depth, albeit slowly compared with versional movements. This review will not examine the mechanisms responsible for generating these movements in any detail, but one aim is to identify candidate sensory control signals for the maintenance or adjustment of binocular vergence position.

Figure–ground segregation

A second important use of binocular input is also unrelated to the perception of depth. This is the use of binocular vision for figure–ground segregation. A particular form of random dot stereogram illustrates this point (see Fig. 2). The stimuli to the left and right eyes are uniform in appearance but the fusion of the two images shows hidden structure. This arises because the central circular region is binocularly correlated between the left and right eyes' images, whereas the surround region is binocularly uncorrelated. In the real 3-D world, these differences of correlation are often associated with differences of depth. In the figure, there is no consistent depth difference between center and surround because the center is arranged to have a disparity of zero. The segregation is brought about purely by the differences in binocular correlation. This is not a new observation psychophysically but it illustrates a point that is important to remember in interpreting neurophysiological experiments: binocular information may contribute to the segmentation of images without the need for an explicit representation of depth.

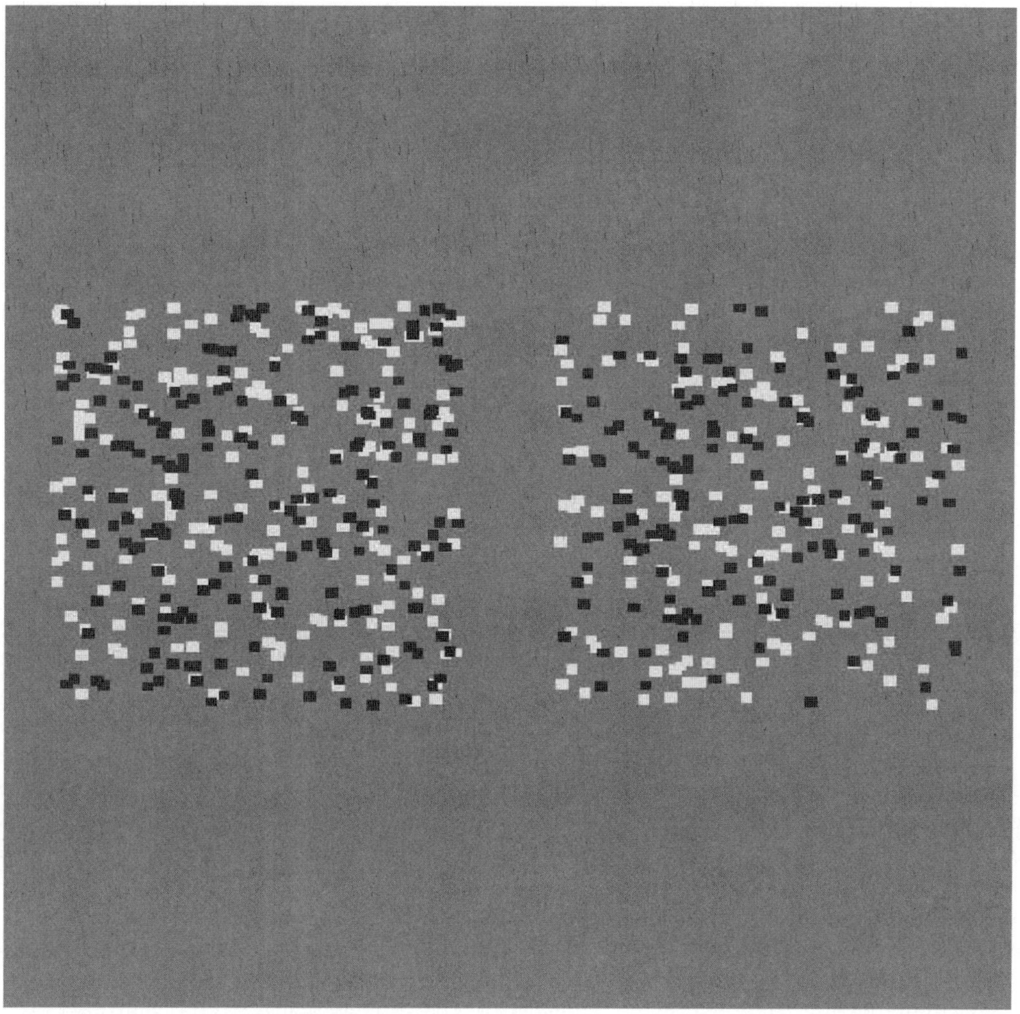

Fig. 2. A binocular pair of random dot pictures. Fusion of the two images results in the segregation of a central region where binocular correlation between right and left images is 100% from a surround region where the eyes' images are uncorrelated, 0%. Note that it does not matter whether these images are viewed with divergent or convergent fusion because the disparity is zero in the centre region and undefined in the surround.

Depth perception

The more immediate reason why the visual system of frontal-eyed animals has special binocular properties is their ability to extract depth from binocular disparities. It is often mistakenly argued that this is only useful in the near workspace (within 0.5–2 m from the viewer). A simple calculation shows that the best human stereo thresholds imply an ability to distinguish between objects that are truly at infinity and those that are over 400 m away. The general principle can be readily verified for yourself by looking out of a window in a building with a good view into the distance. Place a spot or other marker on the window, fixate the distance and open and close the left and right eyes alternately. The binocular parallax of the spot will be readily visible even when you are several meters from the window. Thus binocular vision is capable of contributing significantly to the perception of scene layout as well as discriminating depth in the near workspace.

The conversion of disparity into depth is also a significant issue. When the movement of the eyes changes the point of binocular regard from one depth plane to another, the depth signaled by binocular disparity must be re-evaluated. The most obvious point is that there is a change in the distance from the observer at which objects fall on corresponding points on the left and right retinae. This is implied by bifoveation since the foveae themselves are, of course, corresponding points between the left and right retinae. The necessary readjustment of vergence has long been acknowledged as a potential source of information about distance (Descartes, 1664). Also of significance is the fact that the depth relationship between different disparities must be recalibrated. The same depth difference far away from the observer creates a smaller disparity than the same difference in depth in an object closer to the observer. The source of signals providing this calibration has been studied intensively in recent years (see Mayhew and Longuet-Higgins, 1982; Cumming et al., 1991; Johnston, 1991; Sobel and Collett, 1991; Rogers and Bradshaw, 1993). An elegant recent synthesis is provided by Backus (Backus and Banks, 1999; Backus et al., 1999).

Cortical area V1

The simple picture of the operation of binocular disparity selective neurons in V1 to be advanced here is that they respond primarily to the local disparity of binocular features presented within their receptive fields. The evidence for this is wide-ranging and considerable, but nonetheless there are views incompatible with this simple picture. Here, we initially concentrate on the positive evidence that has led to our conclusions and then attempt to interpret conflicting views in the light of this evidence.

Absolute disparity

Before proceeding any further, it is necessary to make more precise our concept of disparity. Until now, we have referred to binocular stimuli as falling on corresponding or non-corresponding retinal points. Whilst a single point in the dark that falls on non-corresponding retinal points is sufficient to allow a response to the depth of the target, it has been clear since the work of Westheimer in the 1970s that the best binocular performance is achieved when there is more than one point visible within the binocular visual field (Westheimer, 1979). Indeed it appears that the finest stereo judgments are supported by stimulus configurations in which the depth of one feature is judged relative to another.

The diagram in Fig. 3 indicates the distinction that is being made here. In the left-hand diagram, point d alone is at a non-zero disparity but the threshold for detecting that d is not at the fixation plane is made considerably lower by the presence of point f, the visible fixation point (Westheimer, 1979). It is therefore possible to conceive of the binocular disparity of point d in two different ways. With respect to the point of binocular regard of the eyes, it has a measurable disparity, which we refer to as its 'absolute disparity'. With respect to point f, it also has a measurable disparity, which we refer to as its 'relative disparity'. In the left hand figure, the value of absolute and relative disparity is the same: $\alpha + \beta$. Absolute and relative disparity can be distinguished by considering what happens when the eyes move, leaving d and f fixed at their original locations in 3-D space. This is illustrated in the right-hand version of the figure, where it can be appreciated that movement of the eyes changes the absolute disparity of all points in the binocular field, but the relative disparities between pairs of visible points are unaffected. Thus, the relative disparity between d and f remains $\alpha + \beta$, but the absolute disparity of d has decreased, due to the eye movement.

In Cumming and Parker (1999), we investigated how neurons in V1 respond to absolute and relative disparity. The strategy was to add a controlled extra amount of absolute disparity to the receptive field. This simulates the sensory consequences of a change in the vergence state. The extra absolute disparity was held at its target value by means of a feedback loop so that further fluctuations of vergence would have no effect on the added absolute disparity. The result was clear. The co-ordinate system for representing disparity in V1 is linked to absolute disparity. Changes of absolute disparity in the stimulus over the receptive field are the dominant factor in generating the disparity tuning curves of these neurons.

The stimuli used in Cumming and Parker (1999) consisted of a patch of dynamic random dots, which covered the binocular receptive field of the V1 neuron at all disparities tested in the experiment. Surrounding this central patch was an annulus of binoc-

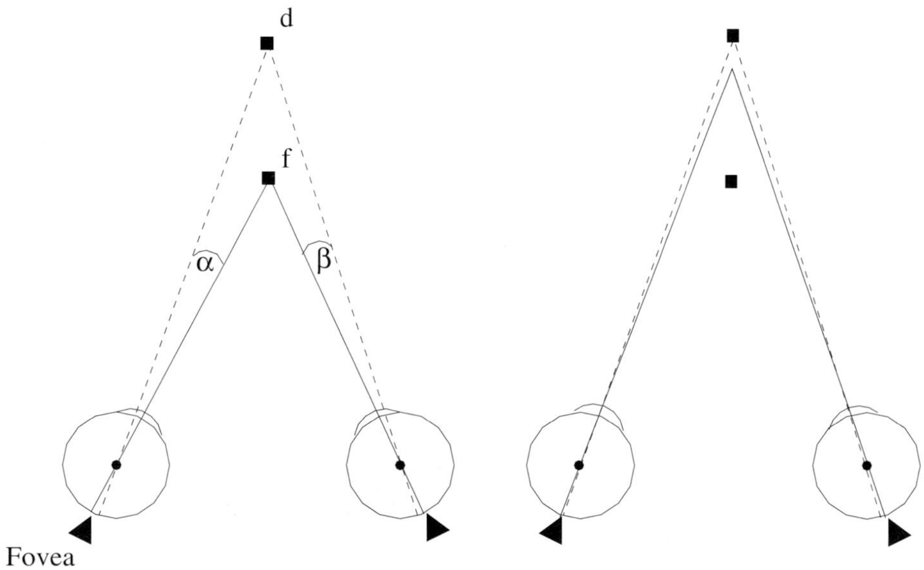

Fig. 3. The distinction between absolute and relative disparities. See text for details.

ular random dots always at zero disparity (same as the fixation point). Thus there is always a relative disparity signal present within the display. It is clear that this relative disparity is perceptually effective because removal of the surround raises the animals' psychophysical thresholds by a factor of 10 (Prince et al., 2000). Nonetheless, the firing of V1 neurons is completely dominated by their response to the absolute disparity of the central region of the display. This suggests that it is necessary to look outside V1, in other cortical visual areas, for signals that are more tightly linked to the perceptual responses of the animal.

We may tentatively assign two functions to the neuronal signals for binocular disparity in V1. First, it is possible to build receptive fields sensitive to relative disparity by combining the signals from several V1 receptive fields. Second, neurons that are sensitive to absolute disparity are potentially useful for controlling changes in the vergence state of the eyes. Therefore the signal from V1 neurons that respond to a target at a non-zero disparity provides a way of estimating the absolute disparity of the target. A signal of this kind would correspond to the sensory control signal that Rashbass and Westheimer (1961) deduced should underlie the generation of vergence eye movements.

There are two recent pieces of evidence that support this proposal of at least a dual function for the disparity-selective neurons in V1. Their potential role in perceptual tasks is emphasized by the fact that they carry highly reliable signals about binocular disparity: the performance of the best neurons approaches that of the psychophysical observer (Prince et al., 2000). The potential role in the control of vergence is highlighted by the fact that there are parallel changes in neuronal signals and fast corrective vergence movements when the contrast of a stimulus is inverted in one eye to form a binocularly anti-correlated stimulus (Cumming and Parker, 1997; Masson et al., 1997).

This comparison between the different stimuli that control vergence and those that control psychophysical judgments of stereoscopic depth makes it clear that the output of V1 may be used in more than one way. In this context, it is significant that earlier investigations established unambiguously that changes of vergence position could be induced by changes in the absolute disparity of random-dot targets, even when the change in disparity did not give rise to a perceived change in stereoscopic depth (Erkelens and Collewijn, 1985). Despite these examples, in general there is relatively little data that directly compare perceptual judgments of binocular depth and the control of vergence movements by assessing their respective sensitivities to different stimulus manipulations. More comparisons of this type will be valuable in delineating the contributions of neural signals to these distinctive binocular functions.

Binocular receptive fields and the energy model

A highly successful account of the responses of binocular neurons in the primary visual cortex has been provided by the energy model (Ohzawa et al., 1990). The energy model describes the responses of complex cells and it is constructed from the outputs of binocular simple cells that themselves summate the input from left and right retinae. The simple cells are generally assumed to have receptive fields that are accurately described by Gabor functions and in the simplest version of the model four such functions are used that differ from each other by $\pi/2$ radians change of phase. The pooling of signals from simple cells to complex cells passes through a 'half-squaring' nonlinearity (a threshold below which the simple cell does not respond and a squaring relationship above the threshold). Since the signals from pairs of simple cells with a π radians difference of phase are added together, this effectively squares the output of this unit-pair. Essentially the same argument applies to the other unit-pair of simple cells, except they are phase-shifted by $\pi/2$ radians. Therefore, the two unit-pairs form a phase-independent energy calculation.

This model had the primary aim of accounting for data derived from recording in the anesthetized, paralyzed cat, but it has proved to be successful in giving an account of the disparity-specific mechanisms in V1 of awake behaving primates. This progress has been fully reviewed by Cumming and DeAngelis (2001), who provide a detailed account of the nature of the disparity-detecting mechanisms in V1 and their reliance on phase and position disparities.

The fact that the energy model is generally applicable is highly informative about the nature of the stereoscopic computations carried out by cortical area V1. Although the model is backed up by a considerable body of evidence, there are some unresolved discrepancies with existing data from V1. A much more serious issue surrounding the energy model is that it fails to provide a complete account of the processing of stereoscopic disparities. The ways in which the model fails are characteristic and arise from the fact that the energy computation is essentially local in nature. Thus it will fail to give an account of stereoscopic depth processing that involve global phenomena.

Limitations of the disparity energy model

The limitations of the disparity energy model are of two forms. The first area of concern is whether all aspects of the neuronal response to disparity within the primary visual cortex are properly characterized by the disparity energy model. In these cases, it may be possible to modify the energy model to make it more faithful to the true picture of neuronal signals, without violating the essential characteristics of the way that the model computes stereo disparity. The second area of concern arises from cases where neither the energy model nor the responses of V1 neurons are sufficient to understand the stereoscopic perception of depth. Strictly speaking, examples of this kind do not really represent failures of the energy model since it was developed primarily to give an account of the physiological responses of V1 cortical neurons. Nonetheless, these limitations on the energy model are provocative and powerful, since they force us to look at the nature of stereo processing outside V1 and to consider how the signals from 'energy-like' disparity-detectors could be further processed to yield responses that better account for stereo depth perception.

Binocularly anti-correlated stimuli

Binocularly anti-correlated stimuli are created by taking a conventional binocular stimulus and inverting the contrast of the stimulus in one eye with respect to the other. Thus in an anti-correlated random dot stereogram, each black dot in one eye's image is partnered with a white dot in the other eye's image and so on (Julesz, 1971). The response of the disparity energy model to this manipulation is an inversion of the disparity-tuning curve. Thus if a Gabor function is used to describe the disparity-tuning curve, then the energy model predicts that the disparity-tuning curve for binocularly correlated stimuli and anti-correlated stimuli should have the same amplitude of response but a complete inversion of phase with respect to one another (Cumming and Parker, 1997).

Experimentally, for both dynamic random-dot stereograms in monkey V1 (Cumming and Parker, 1997) and for the responses of cat V1 neurons calculated by reverse correlation with rapidly presented bar stimuli (Ohzawa et al., 1997), the result is the same. The amplitude of the response to binocularly anti-correlated stimuli is weaker than expected and the range of phases is spread broadly, rather than tightly, around the expected phase inversion of π radians. This discrepancy cannot be repaired by something as simple as an output non-linearity in the relationship between neuronal firing rate and membrane potential within cortical cells. This would leave the range of phase relationships still tightly clustered around π radians. Moreover, an output non-linearity predicts that cortical neurons that show a tuned-inhibitory response to binocularly correlated stimuli should show amplitude ratios *greater* than one in response to binocularly anti-correlated stimuli. It also predicts that neurons with odd-symmetric disparity tuning profiles (so-called 'near' and 'far' cells) should always show amplitude ratios of exactly one. None of these various predictions is fulfilled.

Recently in collaboration with Jenny Read, we have explored the properties of modified energy models that include a monocular non-linear stage prior to binocular combination (Read, Cumming and Parker, in preparation). The monocular stages feed into a binocular simple cell prior to the energy computation on the outputs of multiple simple cells to form a binocular complex neuron. Since the monocular inputs to the binocular simple cell are matched in their response to contrast polarity, the monocular non-linearity has the effect of reducing or eliminating the opportunity for binocular summation when the contrast is inverted in one eye. Models of this type can successfully predict the range of behaviors found in neuronal recordings. However, there is some penalty for these additional stages of processing. The energy model loses some of its elegance and simplicity and it is necessary to add more subunits than the minimum quadrature pairs to maintain the prediction of smooth receptive field profiles for cortical complex neurons. On the whole, the outcome is a successful modification of the energy model that explains the response to binocular anti-correlation without discarding the local nature of the energy computation (see Ohzawa, 1998, for an alternative view of the effects of anti-correlation).

Responses to local binocular stimulation

A more serious limitation of the energy model is illustrated by considering the response of the model to windowed sinusoidal grating stimuli (see Fig. 4). Stimuli of this general type provide an interesting test case for the relationship between the activity of single neurons and perception. As the disparity of the windowed sinusoid is altered, the perception of depth by psychophysical observers is controlled by the disparity of the entire display: thus perceived depth varies linearly with binocular disparity. The situation is rather different for a mechanism with a receptive field of limited spatial extent (as shown by the rectangle superimposed on the grating in Fig. 4). A mechanism of this kind receives a local signal about binocular disparity that is essentially identical for all added disparities that are related by a single period of the grating pattern. Note that this is true even when disparity of the grating pattern is exactly linked to that of the window.

The problem created by this stimulus for a mechanism with limited spatial extent is an example of the aperture problem, which is more typically identified with the processing of motion information (Marr and Ullman, 1981; Wallach: see Würger et al., 1996) but occurs for stereo processing as well (Morgan and Castet, 1997). In order to solve this problem, information about the depth signaled by the sharp boundary of the window needs to be put together with the local contour information given by the gratings. This allows the inherent ambiguity of the grating to be resolved. Perceptually, if there is no window boundary in place, then a spatially extended periodic stimulus is indeed ambiguous and creates the so-called 'wallpaper' effect, in which multiple depth matches are experienced at different times during the viewing of these stimuli (Smith, 1738).

Our recent recordings in cortical area V1 (Cumming and Parker, 2000) show that information from the window boundary fails to influence the firing patterns of V1 neurons. The responses of these neurons

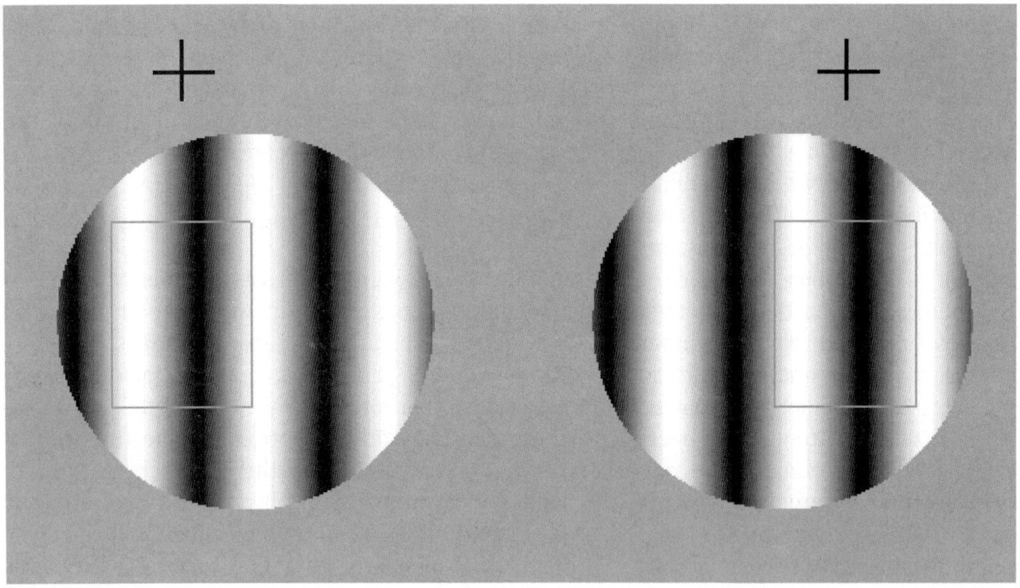

Fig. 4. Windowed sinusoidal grating stimuli used to test whether cortical neurons respond to local disparity or perceived depth. When binocularly fused (without the rectangular box present), the perception is of a single disk of grating at a different depth plane than the fixation point (crosses). A neuron with the receptive field shown by the rectangular box that responds only to local disparity continues to receive stimulation at zero disparity. (The rectangular box over the grating is present for illustrative purposes only and unsurprisingly has an additional effect on the binocular matching process, when attempting to fuse the images in this picture.)

are completely dominated by the visual stimulation created by the local contours within the receptive field. No consistent modulation of V1 responses were linked to the depth percept experienced by the psychophysical observers (either monkeys or humans) in response to these stimuli.

These observations for stereo bear a close analogy to earlier observations (Movshon et al., 1985) on the responses of V1 neurons to moving stimuli that are constructed to contain two component orientations (plaids). The main response of V1 neurons to plaids is dominated by the response of the orientation-selective classical receptive field, which is only sensitive to a component of the plaid that falls within the orientation bandwidth of the receptive field. Consequently, as the orientation and direction of the moving plaid is changed through 360°, the response of a strongly direction-sensitive V1 neuron is bimodal since it responds independently to each component orientation that forms the plaid. Neither of these responses occurs when the plaid is perceived to be moving in a direction similar to the direction-preference of the neuron. Thus the representation of the true direction of motion of the plaid stimulus in the firing patterns of V1 neurons is ambiguous, in much the way that the binocular depth of the windowed grating patch is ambiguously related to the firing patterns of disparity-selective neurons in V1.

This comparison of direction selectivity and disparity selectivity in V1 is made more compelling by the parallel between the responses of computational models of directional and disparity-sensitive detectors. A direction-sensitive motion detector based on the 'motion energy' principle (Adelson and Bergen, 1985) with orientation selective spatial filters has the same ambiguity in response to plaid stimuli as the bulk of V1 neurons. A disparity-selective detector based on the energy principle suffers the same ambiguity as V1 neurons in response to the windowed sinusoidal grating pattern. In the case of motion, there is strong evidence (Movshon et al., 1985) that the ambiguity of response to plaid stimuli is eliminated in the neuronal firing patterns within extrastriate visual cortex (area MT/V5). If this parallel between motion and disparity is correct, then it suggests that the key to disambiguating the windowed-grating stimulus may also be discovered in the extrastriate cortex.

Fidelity of signals

Before turning to a discussion of the extrastriate visual areas, we should attempt to answer more precisely one obvious question: namely, given that the disparity-selective responses of V1 neurons exhibit several discrepancies with the perceptual response to binocular depth, what is the contribution of V1 neurons to the binocular perception of depth? The broad picture is a combination of information derived from studies on binocular responses in anesthetized, paralyzed preparations (where the opportunities for long-duration experiments on single neurons is maximized) and in awake, behaving monkeys (where the opportunity for parallel psychophysical experimentation arises and a natural binocular alignment on the stimuli can be achieved).

The recent years have seen an encouraging convergence of information from these two types of experiment. It now seems clear that V1 neurons respond primarily to absolute disparity of local contours within their receptive fields (Cumming and Parker, 1999, 2000) and it seems likely that some variant of the energy model (Ohzawa et al., 1990) will prove to be a sufficiently accurate description of most features of the neuronal response in V1 to binocular stimuli. The responsiveness to absolute disparity means that V1 neurons provide a sensory signal that is well suited for controlling the disparity-driven components of the vergence eye movement response. Indeed, a signal based on relative disparity would be more closely related to the perceptual response to binocular disparity but would be less suitable for controlling vergence.

In cortical area V1, Prince, Cumming and Parker (manuscript submitted for publication) report that some 40–55% of neurons are disparity selective, depending on the criteria for selectivity that are applied. It is hard to believe that this significant number of disparity-selective neurons is entirely devoted to controlling vergence position. It seems likely that these V1 neurons are also precursors to other binocular neurons whose responses are more closely linked to binocular depth perception. One new line of evidence that is consistent with this is the observation that individual V1 neurons are highly sensitive in signaling binocular disparity. The performance of the best V1 neurons is comparable with the psychophysical performance of the monkeys themselves (Prince et al., 2000). This suggests that the V1 neurons are part of a cortical network that is devoted to the efficient and accurate registration of binocular image differences in preparation for further processing elsewhere, whether it is for vergence eye position or the perception of binocular depth.

The role of extrastriate visual areas

Our knowledge of the responses of extrastriate cortex to binocular disparity is considerably less precise than the statements that we can make about V1. The relevant evidence is patchy and it is entirely conceivable that important and significant features have been completely overlooked. One issue is clear and consistently reported: the overwhelming proportion of visual neurons in extrastriate cortical areas are binocularly driven. Thus the potential for binocular disparity to influence the responses of these neurons is all-pervasive. Moreover, since the incidence of monocular neurons is low in extra-striate cortex, this suggests that the bulk of disparity selectivity observed in these areas derives from the disparity-selective neurons within the striate cortex.

This section will assess briefly some recent advances in three areas: the processing of depth and contour information in cortical area V2; the evidence for a clustered representation of disparities in cortical area V5/MT and the effects of electrical microstimulation within these clusters; the picture of cortical activity provided by recent functional magnetic resonance imaging (fMRI) studies of binocular depth perception.

The diversity of V2

By the standards of visual neuroscience, the study of the processing of binocular disparity in V2 has a long history (Hubel and Wiesel, 1970). Neurons that change their responses systematically with the disparity of isolated bar contours have been associated particularly with the thick cytochrome oxidase stripes of V2 (Hubel and Livingstone, 1987; Peterhans and von der Heydt, 1993). If we consider the responses of V2 neurons in a wider context, it is clear that there are multiple opportunities for interactions between binocular disparity and other visual cues.

For example, there are numerous indications that the processing of texture boundaries, subjective contours, line terminators etc. within V2 is in some way more emphasized than within V1 (Peterhans and von der Heydt, 1993). The mechanisms by which sensitivity to these parameters is achieved have not been clearly elucidated.

It is important to consider the relationship of stereo disparity to these elements that seem to be primarily sensitive to perceptual segregation based on texture boundaries and line terminators. If these mechanisms are truly concerned with perceptual segregation, then one might expect that they will also be sensitive to regional segregation based on binocular disparity (Von der Heydt et al., 2000). This highlights the point that binocular correspondence is used in more than one way by the visual system: it is used for the recovery of depth and distance information, but it is also used for breaking camouflage and achieving segmentation of the visual scene (as illustrated by Fig. 2). Thus there are at least a priori reasons to expect a variety of ways in which disparity might influence the firing patterns of V2 neurons. Not only might there be neurons that change their response systematically with changes of disparity but there might also be neurons whose responses are modulated whenever there is a boundary defined by disparity. Bakin et al. (2000) have recently described modulatory effects of disparity on V2 neurons, using a variety of complex stimulus configurations.

In recent work with Owen Thomas, we have explored how the responses of V2 cortical neurons are modulated by the presence of disparities presented outside the classical receptive field. The stimuli were dynamic random-dot stereograms, arranged so that the depth of a circular central region could be altered independently of the depth of an annular surround. The central region extended just outside the classical receptive field as defined by plotting with bars and edges. In a number of neurons, alteration of the disparity of the surround profoundly affects the responses of the center to the disparity of the stimulus. In these neurons, changing the disparity of the surround alters the disparity preference of the central region. The change is such that the neuron tends to exhibit a consistent preference for the relative disparity between the center and the surround (Thomas et al., 1999; Thomas, Cumming and Parker, in preparation).

In this regard at least, processing of binocular disparity in V2 appears to move closer to neuronal responses that match the perceptual characteristics of binocular depth judgments. In terms of areal dimensions, V2 is obviously a highly significant locus within the cortical visual pathways. For this reason, if no other, it is to be expected that other cortical areas of significant size (such as V4) will also have an important role in regard to binocular depth judgments. We will now turn to other sources of evidence about the role of other extrastriate cortical areas in the processing of binocular depth.

Microstimulation in V5(MT)

Although cortical area V5(MT) is classically associated with the processing of motion information, it has been known for some time that the neurons there are sensitive to binocular disparity (Maunsell and van Essen, 1983). A recent series of studies has revealed a functional organization for disparity within V5(MT). The suggestion is that this has a columnar form, rather like the columnar arrangements in V5(MT) already identified for motion direction (DeAngelis and Newsome, 1999). There are distinct cortical regions within V5(MT) that show common disparity preferences (typically such that a neighborhood of cortex shows a consistent preference for either near or far disparities).

In recent experiments, DeAngelis et al. (1998) exploited this organization to set up a test of whether electrical microstimulation in area V5(MT) might influence judgments of binocular depth, in the same way that earlier studies in V5(MT) had established that electrical microstimulation influences judgments of motion direction (Salzman et al., 1990). The task of the monkey was to indicate whether a patch of dots was at a near or far distance with respect to the fixation plane. The proportion of dots signaling near or far was altered by diluting the dots present with some dots at randomly placed disparities. Thus the task is close in form to the original motion task in which the direction of motion is signaled by the fraction of dots that are moving consistently in one direction against a background of dots that are moving randomly in all directions. Electrical microstimulation in zones of V5(MT) whose neurons preferred near disparities tended to induce the monkey to report more often that the target was near with respect to the fixation plane, with the opposite effect for far disparities. Importantly, the effectiveness of microstimulation was greatest in zones of V5(MT) with a strong rather than weak selectivity for disparity.

Functional magnetic resonance imaging

Recently, functional magnetic resonance imaging has been used in human observers to explore the visual cortical regions that are involved in stereoscopic depth perception. Unsurprisingly, these studies have revealed that there is a widespread activation of visual areas by stimuli whose disparity or degree of interocular correlation is changed systematically. Using a random-dot stereogram stimulus with a central square at a different depth plane, Mendola et al. (1999) reported activation in cortical area V3A, which could be due to activation of either disparity-specific mechanisms or contour-specific mechanisms responsive to the square. In experiments in which a binocular random element stimulus switches from depicting a single plane at the fixation depth to a pair of planes symmetrically disposed either side of the fixation plane, Backus et al. (2001) demonstrate that cortical area V3A is especially sensitive to this manipulation, suggesting a disparity-specific response. It remains to be seen whether other stimulus paradigms will reveal the involvement of other visual areas: notably, in view of the well-characterized disparity sensitivity of V5(MT) neurons, the weakness of evidence for specific activations of this area presents a confusing picture at present.

Conclusions

This is an interesting moment for the study of stereoscopic vision at the cortical level. A number of new paradigms have been added to the neurophysiologists' repertoire. Until recently, the emphasis has been purely on the measurement of disparity selectivity and the characterization of models of how binocular neurons are formed in V1. Such studies have generated fundamental information, but the emphasis is now shifting towards the discovery of cortical sites whose neuronal properties could directly support some of the well-characterized properties of the perception of stereoscopic depth. We are as yet unclear which sites in the extra-striate cortex will eventually prove to be primarily responsible. Nonetheless it is clear that, at the neuronal level, there are interesting differences between cortical areas V2 and V5(MT) in comparison with the striate cortex V1 (see Cumming and DeAngelis, 2001, for a summary). The case of V3A is interesting, since although it has been known for some time (Poggio et al., 1988) that areas V3/V3A in the macaque contain disparity-specific neurons, it is recent human fMRI data that have emphasized its potential specialization. Perhaps this will be a clear case where fMRI data have been able to guide a neurophysiological investigation, rather than the other way round. The next 5–10 years should provide a wealth of new results that will address these questions.

Acknowledgements

This work was supported by the Wellcome Trust. B.G.C. was supported by a Royal Society University Research Fellow.

References

Adelson, E.H. and Bergen, J.R. (1985) Spatiotemporal energy models for the perception of motion. *J. Opt. Soc. Am. A Optics Image Sci. Vis.*, 2: 284–299.

Backus, B.T. and Banks, M.S. (1999) Estimator reliability and distance scaling in stereoscopic slant perception. *Perception*, 28: 217–242.

Backus, B.T., Banks, M.S., van Ee, R. and Crowell, J.A. (1999) Horizontal and vertical disparity, eye position, and stereoscopic slant perception. *Vision Res.*, 39: 1143–1170.

Backus, B.T., Fleet, D.J., Parker, A.J. and Heeger, D.T. (2001) Cortical activity correlates with stereoscopic depth perception. *J. Neurophysiol.*, in press.

Bakin, J.S., Nakayama, K. and Gilbert, C.D. (2000) Visual responses in monkey areas V1 and V2 to three-dimensional surface configurations. *J. Neurosci.*, 20: 8188–8198.

Cumming, B.G. and DeAngelis, G.C. (2001) The physiology of stereopsis. *Annu. Rev. Neuroscience*, 24: 203–238.

Cumming, B.G. and Parker, A.J. (1997) Responses of primary visual cortical neurons to binocular disparity without depth perception. *Nature*, 389: 280–283.

Cumming, B.G. and Parker, A.J. (1999) Binocular neurons in V1 of awake monkeys are selective for absolute, not relative, disparity. *J. Neurosci.*, 19: 5602–5618.

Cumming, B.G. and Parker, A.J. (2000) Local disparity not

perceived depth is signaled by binocular neurons in cortical area V1 of the macaque. *J. Neurosci.*, 20: 4758–4767.

Cumming, B.G., Johnston, E.B. and Parker, A.J. (1991) Vertical disparities and perception of 3-dimensional shape. *Nature*, 349: 411–413.

DeAngelis, G.C. and Newsome, W.T. (1999) Organization of disparity-selective neurons in macaque area MT. *J. Neurosci.*, 19: 1398–1415.

DeAngelis, G.C., Cumming, B.G. and Newsome, W.T. (1998) Cortical area MT and the perception of stereoscopic depth. *Nature*, 394: 677–680.

Descartes, R. (1664) *Tractatus de homine*. Paris.

Erkelens, C.J. and Collewijn, H. (1985) Motion perception during dichoptic viewing of moving random-dot stereograms. *Vision Res.*, 25: 583–588.

Hubel, D.H. and Livingstone, M.S. (1987) Segregation of form, color, and stereopsis in primate area 18. *J. Neurosci.*, 7: 3378–3415.

Hubel, D.H. and Wiesel, T.N. (1970) Cells sensitive to binocular depth in area 18 of the macaque monkey cortex. *Nature*, 225: 41–42.

Johnston, E.B. (1991) Systematic distortions of shape from stereopsis. *Vision Res.*, 31: 1351–1360.

Julesz, B. (1964) Binocular depth perception without familiarity cues. *Science*, 145: 356–362.

Julesz, B. (1971) *Foundations of Cyclopean Perception*. University of Chicago Press, Chicago.

Marr, D. and Ullman, S. (1981) Directional selectivity and its use in early visual processing. *Proc. R. Soc. Lond. B*, 211: 151–180.

Masson, G.S., Busettini, C. and Miles, F.A. (1997) Vergence eye movements in response to binocular disparity without depth perception. *Nature*, 389: 283–286.

Maunsell, J.H.R. and van Essen, D.C. (1983) Functional properties of neurons in middle temporal visual area of the macaque monkey. II. Binocular interactions and sensitivity to binocular disparity. *J. Neurophysiol.*, 49: 1148–1167.

Mayhew, J.E.W. and Longuet-Higgins, H.C. (1982) A computational model of binocular depth-perception. *Nature*, 297: 376–378.

Morgan, M.J. and Castet, E. (1997) The aperture problem in stereopsis. *Vision Res.*, 37: 2737–2744.

Movshon, J.A., Adelson, E.H., Gizzi, M.S. and Newsome, W.T. (1985) The analysis of moving visual patterns. *Pont. Acad. Sci. Scripta Varia*, 54: 118–151.

Mendola, J.D., Dale, A.M., Fischl, B., Liu, A.K. and Tootell, R.B. (1999) The representation of illusory and real contours in human cortical visual areas revealed by functional magnetic resonance imaging. *J. Neurosci.*, 19: 8560–8572.

Ohzawa, I. (1998) Mechanisms of stereoscopic vision: the disparity energy model. *Curr. Opin. Neurobiol.*, 8: 509–515.

Ohzawa, I., Deangelis, G.C. and Freeman, R.D. (1990) Stereoscopic depth discrimination in the visual-cortex — neurons ideally suited as disparity detectors. *Science*, 249: 1037–1041.

Ohzawa, I., DeAngelis, G.C. and Freeman, R.D. (1997) The neural coding of stereoscopic depth. *NeuroReport*, 8: R3–R12.

Peterhans, E. and von der Heydt, R. (1993) Functional organization of area V2 in the alert macaque. *Eur. J. Neurosci.*, 5: 509–524.

Poggio, G.F., Gonzales, F. and Krause, F. (1988) Stereoscopic mechanisms in monkey visual cortex: binocular correlation and disparity selectivity. *J. Neurosci.*, 8: 4351.

Prince, S.J.D., Pointon, A.D., Cumming, B.G. and Parker, A.J. (2000) The precision of single neuron responses in cortical area V1 during stereoscopic depth judgements. *J. Neurosci.*, 20: 3387–3400.

Rashbass, C. and Westheimer, G. (1961) Disjunctive eye movements. *J. Physiol.*, 159: 339–360.

Rogers, B.J. and Bradshaw, M.F. (1993) Vertical disparities, differential perspective and binocular stereopsis. *Nature*, 361: 253–255.

Salzman, C.D., Britten, K.H. and Newsome, W.T. (1990) Cortical microstimulation influences perceptual judgments of motion direction. *Nature*, 346: 174–177.

Smith, R. (1738) *A Complete System of Optics in Four Books*. Cambridge.

Sobel, E.C. and Collett, T.S. (1991) Does vertical disparity scale the perception of stereoscopic depth? *Proc. R. Soc. Lond. B*, 244: 87–90.

Thomas, O.M., Cumming, B.G. and Parker, A.J. (1999) The responses of binocular V2 neurons to relative and absolute disparities. *Soc. Neurosci. Abstr.*, 25: 821.7.

Von der Heydt, R., Zhou, H. and Friedman, H.S. (2000) Representation of stereoscopic edges in monkey visual cortex. *Vision Res.*, 40: 1955–1967.

Westheimer, G. (1979) Cooperative neural processes involved in stereoscopic acuity. *Exp. Brain Res.*, 36: 585–597.

Wheatstone, C. (1838) Contributions to the physiology of vision. I. On some remarkable and hitherto unobserved phenomena of binocular vision. *Phil. Trans. R. Soc.*, 128: 371-394.

Wheatstone, C. (1852) Contributions to the physiology of vision. II. On some remarkable and hitherto unobserved phenomena of binocular vision. *Phil. Trans. R. Soc.*, 142: 1-17.

Würger, S., Shapley, R. and Rubin, N. (1996) 'On the visually perceived direction of motion' by Hans Wallach: 60 years later. *Perception*, 25: 1317–1368.

C. Casanova and M. Ptito (Eds.)
Progress in Brain Research, Vol. 134

CHAPTER 15

Cortical plasticity revealed by circumscribed retinal lesions or artificial scotomas

B. Dreher [1,*], W. Burke [1,2] and M.B. Calford [3]

[1] *Department of Anatomy and Histology, Institute for Biomedical Research, The University of Sydney, Sydney, NSW 2006, Australia*
[2] *Department of Physiology, Institute for Biomedical Research, The University of Sydney, Sydney, NSW 2006, Australia*
[3] *Discipline of Human Physiology, School of Biomedical Sciences, Faculty of Medicine and Health Sciences, University of Newcastle, Callaghan, NSW 2308, Australia*

Abstract: We review the work of others in which the effects of circumscribed, topographically corresponding *binocular* retinal lesions on the topographic organization of the visual cortex revealed that there is a substantial degree of topographical plasticity in the primary visual cortices of adult cats and macaque monkeys. Despite the evidence indicating that the reorganization of the topographic map in primary visual cortices of adult cats and macaques related to the input from one eye could be suppressed for a long time by inputs related to the other eye, we observed a substantial degree of topographical plasticity in the primary visual cortices of adult cats in which we have made circumscribed *monocular* retinal lesions. Overall, in both binocularly and monocularly lesioned adult animals, most cells recorded in the cortical projection zone of the retinal lesion (LPZ), several hours, several weeks or several months after placement of the lesions exhibited 'ectopic' excitatory visual receptive fields (RFs) which were displaced to the normal retina in the immediate vicinity of the lesion. The presence of ectopic RFs in cells recorded in the cortical LPZ, combined with the presence of normal cortical representation of the part of the retina in the vicinity of the lesion, indicate a clear expansion of the cortical representation of the part of the retina surrounding the lesion. When stimulated via the ectopic RFs, cortical cells exhibited normal orientation tuning and in the case of animals with monocular lesions, the orientation tuning of binocular cells when stimulated via ectopic RFs appeared to be very similar to that when the cells were stimulated via the RFs in the normal, unlesioned eye. In both binocularly and monocularly lesioned animals, the responses evoked by optimal visual stimuli from the ectopic RFs were substantially weaker than those evoked from their normal counterparts. Similarly, upper velocity limits were significantly lower when visual stimuli were presented via the ectopic RFs. In contrast to cats in which the retinal lesions were made in adulthood, in cats lesioned monocularly in adolescence (8–11 weeks postnatal), both the peak discharge rates and upper velocity limits of responses to photic stimuli presented via the ectopic RFs were very similar to those to stimuli presented via the normal eye. The intracortical mechanism(s) underlying the long-term cortical plasticity revealed by retinal lesions are likely to be closely linked to the mechanism(s) underlying the short-term reversible enlargement of cortical receptive fields observed with artificial scotomas. Furthermore, a similar putative intracortical mechanism(s) appears to underlie psychophysical phenomena observed in studies of retinal scotomas in humans. Overall, the research reviewed here strongly challenges the view that receptive fields of neurons in mammalian visual cortices are 'hard-wired'.

* Corresponding author: B. Dreher, Department of Anatomy and Histology, Institute for Biomedical Research (F13), The University of Sydney, Sydney, NSW 2006, Australia. Tel.: +61-2-9351-4194; Fax: +61-2-9351-6556;
E-mail: bogdand@anatomy.usyd.edu.au

Introduction

In recent years, we have seen a revolution in our understanding of the concept of the 'receptive field' of individual neurons in the mammalian central nervous system. Until the 1980s, the receptive field (RF) of a sensory neuron was thought as spatially fixed 'forever' and its properties were thought to be 'hard-wired'. In the case of the visual system, the overall responses of a neuron were thought to be determined by the relative degree of activation of the 'center' and 'surround' parts of the RF (e.g. Kuffler, 1953) although it was already well appreciated that the relative strength of the center and surround might vary in time. In the 1960s and 1970s, it was already appreciated that responses of neurons in the mammalian visual system were affected by stimuli falling well outside the cell's 'classical receptive field' (CRF), e.g. suppressive or disinhibitory surrounds in the RFs of the retinal ganglion cells (RGCs; Ikeda and Wright, 1972a; Enroth-Cugell and Jakiela, 1980; Linsenmeier et al., 1982 see for reviews and more recent data Li et al., 1992; Shou et al., 2000), suppressive (Levick et al., 1972; Dreher and Sanderson, 1973; Cleland et al., 1983) or disinhibitory (Maffei and Fiorentini, 1972; Hammond, 1973) surrounds of neurons in the dorsal lateral geniculate nucleus (LGNd), suppressive regions in the RFs of neurons in the superficial layers of the superior colliculus (SC; McIlwain and Buser, 1968; Sterling and Wickelgren, 1969; Dreher and Hoffmann, 1973; Waleszczyk et al., 1999); suppressive regions of neurons in the primary and extrastriate visual cortices (Hubel and Wiesel, 1965a, 1968; Dreher, 1972; Henry et al., 1974a,b; Glezer et al., 1973; Nelson and Frost, 1978; see for reviews and more recent data Allman et al., 1985; Li and Li, 1994; Walker et al., 1999, 2000). With the exception of: (1) the so-called 'periphery effect' (McIlwain, 1964, 1966) and 'shift effect' (Fischer and Krüger, 1974, 1980; Krüger et al., 1975; Krüger, 1977) in the RGCs and LGNd neurons of cats and macaque monkeys; (2) inhibitory effects of remote visual stimuli on the visual responses of cells in the SC of the cat (Rizzolatti et al., 1973, 1974) and (3) inhibitory effects of remote visual stimuli on the visual responses of cells in the lateral suprasylvian cortex of the cat (Rizzolatti and Camarda, 1975) the regions outside the CRF were thought to be strictly spatially confined. However, as a result of studies commencing in the 1980s it gradually became apparent that the RFs of single neurons in mammalian visual cortices (and presumably in other sensory cortices) might not have fixed spatial boundaries and even the boundaries of the CRFs at any given moment could be determined by the interplay of many factors (e.g. Gilbert, 1992, 1993, 1998; Knierim and Van Essen, 1992; Lamme, 1995; Zipser et al., 1996; Polat et al., 1998; Vidyasagar, 1998; Das and Gilbert, 1999; Frégnac and Shulz, 1999; Ito and Gilbert, 1999).

The first direct challenge to the concept of spatially fixed RFs of neurons in neocortices came from studies demonstrating remarkable plasticity in topographic representations in the somatosensory (Rasmusson, 1982; Merzenich et al., 1983), auditory (Robertson and Irvine, 1989) and motor (Sanes et al., 1988) cortices of the adult mammals (see for review Kaas, 1991). At this stage it was not thought that sensory cortices of adult mammals would have any special 'plasticity' capacities, or that the demonstration of such plasticity would have special relevance for the modality concerned. Rather the attraction of studying the plasticity in sensory cortical areas was that the precision of the topographic representations could provide a suitable metric for measuring any induced plasticity.

After the first demonstrations of topographic reorganization in somatosensory and auditory cortices of adult mammals following the removal of a spatially circumscribed input from the periphery it was thought that the underlying basis of reorganization depended on the extent of arborization of thalamocortical afferents and was limited to 1–2 mm across the cortical surface (see Calford, 1991, for a review of this concept). The equivalent experiment on the topographic reorganization in the visual system was an obvious next step, but its implementation was delayed by consideration of the possible mechanism(s) underlying such reorganization as well as the spatial limitations of the proposed mechanism(s). In fact, at that time, many of the researchers involved in those kinds of studies considered it unlikely that the primary visual cortices of mammals would provide a good model for the study of adult plasticity. The reasoning was that the arborization extent of thalamocortical afferents to area V1 (cat: 1–1.5 mm, at most 2–3 mm; Ferster and LeVay, 1978; Gilbert and Wiesel, 1979, 1983; Humphrey et al., 1985; Freund et al., 1985) was less extensive than that in the primary cortices serving other sensory modalities and that the precision of visuotopy (retinotopy), at least in such highly visual mammals as cats and primates, as evidenced in the cortical representational point-spread function (radius of 1.4 mm in cat; Albus, 1975), was around the same as the expected maximum extent of topographic plasticity.

In the present article, we will review some of the functional evidence challenging the concept of the spatially fixed RFs of cells in primary visual cortices of adult and adolescent cats and adult macaque monkeys. Furthermore, this evidence will be linked with some psychophysical data derived from studies of scotomas in humans.

Reorganization of topographic maps in striate cortices of adult mammals following circumscribed retinal lesions

Starting from the first study (Kaas et al., 1990) in which laser lesions of the retina were used to demonstrate plasticity in area V1 (striate cortex, area 17), a number of studies (Heinen and Skavenski, 1991; Gilbert and Wiesel, 1992; Chino et al., 1992, 1995; Darian-Smith and Gilbert, 1995; Schmid et al., 1995, 1996; Calford et al., 1999, 2000) provided unequivocal evidence indicating reorganization of the topographic maps in primary visual cortices of adult cats and macaque monkeys. In all the studies, the basic paradigm was to use a laser to create a circumscribed retinal lesion and subsequently to record activity of single neurons (or neuronal clusters) in primary visual cortices of anesthetized, paralyzed and artificially respired animals. However, the studies differed as to whether the circumscribed retinal lesions were monocular, with (Kaas et al., 1990; Chino et al., 1992) or without (Chino et al., 1992; Schmid et al., 1996; Calford et al., 2000) removal of the other eye, or topographically matched binocular (Heinen and Skavenski, 1991; Gilbert and Wiesel, 1992; Chino et al., 1995; Darian-Smith and Gilbert, 1995). Furthermore, in some studies, lesions were aimed to deactivate only the outer retinal layers (Heinen and Skavenski, 1991; Schmid et al., 1996), while in the others, the lesions were aimed at removing all neural elements in the circumscribed retinal region (Chino et al., 1995; Calford et al., 2000). Despite these variations in the experimental paradigm, the basic findings in all the studies were the same. When adult animals with circumscribed retinal lesions were examined some weeks or months after making the retinal lesions the majority of neurons recorded from the part of striate cortex corresponding to the visuotopic (retinotopic) representation of the lesion (LPZ — lesion projection zone) had distinct RFs displaced from their expected original position to the part of the retina beyond the boundaries of the lesion ('ectopic' receptive fields). Furthermore, a proportion of ectopic RFs had multiple, spatially separated excitatory subregions often located on the opposite sites of retinal lesion (Chino et al., 1992; Gilbert and Wiesel, 1992; Calford et al., 2000). Although both simple and complex cells with spatially distinct ('split') excitatory subregions in their RFs were reported in areas 17, 18 and 19 of normal cats the excitatory discharge subfields of these cells tend to be close to each other and are never separated by more than 4° (cf. Pollen and Ronner, 1975; Feldon et al., 1978; Pollen et al., 1978; Mullikin et al., 1984).

Overall, in all studies in which the circumscribed retinal lesions were made the visuotopic map in the LPZ in area 17 appeared to be altered: the LPZ contained a clear representation of the part of the retina surrounding the lesion and as a result of it there was a clear expansion of the cortical representation of the part of the retina surrounding the lesion.

Substantial physiological and anatomical evidence indicates that in both adult cats and adult macaque monkeys after circumscribed retinal lesions there is no significant sprouting of the retino-geniculate terminals into the lesion projection zone. First, the LGNd neurons in the retinal LPZ cannot be activated by visual stimuli presented through the lesioned eye and the silent zone closely approximates in size to the normal representation of the lesioned retinal area (Eysel et al., 1980, 1981; Eysel, 1982; Eysel and Neubacher, 1984; Eysel and Wolfhard, 1984; Darian-Smith and Gilbert, 1995). Second, the displacements of the RFs observed in the projection zones of retinal lesions in area 17 of cats and macaque monkeys exceed the expected limits of the lateral spread of geniculo-cortical afferent arborizations (Ferster and LeVay, 1978; Gilbert and Wiesel, 1979, 1983; Blasdel and Lund, 1983; Humphrey et al., 1985; Freund et al., 1985, 1989) and the 'jitter' in the normal retinotopic (visuotopic) representation (as evidenced in the point-spread). Indeed, Darian-Smith and Gilbert (1995) demonstrated, using neuroanatomical tracing techniques in cats with binocular topographically corresponding retinal lesions, that the lesion projection zones in area 17 received their geniculate inputs from the LPZ in the LGNd and not from the parts of the LGNd in which cells responsive to the visual stimuli were located. Thus, sprouting of geniculo-cortical projections to area 17 could not account for the topographic reorganization observed at the cortical level. This in turn implicates a cortical mechanism rather than a thalamic mechanism in the topographic reorganization of area 17 (see section on Morphological and physiological basis of the changes in the representation in the lesion projection zones).

Short-term effects of retinal lesions on reorganization of striate cortices in adult cats and macaque monkeys

The studies of 'artificial scotomas' (see further) showing relatively rapid expansion of the extent of the visually responsive area of V1 neurons with partial visual field masking imply that visual cortex may have a capacity for immediate reorganization. There are some difficulties, however, in demonstrating that there is an immediate unmasking component to the plasticity-response induced by retinal lesions. This is because the lesion caused by laser light is based on the heat effect which appears to produce a widespread temporary deactivation precluding the study of the immediate effects. Another factor which has to be taken into consideration is the fact that the laser-lesion procedure, apart from the direct heat damage to the tissue, induces a widespread biochemical activation of a number of retinal cell classes including photoreceptors, Müller cells and ganglion cells (Tassignon et al., 1991; Yamamoto et al., 1996; Humphrey et al., 1997; Chu et al., 1998). Calford et al. (1999) monitored topographic reorganization in the striate cortex of the cat by recording extracellular activity of cells in this area over the 11 h following the creation (with laser) of circumscribed monocular lesions restricted to the outer retinal layers. During the entire period, the animals remained anesthetized and to facilitate comparisons over time, recordings were made repeatedly within the same electrode tracks. In the first hour following the creation of the lesion no neural responses could be elicited within the LPZ by photic stimulation of the lesioned eye. However, in the next 2 h (1–3 h after creation of the lesion) only 39% of the recording sites (a standard grid-pattern method of electrode movement was employed) within the LPZ remained unresponsive to photic stimuli presented via the lesioned eye and in the next few hours the percentage of the recording sites within the LPZ unresponsive to photic stimuli presented via the lesioned eye decreased further: 3–7 h, 31%; 7–11 h, 27%.

An identical recording strategy was employed in experiments involving a less traumatic lesioning procedure (Schmid et al., 1995). In this study, a lower-power laser light was used to make a small lesion in animals which had been preloaded by intravenous infusion with excess fluids. Under these conditions, a retinal detachment 4–5 times larger than the initial lesion can be induced. The detachment takes place rapidly and in most cases was stable after 1 h. Histology did not reveal any obvious damage to neural elements of the detached part of the retina. Nevertheless, the separation of the neural retina from the pigment epithelial layer rendered the detached retina inactive. Indeed, at no stage during the experiment were responses of cortical neurons evident to photic stimuli presented over the detached region of the retina. By contrast, the responses of cortical neurons within the projection zone of the detached part of the retina to photic stimulation of ectopic RFs in the unaffected part of the retina were evident immediately. However, throughout this zone, the overall proportions of responsive recording sites and the time-course of their development, were similar to those for the recording sites in the LPZ after laser lesions (Calford et al., 1999). In both paradigms, the final proportions of recording sites at which neural responses could be evoked by photic stimulation of ectopic RFs were similar to those obtained, in the same laboratory, for cases with post-lesion survival times of 2 weeks to 3 months (Schmid et al., 1996).

Three studies have reported observations of a limited short-term topographic plasticity in cats and/or macaque monkeys following topographically matched binocular retinal lesions (Heinen and Skavenski, 1991; Gilbert and Wiesel, 1992; Darian-Smith and Gilbert, 1995). In all three studies, a central silent zone was found immediately following the retinal lesions, but evidence of unmasking was also apparent. In particular, for cortical sites located close to or just inside the LPZ, cortical cells showed a substantial increase in their RF sizes. Indeed, the RF sizes fell well "outside the range for neurons at these depths and eccentricities" (Darian-Smith and Gilbert, 1995). Furthermore, the largest ectopic RFs (displaced centrifugally to the region just outside the lesion) were characteristic of cells located just inside the boundary of the LPZ (Darian-Smith and Gilbert, 1995). Although cortical cells with ectopic RFs, like cells recorded from normal cortices, tended to be binocular, orientation-selective and frequently direction-selective, their responses were weak and sluggish and habituated quickly (Darian-Smith and Gilbert, 1995).

Similarly, in the monocularly lesioned cats, the ectopic RFs of cells recorded from the LPZ of striate cortices within a few hours after placement of the retinal lesions were substantially (up to 10-fold) larger than their normal counterparts revealed by stimulation of the same cells via the unlesioned eye (Calford et al., 1999).

It is also important to point out that overall, in 'retinally deafferented' (LPZ) regions of striate cortices of adult cats, 1–2 weeks after placement of bilateral homonymous retinal lesions, both the spontaneous activity and the visually evoked activity are reported to be significantly reduced (Eysel et al., 1999). This reduction in spontaneous and visually evoked activity in the LPZ was associated with a clear (15–26%) reduction in the number of glutamate-immunoreactive neurons in both the supra- and infragranular layers. At the same time, both spontaneous and visually evoked activities are reported to be significantly increased in the regions of the cortex immediately adjacent to the LPZ (Eysel et al., 1999). Again, the increase in spontaneous and visually evoked activity was associated with a sharp increase (50–100%) in glutamate immunoreactivity in layers II–VI just outside the LPZ.

There is some difficulty in equating the extent of topographic reorganization evident in these studies of the cells in the LPZ in striate cortices of binocularly lesioned cats or macaque monkeys with those of cells in the LPZ in striate cortices of monocularly lesioned cats. The more extensive cortical reorganization reported in the cat may be related to the different method of producing the retinal lesions and/or the criteria used to define the cortical projection zone of the lesion. Additionally, the temporal and geometrical extent of any transient surrounding retinal deactivation, and hence the delay in responses becoming evident, may depend on the strength of the laser. Definition of the affected cortical area in the Heinen and Skavenski's (1991) study, which was primarily designed to examine oculomotor effects, differed from that in the other studies of retinal lesions. Thus, Heinen and Skavenski (1991) described a partially responsive cortical region (1–2 mm wide) surrounding a zone of unresponsiveness but it is not clear how this zone relates to the LPZ and whether this was an area of cortex in which neurons had reorganized RFs, or an area corresponding to regions of the retina which were indirectly affected by the laser.

Monocular vs. binocular retinal lesions

Suppression of cortical reorganization by inputs from the unlesioned eye?

Chino et al. (1992) recorded activity of neuronal clusters in area 17 of anesthetized, paralyzed and artificially respired cats in which the circumscribed lesions in the contralateral superior nasal retinae were made by photocoagulation with argon laser either immediately before the cortical mapping (immediate group) or two months before the cortical mapping (delayed group). Lesions involved all retinal layers. In both immediate and delayed groups no neuronal clusters within the LPZ responded to visual stimulation via the lesioned eye. However, in both groups of animals after removal of the other, unlesioned eye, there was an immediate 'unmasking' of responsiveness of neuronal clusters in the LPZ to the stimuli presented via the lesioned eye. Thus, Chino and colleagues concluded that the reorganization of the topographic map related to the input from one eye can be suppressed for a long time by inputs related to the other eye. Similar conclusions were made by Murakami et al. (1997) who recorded multiunit activity from the striate cortices of anesthetized, paralyzed and artificially respired monkeys 9 months after monocular circumscribed argon laser photocoagulations of the outer retinal layers were made in the proximity of the fovea. In this animal, cells in the LPZ of striate cortices were all monocular and responded only to visual stimuli presented via the unlesioned eye. Indeed, several earlier reports indicate that the input from one retina might contribute to a cortical process inhibiting the responses to stimuli presented through the other eye. Thus, iontophoretic application of bicuculline (selective blocker of $GABA_A$ receptors) into area 17 of cats monocularly deprived of pattern vision during the critical period of development (see section on Reorganization of topographic map in adult striate cortex following circumscribed monocular lesions of all retinal layers in adolescence) results in transient partial reversal of deprivation amblyopia, that is, many area 17 cells responded not only to stimuli presented via the nondeprived eye, but also (albeit usually rather weakly) to stimuli presented via the deprived eye (Burchfiel and Duffy, 1981; Sillito et al., 1981; see also Duffy et al., 1976). Similarly, in area 17 of monocularly pattern vision-deprived young cats, removal of the nondeprived eye results in a rapid, dramatic and permanent increase in the proportion of cells responding to visual stimuli presented via the remaining originally deprived eye (Kratz et al., 1976; Hoffmann and Cynader, 1977; Smith et al., 1978). Furthermore, microiontophoretic application of bicuculline into area 17 of cats reared during the early postnatal period with surgically induced squint, results in reversible restoration of binocularity in a high proportion of area 17 neurons (Mower et al., 1984). It is worth pointing out, that when bicuculline was applied iontophoretically in area 17 of normal cats a high proportion of apparently monocular cells became binocular and that both the absolute and relative strength of responses of some binocular cells to stimuli presented through either eye was also reversibly affected by iontophoretic application of bicuculline (Sillito et al., 1980).

On the other hand, Schmid et al. (1996), using a very similar experimental design, obtained quite different results. Thus, weeks to months after placement of a discrete laser lesion in the superior nasal retina of one eye (lesion was restricted to the outer layers of the retina) the activity of area 17 neurons of the anesthetized, paralyzed and artificially respired cats was studied with extracellular recording and this procedure was immediately repeated following removal (by laser coagulation of the optic nerve head) of the retinal input from the other eye. However, unlike Chino's group (1992), Schmid's group (1996) reported that removal of the retinal input from the other eye had no effect on the proportion of neurons responding to visual stimuli presented via the originally lesioned eye. Indeed, both before and after the removal of retinal input from the unlesioned eye recordings from the LPZ revealed reorganized RFs for neurons at 50–60% of sites within the LPZ.

Ectopic cortical RFs vs. retinal modulated 'periphery effect' or 'shift effect'

One interpretation of the apparent discrepancy between the results obtained by Chino's group and those obtained by Schmid's group relates to the fact that retinal lesions made by Schmid's group, unlike those made by Chino's group, were restricted to the outer retinal layers and presumably functional RGCs, albeit deprived of their input from the underlying photoreceptors, were left in situ. Thus, it has been suggested that the responsiveness of the neurons in the LPZ of area 17 of cats with monocular retinal lesions restricted to the outer retinal layers relates to the presence of RGCs in the lesioned part of the retina rather than to reorganization occurring at the cortical level (Chino et al., 1995; Horton and Hocking, 1998). According to this suggestion, the RGCs left in situ after the lesioning of the outer retinal layers might be activated by visual stimuli presented in the unlesioned parts of the retina. Indeed, in normal cats and macaques, many RGCs respond to the sudden movement of large, especially fast-moving contours well outside the cells' CRFs (McIlwain, 1966; Ikeda and Wright, 1972b; Krüger and Fischer, 1973; Krüger et al., 1975). This so-called modulated 'periphery effect' (McIlwain, 1966) or 'shift effect' (Krüger and Fischer, 1973; Fischer et al., 1975) are not due to light scattered on the cell's CRF (McIlwain, 1964; Levick et al., 1965; Barlow et al., 1977) and are especially pronounced in Y-type retinal ganglion cells (Ikeda and Wright, 1972b; Krüger and Fischer, 1973; Fischer et al., 1975; Derrington et al.,

1979). The 'modulated periphery effects' and 'shift effects' appear to be mediated by the amacrine cells (Dowling and Boycott, 1966; Werblin and Copenhagen, 1974). Both the modulated periphery effect and shift effect are also detectable in the LGNd neurons of both cats (McIlwain, 1964, 1966; Fischer and Krüger, 1974; Derrington and Fuchs, 1979; Funke et al., 1996) and macaque monkeys (Krüger, 1977). A strong periphery effect could be evoked by stimuli located as far as 30–40° away from the CRFs of the RGCs under examination, and in the case of LGNd neurons, by stimuli located in the visual field ipsilateral to the LGNd under examination (McIlwain, 1964). Thus, the ectopic RFs of neurons in the LPZ of the striate cortices of cats with monocular lesions of the outer retinal layers observed by Schmid group might represent the modulated periphery effect or shift effect of the RGCs (remaining in situ after lesion of the underlying photoreceptors and bipolar cells) and relayed to the cortex via the LGNd rather than genuine ectopic cortical RFs based on the cortico-cortical connections (Chino et al., 1995; Horton and Hocking, 1998). Following the same line of reasoning, one might interpret reported (Murakami et al., 1997) paucity of cells with ectopic RFs in the LPZ in striate cortices of macaque monkey with circumscribed monocular lesion restricted to the outer retinal layers as indicating a lack of transferability of modulated periphery or shift effects from the LGNd of macaque monkeys to the striate cortex. In particular, since the clear excitatory shift effect in monkey's LGNd is virtually restricted to the magnocellular cells (Krüger, 1977), Murakami et al. (1997) were presumably unable to detect the contribution of the magnocellular LGNd layers to the multiunit activity of cells in the LPZ in the striate cortex of the monkey examined by them.

However, several lines of evidence argue against this proposal. Thus, in animals with lesions restricted to the outer retinal layers the ectopic cortical RFs although quite large, unlike the RFs of RGCs or LGNd cells due to the periphery effect could be clearly spatially delineated (Gilbert and Wiesel, 1992; Schmid et al., 1996; Calford et al., 1999). The lack of responses of cortical neurons to photic stimuli presented over the detached region of the retina (Schmid et al., 1995) also argues against the modulated retinal periphery effect or shift effect underlying the ectopic RFs of cortical cells recorded from the projection zone of retinal detachment.

Overall, we believe it is rather unlikely that the ectopic RFs observed in animals with monocular lesions restricted to the outer layers of the retina reflect the retinal modulated periphery effect or shift effect. Nevertheless, a definitive measure of the function of surviving ganglion cells is yet to be made in retina with outer retinal lesions.

Reorganization of topographic map of one retina in adult striate cortex following circumscribed monocular lesions of all retinal layers

In our recent study (Calford et al., 2000), we obtained strong evidence indicating that cortical mechanisms rather than a retinal periphery effect underlie the topographic reorganization of area 17 following chronic monocular retinal lesions. In this series of experiments, young adult (minimum age 24 weeks at the time of lesion placement) cats were anesthetized with ketamine (40 mg/kg i.m. in Ketalar) and xylazine (4 mg/kg i.m., Rompun) and discrete retinal lesions of approximately 10–12° diameter were placed in the upper nasal retina of the left eye. The lesions were produced with an argon-green laser (see Schmid et al., 1996 for details of delivery system) focussed to approximately 300 μm at an intensity of 450–650 mW. In the lesioned regions of all eight animals, all retinal layers had been destroyed (Fig. 1A–C). In addition, in four animals, the photocoagulation also destroyed the innermost nerve fiber layer of the retina resulting in retrograde degeneration of RGCs in a large radial segment of the retina beyond the confines of the lesion (Fig. 1 A,D,E).

Two to 24 weeks after placement of the lesions, extracellular recordings were made from the part of area 17 corresponding to and surrounding the projection zone of the lesion (LPZ). The responses to visual stimuli were characterized both qualitatively (with hand-held stimuli) and quantitatively (with computer-operated stimuli). During the recording sessions, animals were anesthetized with a gaseous mixture of N_2O/O_2 (67%/33%) and halothane (0.5–0.8%). In order to minimize eye movements, animals were paralyzed with either pancuronium bromide (Pavulon 0.15 mg/kg/h i.v.) or paralysis was induced with gallamine triethiodide (7.5 mg/kg/h

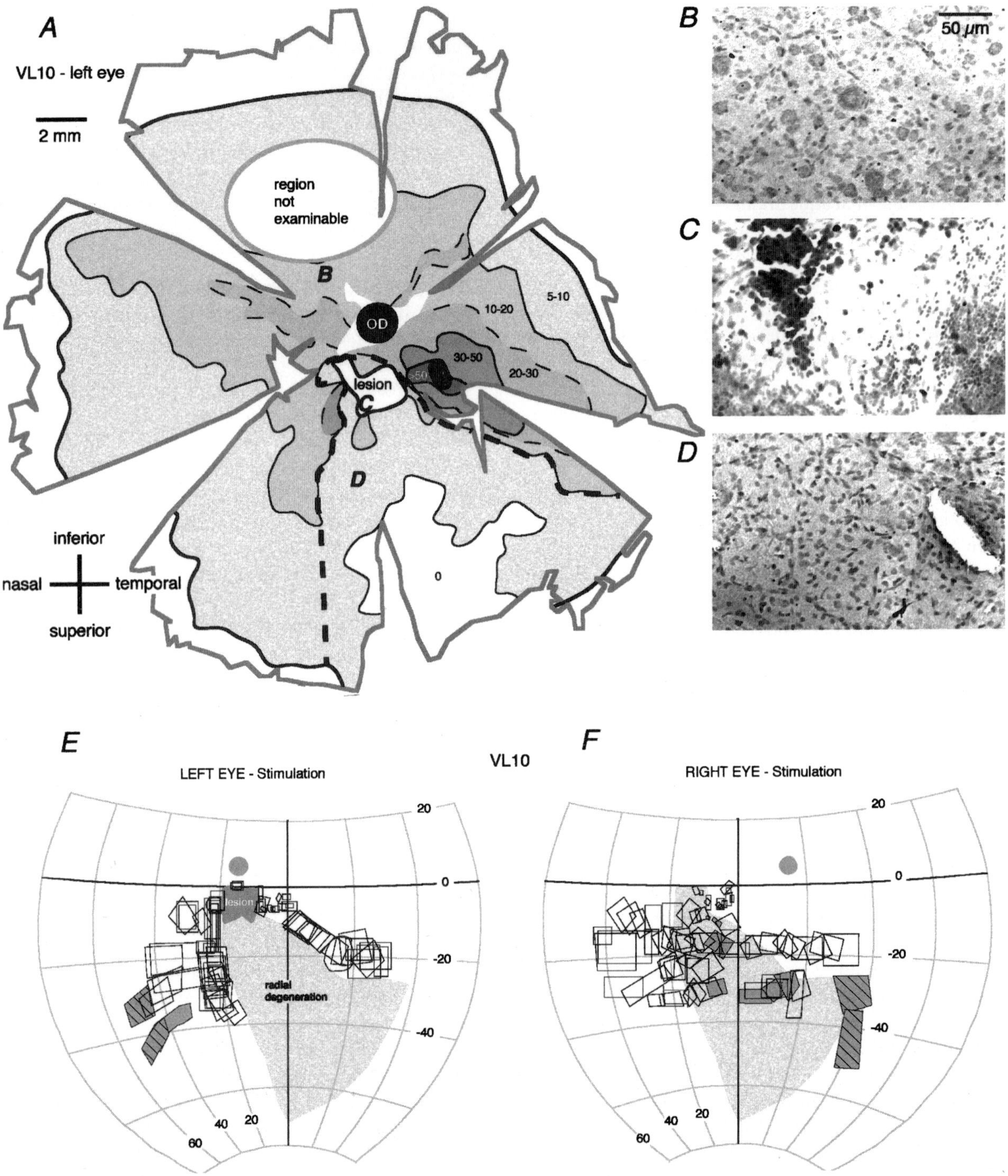
A
VL10 - left eye
2 mm
region
not
examinable
B
OD
10-20
5-10
30-50
20-30
>50
lesion
C
D
0
inferior
nasal
temporal
superior
B
50 µm
C
D
E
LEFT EYE - Stimulation
VL10
F
RIGHT EYE - Stimulation
20
0
-20
-40
lesion
radial
degeneration
60
40
20

i.v.) combined with bilateral sympathectomy. Heart rate and electro-encephalogram (EEG) were monitored continuously. By adjusting the concentration of halothane in the gaseous mixture the EEG maintained a slow wave record while heart rate was kept below 180 beats per minute.

Unlike in the report of Chino et al. (1992) cited above, despite the fact that the normal, unlesioned eye had not been removed, we have found unequivocal evidence of extensive reorganizational plasticity in the striate cortices of these animals (cf. also Rosa et al., 1995; Schmid et al., 1996; Calford et al., 1999). With visual stimulation via the lesioned (contralateral) eye about 75% of single area 17 neurons in the LPZ had ectopic visual discharge fields which were displaced to normal retina in the immediate vicinity of the lesion (Figs. 1E and 2B) or just outside the radial segment of the retina in which, due to involvement of the fibers passing through the lesioned part of the retina, the RGCs had degenerated (Fig. 1E). Thus, unlike in normal cats, in cats with monocular retinal lesions, cortical neurons recorded from the LPZ have their RFs in heterotopic parts of the visual field. The topographic map of the retina in the LPZ was reorganized only in relation to the lesioned retina.

Consistent with the fact that the retinal lesion involved all retinal layers and RGCs were absent from the lesioned region, several RF properties of cells recorded from the LPZ were clearly inconsistent with the periphery effect. Thus: (1) for binocular neurons recorded from the LPZ the sizes of the ectopic discharge fields were not significantly different from the sizes of their normal counterparts (Fig. 2C) and (2) binocular cells recorded from the LPZ when stimulated via the ectopic RFs exhibited not only normal orientation-tuning (Fig. 3A), but the preferred orientations for stimuli presented via the lesioned eye were virtually the same or very similar to the preferred orientations for stimuli presented via the normal eye (Fig. 3B). Normal orientation tuning of cells recorded from the LPZ for stimuli presented via the lesioned eye is consistent with earlier findings of Chino et al. (1995) who reported that neurons in the LPZ of striate cortices of adult cats with topographically matching lesions in two retinae exhibited strikingly normal orientation tuning (cf. also Darian-Smith and Gilbert, 1995).

Overall, most cells recorded from the LPZ were binocular, that is, they could be activated through either eye and the proportion of monocular cells in the LPZ which could be activated exclusively via the normal, ipsilateral, unlesioned eye was virtually the same as the proportion of monocular cells which could be activated exclusively via the ipsilateral eye in normal animals (Fig. 4). On the other hand: (1) the proportion of binocular cells in the LPZ dominated by the unlesioned ipsilateral eye (class 4 cells) was substantially higher (50%) than the proportion of class 4 cells in area 17 of normal cats (26.5%); (2) the proportion of monocular cells which could be activated exclusively via the lesioned, contralateral eye was substantially lower in the LPZ than the proportion of monocular cells which could be activated exclusively via the contralateral eye in area 17 of normal animals (Fig. 4); (3) in the LPZ the

Fig. 1. Anatomy of retinal lesions and displacements of cortical RFs. (A) Density contours of ganglion cells (mm^{-2}) as determined by extrapolating from the density at 410 sampled sites, each of 0.40 mm^2, on the wholemounted left retina of cat VL10. The retinal lesion produced a degeneration of ganglion cells in a radial segment (inside dashed contour) due to damage to the nerve fibre layer at the lesion site. Positions marked B, C and D indicate respectively the centers of the photomicrographs shown at the right. Micrograph C is from the edge of the lesion and reveals no surviving neurons. Micrographs B and D are of the ganglion cell layer and are from regions that would normally have similar densities of ganglion cells. Note that micrograph D from the area distal to the lesion shows clear indications of microglia activation and contains no ganglion cells. This retina was removed 15 days after production of the lesion. (E, F) Projection of all the RFs of single units and multiunit clusters recorded from area 17 of cat VL10 for stimuli presented separately through each eye (Lambert projection, 20° grid, optic disks are indicated as shaded circles), recorded from areas 17 of both hemispheres. Monocular RFs are shaded — those with a hatch pattern are probably beyond the area of binocular overlap. A laser lesion was made in the left eye, as indicated, and this produced a large segment of visual space at which neurons were unresponsive to photic stimulation. This segment of visual space corresponds to the segmental degeneration of ganglion cells shown in A. The projection of the lesion plus projection of segment of the retina in which retinal ganglion cells degenerated due to the severance of the axons in the nerve fibre layer are reproduced in F. It is apparent that many recordings were made from single units and multiunit clusters which had a normally positioned right eye RFs and displaced (ectopic) left eye RFs. (From Calford et al. (2000) with permission.)

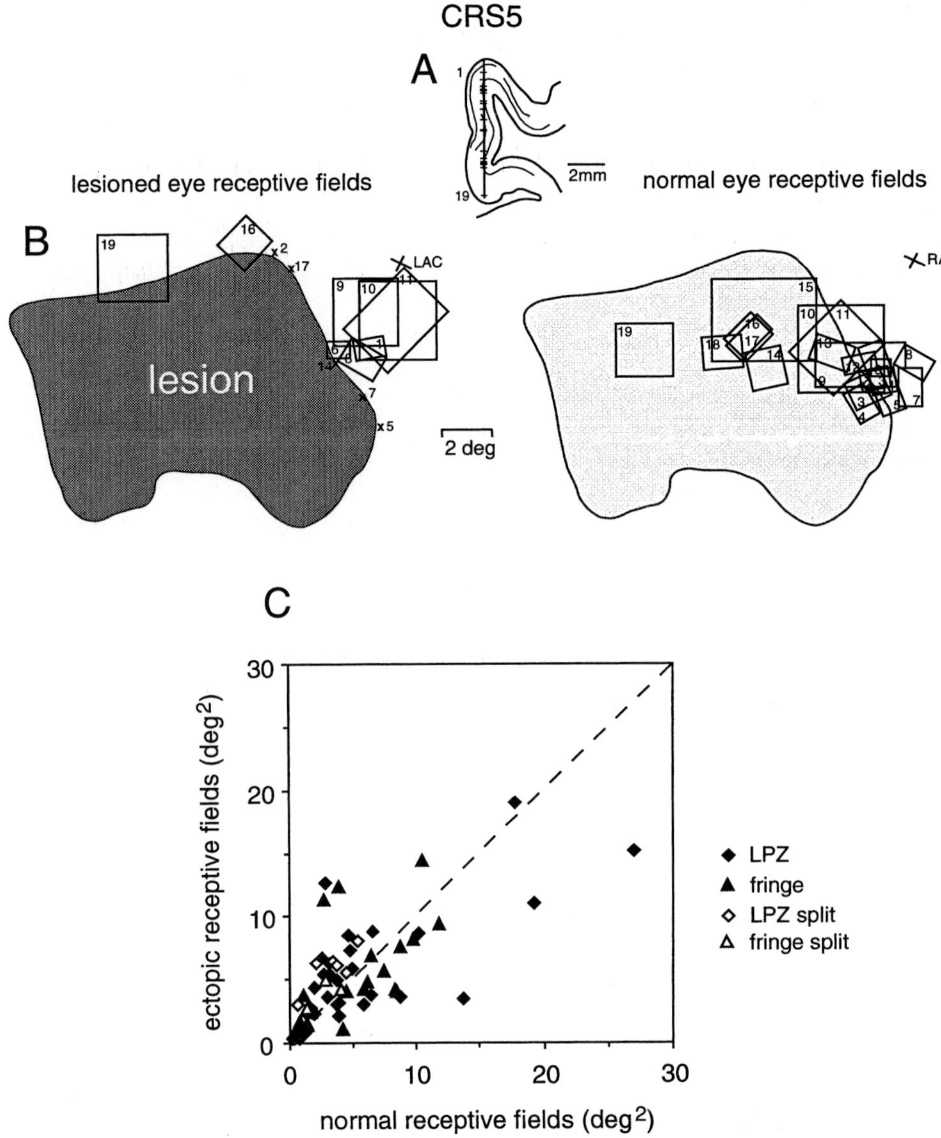

Fig. 2. Ectopic and normal RF positions and areas of cells recorded from the lesion projection zone. (A) Outline drawing of frontal section through occipital cortex of cat CRS5 to show the positions at which recordings were made. (B) Tangent screen projection of the RFs of single neurons obtained by stimulation of the lesioned eye on the left (region occupied by lesion shaded) and by stimulation of the non-lesioned eye on the right (outline of lesion included to show relative position). Left and right areae centrales are indicated by crosses and LAC, RAC, respectively. The boundaries of some RFs (visual stimuli presented via lesioned eye) could not be accurately determined and the approximate centers of these RFs are indicated by small crosses. (C) Graph of ectopic RF area versus RF area from the non-lesioned eye for 62 neurons. LPZ, lesion projection zone; fringe, border region of LPZ (1.5 mm inside the boundary); LPZ split, neurons in LPZ with split RFs (multiple excitatory discharge fields); fringe split, neurons from the border region of LPZ with split RFs. For split RFs the areas of the separate excitatory discharge subregions have been combined. Note that the LPZ split and the FPZ split cells constituted almost 15% of the sample (9/62). For neurons with single RFs to stimulation of the lesioned eye, the areas of the ectopic and normal RFs were not significantly different ($P > 0.05$) and were significantly correlated for locations both in the center of the LPZ ($r^2 = 0.53$, $P < 0.001$) and in the fringe region ($r^2 = 0.32$, $P < 0.001$). (Modified from Calford et al. (2000) with permission.)

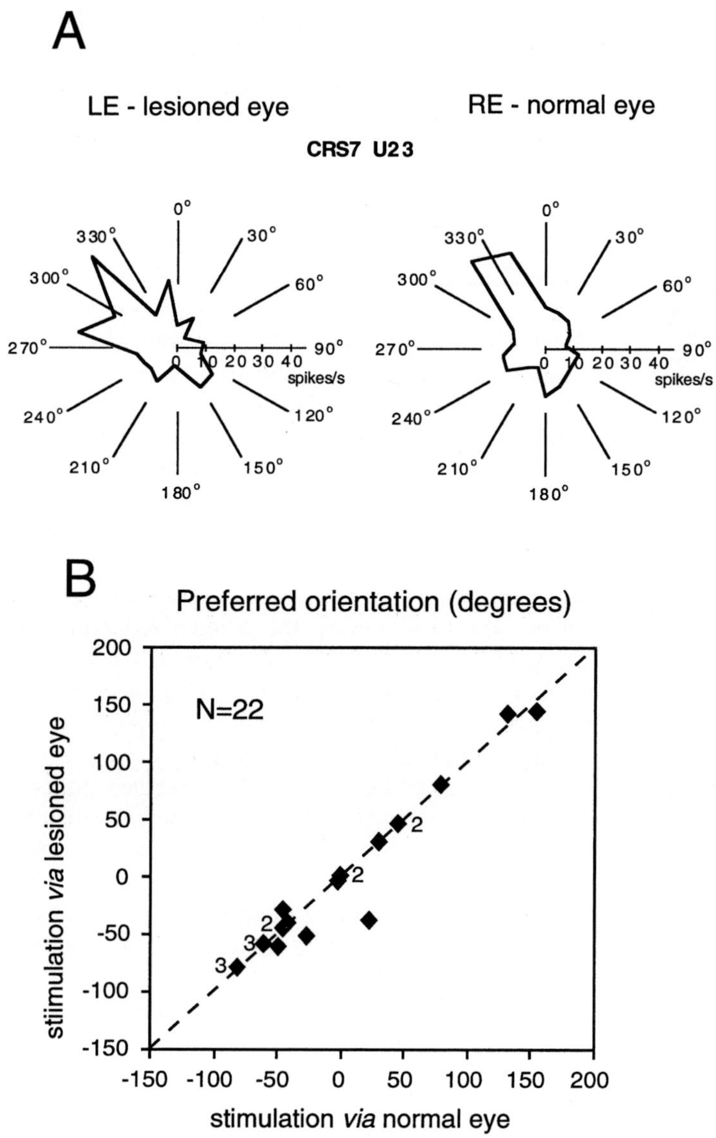

Fig. 3. Orientation tuning for ectopic and normal RFs of cells recorded from the lesion projection zone in area 17. (A) Polar plots of the orientation tuning of the peak excitatory response of a neuron recorded from the lesion projection zone (LPZ) to stimulation of each eye with bars of optimal size moving at preferred velocity. Note the similarity of preferred orientations and direction selectivities. (B) Graph of preferred orientations for 22 neurons recorded from the LPZ of adult cats with monocular circumscribed lesions of the retinae made in adulthood. Note that preferred orientations for stimuli presented through the normal and through lesioned eye are almost perfectly matched. (Modified from Calford et al. (2000) with permission.)

proportion of binocular cells dominated by the input from the lesioned, contralateral eye (class 2 cells) was substantially lower than the proportion of class 2 cells in area 17 of normal cats; and (4) over a third (38.5%) of class 4 cells recorded from the LPZ responded so poorly to photic stimulation via the lesioned eye that we were unable to fully delineate the extent of their ectopic RFs (see Fig. 2B).

Indeed, despite the fact that the great majority of cells recorded from the LPZ responded to stimuli presented via the lesioned eye, the responses to optimal stimuli (optimal orientation, optimal velocity,

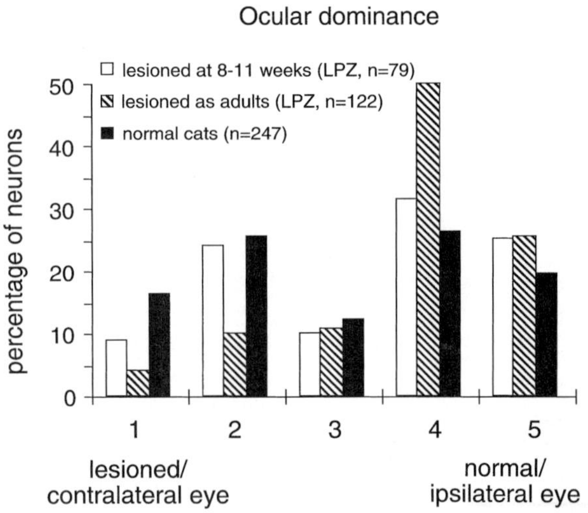

Fig. 4. Ocular dominance of area 17 cells in adult normal cats and from LPZ of cats with circumscribed retinal lesions. Neurons were divided into five groups: 1 and 5 comprised monocular neurons which could be activated only by visual stimuli presented via the contralateral (lesioned) and ipsilateral (normal) eyes respectively; 2 and 4 comprised binocular neurons with stronger response to visual stimuli presented via the lesioned and non-lesioned eyes respectively; group 3 cells responded about equally strongly to stimuli presented via either eye. Data from normal cats shown in black (Burke et al., 1992); from cats lesioned as adults, hatched (Calford et al., 2000); and from cats lesioned in adolescence, white (Dreher et al., 2000). There was a significant difference in the distribution of groups between normal cats and adult-lesioned cats ($\chi^2 = 447$; $P < 0.001$) but not between normal cats and cats lesioned in adolescence.

etc.) presented via ectopic discharge fields were generally weaker (lower peak discharge rates) than those to optimal stimuli presented via normal discharge fields. Furthermore, despite the fact that preferred stimulus velocities when cells were stimulated via the ectopic RFs (Fig. 5A) were indistinguishable from those found when the cells were stimulated via the normal eyes, their upper-velocity limits were usually substantially lower than normal (Figs. 5B and 6). These findings are consistent with the findings of Chino et al. (1995) who reported that neurons in the LPZ of striate cortices of adult cats with topographically matching lesions in two retinae have abnormally elevated contrast thresholds and their response magnitudes under optimal stimulus conditions were significantly reduced.

Our observations that, several weeks or months following the monocular retinal lesions, the ectopic discharge fields revealed by photic stimulation via the lesioned eyes were not significantly larger than the corresponding discharge fields revealed by stimulation via the normal unlesioned eyes seem to be in conflict with earlier reports indicating that both in cats (Gilbert and Wiesel, 1992; Chino et al., 1995; Darian-Smith and Gilbert, 1995) and macaques (Gilbert and Wiesel, 1992; Darian-Smith and Gilbert, 1995) the RFs of neurons recorded from the LPZs of area 17 several months after the topographically matched binocular retinal lesions, were slightly but significantly larger than the RFs of cells recorded from the same region of the cortex *before the retinal lesions*. However, the RFs of neurons recorded from the LPZs of area 17 of cats and macaques, several months after the topographically matched binocular retinal lesions, were substantially smaller than the receptive fields of cells recorded from the LPZs of area 17 *immediately after placement of the retinal lesions*. Thus, the trend toward the gradual reduction with time of the ectopic RF sizes in mammalian area 17 is apparent not only in animals with monocular retinal lesions, but also in animals with the topographically matched binocular retinal lesions.

Our data combined with those obtained from cats and macaque monkeys with topographically matched binocular retinal lesions (Gilbert and Wiesel, 1992; Chino et al., 1995; Darian-Smith and Gilbert, 1995) suggest that the general trend towards shrinkage of the ectopic RFs might be strengthened by some sort of suppressive effect exerted on the ectopic RFs by the presence of input from the unlesioned eye from the part of the retina topographically corresponding to the lesion.

Reorganization of topographic map in adult striate cortex following circumscribed monocular lesions of all retinal layers in adolescence

As we have mentioned above, the relative weakness of the responses of cells in the LPZ to stimuli presented via the ectopic RFs is apparent not only in adult cats with monocular retinal lesions involving all retinal layers (Calford et al., 2000), but also in adult cats with topographically matching lesions in both retinae (Chino et al., 1995). Thus, postulated suppression of the reorganization of the topographic map related to the input from one eye by inputs

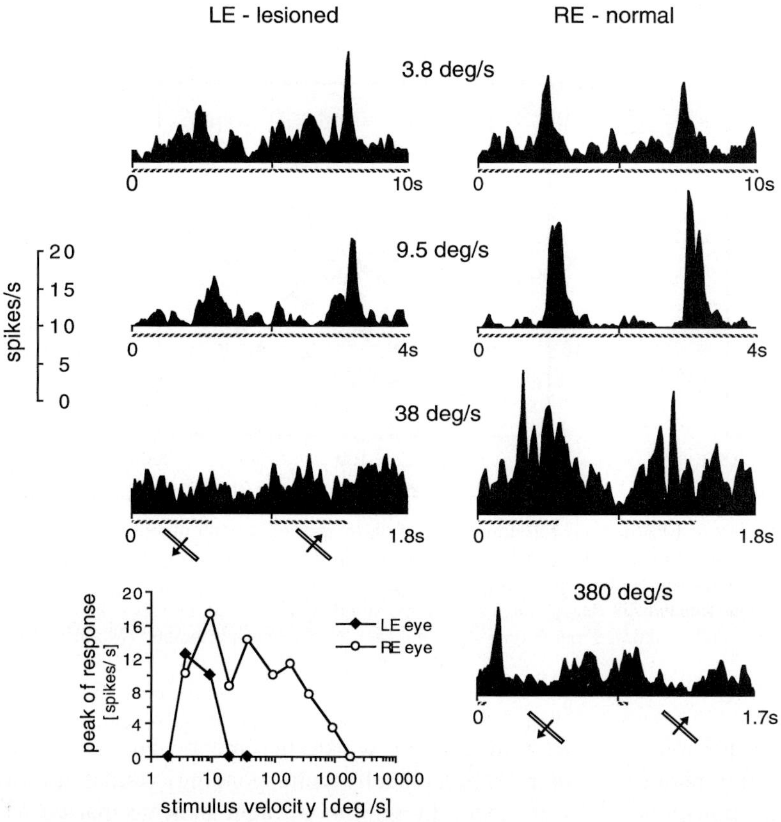

Fig. 5. Velocity tuning for ectopic and normal RFs in adult-lesioned cats. Upper, peristimulus response–time histograms to a horizontal light bar (5.5 × 0.6°) moving at the indicated velocities (center) and presented via the right (normal, ipsilateral) or the left (lesioned, contralateral) eye. The RF revealed by photic stimulation of the right (normal) eye was located in the region corresponding to the projection of the retinal lesion in the left eye; the RF of the left eye was located just outside the lesion projection. Lower left, velocity selectivity curves for the peak responses of this neuron. The records are typical in showing that there are responses at higher velocities for stimulation of the normal eye than for stimulation of the lesioned eye. Each histogram was compiled from 30 stimulus sweeps; hatched lines under the timebase indicate the duration of bar movement. (Modified from Calford et al. (2000) with permission.)

related to the other eye cannot be the only factor underlying the relative weakness of responses to stimuli presented via the ectopic RFs.

It has been well documented that when one eye of a cat or macaque monkey is deprived of form vision during early postnatal life, this eye becomes amblyopic. Indeed, the great majority of neurons in the striate cortices of cats or monkeys monocularly deprived of form vision during the early postnatal period can be excited only by photic stimuli presented via the non-deprived eye (Wiesel and Hubel, 1963, 1965; Hubel and Wiesel, 1970; Shatz and Stryker, 1978; LeVay et al., 1980; see for reviews Movshon and Van Sluyters, 1981; Wiesel, 1982; Sherman and Spear, 1982). The proportion of cells which could be activated by visual stimuli presented via the deprived eye is highest in layer 4 (e.g. Shatz and Stryker, 1978) and after a brief (24 h) period of monocular deprivation, normal binocularity in layer 4 is preserved, while in the extragranular layers, virtually all cells respond only to stimuli presented via the non-deprived eye (Trachtenberg et al., 2000). This in turn suggests that monocular deprivation affects mainly cortico-cortical synapses rather than geniculo-cortical synapses. Indeed, monocular deprivation during the critical postnatal period results in great reduction of functional cortico-cortical interactions as indicated by paucity of the slow-distributed component of field potentials when non-retinotopic loci are stimulated via the deprived eye (Kasamatsu et al., 1998).

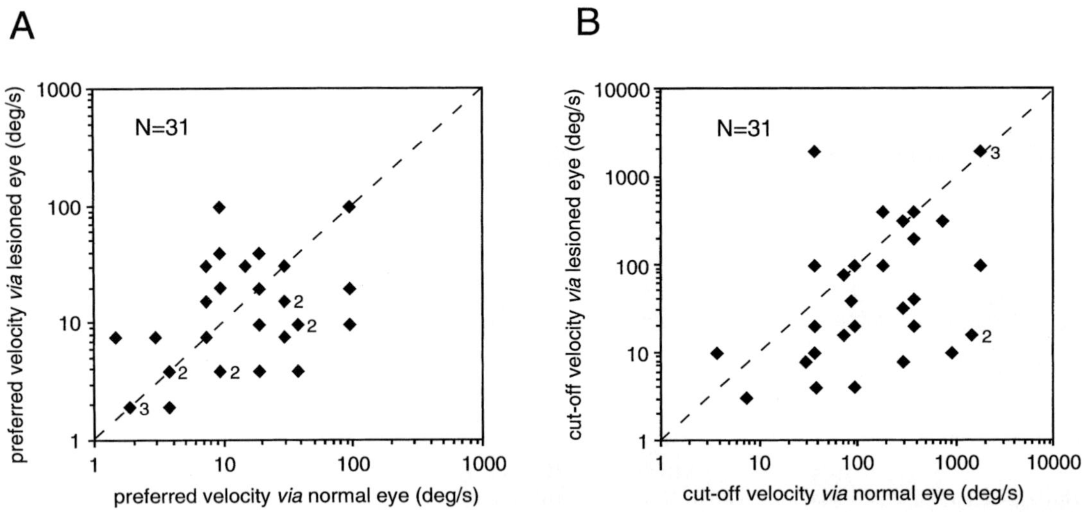

Fig. 6. Pairwise comparisons of the velocity sensitivity of LPZ neurons for stimulation of either eye. (A) Graph of velocity giving the maximal response to stimulation of each eye (preferred velocity). (B) Graph of upper velocity limit of excitatory responsiveness to stimulation of each eye (cut-off velocity). Stimuli were at optimal orientation for each RF. The velocity cut-off for normal eye stimulation (median 190 deg/s) was significantly higher than that (median 38 deg/s) for lesioned eye stimulation ($P < 0.004$), but there was no significant difference between the preferred velocities ($P > 0.05$). Figures on graphs indicate double or triple points. (Modified from Calford et al. (2000) with permission.)

Similarly, when kittens or young macaque monkeys are reared during the early postnatal period with artificial (surgically induced) squint, binocular interactions in the striate cortices are dramatically disrupted and virtually all cells become monocular, that is, they could be activated only via one eye, either the normal or the squinting eye (Hubel and Wiesel, 1965b; Baker et al., 1974; see for reviews Movshon and Van Sluyters, 1981; Wiesel, 1982). A similar loss of binocularity in striate cortices is apparent if each eye of the 1–10-week-old kittens is deprived of contour vision on alternative days (Hubel and Wiesel, 1965b).

The susceptibility to form deprivation appears to be largely restricted to the relatively well defined short period (from 1 to 4 postnatal months in kittens and about the first year of postnatal life in macaque monkeys) and prolonged monocular deprivation of pattern vision after this critical period induces only very moderate plastic changes in the visual cortices (Wiesel and Hubel, 1963; Hubel and Wiesel, 1970; Blakemore and Van Sluyters, 1974; LeVay et al., 1980; Olson and Freeman, 1980; Blakemore et al., 1978, 1981).

We wondered if the relative weakness of responses to visual stimuli presented via the ectopic RFs in cats in which the monocular (or binocular topographically corresponding) retinal lesions were made in adulthood might indicate that the lesion-induced topographic reorganization of striate cortex in adult animals represents only the tail end of cortical plasticity. To test this idea, intense monocular laser lesions were made in a number of adolescent 8–11-week-old kittens (Burke et al., 2000; Dreher et al., 2000). The lesions removed all cellular layers in a circumscribed region (~12° in diameter) in the superior nasal retina. Six to 12 months later, the striate cortices of these animals were studied electrophysiologically (for details of experimental procedures see section on Reorganization of topographic map of one retina in adult striate cortex following circumscribed monocular lesions of all retinal layers). In these animals, as in the cats in which circumscribed monocular retinal lesions were made in adulthood (Calford et al., 2000), visual stimulation via the lesioned (contralateral eye) resulted in activation of about 75% of single neurons in the LPZ and their ectopic visual discharge fields were displaced to normal retina in the immediate vicinity of the lesion. Furthermore, as in cats with retinal lesions made in adulthood (Calford et al., 2000), in these cats: (1) the sizes of the ectopic discharge fields of binocular neurons recorded from the LPZ were not significantly different from the sizes of their normal counterparts; and (2) binocular cells recorded from the LPZ when stimulated via the ectopic RFs exhibited orientation-tuning and preferred stimulus velocities which were indistinguishable from those found when the cells were stimulated via the normal eyes.

However, in contrast to cats in which the retinal lesions were made in adulthood, in cats lesioned in adolescence the ocular dominance distribution of cells recorded from the LPZ of striate cortex did not differ significantly from that of cells recorded from the striate cortices of cats without retinal lesions (Fig. 4). Indeed, many binocular cortical neurons recorded from the LPZ of cats operated on in adolescence responded more vigorously when visual stimuli were presented via the lesioned eye (Fig. 7) and overall the peak discharge rates of binocular cells to photic stimuli presented via the ectopic RFs were not significantly different from those to stimuli presented via their normal counterparts.

Thus, despite the fact that we have made the retinal lesions in adolescent cats at the time when the susceptibility to monocular deprivation of pattern vision is past its peak (4–6 weeks postnatally; Blakemore and Van Sluyters, 1974; Olson and Freeman, 1978, 1980), it appears that in cats operated at 8–11 weeks postnatal, the presumed cortical mechanism(s) underlying the topographic reorganization of area 17 following monocular retinal lesions, as far as the strength of the response is concerned, is capable of full compensation for the loss of the retinal input relayed directly to the cortex via the dorsal thalamus.

Artificial scotomas

The use of 'artificial scotomas' has proved very useful for understanding the perceptual changes that result from retinal lesions. The term 'artificial scotoma' is not always used in the same way. Thus, Gerrits et al. (1966) use it to describe the disappearance of a stabilized retinal image. It had previously been shown by Ditchburn and Ginsborg (1952) that there is a transient fading of an image when micro-saccades are nullified. There is a long history of demonstrations of disappearances of peripheral targets displayed on a uniform field. Thus, even when micro-saccades are occurring normally, small, low-contrast objects in the periphery of the visual field can become indistinguishable from the background, provided fixation is well maintained (the Troxler effect). Troxler (1804) found that his target reappeared if it moved or if there were eye movements or blinks. An important feature that emerged from subsequent work was the nature of the background to the target. Anstis (1989) showed that a target of drifting dots disappeared if the surround consisted of dynamic noise, but not if it was stationary. Spillman and Kurtenbach (1992) used a small uniform target of medium contrast placed at 10° eccentricity and showed that it faded much more quickly if the background consisted of dynamic noise than if the background consisted of static noise or uniform texture; fading was also faster with static noise than with uniform background. Overall, all these findings can be summarized by saying that movement of the target opposes fading, whereas movement of the background facilitates fading.

It is uncertain where in the visual pathways these effects occur. Although center–surround interactions and interactions with surrounds outside the CRFs can be demonstrated in RGCs and in the LGNd (see references in Introduction), it is probable that major effects occur in the visual cortex, especially in areas V2 or V3 of the macaque monkey where neurophysiological correlates of the filling-in process have been described (De Weerd et al., 1995).

More recently 'artificial scotoma' is taken to mean a region of retina that is shielded from photic stimulation, while at the same time the surrounding region is exposed to such stimulation. Using this method, several authors (Fiorani et al., 1992; Pettet and Gilbert, 1992; DeAngelis et al., 1995) carried the study of the interactions between target and surround an important step further. Thus, Pettet and Gilbert (1992) recorded from single cells in area 17 of the cat and stimulated the retina with a pattern of moving lines, while masking out the region corresponding to the CRF of the cell. After a conditioning period of 15 min, this artificial scotoma resulted in an average 5-fold expansion in RF area. Stimulation of the CRF caused a shrinkage of the RF back to its original size. Further surround stimulation led to an additional increase in area and the sequence of RF expansion and contraction could be repeated in-

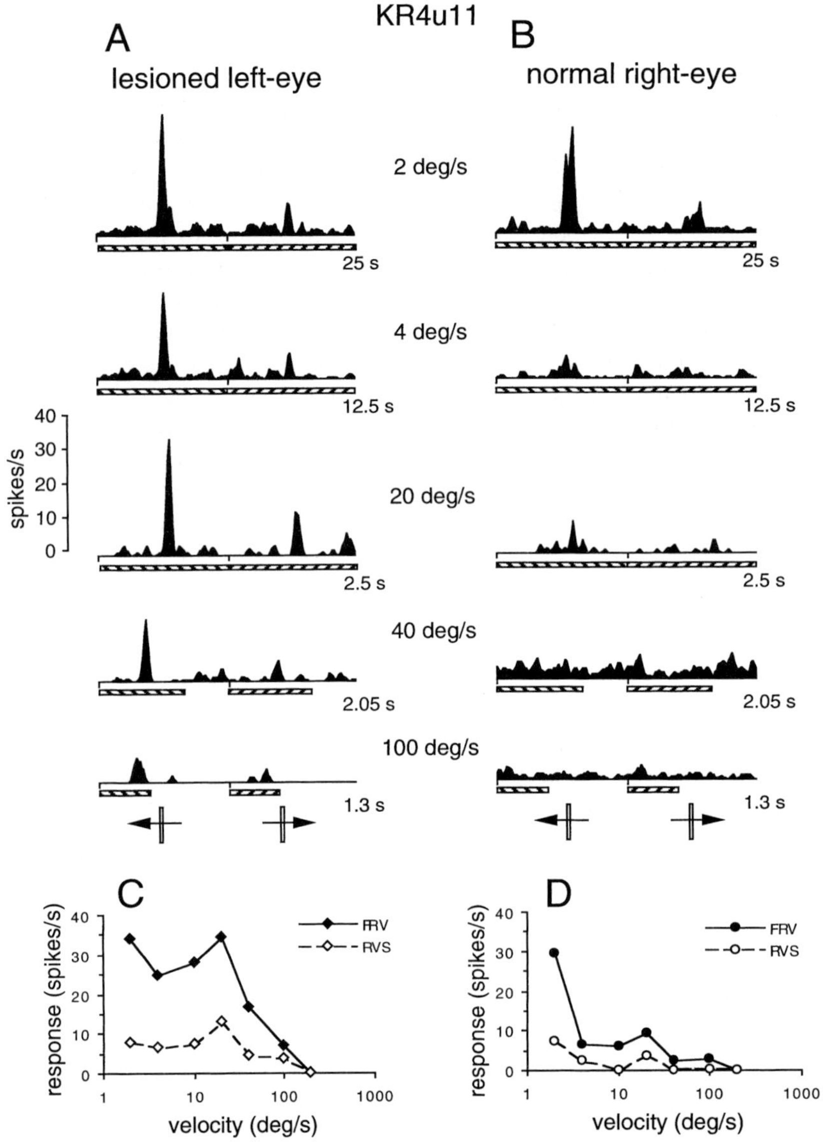

Fig. 7. Velocity tuning for ectopic and normal RFs in kitten-lesioned cats. (A, B) Peristimulus response–time histograms to a vertical light bar (8.5 × 0.5°) moving at the indicated velocities (center). Hatched lines under the timebase indicate the duration of bar movement. The RF of the right eye was in a region corresponding to the lesioned part of the left eye. (C, D) Graphs of response versus velocity for the left eye (C) and right eye (D). FRV, responses for the forward (preferred) direction; RVS, responses for the reverse direction. Note the similarity of the preferred and cut-off velocities for the two eyes: compare and contrast with Fig. 5.

definitely, although with longer-lasting effects on expansion as time progressed. DeAngelis et al. (1995) performed similar experiments, but interpreted their results as indicating a change in gain rather than a change in RF size. Pettet and Gilbert (1992) used their results to propose a way in which 'filling-in' of scotoma, or, indeed, any other non-stimulated region of retina, can occur. RFs of cortical cells receiving input from a 'silent' region of retina increase in size to encompass regions of retina outside the scotoma (or unstimulated region). Thus, these cortical cells are now getting input from outside the scotoma and therefore signal a 'filling-in' or disappearance of the scotoma or target. This explains also why fading is slower if there is no pattern or no movement in the region outside the scotoma (Ramachandran et al., 1993). Finally, Pettet and Gilbert (1992) suggest that the same process may account for the completion of the so-called illusory contours (Von der Heydt et al., 1984; Peterhans and von der Heydt, 1989; Von der Heydt and Peterhans, 1989), although why this type of filling-in is quite common in area V2 of macaque monkeys (Von der Heydt et al., 1984; Peterhans and von der Heydt, 1989; Von der Heydt and Peterhans, 1989; Leventhal et al., 1998) and area V2 (area 18) of cats (Leventhal et al., 1998), but much less common in area V1 (area 17) of macaques (Grosof et al., 1993; Leventhal et al., 1998) or cats (Leventhal et al., 1998), is not clear.

It would follow from the above discussion that unequal stimulation of parts of the retina might result in confusion about the position of certain features in the visual field. Such mislocation, albeit to a minor degree, has been demonstrated by Kapadia et al. (1994) who studied spatial localization around an artificial scotoma in human subjects. After experiencing an artificial scotoma similar to that used by Pettet and Gilbert (1992), the subject made an error in locating the position of a target bar, the bar appearing to be shifted towards the interior of the scotoma. Kapadia et al. (1994) were able to explain the shift by making two assumptions. First, that the position of a target is estimated by integration of all the discharges in the afferent sensory neurons stimulated by the target, due regard being paid to the position signaled by each of the neurons. Second, the RFs of the 'silent' neurons are enlarged as in the Pettet and Gilbert (1992) experiment. Thus, in the test run, stimuli outside the target are able to excite neurons whose labeled positions are inside the scotoma. The estimation of the target's position is therefore biased towards the scotoma.

As indicated above, some adaptive changes occur in the retina and the LGNd, but it is generally agreed that the major change occurs in visual cortex. Strong evidence in support of this belief was the demonstration by Volchan and Gilbert (1994) that for neurons in area 17 of the cat conditioning one eye with an artificial scotoma causes an expansion of their RF irrespective of the eye through which the conditioning stimuli were presented and the eye through which the effects of conditioning were tested.

Consistent with this, it has been recently demonstrated in humans that light deprivation for 45–60 min leads to a significant (reversible) increase in excitability in visual cortex, measured by transcranial magnetic stimulation and functional magnetic resonance imaging, a change that was absent at LGNd level (Boroojerdi et al., 2000).

A further indication that the changes occur in the visual cortex and to only a minor degree or not at all in the retina or LGNd is the result obtained by De Weerd et al. (1995). These authors recorded from single cells in areas V1, V2 and V3 of macaque monkeys and found that if the CRF of the cell was not stimulated, but the surrounding region was stimulated by a large textured surround, the cell exhibited 'climbing activity' defined as a gradually increasing level of activity. The increase in activity was significant for neurons recorded from areas V2 and V3, but not for those recorded from area V1. The activity of neurons in area V3 increased to a value not significantly different from that obtained when the RFs were covered by the textured field. The increase in activity of neurons in area V2 did not reach this level. The time course of the increases in activity was similar to that of the filling-in process recorded by human subjects viewing the same stimulus. De Weerd et al. (1998) believe that the time taken for filling-in is related to the time required for figure–ground segregation to fail rather than for the spread of background across the target because it is proportional to the length of contour or the area of profile filled in.

A further important feature of the expansion of RFs resulting from artificial scotomas is that cells in area 17 that are already closely linked (substantial RF overlap, similar orientation preferences and direction selectivities, strongly binocular) become even more closely linked, as evidenced by increases in area of cross-correlogram peaks (Das and Gilbert, 1995). Thus, excitation of the common RF surround of cells tends to synchronize their subsequent responses. This might have a strong influence on perception.

In spite of the similarities between filling-in of profiles and enlargement of RFs in artificial scotomas, there is also a fundamental difference in that only seconds are required for the former whereas, several minutes are needed for the latter. Also, the former process can be mimicked in areas V2 and V3, but not in area V1 (De Weerd et al., 1995), whereas the latter can be demonstrated in area V1. Although the effect of lesions seems similar to that of artificial scotomas, there is the difference that the latter transfers to the unconditioned eye, whereas this is not so for lesions.

Perceptual consequences of retinal lesions in human

Patients with degenerative eye disease experience a variety of perceptual distortions, including, in some cases, visual hallucinations and illusions (for a recent review see ffytche and Howard, 1999). One of the commonest distortions is termed metamorphopsia. Very often a patient with a central retinal lesion does not present with a scotoma, but complains that objects appear distorted or fragmented (Morgan and Schatz, 1985; Smith et al., 1990). For example, when a patient with central retinal lesion involving the fovea views an Amsler Chart (Fig. 8A) the lines appear bent (Fig. 8B). Depending on the position and extent of the retinal lesion, the distortion takes many forms. The smaller the lesion and the more peripheral it is, the greater the chance that the perception of any different appearance will disappear — the scotoma is 'filled in'. Even a large scotoma such as the optic disc, less than 20° from the fovea, is normally not distinguishable from the background (Ramachandran, 1992).

The time course of the 'filling-in' process for a retinal scotoma was first determined by Gerrits and Timmerman (1969). In their patients a scotoma was 'filled in' immediately by the color of a surrounding colored patch. They contrast this with the time for fading of a stabilized image (Gerrits et al., 1966) which takes several seconds.

The peripheral placement of scotomas makes a true description of the filling-in details difficult because of the reduced acuity. Craik (1966) inflicted a foveal scotoma on his right eye by fixating the sun for 2 min. He reported that 6 h later, the scotoma was subjectively filled in with the color of the adjacent background: small objects (less than 1°) within the scotoma were not seen: wires were seen as thinner.

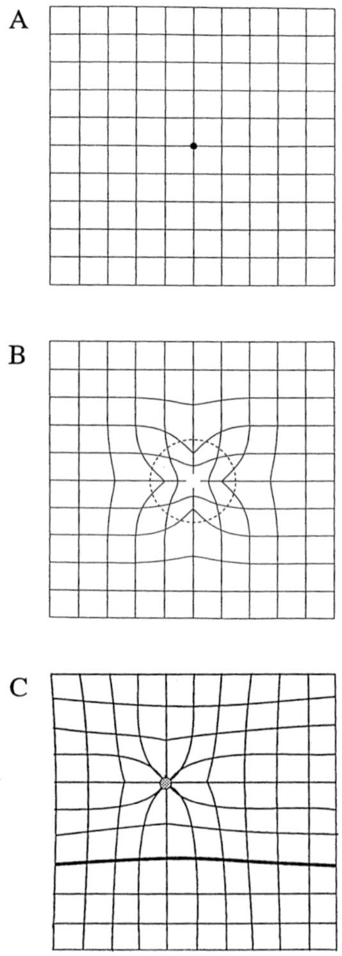

Fig. 8. Distortion of perception due to retinal lesion. (A) Amsler Chart, a Cartesian grid used as a test for metamorphopsia in patients with retinal lesions. (B) Appearance of Amsler Chart viewed at a distance such that the lines are 0.5° apart, as seen by eye with macular hole. The dashed circle indicates the size of the scotoma in this eye. Note the radial distortion extending well outside the scotoma (Burke et al., 1999). (C) Diagram presented by Gilbert (1992, 1993) to represent the distorted topography in the primary visual cortex of a monkey 2 months after a laser lesion in the retina of one eye, as inferred from electrophysiological observations. Allowing for differences in the sizes of the lesions, their positions on the retina and the scaling of the chart, B and C are remarkably similar.

Other observations indicated a radial distortion. For example, a black ring held at such a distance that it just overlapped the edges of the scotoma appeared as a uniform dark-gray disk: a ring of white spots appeared as a white disc. Craik reported that movement over the scotoma prevented the filling in. A month after inflicting the lesion, Craik found distortion of perception over an area about 2° in diameter centered on the fovea, involving curving of straight lines. He ascribed this distortion to changes in the retina, although he admitted the possibility of effects within central visual nuclei. Lewis et al. (1986) also reported inward bending of horizontal paracentral lines.

A more complete description of the distortion experienced following a central retinal lesion was provided by one of us (W. Burke, 1999) who recently experienced a macular hole, that is, a scotoma due to a localized detachment of the retina at the fovea (Gass, 1997). The detached retina may remain viable for some time at least; it is, however, non-functional, probably because of separation from the pigment epithelium. Although there is a popular belief that the filling-in process involves a copying of the surround region onto the scotomatous region, this is a mistaken idea, partly due to the use of homogeneous colored backgrounds or surrounds containing random elements. The perceptual distortion observed by W.B. is most simply illustrated by the appearance of the Amsler Chart (Fig. 8B). Whatever elements lie outside the scotoma are displaced radially inwards. In agreement with Gerrits and Timmerman (1969), this filling-in is always present: at no time is there a distortion-free image. It is interesting to compare the appearance of the Amsler Chart (Fig. 8A) as viewed by the lesioned eye (Fig. 8B) with the distorted projection of the visual field onto the visual cortex as inferred from animal experiments (Fig. 8C; Gilbert, 1992, 1993). Allowing for differences in size and position of the lesion on the retina and the scaling of the Chart, there is a striking similarity in the two diagrams. This reinforces the suggestion that the significant changes leading to the 'metamorphopsia' occur in the cortex.

Nevertheless, topographic post-lesion changes in the retina have been also reported. For example, according to Busch et al. (1999) following a circumscribed retinal lesion in the rat there is a slight movement of the surviving retina (around the lesion) inwards, the outer segments of the photoreceptors moving most (up to 200 μm). If such inward movement of the retina into the lesion occurs in the human it would have the opposite perceptual effect to that observed, i.e. there would be a radial distortion *outwards*. Patients with central scotomas tend to form new fixation points (Craik, 1966) and, with practice and good viewing conditions, can develop adequate reading skills with high accuracy albeit reduced speed (Cummings et al., 1985). Some patients use more than one fixation point (Duret et al., 1999). These adaptations should reduce the distortion.

Morphological and physiological basis of the changes in the representation in the lesion projection zones

The changes that occur during artificial scotomas and as a result of retinal lesions have led to a discussion about the underlying morphology. A basic fact that must be explained is that an ectopic RF can be sited at a considerable distance from the original RF of the neuron. Although to our knowledge so far the maximal extent of the limits of displacement from the original RFs for the cells recorded from within the LPZ in striate cortices has not been adequately explored, some estimate of the extent of displacements can be gleaned from the figures presented in relevant papers. Thus, in macaque monkeys with binocular parafoveal lesions Gilbert and Wiesel (1992) show displaced RFs which would normally be represented at sites at least 6 mm away (parallel to the cortical surface). Although Heinen and Skavenski (1991) do not present comparable receptive-field displacement data in striate cortices for their case of binocular foveal lesion in macaque monkey, based on the size of their lesions and the extent of a centrally projecting unresponsive zone it can be estimated that the reorganized zone extends around 5 mm from the LPZ boundary. Similarly, in the studies involving recording from the striate cortices of the cats in which retinal lesions were made several months earlier, examples of RF displacements greater than 6–8 mm have been presented (Kaas et al., 1990; Gilbert and Wiesel, 1992; Darian-Smith and Gilbert, 1994, 1995; Schmid et al., 1996). By contrast, the reorganization of the LPZ observed immediately after the placements of monocular retinal lesion and enucleation of the non-lesioned eye extended only over 2–3 mm of the cortex (Chino et al., 1992). For long-term human foveal lesions, the observed deflection of a straight line can be up to 0.8° (Burke, 1999), equivalent to 8 mm in the human primary visual cortex (Virsu and Hari, 1996).

As we have mentioned earlier (see section on Reorganization of topographic maps in striate cortices of adult mammals following circumscribed retinal lesions) there is no significant sprouting of the retinogeniculate terminals into the lesion projection zone and sprouting of geniculocortical projections to area 17 could not account for the topographic reorganization observed at the cortical level. Indeed, the widespread horizontal cortico-cortical connections appear to provide the anatomical basis for a number of functional findings indicating integration of signals over wide areas of visual cortex. First, in the cat at least, the synaptic integration fields of area 17 neurons are much larger than the CRFs (Bringuier et al., 1999). Second, the nonretinotopic slow component of field potentials evoked from recording sites within cat's area 17 by contrast reversal of oriented bar gratings indicates the presence of RFs encompassing wide areas of the visual field (Kitano et al., 1994). Third, in adult cats whose visual experience was restricted to vertically oriented grating moving unidirectionally at fixed distance in front of the restrained animals, a substantial proportion (over 10%) of neurons in areas 17 and 18 has excitatory receptive fields extending over as much as 15° and containing multiple spatially separated (more than 4°) excitatory discharge regions (Singer and Tretter, 1976a). Such cells, albeit less common, are also present in areas 17 and 18 of adult cats binocularly deprived (from birth) of contour vision as well as in areas 17 of the young kittens studied at the beginning of the critical period (Singer and Tretter, 1976b). Cells with such large receptive fields containing widely spatially separated excitatory discharge regions are intermingled with small conventional receptive fields located in the visuotopically appropriate parts of the contralateral visual field (Singer and Tretter, 1976a,b). Fourth, in adult cats with topographically corresponding binocular retinal lesions (Chino et al., 1992; Gilbert and Wiesel, 1992) or monocular retinal lesions (Calford et al., 2000) a substantial proportion of ectopic receptive fields contains widely separated excitatory discharge regions ('split' receptive fields). Presumably, a dynamic balance between excitatory inputs tending to enlarge RFs and more localized inhibitory interconnections tending to restrict RFs accounts for the fact that normally the RF of a visual cortical cell is restricted to an area much less than might be inferred from the extent of horizontal connections (e.g. Hirsch and Gilbert, 1991). This balance, ever changing with the current visual scene, is temporarily disrupted by artificial scotomas while retinal lesions, restricted visual experience or deprivation of contour vision produce more radical and permanent disruptions.

It has been suggested in the past (see Chino, 1995; Darian-Smith and Gilbert, 1995) that topographic reorganization in the lesion projection zone of striate cortices following circumscribed retinal lesions might reflect 'feedback' signals originating in the extrastriate visual cortices. Indeed, at any given eccentricity the RFs of cells in the extrastriate cortices of both cats and macaque monkeys are substantially larger than those of cells in striate cortices (Tusa et al., 1981; Dreher, 1986; Kaas, 1986). Furthermore, the 'composite receptive fields' of extrastriate afferents (e.g. area 18) to a given region of area 17 are much larger than those of the 'composite receptive fields' of target cells in area 17 (Salin et al., 1993; Salin and Bullier, 1995). Following this line of logic, ectopic RFs of cells in the LPZ in area 17 might represent the parts of normal RFs of cells in the extrastriate cortices which project to the LPZ in the striate cortices. However, so far, there is no experimental support for this proposal.

At the moment, the most likely source of the capacity for reorganization in area 17 appears to be the extensive network of intrinsic interconnections within area V1 — including the long-range horizontal, associational collaterals of pyramidal cells (Fisken et al., 1973, 1975; Gilbert and Wiesel, 1979, 1983, 1989; LeVay, 1988; Matsubara et al., 1985; Gilbert et al., 1990; LeVay and Nelson, 1991; Gilbert, 1992, 1993, 1998; cf. also horizontal connections within primary auditory and somatosensory cortices — Imig and Brugge, 1978; Jones et al., 1978). Indeed, in the cat, injection of retrograde tracers demonstrated connections between columns of similar orientation selectivity across 8 mm of area 17 (Gilbert and Wiesel, 1989).

Direct experimental support for the proposal that the capacity for reorganization in area 17 is based on the extensive network of intrinsic interconnections within striate cortex comes from a recent study of

Calford's group (Wright et al., 1999). In adult cats, they made monocular circumscribed retinal lesions with an argon green laser. Three to 13 weeks after placement of the lesions animals were anesthetized with a gaseous mixture of N_2O/O_2 (67%/33%) and halothane (0.5–1%) and paralyzed with pancuronium bromide (Pavulon 0.15 mg/kg/h i.v.). Extracellular recordings were made from area 17. When stimulated via the lesioned eye cells in the lesion projection zone exhibited ectopic RFs. The magnitude of the responses evoked by visual stimuli presented at ectopic RFs was substantially reduced when the neurotoxin kainic acid was microinjected into the part of area 17 which received its retinal input (via relays in the LGNd) from the retinal ganglion cells located in the area of the ectopic RFs. At the same time, the responses of cells in the LPZ to visual stimuli presented via the unlesioned eye were unaffected by injections of kainic acid.

We are at a stage when we do not have all the data to give a comprehensive explanation for all the results. Nevertheless, it may stimulate further research if we tentatively suggest a neural circuit which satisfies some of the findings. Fig. 9A shows a region of visual cortex in which the region between the vertical dashed lines is the lesion projection zone, i.e. it is effectively deafferented with respect to the retina. The neuron P1 no longer receives input from the A region of retina, whereas neuron P2 in normal cortex receives input from normal retina at B. We suppose that branches of geniculo-cortical fibers extend to adjacent regions of cortex where they would be capable of exciting other neurons were it not for the fact that they are prevented from doing so by the action of inhibitory interneurons (I) which in turn are kept active by strong volleys in the dominant input to that region. In the absence of such input, the interneuron falls silent and now the branch of the input from B can excite neuron P1. If input from the A region of retina is restored, for a short time neuron P1 will appear to have an enlarged RF. If we suppose that discharges of interneuron I do not immediately cease in the absence of geniculo-cortical input but decline slowly over minutes, then the diagrammatically illustrated model will explain the enlargement of RFs observed following artificial scotomas. If input from the A region of retina resumes, interneuron I will be reactivated and the size of the RF will shrink back to its original size. If input from the A region of retina is interrupted permanently, as with a retinal lesion, cell P1 will remain excitable from retinal sites outside the scotoma. Consistent with the proposed model, in adult cats and macaque monkeys the RFs of area 17 neurons in the LPZ are dramatically enlarged shortly after the infliction of the retinal lesion (Gilbert and Wiesel, 1992; Darian-Smith and Gilbert, 1995; Schmid et al., 1995; Calford et al., 1999; see section on the Short-term effects of retinal lesions), although after several months, the size of the ectopic RFs seems to have returned to more or less normal values (Chino et al., 1995; Darian-Smith and Gilbert, 1995; Calford et al., 2000). Undoubtedly slow adaptive changes are occurring. Apart from this, it seems that the 'true' RF of the cell must be greater than that measured because the cell is no longer receiving its normal input to which it presumably could still respond if it could be activated.

However, the model outlined in Fig. 9A will not account for many of the reported changes. In particular, the branching of geniculo-cortical afferents in the visual cortex is not great enough nor do these branches sprout to a sufficient extent under the stimulus of deafferentation to account for the observed enlargements of RFs of cortical neurons and the spatial extent of distortions of perception reported following circumscribed retinal lesions in humans. Several mechanisms have been proposed to account for the long-term changes in topographic organization of striate cortex following retinal lesions. One possibility involves changes in the synaptic strength of the existing cortico-cortical connections (e.g. Hirsch and Gilbert, 1993). Presumably the modifiability of RF sizes of neurons in visual cortices of the adult anesthetized cats following 10–60 min visual co-stimulation of excitatory RF and adjacent to it unresponsive regions observed by Eysel et al. (1998) is based on such changes. A complementary mechanism based on sprouting of the axonal collaterals of pyramidal cells and strengthening their synaptic efficacy has been proposed by Darian-Smith and Gilbert (1995). Indeed, these researchers have shown that the axon collaterals of pyramidal neurons in the striate cortex of adult cats sprout extensively in the 'retinally deafferented' cortex, although they seem not to increase in length; the sprouting probably develops over weeks or months and so the

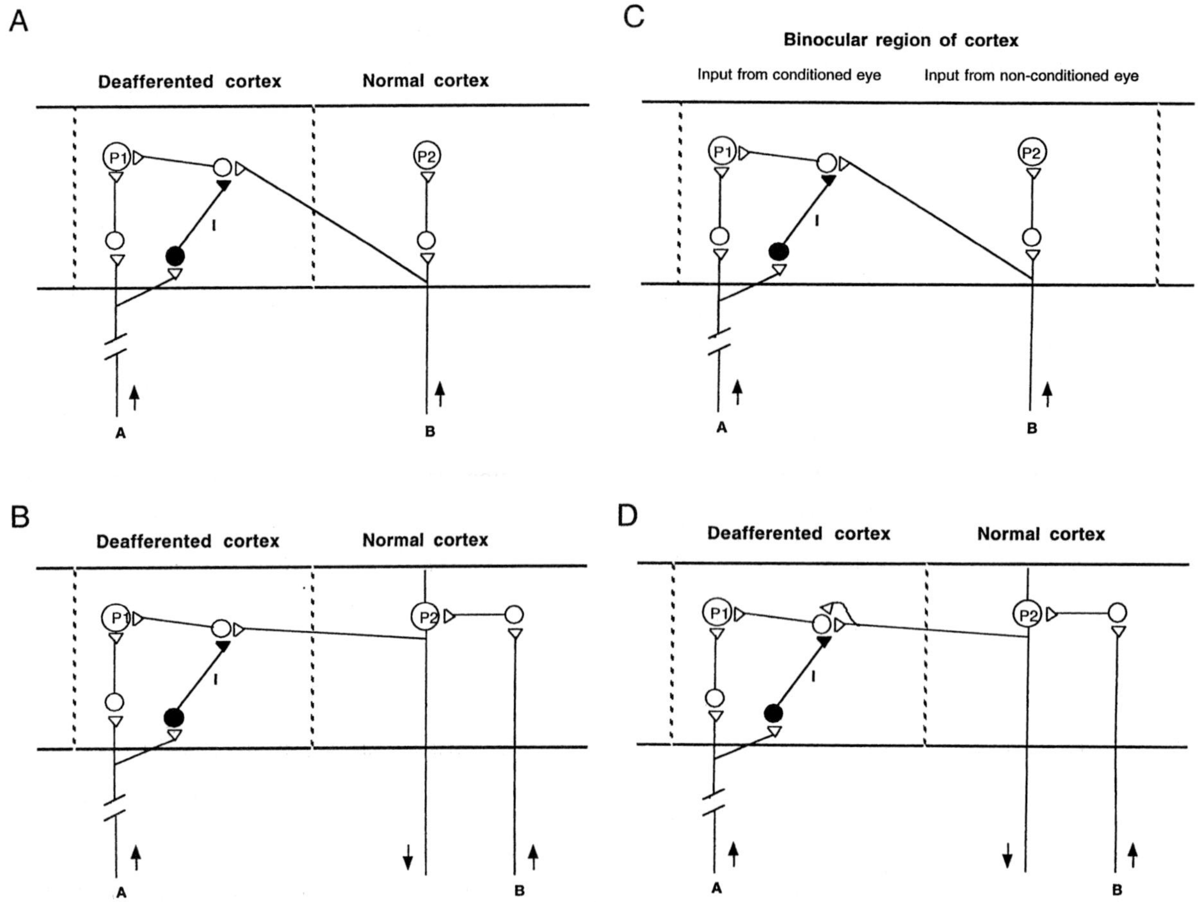

Fig. 9. Possible neural circuits underlying reorganization of striate cortex following circumscribed retinal lesions. (A) Enlargement of RFs of neurons in deafferented cortex (produced by lesion or artificial scotoma) may be due to loss of activity in inhibitory interneuron (I), allowing activation of neuron P1 by input from normal retina at B. (B) The circuit in A is inadequate to explain the chronic changes following a retinal lesion, when stimulation of normal retina is effective at long distances (e.g. equivalent to 8 mm in the cortex) and for which activity in axon collaterals of pyramidal cells (e.g. P2) is postulated. (C) Circuit, similar to that in A, to explain how the change in RF size due to an artificial scotoma (reduced input from retina at A) could transfer to the non-conditioned eye (input from B). Neuron P1 has normal strong input from B (not shown) as well as inputs from B normally held off by activity in the interneuron (I). When this neuron falls silent, these weaker inputs then become effective. (D) The stronger ectopic RFs resulting from retinal lesions in adolescence might be due to a greater growth in the terminal arborization of axon collaterals in the deafferented zone (symbolized by an increase in number of boutons from 1 to 2). In all these circuits, many neurons are involved, each with a different level of activity and effectiveness; a complete explanation of the various phenomena must take into account such population effects.

connections they form become more and more effective. Diagram B in Fig. 9 is similar to diagram A except that the axon collateral of the geniculo-cortical input has been replaced by that of the P2 cell. The axon collateral will account for the displacement of RFs of cortical neurons in the LPZ observed after the retinal lesion, although it does not account for the later decrease in RF size (Gilbert and Wiesel, 1992; Chino et al., 1995; Calford et al., 2000). Split ectopic RFs with more than one discrete regions of the visual field which were often observed following circumscribed retinal lesions (Chino et al., 1992; Gilbert and Wiesel, 1992; Calford et al., 2000) might be due to activation of the cell by axon collaterals projecting from several sites around the LPZ.

To explain how, following conditioning with an artificial scotoma, there is increase in RF size, not only by stimulation of the conditioned eye, but also via the non-conditioned eye, we propose the circuit in Fig. 9C. This is essentially the same circuit as in Fig. 9A but we are now looking at the interaction between the two eyes. We suppose that neuron P1 normally gets a strong input from the retina at B (not shown). As in Fig. 9A it is assumed that the lack of stimulation from the retina at A leads to decreased activity in interneuron I. This allows input from the retina at B, normally subthreshold, to now reach threshold and become effective.

It is interesting that no increase in RF size of cells in the LPZ to stimuli presented via the non-lesioned eye has been reported. It is likely that in the long term, there will be adaptive effects such as recovery of activity in interneuron I which would account for the decrease in RF size for stimuli presented via the lesioned eye and would nullify any changes in the RFs for stimuli presented via the non-lesioned eye. RFs from the non-lesioned eye have not been examined at times less than 1 h after the lesion. If the adaptive process occurred within this time, a change in RF size via the non-lesioned eye would be missed. However, at this time (1 h), there is a strong effect for stimuli presented via the lesioned eye, so there is a difference between the two eyes which circuit C does not explain.

The greater responsiveness of area 17 cells in the LPZ to stimuli presented via the lesioned eye when the retinal lesion has been made in kittens (Burke et al., 2000; Dreher et al., 2000) may reflect a more robust change in adolescent animals in the synaptic strength of the existing cortico-cortical connections as well as more robust growth in the pyramidal cell axon collaterals (e.g., Trachtenberg, and Stryker, 2001; either in length of axons or in terminal arborization so that synaptic effectiveness increases). We have symbolized this growth by increase in the number of synaptic boutons from 1 to 2 in Fig. 9D.

Finally, the close matching of orientation preferences and selectivities of ectopic and normal RFs is consistent with the demonstrated presence of substantial interconnections between columns of similar orientation selectivity across wide expanses of area 17 (see for reviews LeVay and Nelson, 1991; Gilbert, 1992, 1993, 1998; Malach et al., 1993).

Although there is morphological evidence for all the elements in the circuits in Fig. 9, the circuits have not been functionally validated. Probably this would be best attempted in a brain slice incorporating the deafferented region. In such a preparation, single neuron activity is initially suppressed in the deafferented zone and there is increased activity in the surround region in the 1–2 weeks after the lesion (Eysel et al., 1999). This approach is likely to be most rewarding when combined with in vivo studies.

It is also important to point out that permanent disruptions in flow of visual information appears to result in topographic reorganization not only in area 17, but also in other visual cortical areas. Thus, Kaas et al. (1990) reported topographic reorganization in the lesion projection zones in both areas 17 and 18 of primary visual cortices following binocular, topographically matched lesions of the contralateral and ipsilateral retina of adult cats. Furthermore, a recent study of Rosa et al. (2000) provides evidence of topographic reorganization in the so-called 'higher-order' visual cortical areas of adult mammals. Thus, several weeks after ablations of large sections of the striate cortices of the New-World diurnal monkeys, marmosets (*Callithrix jacchus*), Rosa and his colleagues recorded single neuron activity in the higher-order motion processing area, the middle temporal area (MT). The majority of the MT neurons recorded from the striate cortex projection zone had ectopic RFs displaced to the part of the visual field immediately surrounding the part of the visual field which had lost its representation in the striate cortex. Presumably, destruction of the principal cortical input to area MT triggers a process of topographic reorganization based on the potentiation of intrinsic horizontal connections within area MT.

Distortion of perception outside the lesion projection zone

It is also evident from human psychophysics that there is a perceptual distortion of the visual field projected onto the intact part of the retina just outside the lesion. Put another way, the scotoma is not only filled in from the background, it draws the background inwards, thereby distorting it. The neural basis for this inwards movement is demonstrated in the animal experiments by the appearance of ectopic RFs around the borders of the lesion. However, this is still an incomplete explanation. According to present ideas (see above) the neurons within the deafferented zone (LPZ) of the cortex receive an input from outside the zone, probably via axon collaterals of neurons lying in normal cortex. These normal neurons are receiving an input from the intact retina lying outside the lesion. Thus, two sets of neurons (one inside, the other outside, the LPZ) are receiving input from the same part of the retina. How does the brain interpret this? If we follow the argument of Kapadia et al. (1994) (see section on Artificial scotomas) the position of an object is determined by the integrated discharges of all neurons stimulated by the object with due regard for the position label of each neuron. If we accept this argument, we must account for the large deflections of a line observed psychophysically (e.g. 0.8°; see Fig. 8B; cf. Burke, 1999) as dependent upon either a very high rate of discharge in cells within the LPZ or by supposing that many such cells are discharging (at more moderate rates). Neither in cats in which the retinal lesion were made in adulthood (Calford et al., 2000) nor in the cats in which the retinal lesions were made in adolescence (Dreher et al., 2000) did we observe cells in the LPZ discharging at rates different to those of cells located outside the LPZ, so the latter possibility seems more reasonable.

Nevertheless, even if this is so, there still remains a problem because there is a distortion of perception extending well outside the scotoma. As indicated in Fig. 8B lines up to 1° or more outside the border of the scotoma appear bent (in W.B.'s right eye, distortions now extend up to 3° from the border of the macular hole). At the present time there is no clear explanation for this effect.

Conclusions

The research described in this review has changed our view of receptive fields of neurons in mammalian visual cortices from the classical 'hard-wired' model to a more flexible dynamic one. This has also influenced our ideas about visual perception, both normal and pathological. The fact that the major changes resulting from retinal lesions occur in the visual cortex and not in the retina will influence the practice of ophthalmology and may eventually lead to appropriate remediation. It is probable that visual distortions resulting from lesions of the cerebral cortex (e.g. Charles Bonnet syndrome, the hemi-neglect syndrome) will find an explanation in the loss of original RFs and the emergence of ectopic ones. This is an exciting area of research which is only just beginning (e.g. Eysel et al., 1999; Rosa et al., 2000).

Acknowledgements

This work was supported by grants from the Australian Research Council and the National Health and Medical Research Council of Australia. We thank Drs. Wioletta J. Waleszczyk, Chun Wang, Layne L. Wright, Andrew B. Metha and Mr Joshua Young for their collaboration in the series of experiments conducted recently in our laboratories. So far, the results of these experiments have been published only in forms of abstracts (Burke et al., 2000; Dreher et al., 2000) and in the present review.

References

Albus, K. (1975) A quantitative study of the projection area of the central and the paracentral visual field in area 17 of the cat. I. The precision of the topography. *Exp. Brain Res.*, 24: 159–179.

Allman, J., Miezin, F. and McGuiness, E. (1985) Stimulus specific responses from beyond the classical receptive field: Neurophysiological mechanisms for local–global comparisons in visual neurons. *Annu. Rev. Neurosci.*, 8: 407–430.

Anstis, S. (1989) Kinetic edges become displaced, segregated and invisible. In: D.M.-K. Lam and C.D. Gilbert (Eds.), *Neuronal Mechanisms of Visual Perception*. Gulf, Houston, TX, pp. 247–260.

Baekelandt, V., Arckens, L., Annaert, W., Eysel, U.T., Orban, G.A. and Vandesande, F. (1994) Alterations in GAP-43 and synapsin immunoreactivity provide evidence for synaptic reorganization in adult cat dorsal lateral geniculate nucleus following retinal lesions. *Eur. J. Neurosci.*, 6: 754–765.

Baker, F.H., Grigg, P. and von Norden, G.K. (1974) Effects of visual deprivation and strabismus on the response of neurons in the visual cortex of the monkey, including studies on the striate and prestriate cortex in the normal animal. *Brain Res.*, 66: 185–208.

Barlow, H.B., Derrington, A.M., Harris, L.R. and Lennie, P. (1977) The effects of remote retinal stimulation on the responses of cat retinal ganglion cells. *J. Physiol. (Lond.)*, 269: 177–194.

Blakemore, C. and Van Sluyters, R.C. (1974) Reversal of the physiological effects of monocular deprivation in kittens: further evidence for a sensitive period. *J. Physiol. (Lond.)*, 237: 195–216.

Blakemore, C., Garey, L.J. and Vital-Durand, F. (1978) The physiological effects of monocular deprivation and their reversal in the monkey's visual cortex. *J. Physiol. (Lond.)*, 283: 223–262.

Blakemore, C., Vital-Durand, F. and Garey, L.J. (1981) Recovery from monocular deprivation in monkey. I. Recovery of physiological effects in the visual cortex. *Proc. R. Soc. Lond. B*, 213: 399–423.

Blasdel, G.G. and Lund, J.S. (1983) Termination of afferent axons in macaque striate cortex. *J. Neurosci.*, 3: 1389–1413.

Boroojerdi, B., Bushara, K.O., Corwell, B., Immisch, I., Battaglia, F., Muellbacher, W. and Cohen, L.G. (2000) Enhanced excitability of the human visual cortex induced by short-term light deprivation. *Cereb. Cortex*, 10: 524–534.

Bringuier, V., Chavane, F., Glaeser, L. and Frégnac, Y. (1999) Horizontal propagation of visual activity in the synaptic integration field of area 17 neurons. *Science*, 283: 695–699.

Burchfiel, J.L. and Duffy, F.H. (1981) Role of intracortical inhibition in deprivation amblyopia: reversal by microiontophoresis of bicuculline. *Brain Res.*, 206: 479–484.

Burke, W. (1999) Psychophysical observations concerned with a foveal lesion (macular hole). *Vision Res.*, 39: 2421–2427.

Burke, W., Dreher, B., Michalski, A., Cleland, B. and Rowe, M.H. (1992) Effects of selective pressure block of Y-type optic nerve fibres on receptive-field properties of neurons in the striate cortex of the cat. *Vis. Neurosci.*, 9: 47–64.

Burke, W., Waleszczyk, W.J., Wang, C., Dreher, B. and Calford, M.B. (2000) Reorganization of neural circuits in area 17 of the cat following retinal lesions in adolescent kittens. *J. Physiol. (Lond.)*, 528: 75P.

Busch, E.-M., Gorgels, T.G.M.F. and van Norren, D. (1999) Filling-in after focal loss of photoreceptors in rat retina. *Exp. Eye Res.*, 68: 485–492.

Calford, M.B. (1991) Curious cortical change (news and views). *Nature*, 352: 759–760.

Calford, M.B., Schmid, L.M. and Rosa, M.G.P. (1999) Monocular focal retinal lesions induce short-term topographic plasticity in adult visual cortex. *Proc. R. Soc. Lond. B*, 266: 499–507.

Calford, M.B., Wang, C., Taglianetti, V., Waleszczyk, W.J., Burke, W. and Dreher, B. (2000) Plasticity in adult cat visual cortex (area 17) following circumscribed monocular lesions of all retinal layers. *J. Physiol. (Lond.)*, 524: 587–602.

Chino, Y.M. (1995) Adult plasticity in the visual system. *Can. J. Physiol. Pharmacol.*, 73: 1323–1338.

Chino, Y.M., Kaas, J.H., Smith III, E.L., Langston, A.L. and Cheng, H. (1992) Rapid reorganization of cortical maps in adult cats following restricted deafferentation in retina. *Vision Res.*, 32: 789–796.

Chino, Y.M., Smith III, E.L., Kaas, J.H., Sasaki, Y. and Cheng, H. (1995) Receptive-field properties of deafferentated visual cortical neurons after topographic map reorganization in adult cats. *J. Neurosci.*, 15: 2417–2433.

Chu, Y., Humphrey, M.F., Alder, V.V. and Constable, I.J. (1998) Immunocytochemical localization of basic fibroblast growth factor and glial fibrillary acidic protein after laser photocoagulation in the Royal College of Surgeons rat. *Aust. N. Z. J. Ophthalmol.*, 26: 87–96.

Cleland, B.G., Lee, B.B. and Vidyasagar, T.R. (1983) Response of neurons in the cat's lateral geniculate nucleus to moving bars of different length. *J. Neurosci.*, 3: 108–116.

Craik, K.J.W. (1966) On the effects of looking at the sun. In: S.L. Sherwood Jr. (Ed.), *The Nature of Psychology*. Cambridge University Press, Cambridge, pp. 98–101.

Cummings, R.W., Whittaker, S.G., Watson, G.R. and Budd, J.M. (1985) Scanning characters and reading with a central scotoma. *Am. J. Optom. Physiol. Opt.*, 62: 833–843.

Darian-Smith, C. and Gilbert, C.D. (1994) Axonal sprouting accompanies functional reorganization in adult cat striate cortex. *Nature*, 368: 737–740.

Darian-Smith, C. and Gilbert, C.D. (1995) Topographic reorganization in the striate cortex of the adult cat and monkey is cortically mediated. *J. Neurosci.*, 15: 1631–1647.

Das, A. and Gilbert, C.D. (1995) Receptive field expansion in adult visual cortex is linked to dynamic changes in strength of cortical connections. *J. Neurophysiol.*, 74: 779–792.

Das, A. and Gilbert, C.D. (1999) Topography of contextual modulations mediated by short-range interactions in primary visual cortex. *Nature*, 399: 655–661.

De Weerd, P., Gattass, R., Desimone, R. and Ungerleider, L.G. (1995) Responses of cells in monkey visual cortex during perceptual filling-in of an artificial scotoma. *Nature*, 377: 731–734.

De Weerd, P., Desimone, R. and Ungerleider, L.G. (1998) Perceptual filling-in: a parametric study. *Vision Res.*, 38: 2721–2734.

DeAngelis, G.C., Anzai, A., Ohzawa, I. and Freeman, R.D. (1995) Receptive field structure in the visual cortex: does selective stimulation induce plasticity? *Proc. Natl. Acad. Sci. USA*, 92: 9682–9686.

Derrington, A.M. and Fuchs, A.F. (1979) Spatial and temporal properties of X and Y cells in the cat lateral geniculate nucleus. *J. Physiol. (Lond.)*, 293: 347–364.

Derrington, A.M., Lennie, P. and Wright, M.J. (1979) The mechanism of peripherally evoked responses in retinal ganglion cells. *J. Physiol. (Lond.)*, 289: 299–310.

Ditchburn, R.W. and Ginsborg, B.L. (1952) Vision with a stabilized retinal image. *Nature (Lond.)*, 170: 36–37.

Dowling, J.E. and Boycott, B.B. (1966) Organization of the primate retina; electron microscopy. *Proc. R. Soc. Lond. B*, 166: 80–111.

Dreher, B. (1972) Hypercomplex cells in the cat's striate cortex. *Invest. Ophthalmol.*, 11: 355–356.

Dreher, B. (1986) Thalamocortical and corticocortical interconnections in the cat visual system: Relation to the mechanisms of information processing. In: J.D. Pettigrew, K.J. Sanderson and W.R. Levick (Eds.), *Visual Neuroscience*. Cambridge University Press, Cambridge, pp. 290–314.

Dreher, B. and Hoffmann, K.-P. (1973) Properties of excitatory and inhibitory regions in the receptive fields of single units in the cat's superior colliculus. *Exp. Brain Res.*, 16: 333–353.

Dreher, B. and Sanderson, K.J. (1973) Receptive field analysis: responses to visual contours by single lateral geniculate neurones in the cat. *J. Physiol. (Lond.)*, 234: 95–118.

Dreher, B., Waleszczyk, W.J., Wang, C., Burke, W. and Calford, M.B. (2000) Topographic reorganization of area 17 of adult cats following circumscribed monocular retinal lesions in adolescence. *Proc. Aust. Neurosci. Soc.*, 11: 219.

Duret, F., Issenhuth, M. and Safran, A.B. (1999) Combined use of several preferred retinal loci in patients with macular disorders when reading single words. *Vision Res.*, 39: 873–879.

Duffy, F.H., Snodgrass, S.R., Burchfiel, J.L. and Conway, J.L. (1976) Bicuculline reversal of deprivation amblyopia in the cat. *Nature*, 260: 256–257.

Enroth-Cugell, C. and Jakiela, H.G. (1980) Suppression of cat retinal ganglion cell responses by moving patterns. *J. Physiol. (Lond.)*, 302: 49–72.

Eysel, U.T. (1982) Functional reconnections without new axonal growth in a partially denervated visual relay nucleus. *Nature*, 299: 442–444.

Eysel, U.T. and Neubacher, U. (1984) Recovery of function is not associated with proliferation of retinogeniculate synapses after chronic deafferentation in the dorsal lateral geniculate nucleus of the adult cat. *Neurosci. Lett.*, 49: 181–186.

Eysel, U.T., Gonzalez-Aguilar, F. and Mayer, U. (1980) A functional sign of reorganization in the visual system of adult cats; lateral geniculate neurons with displaced receptive fields after lesions of the nasal retina. *Brain Res.*, 181: 285–300.

Eysel, U.T., Gonzalez-Aguilar, F. and Mayer, U. (1981) Time-dependent decrease in the extent of visual deafferentation in the lateral geniculate nucleus of adult cats with small retinal lesions. *Exp. Brain Res.*, 41: 256–263.

Eysel, U.T., Eyding, D. and Schweigart, G. (1998) Repetitive optical stimulation elicits fast receptive field changes in mature visual cortex. *NeuroReport*, 9: 949–954.

Eysel, U.T., Schweigart, G., Mittmann, T., Eyding, D., Qu, Y., Vandesande, F., Orban, G. and Arckens, L. (1999) Reorganization in the visual cortex after retinal and cortical damage. *Restor. Neurol. Neurosci.*, 15: 153–164.

Eysel, U.T. and Wolfhard, U. (1984) The effects of partial retinal lesions on activity and size of cells in the dorsal lateral geniculate nucleus. *J. Comp. Neurol.*, 229: 301–309.

Feldon, S.E., Andrews, B.W. and Pollen, D.A. (1978) Periodic complex cells in cortical area 19 of the cat. *Vision Res.*, 18: 347–350.

Ferster, D. and LeVay, S. (1978) The axonal arborization of lateral geniculate neurons in the striate cortex of the cat. *J. Comp. Neurol.*, 182: 923–944.

ffytche, D.H. and Howard, R.J. (1999) The perceptual consequences of visual loss: 'positive' pathologies of vision. *Brain*, 122: 1247–1260.

Fiorani Jr., M., Rosa, M.G.P., Gattass, R. and Rocha-Miranda, C.E. (1992) Dynamic surrounds of receptive fields in primate striate cortex: a physiological basis for perceptual completion? *Proc. Natl. Acad. Sci. USA*, 89: 8547–8551.

Fischer, B. and Krüger, J. (1974) The shift-effect in the cat's lateral geniculate neurons. *Exp. Brain Res.*, 21: 225–227.

Fischer, B. and Krüger, J. (1980) Continuous movement of remote patterns and shift-effect of cat retinal ganglion cells. *Exp. Brain Res.*, 40: 229–232.

Fischer, B., Krüger, J. and Droll, W. (1975) Quantitative aspects of the shift-effect in cat retinal ganglion cells. *Brain Res.*, 83: 391–403.

Fisken, R.A., Garey, L.J. and Powell, T.P.S. (1973) Patterns of degeneration after intrinsic lesions of the visual cortex (area 17) of the monkey. *Exp. Brain Res.*, 53: 208–213.

Fisken, R.A., Garey, L.J. and Powell, T.P.S. (1975) The intrinsic, association and commissural connections of area 17 of the visual cortex. *Biol. Sci.*, 272(Suppl. 919): 487–536.

Frégnac, Y. and Shulz, D.E. (1999) Activity-dependent regulation of receptive field properties of cat area 17 by supervised Hebbian learning. *J. Neurobiol.*, 41: 69–82.

Freund, T., Martin, K.A.C. and Whitteridge, D. (1985) Innervation of cat visual areas 17 and 18 by physiologically identified X- and Y-type thalamic afferents. I. Arborization patterns and quantitative distribution of postsynaptic elements. *J. Comp. Neurol.*, 242: 263–274.

Freund, T., Martin, K.A.C., Soltesz, I., Somogyi, P. and Whitteridge, D. (1989) Arborization pattern and postsynaptic targets of physiologically identified thalamocortical afferents in striate cortex of the macaque monkey. *J. Comp. Neurol.*, 289: 315–336.

Funke, K., Meller, P., Pape, H.-C. and Eysel, U.T. (1996) Linear and non-linear components in the centre-surround response of X- and Y-cells in the cat lateral geniculate nucleus. *Brain Res.*, 742: 50–62.

Gass, J.D.M. (1997) Macular disfunction caused by vitreous and vitreoretinal interface abnormalities. In: J.D.M. Gass (Ed.), *Stereoscopic Atlas of Macular Diseases*, Vol. 2, *Diagnosis and Treatment*, 4th edn. Mosby, St. Louis, pp. 903–973.

Gerrits, H.J., De Haan, B. and Vendrik, A.J. (1966) Experiments with retinal stabilized images. Relations between the observations and neural data. *Vision Res.*, 6: 427–440.

Gerrits, H.J.M. and Timmerman, G.J.M.E.N. (1969) The filling-in process in patients with retinal scotomata. *Vision Res.*, 9: 439–442.

Gilbert, C.D. (1992) Horizontal integration and cortical dynamics. *Neuron*, 9: 1–13.

Gilbert, C.D. (1993) Circuitry, architecture, and functional dynamics of visual cortex. *Cereb. Cortex*, 3: 373–386.

Gilbert, C.D. (1998) Adult cortical dynamics. *Physiol. Rev.*, 78: 467–485.

Gilbert, C.D. and Wiesel, T.N. (1979) Morphology and intracortical projections of functionally characterised neurones in the cat visual cortex. *Nature*, 280: 120–125.

Gilbert, C.D. and Wiesel, T.N. (1983) Clustered intrinsic connections in cat visual cortex. *J. Neurosci.*, 3: 1116–1133.

Gilbert, C.D. and Wiesel, T.N. (1989) Columnar specificity of intrinsic horizontal and corticocortical connections in cat visual cortex. *J. Neurosci.*, 9: 2432–2442.

Gilbert, C.D. and Wiesel, T.N. (1992) Receptive field dynamics in adult primary visual cortex. *Nature*, 356: 150–152.

Gilbert, C.D., Hirsch, J.A. and Wiesel, T.N. (1990) Lateral interactions in visual cortex. In: *Cold Spring Harbor Symposia of*

Quantitative Biology, Vol. LV. Cold Spring Harbor Laboratory Press, Cold Spring Harbor, NY, pp. 663–677.

Glezer, V.D., Ivanoff, V.A. and Tscherbach, T.A. (1973) Investigation of complex and hypercomplex receptive fields of visual cortex of the cat as spatial frequency filters. *Vision Res.*, 13: 1875–1904.

Grosof, D.H., Shapley, R.M. and Hawken, M.J. (1993) Macaque V1 neurons can signal 'illusory contours'. *Nature*, 365: 550–552.

Hammond, P. (1973) Contrasts in spatial organization of receptive fields at geniculate and retinal levels: Centre, surround and outer surround. *J. Physiol. (Lond.)*, 228: 115–137.

Heinen, S.J. and Skavenski, A.A. (1991) Recovery of visual responses in foveal V1 neurons following bilateral foveal lesions in adult monkey. *Exp. Brain Res.*, 83: 670–674.

Henry, G.H., Bishop, P.O. and Dreher, B. (1974a) Orientation, axis and direction as stimulus parameters for striate cells. *Vision Res.*, 14: 767–777.

Henry, G.H., Dreher, B. and Bishop, P.O. (1974b) Orientation specificity of cells in cat striate cortex. *J. Neurophysiol.*, 37: 1394–1409.

Hirsch, J.A. and Gilbert, C.D. (1991) Synaptic physiology of horizontal connections in the cat's visual cortex. *J. Neurophysiol.*, 11: 1800–1809.

Hirsch, J.A. and Gilbert, C.D. (1993) Long-term changes in synaptic strength along specific intrinsic pathways in the cat's visual cortex. *J. Physiol. (Lond.)*, 461: 247–262.

Hoffmann, K.-P. and Cynader, M. (1977) Functional aspects of plasticity in the visual system of adult cats after early monocular deprivation. *Phil. Trans. R. Soc. Lond. B*, 278: 411–424.

Horton, J.C. and Hocking, D.R. (1998) Monocular core zones and binocular border strips in primate striate cortex revealed by the contrasting effects of enucleation, eyelid suture, and retinal laser lesions on cytochrome oxidase activity. *J. Neurosci.*, 18: 5433–5455.

Hubel, D.H. and Wiesel, T.N. (1965a) Receptive fields and functional architecture in two nonstriate visual areas (18 and 19) of the cat. *J. Neurophysiol.*, 28: 229–289.

Hubel, D.H. and Wiesel, T.N. (1965b) Binocular interaction in striate cortex of kittens reared with artificial squint. *J. Neurophysiol.*, 28: 1041–1059.

Hubel, D.H. and Wiesel, T.N. (1968) Receptive fields and functional architecture of monkey striate cortex. *J. Physiol. (Lond.)*, 195: 215–243.

Hubel, D.H. and Wiesel, T.N. (1970) The period of susceptibility to the physiological effects of unilateral eye closure in kittens. *J. Physiol. (Lond.)*, 206: 419–436.

Humphrey, A.L., Sur, M., Ulrich, D.J. and Sherman, S.M. (1985) Projection patterns of individual X- and Y-cell axons from the lateral geniculate nucleus to cortical area 17 in the cat. *J. Comp. Neurol.*, 233: 159–189.

Humphrey, M.F., Chu, Y., Mann, K. and Rakoczy, P. (1997) Retinal GFAP and bFGF expression after multiple argon laser photocoagulation injuries assessed by both immunoreactivity and mRNA levels. *Exp. Eye Res.*, 64: 361–369.

Ikeda, H. and Wright, M.J. (1972a) The outer disinhibitory surround of the retinal ganglion cell receptive field. *J. Physiol. (Lond.)*, 226: 511–544.

Ikeda, H. and Wright, M.J. (1972b) Functional organization of the periphery effect in retinal ganglion cells. *Vision Res.*, 12: 1857–1879.

Imig, T.J. and Brugge, J.F. (1978) Sources and terminations of callosal axons related to binaural and frequency maps in primary auditory cortex of the cat. *J. Comp. Neurol.*, 182: 637–660.

Ito, M. and Gilbert, C.G. (1999) Attention modulates contextual influences in the primary visual cortex of alert monkeys. *Neuron*, 22: 593–604.

Jones, E.G., Coulter, J.D. and Hendry, S.H.C. (1978) Intracortical connectivity of architectonic fields in the somatic sensory, motor and parietal cortex of monkeys. *J. Comp. Neurol.*, 181: 291–348.

Kaas, J.H. (1986) The structural basis for information processing in the primate visual system. In: J.D. Pettigrew, K.J. Sanderson and W.R. Levick (Eds.), *Visual Neuroscience*. Cambridge University Press, Cambridge, pp. 315–340.

Kaas, J.H. (1991) Plasticity of sensory and motor maps in adult mammals. *Annu. Rev. Neurosci.*, 14: 137–167.

Kaas, J.H., Krubitzer, L.A., Chino, Y.M., Langston, A.L., Polley, E.H. and Blair, N. (1990) Reorganization of retinotopic cortical maps in adult mammals after lesions of the retina. *Science*, 248: 229–231.

Kapadia, M.K., Gilbert, C.D. and Westheimer, G. (1994) A quantitative measure for short-term cortical plasticity in human vision. *J. Neurosci.*, 14: 451–457.

Kasamatsu, T., Kitano, M., Sutter, E.E. and Norcia, A.M. (1998) Lack of lateral inhibitory interactions in visual cortex of monocularly deprived cats. *Vision Res.*, 38: 1–12.

Kitano, M., Niiyama, K., Kasamatsu, T., Sutter, E.E. and Norcia, A.M. (1994) Retinotopic and nonretinotopic field potentials in cat visual cortex. *Vis. Neurosci.*, 11: 953–977.

Knierim, J.J. and Van Essen, D.C. (1992) Neuronal responses to static texture patterns in area V1 of the alert macaque monkey. *J. Neurophysiol.*, 67: 961–980.

Kratz, K.E., Spear, P.D. and Smith, D.C. (1976) Postcritical-period reversal of effects of monocular deprivation on striate cortex cells in the cat. *J. Neurophysiol.*, 39: 501–511.

Krüger, J. (1977) The shift-effect in the lateral geniculate body of the rhesus monkey. *Exp. Brain Res.*, 29: 387–392.

Krüger, J. and Fischer, B. (1973) Strong periphery effect in cat retinal ganglion cells. Excitatory responses in on- and off-centre neurones to single grid displacements. *Exp. Brain Res.*, 18: 316–318.

Krüger, J., Fischer, B. and Barth, R. (1975) The shift-effect in retinal ganglion cells in the rhesus monkey. *Exp. Brain Res.*, 23: 443–446.

Kuffler, S.W. (1953) Discharge patterns and funtional organization of mammalian retina. *J. Neurophysiol.*, 16: 37–68.

Lamme, V.A.F. (1995) The neurophysiology of figure–ground segregation in primary visual cortex. *J. Neurosci.*, 15: 1605–1615.

LeVay, S. (1988) The patchy intrinsic projections of visual cortex. *Prog. Brain Res.*, 75: 147–161.

LeVay, S. and Nelson, S.B. (1991) Columnar organization of the visual cortex. In: J. Cronly-Dillon (Ed.), *Vision and Visual Dysfunction*, Vol. 4. In: A.G. Leventhal (Ed.), *The Neural Basis of Visual Function*. Macmillan Press, Houndmills, pp. 266–315.

LeVay, S., Wiesel, T.N. and Hubel, D.H. (1980) The development of ocular dominance columns in normal and visually deprived monkeys. *J. Comp. Neurol.*, 191: 1–51.

Leventhal, A.G., Wang, Y.-C., Schmolesky, M.T. and Zhou, Y.-F. (1998) Neural correlates of boundary perception. *Vis. Neurosci.*, 15: 1107–1118.

Levick, W.R., Cleland, B.G. and Dubin, M.W. (1972) Lateral geniculate neurons of cat: Retinal inputs and physiology. *Invest. Ophthalmol.*, 11: 302–310.

Levick, W.R., Oyster, C.W. and Davies, D.L. (1965) Evidence that McIlwain's periphery effect is not a stray light artefact. *J. Neurophysiol.*, 28: 555–559.

Lewis, H., Cowan, G.M. and Straatsma, B.R. (1986) Apparent disappearance of a macular hole associated with development of an epiretinal membrane. *Am. J. Ophthalmol.*, 102: 172–175.

Li, C.-Y. and Li, W. (1994) Extensive integration field beyond the classical receptive field of cat's striate cortical neurons: classification and tuning properties. *Vision Res.*, 34: 2337–2355.

Li, C.-Y., Zhou, Y.X., Pei, X., Qiu, F.T., Tang, C.Q. and Xu, X.Z. (1992) Extensive disinhibitory region beyond the classical receptive field of cat retinal ganglion cells. *Vision Res.*, 32: 219–228.

Lin, L.H., Bock, S., Carpenter, K., Rose, M. and Norden, J.J. (1992) Synthesis and transport of GAP-43 in entorhinal cortex neurons and perforant pathway during lesion-induced sprouting and reactive synaptogenesis. *Mol. Brain Res.*, 14: 147–153.

Linsenmeier, R.A., Frishman, L.J., Jakiela, H.G. and Enroth-Cugell, C. (1982) Receptive field properties of X and Y cells in the cat retina derived from contrast sensitivity measurements. *Vision Res.*, 22: 1173–1183.

Maffei, L. and Fiorentini, A. (1972) Retinogeniculate convergence and analysis of the contrast. *J. Neurophysiol.*, 35: 65–72.

Maffei, L. and Fiorentini, A. (1976) The unresponsive regions of visual cortical receptive fields. *Vision Res.*, 16: 1131–1139.

Malach, R., Amir, Y., Harel, M. and Grinvald, A. (1993) Relationship between intrinsic connections and functional architecture revealed by optical imaging and in vivo targeted biocytin injections in primate striate cortex. *Proc. Natl. Acad. Sci. USA*, 90: 10469–10473.

Matsubara, J., Cynader, M., Swindale, N.V. and Stryker, M.P. (1985) Intrinsic projections within visual cortex: evidence for orientation-specific local connections. *Proc. Natl. Acad. Sci. USA*, 82: 935–939.

McIlwain, J.T. (1964) Receptive fields of optic tract axons and lateral geniculate cells: peripheral extent and barbiturate sensitivity. *J. Neurophysiol.*, 27: 1154–1173.

McIlwain, J.T. (1966) Some evidence concerning the physiological basis of the periphery effect in the cat's retina. *Exp. Brain Res.*, 1: 265–271.

McIlwain, J.T. and Buser, P. (1968) Receptive fields of single cells in the cat's superior colliculus. *Exp. Brain Res.*, 5: 314–325.

Merzenich, M.M., Kaas, J.H., Wall, J., Nelson, R.J., Sur, M. and Felleman, D. (1983) Topographic reorganization of somatosensory cortical areas 3b and 1 in adult monkeys following restricted deafferentation. *Neuroscience*, 8: 33–55.

Morgan, C.M. and Schatz, H. (1985) Idiopathic macular holes. *Am. J. Ophthalmol.*, 99: 437–444.

Movshon, J.A. and Van Sluyters, R.C. (1981) Visual neuronal development. *Annu. Rev. Psychol.*, 32: 477–522.

Mower, G.D., Christen, W.G., Burchfiel, J.L. and Duffy, F.H. (1984) Microiontophoretic bicuculline restores binocular responses to visual cortical neurons in strabismic cats. *Brain Res.*, 309: 168–172.

Mullikin, W.H., Jones, J.P. and Palmer, L.A. (1984) Periodic simple cells in cat area 17. *J. Neurophysiol.*, 52: 372–387.

Murakami, I., Komatsu, H. and Kinoshita, M. (1997) Perceptual filling-in at the scotoma following a monocular retinal lesion in the monkey. *Vis. Neurosci.*, 14: 89–101.

Nelson, J.I. and Frost, J. (1978) Orientation selective inhibition from beyond the classic visual receptive field. *Brain Res.*, 139: 359–365.

Olson, C.R. and Freeman, R.D. (1978) Monocular deprivation and recovery during sensitive period in kittens. *J. Neurophysiol.*, 41: 65–74.

Olson, C.R. and Freeman, R.D. (1980) Profile of the sensitive period for monocular deprivation in kittens. *Exp. Brain Res.*, 39: 17–21.

Peterhans, E. and von der Heydt, R. (1989) Mechanisms of contour perception in monkey visual cortex. II. Contours bridging gaps. *J. Neurosci.*, 9: 1749–1763.

Pettet, M.W. and Gilbert, C.D. (1992) Dynamic changes in receptive-field size in cat primary visual cortex. *Proc. Natl. Acad. Sci. USA*, 89: 8366–8370.

Polat, U., Mizobe, K., Pettet, M.W., Kasamatsu, T. and Norcia, A.M. (1998) Colinear stimuli regulate visual responses depending on cell's contrast threshold. *Nature*, 391: 580–584.

Pollen, D.A. and Ronner, S.F. (1975) Periodic excitability changes across the receptive fields of complex cells in the striate and parastriate cortex of the cat. *J. Physiol. (Lond.)*, 245: 667–697.

Pollen, D.A., Andrews, B.W. and Feldon, S.E. (1978) Spatial frequency selectivity of periodic complex cells in the visual cortex of the cat. *Vision Res.*, 18: 665–682.

Ramachandran, V.S. (1992) Blind spots. *Sci. Am.*, 266: 85–91.

Ramachandran, V.S., Gregory, R.L. and Aiken, W. (1993) Perceptual fading of visual texture borders. *Vision Res.*, 33: 717–721.

Rasmusson, D.D. (1982) Reorganization of raccoon somatosensory cortex following removal of the fifth digit. *J. Comp. Neurol.*, 205: 313–326.

Rizzolatti, G., Camarda, R., Grupp, L.A. and Pisa, M. (1973) Inhibition of visual responses of single units in the cat superior colliculus by the introduction of a second visual stimulus. *Brain Res.*, 61: 390–394.

Rizzolatti, G., Camarda, R., Grupp, L.A. and Pisa, M. (1974)

Inhibitory effect of remote visual stimuli on visual responses of cat superior colliculus: spatial and temporal factors. *J. Neurophysiol.*, 37: 1262–1275.

Rizzolatti, G. and Camarda, R. (1975) Inhibition of visual responses of single units in the cat visual area of the lateral suprasylvian gyrus (Clare-Bishop area) by the introduction of the second visual stimulus. *Brain Res.*, 88: 357–361.

Robertson, D. and Irvine, D.R.F. (1989) Plasticity of frequency organization in auditory cortex of guinea pigs with partial unilateral deafness. *J. Comp. Neurol.*, 282: 456–471.

Rosa, M.G.P., Schmid, L.M. and Calford, M.B. (1995) Responsiveness of cat area 17 after monocular inactivation; limitation of topgraphic plasticity in adult cortex. *J. Physiol. (Lond.)*, 482: 589–608.

Rosa, M.G.P., Tweedale, R. and Elston, G.N. (2000) Visual responses of neurones in the middle temporal area of new world monkeys after lesions of striate cortex. *J. Neurosci.*, 20: 5552–5563.

Salin, P.A., Girard, P. and Bullier, J. (1993) Visuotopic organization of corticocortical connections in the visual system. *Prog. Brain Res.*, 95: 169–178.

Salin, P.A. and Bullier, J. (1995) Corticocortical connections in the visual system: structure and function. *Physiol. Rev.*, 75: 107–154.

Sanes, J.N., Suner, S., Lando, J.F. and Donoghue, J.P. (1988) Rapid reorganization of adult rat motor cortex somatic representation patterns after motor nerve injury. *Proc. Natl. Acad. Sci. USA*, 85: 2003–2007.

Schmid, L.M., Rosa, M.G.P. and Calford, M.B. (1995) Retinal detachment induces massive immediate reorganization in visual cortex. *NeuroReport*, 6: 1349–1353.

Schmid, L.M., Rosa, M.G.P., Calford, M.B. and Ambler, J.S. (1996) Visuotopic reorganization in the primary visual cortex of adult cats following monocular and binocular retinal lesions. *Cereb. Cortex*, 6: 388–405.

Shatz, C.J. and Stryker, M.P. (1978) Ocular dominance in layer IV of the cat's visual cortex and the effects of monocular deprivation. *J. Physiol. (Lond.)*, 281: 267–283.

Sherman, S.M. and Spear, P.D. (1982) Organization of visual pathways in normal and visually deprived cats. *Physiol. Rev.*, 62: 738–855.

Shou, T., Wang, W. and Yu, H. (2000) Orientation biased extended surround of the receptive field of cat retinal ganglion cells. *Neuroscience*, 98: 207–212.

Sillito, A.M., Kemp, J.A. and Patel, H. (1980) Inhibitory interactions contributing to the ocular dominance of monocularly dominated cells in the normal cat striate cortex. *Exp. Brain Res.*, 41: 1–10.

Sillito, A.M., Kemp, J.A. and Blakemore, C. (1981) The role of GABAergic inhibition in the cortical effects of monocular deprivation. *Nature*, 291: 318–320.

Singer, W. and Tretter, F. (1976a) Unusually large receptive fields in cats with restricted visual experience. *Exp. Brain Res.*, 26: 171–184.

Singer, W. and Tretter, F. (1976b) Receptive-field properties and neuronal connectivity in striate and parastriate cortex of contour-deprived cats. *J. Neurophysiol.*, 39: 613–630.

Smith, D.C., Spear, P.D. and Kratz, K.E. (1978) Role of visual experience in postcritical period reversal of effects of monocular deprivation in cat striate cortex. *J. Comp. Neurol.*, 178: 313–328.

Smith, R.G., Lea, S.J.H. and Galloway, N.R. (1990) Visual performance in idiopathic macular holes. *Eye*, 4: 190–194.

Spillman, L. and Kurtenbach, A. (1992) Dynamic noise backgrounds facilitate target fading. *Vision Res.*, 32: 1941–1946.

Sterling, P. and Wickelgren, B.G. (1969) Visual receptive fields in the superior colliculus of the cat. *J. Neurophysiol.*, 32: 1–15.

Tassignon, M.J., Stempels, N., Nguyen, L.J., De, W.F. and Brihaye, M. (1991) The effect of wavelength on glial fibrillary acidic protein immunoreactivity in laser-induced lesions in rabbit retina. *Graefes Arch. Clin. Exp. Ophthalmol.*, 229: 380–388.

Trachtenberg, J.T. and Stryker, M. (2001) Rapid anatomical plasticity of horizontal connections in the developing visual cortex. *J. Neurosci.*, 21: 3476–3482.

Trachtenberg, J.T., Trepel, C. and Stryker, M. (2000) Rapid extragranular plasticity in the absence of thalamocortical plasticity in the developing primary visual cortex. *Science*, 287: 2029–2032.

Troxler, D. (1804) Über das Verschwinden gegebener Gegenstände innerhalb unseres Gesichtskreises. In: K. Himly and A. Schmidt (Eds.), *Ophthalmologie Bibliothek*. Springer, Jena, pp. 431–573.

Tusa, R.J., Palmer, L.A and Rosenquist, A.C. (1981) Multiple cortical visual areas: visual field topography in the cat. In: C.N. Woolsey (Ed.), *Cortical sensory organization*, Vol. 2, *Multiple Visual Areas*. Humana Press, Clifton, NJ, pp. 1–31.

Vidyasagar, T.R. (1998) Gating of neuronal responses in macaque primary visual cortex by an attentional spotlight. *NeuroReport*, 9: 1947–1952.

Virsu, V. and Hari, R. (1996) Cortical magnification, scale invariance and visual ecology. *Vision Res.*, 36: 2971–2977.

Volchan, E. and Gilbert, C.D. (1994) Interocular transfer of receptive field expansion in cat visual cortex. *Vision Res.*, 35: 1–6.

Von der Heydt, R., Peterhans, E. and Baumgartner, G. (1984) Illusory contours and cortical neuron responses. *Science*, 224: 1260–1262.

Von der Heydt, R. and Peterhans, E. (1989) Mechanisms of contour perception in monkey visual cortex. I. Lines of pattern discontinuity. *J. Neurosci.*, 9: 1731–1748.

Waleszczyk, W.J., Wang, C., Burke, W. and Dreher, B. (1999) Velocity response profiles of collicular neurons: parallel and convergent visual information channels. *Neuroscience*, 93: 1063–1076.

Walker, G.A., Ohzawa, I. and Freeman, R.D. (1999) Asymmetric suppression outside the classical receptive field of the visual cortex. *J. Neurosci.*, 19: 10536–10553.

Walker, G.A., Ohzawa, I. and Freeman, R.D. (2000) Suppression outside the classical receptive field. *Vis. Neurosci.*, 17: 369–379.

Werblin, F.S. and Copenhagen, D.R. (1974) Control of retinal sensitivity. III. Lateral interactions at the inner plexiform layer. *J. Gen. Physiol.*, 63: 88–110.

Wiesel, T.N. (1982) Postnatal development of the visual cortex and the influence of environment. *Nature*, 299: 583–592.

Wiesel, T.N. and Hubel, D.H. (1963) Single-cell responses in striate cortex of kittens deprived of vision in one eye. *J. Neurophysiol.*, 26: 1003–1017.

Wiesel, T.N. and Hubel, D.H. (1965) Comparison of the effects of unilateral and bilateral eye closure on cortical unit responses in kittens. *J. Neurophysiol.*, 28: 1029–1040.

Wright, L.L., Metha, A.B. and Calford, M.B. (1999) A quantitative study of horizontal interactions in primary visual cortex in response to retinal-lesion-induced plasticity. *Proc. Aust. Neurosci. Soc.*, 10: 186.

Yamamoto, C., Ogata, N., Yi, X., Takahashi, K., Miyashiro, M., Yamada, H., Uyama, M. and Matsuzaki, K. (1996) Immunolocalization of basic fibroblast growth factor during wound repair in rat retina after laser photocoagulation. *Graefes Arch. Clin. Exp. Ophthalmol.*, 234: 695–702.

Zipser, K., Lamme, V.A.F. and Schiller, P.H. (1996) Contextual modulation in primary visual cortex. *J. Neurosci.*, 16: 7376–7389.

C. Casanova and M. Ptito (Eds.)
Progress in Brain Research, Vol. 134

CHAPTER 16

Neural analysis of visual information during locomotion

Helen Sherk * and Garth A. Fowler

Department of Biological Structure, Box 35-7420, University of Washington, Seattle, WA 98195, USA

Abstract: For most vertebrate species, vision is critical during locomotion. In this review, we survey what is known about neural mechanisms that might be involved in this visual analysis. Problems that such mechanisms are likely to solve include: (1) determination of heading (the discrepancy between an observer's direction of motion and direction of gaze); (2) detection of course changes; (3) setting of courses using goals and landmarks; (4) obstacle avoidance; (5) accurate foot placement. To understand how the visual system handles these tasks, we must first consider what neurons 'see' during locomotion: this is determined both by an observer's motion and by his gaze. We then review response properties of neurons in the cortical 'motion pathways' of the monkey and cat as they relate to problems encountered during locomotion. The most studied areas are the medial superior temporal area in the monkey, which has been linked to heading determination, and the lateral suprasylvian area in the cat, where many cells are sensitive to motion in depth, and some are selective for optic flow patterns generated during locomotion. A few subcortical populations have also been linked to visual analysis during locomotion. Most notable are cells in the pigeon's nucleus rotundus: these respond selectively to looming stimuli, some firing at a specific time before the stimulus collides with the bird. Another intriguing population is in the cat's visual pontine nucleus, where cells respond to large displays suggestive of optic flow during locomotion.

How is vision used during locomotion?

To get around in the world, most terrestrial animals depend on vision. A locomoting observer must deal with various problems not faced by an observer at rest, and many investigators have thus suggested that specialized neural mechanisms are called into play. What problems confront a locomoting visual system? Here is a list of those we think most important:

- Heading determination
- Detection of course changes
- Course setting using goals and landmarks
- Obstacle avoidance
- Foot placement.

The first task, heading determination, has received the lion's share of attention in studies of neural mechanisms involved in visual guidance. The 'heading problem' concerns the discrepancy between the direction one is going and the direction one is looking. Visual images are seen in retinal coordinates, but to take appropriate action — to avoid walking into a chair, for example — one must know the location of an object in body-centered coordinates.

Is there really a 'heading problem'? A locomoting observer could solve the problem by continuously fixating his heading point so that his retinal and body-centered coordinate systems remain aligned — thus, for example, when walking along a sidewalk, an observer would keep his gaze centered and fixed on the horizon. Readers may suspect from their own experience that humans, at least, do not always behave this way. Indeed, while this might be a workable strategy for a flying observer[1], when walking

* Corresponding author: H. Sherk, Department of Biological Structure, Box 35-7420, University of Washington, Seattle, WA 98195, USA. Tel.: +1-206-543-4851; Fax: +1-206-543-1524; E-mail: has@u.washington.edu

[1] Clearly some birds do not follow this strategy. One species that is particularly easy to observe is the short-eared owl, which hunts by day, flying over open fields. Because owls are virtually incapable of making eye movements, they move their heads to shift their gaze, and it is readily apparent that short-eared owls look around while in flight.

or running it is a poor strategy because it would keep the observer's gaze at eye level, while the region of interest is generally on or near the ground. In practice, terrestrial vertebrates probably seldom fixate their heading points when walking or running, and so they indeed must solve the 'heading problem'. Just what observers do with their gaze when locomoting is an issue that is only now beginning to receive experimental attention; in the next section (What does a locomoting observer see?) we describe some observations on cats and humans.

The 'heading problem' is really an instance of a general problem that must be solved by any observer who relies on vision to interact with his surroundings. A locomoting observer has the advantage that abundant visual information specifies his direction of heading. Images move in a stereotyped 'optic flow field' (Gibson, 1950, 1979), approximately radially outward from the heading point, with each image accelerating and expanding as it moves (see Fig. 1A). Psychophysical work suggests that humans can accurately specify the location of their heading point based on the pattern of motion in an optic flow field (Warren and Hannon, 1988; Warren et al., 1988). In these experiments, we should note, observers were seated and stationary, and attempted to localize a simulated heading point in a display of moving dots. Experiments on heading determination in locomoting subjects, animal or human, have not been attempted. Nonetheless, these psychophysical experiments demonstrated that humans can make use of 'optic flow' cues to localize a simulated heading point. In the third section (Medial superior temporal area (MST) and heading determination) we discuss cells in one cortical area in macaque monkeys that may play a key role in this computation.

The second item on our list, detection of course changes, could be accomplished by neurons that distinguish between different patterns of optic flow. The optic flow generated by locomotion along a straight path (as in Fig. 1A) has been widely described. Less often discussed is the pattern of optic flow that occurs when the locomoting observer turns (for example, see Fig. 1B). The image of a particular object in the optic flow field can change directions during a turn, even reversing course, because a new vector of motion is added to its 'optic flow' vector. The 'optic flow' vector is generated by the observer's forward movement, while the new vector is horizontal and opposite to the direction of the turn. This altered optic flow provides potent feedback about the observer's change of course. In the fourth section (Dectecting course changes during locomotion) we discuss neurons that might detect such changes.

Cells used for solving either of these first two tasks presumably respond to global patterns of motion rather than to a particular image in an optic flow field. Cells have been found in several studies that respond to global motion, but whose behavior is not clearly related to either of our first two proposed tasks. These neurons are described in the fifth section (Other cells responsive to global patterns of motion).

The third task, course-setting using goals, was explored in some early psychophysical studies, but has not been the focus of any neurophysiological work. Thomson (1983) found that observers who view a goal (a post in the middle of an open field) while standing still do not need any subsequent visual feedback to walk accurately to it (see also Elliot, 1986; Steenhuis and Goodale, 1988; Rieser et al., 1990). Does this mean that visual feedback during locomotion is unnecessary for choosing and then approaching a goal? No — in many situations, a *locomoting* observer chooses a goal and sets a course towards it. A flying bird needs to pick out a suitable branch for landing; a mouse fleeing from a cat must locate a hole to hide in; a cat fleeing from a dog seeks a telephone pole or tree to climb.

Equally common may be the use of visual cues (landmarks) to make continuous course corrections. By landmark we mean any fixed object, distant or close, whose position is used as a reference for one's motion. Thus, for example, when walking along a trail through a meadow, the grass on either side of the trail serves as a landmark to keep one centered on the trail. In the sixth section (Use of goals and landmarks to set a course, and obstacle avoidance) we discuss cells that respond to specific objects in simulated optic flow fields that might represent landmarks.

The fourth item on our list, obstacle avoidance, is closely related to goal-directed locomotion. In both cases the visual system must recognize that there is an object in the observer's path. The observer's response to the object may be quite different depend-

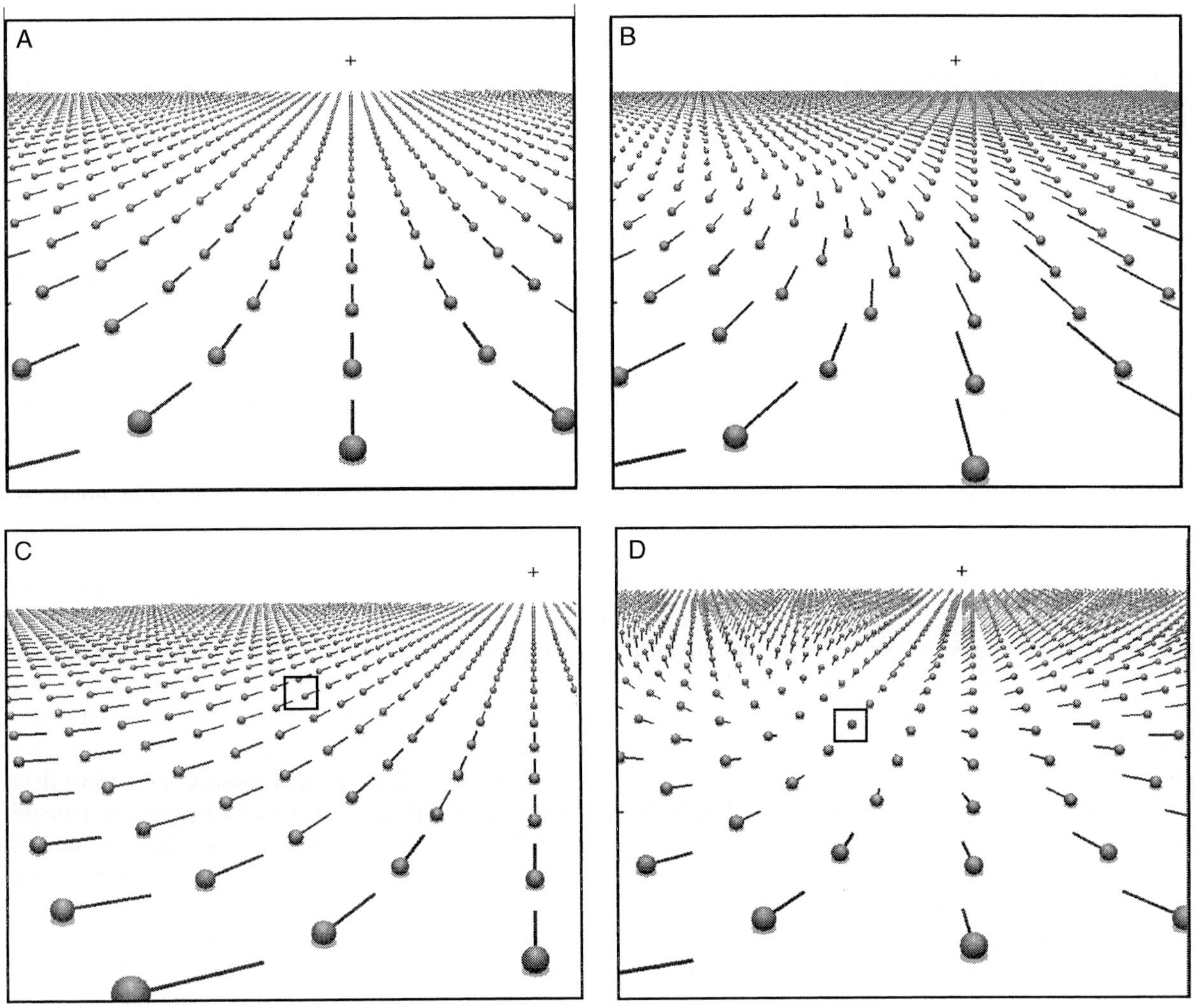

Fig. 1. Optic flow fields and retinal flow fields, illustrated by the motion of small balls distributed across a substrate. Each ball is attached to the head of a vector showing its direction and speed; the cross represents the observer's heading point. (A) Optic flow generated by motion along a straight path. (B) Optic flow generated by forward motion at 80 cm/s combined with a left turn at 30 deg/s. (C) Retinal flow pattern generated by locomotion along a straight path while maintaining gaze down and to the left of the heading point (box). (D) Retinal flow generated by locomotion along a straight path while tracking one of the balls (enclosed in box).

ing on circumstances — thus a tree may represent an obstacle to be avoided by a cat strolling in the garden, but signify a haven to be climbed when the cat is pursued by a dog. Nonetheless, the visual stimulus in both cases is identical. Cells that might respond to objects in the observer's path are described in the sixth section (Use of goals and landmarks to set a course, and obstacle avoidance).

The final item on our list is visual guidance of foot placement. In our artificial environment of smooth floors, pavement, lawns, and paths, we only occasionally have to pay attention to how we place our feet. In a natural environment, however, the ground is generally uneven and populated with hazards such as stones, holes, and roots. To avoid stumbling, an observer moving across natural terrain must place his feet with care. The seventh section (Foot placement) deals with cells that might detect small objects or irregularities and lead to alterations in foot placement.

What does a locomoting observer see?

Walking or running give rise to predictable optic flow fields like those in Fig. 1A and B. But, because an observer is free to look at different parts of an optic flow field, or to track particular images in it, the pattern of motion that falls on his retina — what we might refer to as *retinal flow* — is less predictable. To understand what kind of stimulation a given neuron is exposed to we need to know something about the gaze strategies that locomoting observers employ. Based on the behavior of stationary observers, we might predict two strategies. (1) The observer might maintain a relatively constant angle of gaze, so that the discrepancy between direction of heading and direction of gaze remains constant. Fig. 1C shows the retinal flow seen by an observer walking along a straight path and maintaining an angle of gaze that is 39° to the left of his heading point. (2) The observer might fixate a stationary object in the environment and track it as he locomotes, using some combination of eye and head movements. Fig. 1D shows the retinal flow that an observer sees when he tracks a small ball on the ground that is 60 cm away and 20 cm to the left of his path.

A tracking strategy seems particularly likely for species like primates and cats that have a highly mobile gaze (at least when standing still). One might even argue that they would *always* track because it is well known that, when there is motion across the entire visual field (as when a subject, either animal or human, is placed inside a rotating striped drum), an observer tracks that motion — that is, they display an optokinetic reflex. But the motion in an optic flow field is quite different from the uniform motion seen inside a rotating drum — images move in many different directions and at many different speeds. Tracking an object that one is approaching is also a challenge to the oculomotor system because the observer must converge his eyes as he approaches it. Primates appear capable of such tracking at walking speeds (Miles, 1998); other species have not been tested.

What, then, do locomoting observers actually do with their gaze? This is difficult to measure. Stationary monkeys viewing a cloud of dots simulating an optic flow field appear at times to track the motion of some dots, though at such a low gain that images still move fairly briskly across the fovea (Lappe et al., 1998). In the only study done on locomoting monkeys, Solomon and Cohen (1992) found that a macaque monkey walking in a tight circle tended to repeatedly fixate a stable object. In this experimental situation, however, no visual guidance was necessary — the monkey was attached to a rigid arm that rotated around a central post and constrained its path. At the opposite extreme in terms of visual guidance, in a test situation in which precise foot placement was demanded for each step, human subjects appeared to fixate each target 'stepping stone' until foot contact (Hollands et al., 1995). This situation was highly unusual — as readers know from their own experience, we do not normally watch each foot as it contacts the ground. Using a more natural task (subjects walked down a runway and stepped over an obstacle) Patla and Vickers (1997) found that subjects used both of the strategies proposed above — they fixated the obstacle for about 33% of the time, and they maintained an approximately constant angle of gaze for about 20% of the time. We have found that cats show similar behavior. Cats walking down an alley and relying on vision to avoid stepping on numerous small objects maintain a constant angle of gaze about half the time (Fowler et al., 2000). However, these episodes of constant gaze are generally short (<500 ms), so the cat spends a considerable amount of time shifting its gaze. During episodes of constant gaze the cat keeps its gaze close to its own midsagittal plane (within about 15°) and directed downward, a strategy that seems sensible for an observer who needs to pay close attention to the path in front of its feet. Cats also occasionally track objects in the alley as they walk, and in addition may glance to one side or up. When the walking cat makes a turn, its gaze anticipates the turn by rotating in the direction of the turn before the cat actually changes course. Similar behavior is shown by humans driving cars on a winding road (Land and Lee, 1994): when approaching a turn, a driver's gaze shifts to a point in advance of the car's current heading point.

What, then, can we conclude about the pattern of retinal flow that neurons may see during visually guided locomotion? For cats walking across a cluttered substrate, the most common retinal flow pattern appears to resemble that in Fig. 1A, with the center of gaze some 10–20° below the horizon and fairly close to the midline. Cats thus do face a 'heading problem', although the discrepancy between direction of gaze and direction of heading is generally modest. Humans likewise shift their gaze frequently when walking. We would like to know what gaze strategy monkeys commonly follow, since so much physiological work has been done on the macaque, but experiments on locomoting monkeys who are using visual cues remain to be done. We should note, however, that arboreal monkeys might employ rather different gaze strategies since their common mode of locomotion — leaping and hopping through a tree canopy (Fleagle, 1978) — differs from that of ground-dwelling species.

Medial superior temporal area (MST) and heading determination

A cell that signals the discrepancy between direction of gaze and direction of heading might be expected to respond to a global pattern of motion rather than to individual elements within such a pattern. Attention focused on area MST in the macaque monkey (shown in Fig. 2) when Saito et al. (1986) discovered that some cells (11% of their sample from dorsal MST) responded preferentially to a large field of dots that were moving radially outward and increasing in size. They pointed out that such a pattern occurs naturally only when an observer moves through the environment.

Subsequent early studies focused on two issues. First was the idea that any optic flow field can be decomposed into four basic elements: motion in a frontoparallel plane ('planar motion'), radial motion outward or inward, circular motion, and shear (Koenderink, 1986). Shear here refers to the deformation of image shape as an object's position relative to the observer changes. It was suggested (Tanaka and Saito, 1989; Orban et al., 1992) that distinct populations of neurons respond specifically to each component, and their combined outputs then describe the optic flow field. Later work (Duffy and Wurtz, 1991a; Graziano et al., 1994) indicated that these populations were less distinct than originally thought. An equally serious problem for the decomposition model is that the behavior of cells in MST is far from linear, so that even a cell that is selective for a single motion component (for example, radial motion) fails to reliably extract information about that motion component from a complex stimulus such as an optic flow field (Orban et al., 1992).

A second issue raised in early studies was that of response constancy across spatial displacements of the stimulus pattern. Two kinds of motion — radial and circular — have a unique center of motion or focus of expansion (FOE). Investigators asked whether a cell selective for such motion responds equally well no matter where in the receptive field the FOE is located. They reasoned that a cell that extracts one component of motion should not confound the type of motion with the position of the FOE. Several investigators (Saito et al., 1986; Duffy and Wurtz, 1991b; Orban et al., 1992) found that a substantial number of cells did in fact respond in a position-invariant fashion.

Although in early studies investigators had a well-defined hypothesis about how cells in MST might decompose an optic flow field into components of motion, they were less clear about how this would be useful for guiding locomotion. It was suggested, for example, that the monkey could use this information "to perceive the mode, direction, and speed of the relative movement between the self and external space" (Tanaka and Saito, 1989, p. 639) or to determine the monkey's 'direction and path of self-motion' (Duffy and Wurtz, 1991a, p. 1343). The pattern of optic flow does indeed provide information about one's path — that is, whether one is going straight or turning (e.g. Fig. 1) — but no studies on MST have asked whether cells are sensitive to these different patterns. Information about one's own direction of motion relative to the environment is more problematic. The image motion generated by a particular object could inform a monkey whether it was heading directly towards the object or to one side of it. However, cells in MST are reportedly not concerned with the motion of particular objects, but rather with the global pattern of motion generated by all elements in the environment. For an observer moving in a straight line, this global pattern will be the same for all directions of travel relative to the environment, whether up or down, north or south. Nor can observer speed be extracted solely from optic flow information since image speed depends both on the observer's speed and on the distance of objects from the observer.

More recent studies on MST have turned to its possible role in determining heading. Lagae et al. (1994)

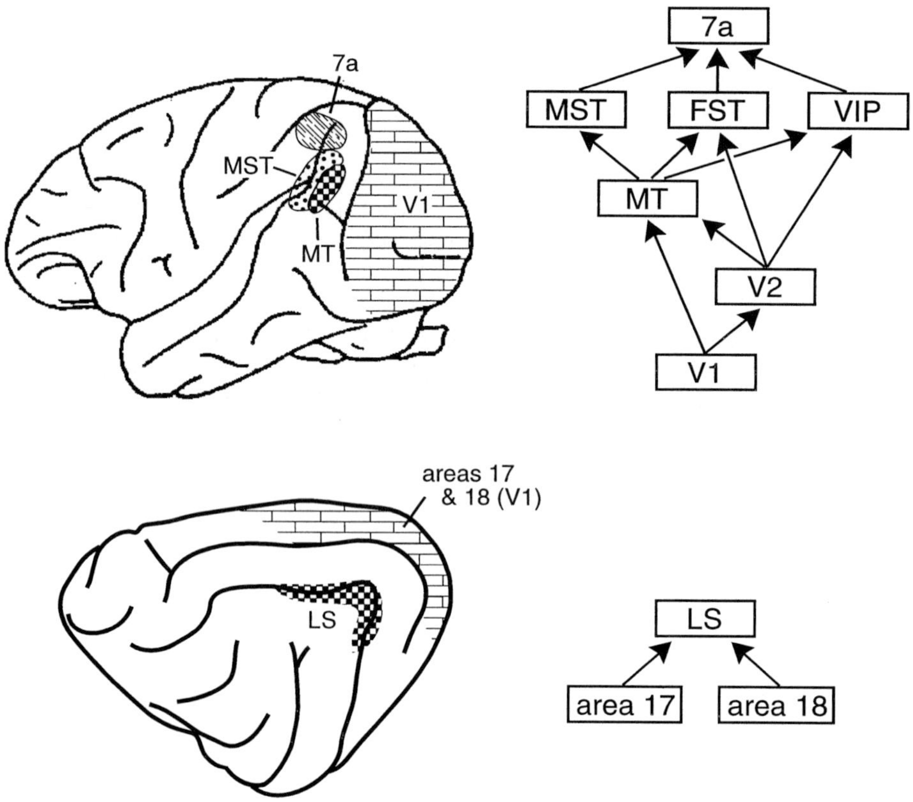

Fig. 2. Cortical areas of the 'motion streams' of the macaque monkey (top) and cat (bottom). In the brains on the left, only those areas are shown that we discuss. In the diagrams on the right, a few additional areas have been added for the monkey. Feedback connections are not drawn, nor are connections that link areas that appear to be at the same hierarchical level. Data for monkey are based on Ungerleider and Desimone (1986) and Felleman and Van Essen (1991).

pointed out that cells that respond well to radial-out motion might be involved in this calculation. They also noted that a cell that responds equally well no matter where the FOE is located cannot very well provide useful information about heading, and subsequently interest in this kind of constancy has waned. Instead, investigators began to ask whether cells in MST are selective for the location of the FOE within their receptive fields. Duffy and Wurtz (1995) tested cells with radial-outward moving fields of dots that were either centered, or offset 45° from the fovea in one of eight different directions. They found that 65% of cells had a significant preference for FOE position, although their tuning was often quite broad. Although the single most commonly preferred location of the FOE was at the center of gaze, many cells preferred locations with eccentricities of 45°. Does this mean that monkeys commonly keep their gaze directed 45° away from their heading point during locomotion? This behavior seems unlikely and, in an arboreal animal, downright dangerous. Lappe et al. (1996) suggested how the puzzling preference for very eccentric FOE locations might be resolved. Instead of determining heading by asking which cells respond most strongly, the system could take a weighted average of the activity of all cells that are selective for FOE location. These investigators tested this hypothesis by generating fine-grained maps of sensitivity to FOE location for a sample of MST cells. Unlike Duffy and Wurtz, they found that cells preferring a centered FOE were rare. More typical were ones that showed a gradient of response to a given pattern such as radial-outward motion, with response being maximal when the FOE was placed near one edge of the large stimulus display, and response being minimal when the FOE was placed near the opposite edge. Fig. 3

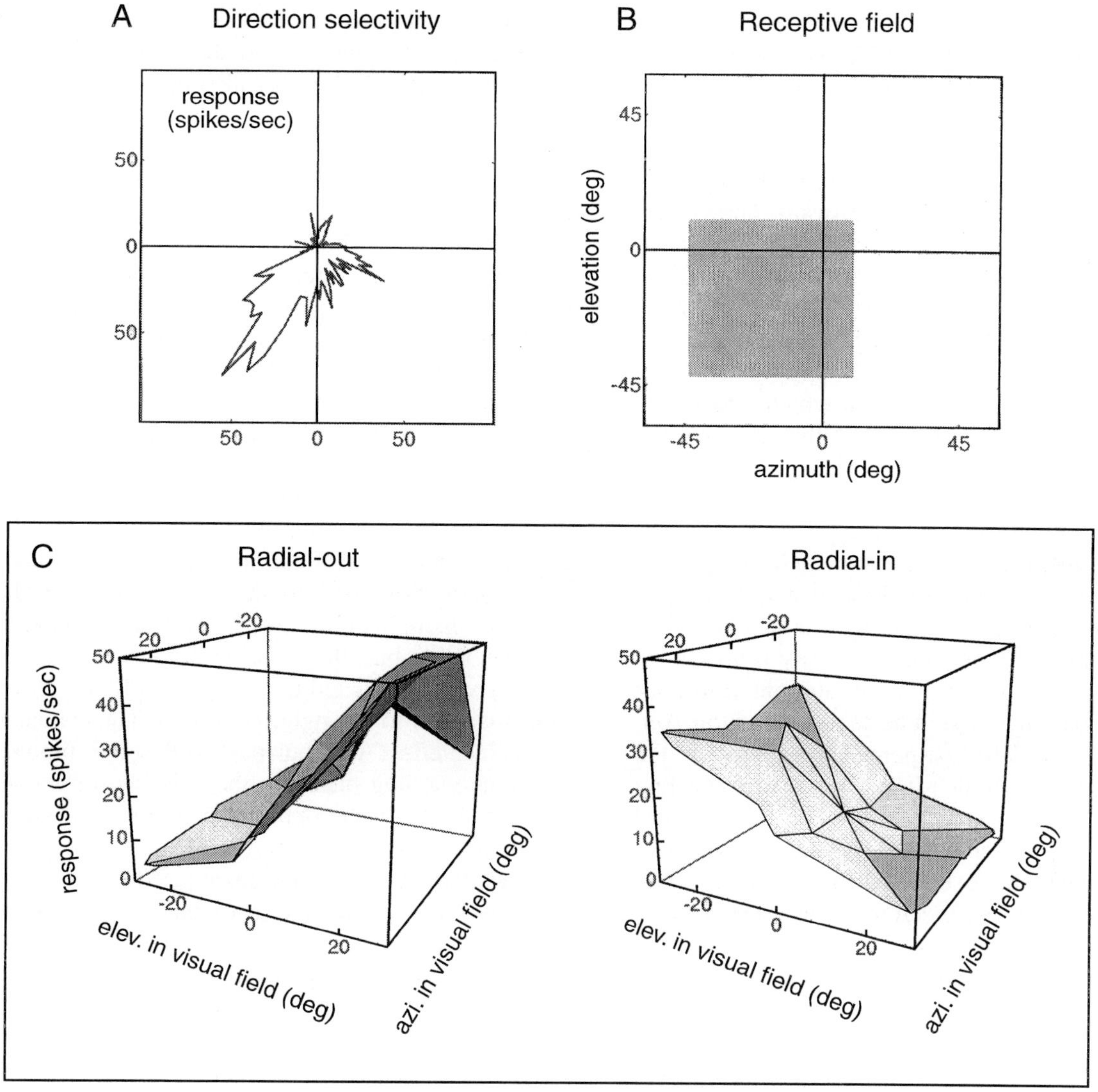

Fig. 3. Responses of a cell in area MST showing selectivity for location of the FOE. (A) Direction tuning for a large display of dots moving in a frontoparallel plane, plotted in polar coordinates. (B) Receptive field — like most in MST, it is large and includes the fovea. (C) Three-dimensional plot of responses to large displays of dots moving radially outward (on left) or inward (on right). Seventeen different locations of the FOE were tested. The cell responded best when the FOE was far up in the visual field and dots moved radially outward, but it preferred FOE locations in the lower hemifield when dots moved radially inward. (After Lappe et al., 1996, with permission.)

illustrates the behavior of one such cell. The tuning of any given cell for FOE position was broad, but the population response (using a sample of only 31 cells) yielded a surprisingly accurate estimate of FOE position, within 4.3° of the correct location.

So far we have considered the evidence suggesting that the function of MST is to determine heading. There are, however, difficulties with this interpretation. For one thing, cells that are selective for the location of the FOE might well give unreliable information when the monkey tracks a fixed point in the environment. In this case, as we have seen in Fig. 1D, the FOE does not tell the monkey where its heading point is located (Regan and Beverley, 1982).

The same problem arises when the monkey turns (e.g. Fig. 1B). Bradley et al. (1996) have investigated cell behavior in a paradigm that at first glance appears to be similar to the first of these situations: a monkey tracked a target moving in a straight line at constant speed, superimposed against a background display of dots moving radially outward. They found that some cells that responded to specific visual field locations of the FOE appeared to compensate for shifting gaze — that is, they reported on FOE location in head-centered, not retinal-centered, coordinates. Note, however, that Bradley et al.'s test situation was simpler than that in which a locomoting monkey tracks a fixed point in the environment, in which case its gaze is accelerating, and, during turns, following a curving trajectory.

Another difficulty is that many cells in MST appear to be ill-suited for determining heading. It is hard to think of a role for those that respond primarily or exclusively to planar motion — only when a locomoting observer looks 90° away from his direction of heading (straight up, straight down, or directly to one side) would he see such motion. Yet, as Saito et al. (1986) first pointed out, these are the most abundant cells in MST. Even more puzzling are cells that are strongly selective for radial-inward motion — a smaller population than those selective for radial-out, to be sure (Saito et al., 1986; Tanaka and Saito, 1989), but a cell type observed in many studies of MST. Such a pattern indicates that the observer is looking backward while locomoting forward. (Alternatively, the observer might simply be walking backward.) In either case, the visual information would be useless for guidance since the observer would be looking where he had been, rather than where he was going. Similarly, cells that are selective for circular motion have no clear role in optic flow analysis. No mode of locomotion gives rise to a global pattern of rotation. Spiral motion contains a rotational component and, when filling the receptive field, can drive some cells in MST (Graziano et al., 1994). However, the spiral motion occurring during turns is limited to a small part of the visual field (e.g. Fig. 1C), and the response of MST cells to such simulations is unknown.

Another mysterious subset of cells in MST are those that respond to vestibular stimulation. There seems to be no systematic agreement between the direction of physical movement of a monkey that drives such cells, and the simulated heading direction in a visual display that also drives these cells (Duffy, 1998; Bremmer et al., 1999). How vestibular input might contribute to heading perception is thus puzzling. Finally, many cells in MST fire vigorously either to small stimuli that bear no resemblance to optic flow fields, or in conjunction with smooth pursuit eye movements (Tanaka et al., 1986; Komatsu and Wurtz, 1988).

Obviously, it would be of great interest to link neural activity in MST with heading perception, but doing so is not easy. Britten and van Wezel (1998) made an attempt by electrically stimulating sites in MST during a behavioral task. As one cannot ask a stationary monkey where it perceives its heading direction to be, these investigators instead asked the monkey whether the FOE in a dot display simulating optic flow was to the left or right of the monkey's fixation point. Electrical stimulation might be expected to bias the monkey's choice if a cluster of cells was stimulated that, for example, preferred FOE locations to the right of fixation. The evidence for such an effect was equivocal, with some stimulus locations yielding biases in the expected direction, other locations in the opposite direction, and many having no consistent effect. Another perplexing finding was that the same experiment performed on area MT had a similar outcome (Nace and Britten, 1997), even though MT is generally not thought to play any special role in heading perception.

Considering this array of results, it seems possible that MST plays a major role in determining heading during locomotion, but this conclusion should be tempered with some cautionary notes. First, no direct evidence yet exists to support this conclusion, and indeed such evidence may remain elusive since it is difficult to think how one might test heading determination in a locomoting monkey. Second, many cells in MST appear to be poorly suited for this task, suggesting that this area is also involved in other kinds of analysis (e.g. Saito et al., 1986; Komatsu and Wurtz, 1988).

Detecting course changes during locomotion

Another role that cells with a strong preference for global patterns of motion might play is to detect a change in the direction of locomotion. The entire optic flow pattern changes abruptly when a locomoting observer begins to turn. A cell that detects unintended turns might respond when the pattern of optic flow changes from that generated by motion along a straight path (Fig. 1A) to that generated by a turn (Fig. 1B). We have looked for such cells in an extrastriate cortical area in the cat, the lateral suprasylvian visual area (LS) (Sherk et al., 1996). LS is the lateral suprasylvian region that receives direct input from striate cortex, and, because of its anatomical, physiological and retinotopic similarities, has often been considered analogous to the primate area MT (Zeki, 1974; Sherk and Mulligan, 1993). Cells that signal a turn, we hypothesized, would respond weakly or not at all to optic flow simulating travel along a straight path, and strongly to optic flow simulating a turn. Our stimuli simulated this sequence of events for turns of various sizes to the left or right. About 21% of the sample responded specifically to the optic flow generated when a turn began. Fig. 4 shows a cell that was selective not only for turn direction (to the left), but also for the rate of turn (30 deg/s).

The displays that we tested simulated what a cat would see if it looked at a point 8° below its heading point while turning. This pattern of retinal flow mimics what a cat might experience if it were following a straight path and inadvertently veered to one side. But if the cat made an intentional turn, we would expect a cell to see a different pattern because turning cats look ahead in the direction of their turn before they actually begin turning (see What does a locomoting observer see?). How cells in LS (or anywhere else) might respond to the retinal flow generated by this sequence of events is unknown.

Other cells responsive to global patterns of motion

Cells in some locations other than MST and LS have been identified that respond strongly to global patterns of motion suggestive of optic flow. One might expect to find such cells in the 'motion' stream of visual cortical processing (see Fig. 2). However, experiments in macaque monkeys on the first stage in this pathway, area MT, have yielded only equivocal evidence. MT cells respond relatively poorly to large displays of dots moving in a fronto-parallel plane, probably because many have suppressive surrounds (Allman et al., 1985; Tanaka et al., 1986). Looking at absolute levels of response, however, Lagae et al. (1994) found that MT cells respond on the whole significantly more strongly than MST cells to such displays. We should not discount the possibility that MT cells play a role in optic flow analysis independent of MST, which is only one of several targets of its output (Ungerleider and Desimone, 1986). Investigating what may be the top level of the macaque's 'motion' pathway, area 7a, Siegel and Read (1997) found just a tiny number of cells to be selective for dot displays with radial-outward motion. Whether cells specialized for analysis of global optic flow are confined in the macaque to intermediate stages of the motion pathway, or whether they might be discovered in MT or area 7 by the use of alternative stimuli, remains to be seen.

One might expect that the cat's LS, since it seems to be analogous to MT, would lack cells that respond strongly to large-field optic flow displays. But, as we have seen in the previous section, a subset of cells in LS do respond selectively to particular patterns of global motion. In addition to cells that prefer simulations of optic flow during turns, we found cells that prefer optic flow simulating travel along a straight path (Kim et al., 1997). For a small number of cells, such optic flow was the best stimulus that we could find (see cell in Fig. 5). Among the general population, we found a striking bias for optic flow that simulated the cat's forward motion compared to optic flow simulating backward motion. These findings suggest that some (and perhaps many) cells in LS are involved in visual analysis during locomotion, though exactly what role they play is unknown.

In the cat, nothing is known about optic flow analysis in the cortical 'motion' pathway beyond LS. Interestingly, however, one of the major subcortical targets of LS, the visual pontine region, contains neurons that have long been linked to analysis of optic flow fields. Located in the ventromedial visual pontine region, these cells have huge receptive fields and respond preferentially to large moving dot patterns (Baker et al., 1976). They are direction selective, and as a population prefer downward and outward motion (that is, away from the vertical

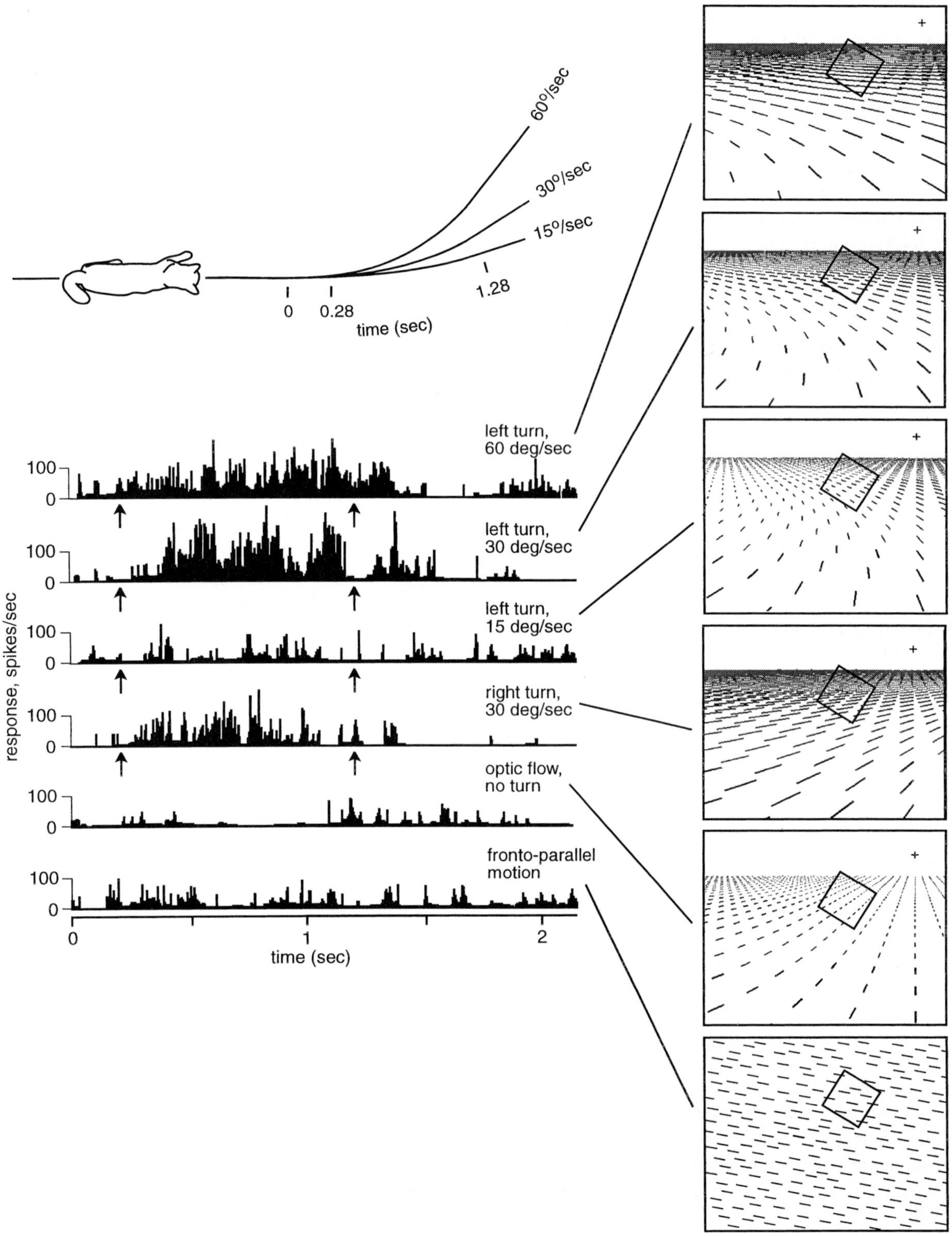
60°/sec
30°/sec
15°/sec
0
0.28
1.28
time (sec)
left turn,
60 deg/sec
left turn,
30 deg/sec
left turn,
15 deg/sec
right turn,
30 deg/sec
optic flow,
no turn
fronto-parallel
motion
response, spikes/sec
100
0
0
1
2
time (sec)

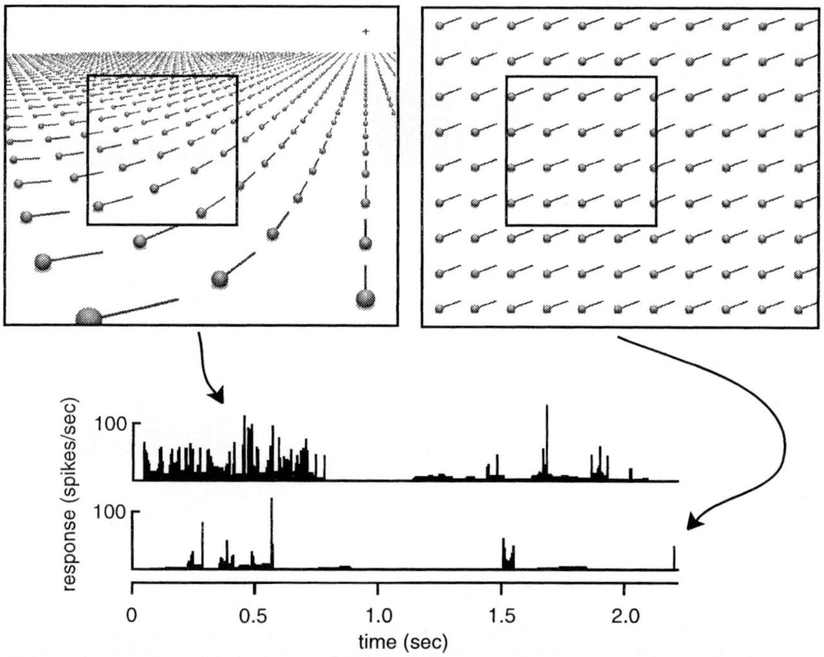

Fig. 5. Responses of a cell in area LS that responded only to optic flow generated by locomotion along a straight path. Vector representation of the retinal flow stimulus is at the top left (the actual stimulus simulated a carpet of small balls of varying shades of gray, across which the cat moved at 80 cm/s, maintaining its gaze 12° below its heading point). The cell had almost no response to frontoparallel motion with a direction and speed matched to that at the center of the receptive field in the retinal flow stimulus (righthand vector drawing, and bottom PSTH). Squares in the vector drawings represent the receptive field, located on the horizontal meridian at an azimuth of 34°.

meridian), the directions that predominate in the optic flow seen by terrestrial observers (e.g. Fig. 1A). Although these properties are quite different from those described for primary visual cortex (Hubel and Wiesel, 1962, 1965), Gibson et al. (1978) demonstrated that the small subpopulation in area 18 that projects to the visual pontine nuclei have anomalous response properties that are strikingly similar to those of visual pontine cells. We might thus picture a pathway that routes visual information from areas 18 and LS through the visual pontine nuclei and thence to the cerebellum, providing a mechanism for the rapid modulation of motor output during locomotion.

Use of goals and landmarks to set a course, and obstacle avoidance

So far we have discussed cells that are selective for the global pattern of motion over a large region

---

Fig. 4. Responses of a cell in area LS to retinal flow simulating locomotion along a straight path and then turning to the left or right, with gaze 8° below the heading point. Simulated paths are shown at the top. Responses to three rates of leftward turn are illustrated in the top three PSTHs (the turn portion of the stimulus lies between the arrows). Responses are also shown for one rightward turn, and no turn (4th and 5th PSTHs). Finally, the response to frontoparallel motion is shown (bottom PSTH); in it, speed and direction matched that at the center of the receptive field during the 30 deg/s left turn. Vector diagrams at the right illustrate the motion seen in the retinal flow simulations. Box represents the receptive field, cross is the simulated heading point. The actual stimulus simulated an environment in which the substrate was densely carpeted with small balls in different shades of gray, with similar balls hovering in air; the balls' motion accurately reproduced that seen by a cat walking at 80 cm/s and turning. This cell responded best to optic flow simulating a 30 deg/s left turn. It failed to respond either to optic flow simulating 'straight path' locomotion or to frontoparallel motion matched in speed and direction to the 30 deg/s turn.

of visual field. To accomplish the remaining three tasks on our list, however, a locomoting observer needs to detect individual objects that are part of an optic flow field. Thus, for example, a monkey leaping or hopping through a tree canopy must select a goal (a tree branch) for its next foot placement (Fleagle, 1978). The monkey must also plan its leaps to avoid colliding with tree trunks. How does the visual system extract information about a single critical object from a complex optic flow field? In one particular situation, that of an object that lies directly in an observer's path and is close to eye level, a unique and powerful cue is available: the image of the object moves in opposite directions in the two eyes[2]. Because such motion occurs only when an object is on a collision course with the observer's head, it seems plausible that there are neurons specialized for its detection. These have been termed 'approach' cells.

Such cells have been observed in various locations. In the cat's area 18, Cynader and Regan (1978) found a few cells that responded to opposing horizontal directions of motion in the two eyes, but showed some inhibition when stimuli moved in the same direction in both eyes. The majority of these cells actually responded to motion away from, not towards, the cat and thus would not be useful during locomotion. Rare observations of similar cells have been made in other studies of primary visual cortex (see, for example, the study of macaque monkey's V1 by Poggio and Fischer, 1977).

In contrast to these reports, Toyama and colleagues (Toyama and Kozasa, 1982; Toyama et al., 1986a,b; Akase et al., 1998) found abundant cells (as many as 60%) that appeared to be selective for motion in depth in the cat's area LS. In early experiments these investigators tested responses to a 3-dimensional disk that started out centered in the receptive field and physically moved directly towards the cat's nose, and then away. They also used stereoscopic displays that simulated such motion, generally by presenting stimuli that moved in opposite directions in the two eyes. The largest subset

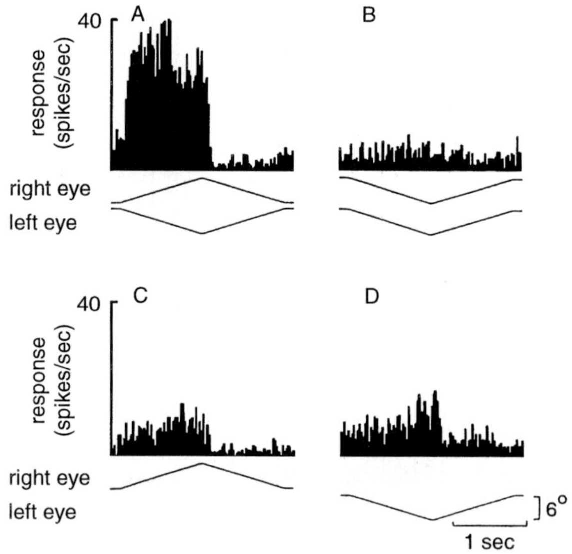

Fig. 6. Responses of an 'approach' cell in LS to simulated motion in depth. A spot stimulus, 4° in diameter and moving horizontally, was presented independently to each eye; the traces below the PSTHs indicate its direction of motion (up signifies rightward motion, and down, leftward motion). Receptive field azimuth = 6.4°, elevation = −6, and diameter = 1°. (A) The spot moved in opposite directions in the two eyes, simulating motion in depth starting in the receptive field and 57 cm distant, approaching to 22 cm, and then retracing its path (simulating a speed of 35 cm/s). (B) The spot had identical motion in two eyes. (C) Monocular presentation, right eye only. (D) Monocular presentation, left eye only. (After Toyama et al., 1986a, with permission.)

(~36%) of cells responded selectively to object trajectories that would end in collisions with the cat's nose ('approach' cells), like the cell illustrated in Fig. 6. They were often quite selective, discriminating between motion towards the nose and motion towards one eye.

Would 'approach' cells warn a locomoting cat about an impending collision? Not necessarily — because of suppression by their receptive field surrounds, during locomotion, when images move throughout the visual field, these cells might fail to respond to *any* object. Many cells in LS have large surrounds that profoundly depress cell responses when they 'see' motion in the cell's preferred direction (Von Grunau and Frost, 1983). We have observed, however, that optic flow motion, which is a complex pattern containing a range of directions, does not suppress responses to the same extent as

[2] An observer can, of course, suppress this motion by continuously tracking the object with converging eye movements.

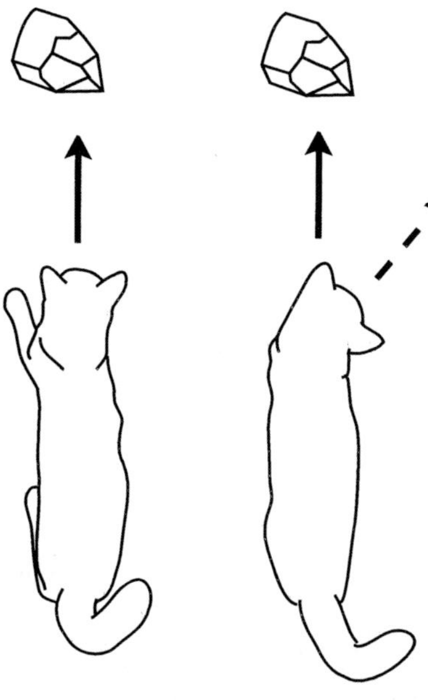

Fig. 7. Walking cats on a collision course with an object. For the cat on the left, cells with receptive fields within a few degrees of the vertical meridian would see the object. For the cat on the right, which is maintaining its gaze 40° to the right of its heading point, cells with receptive fields ~40° to left of the vertical meridian would see the object.

a pattern in which motion is uniform in direction and speed (Sherk and Kim, 1997). Supposing, then, that 'approach' cells do respond to objects that are part of optic flow fields, would they be useful to the cat? The answer probably depends on their receptive field locations. In order for an 'approach' cell to see an object move from its receptive field towards the cat's nose, the receptive field must be aligned with the cat's heading point (see Fig. 7). Receptive fields centered close to the vertical meridian, and near or above the center of gaze, are likely to experience image motion from the receptive field towards the nose because cats tend to look downward and close to the midline as they walk, as discussed above. A peripheral receptive field, on the other hand, might never see a stationary object on a collision course with the cat since cats do not, like the righthand cat in Fig. 7, gaze far off to one side as they walk. 'Approach' cells have receptive fields ranging from central to peripheral (Toyama et al., 1986a), but many are probably appropriate for detecting objects in the cat's path under some circumstances. A more problematic (and less numerous) population described by Toyama and colleagues are 'receding' cells. These respond best to objects moving directly away from the cat's nose, a situation that does not normally occur when walking or running [3].

Like the cat's 'approach' cells, some cells in the pigeon's nucleus rotundus (a tectorecipient thalamic nucleus) respond selectively to objects on a collision course with the bird (Wang and Frost, 1992; Sun and Frost, 1998). These so-called 'looming' cells differ from 'approach' cells in a number of ways, however. Their receptive fields are huge, and they have strong and selective monocular responses. Their responses are not tied to a particular direction of image motion, since they can respond to a looming object originating anywhere in their large receptive fields. Perhaps their most interesting feature (true at least for a subset of cells) is that they begin responding to an approaching object at a particular time, typically about 1 s, before it strikes the bird. Such cells thus provide the pigeon with 'time to collision', which Lee (1976) pointed out is the crucial information that a locomoting observer needs in order to take appropriate action (see also Lee and Reddish, 1981; Lee, 1994). Frost and colleagues surmised that 'looming' cells detect objects such as predators approaching a stationary bird, rather than detecting fixed objects when the bird is walking or flying. When Wang and Frost (1992) simulated an approach to a wall by using a 'looming' stimulus that filled the entire receptive field, cells responded poorly. When they simulated a situation in which their normal 'looming' stimulus (a black-and-white checked soccer ball) was positioned in front of a black-and-white checked wall, with both ball and wall moving towards the pigeon, cells again failed to respond (Frost and Sun, 1997). But they might still respond to an object in the path of a flying pigeon in a more natural situation, when the object is well distinguished from its surroundings (as, for example, when a pigeon approaches a roof top prior to landing).

What about detection of objects that are not directly in the path of the locomoting observer? Such

[3] One might think that a cat pursuing a mouse would see the mouse as a receding target, but in practice cats capture mice by stalking and pouncing, not by running after their prey.

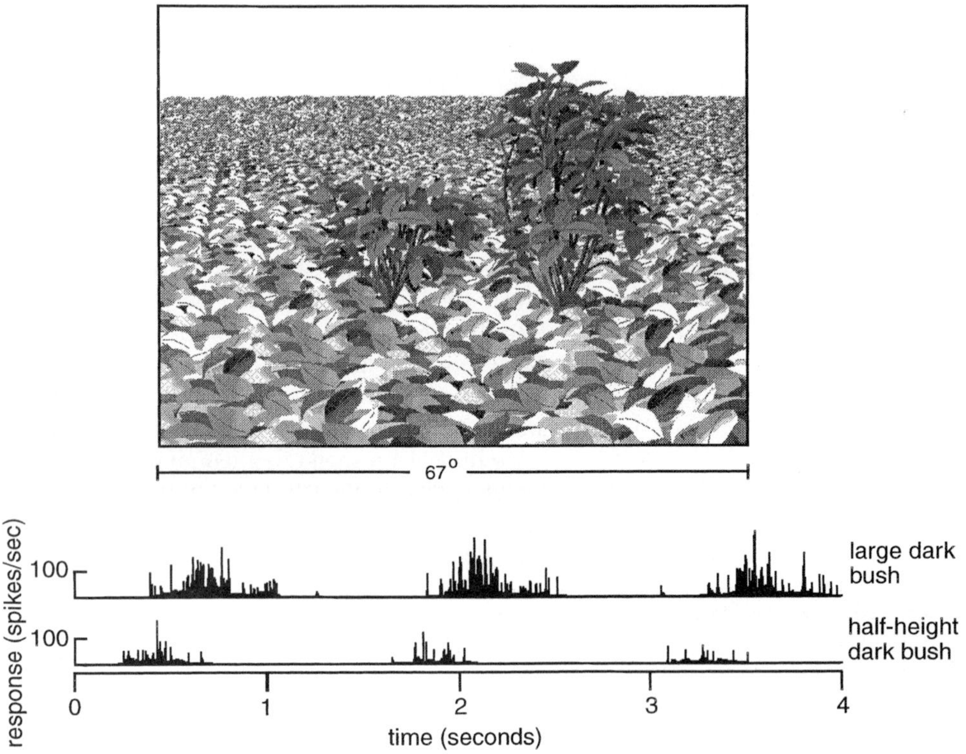

Fig. 8. Cell in LS that responded strongly to a large bush that was part of an optic flow display simulating locomotion along a straight path. The bush appeared three times during the display. In contrast, the cell responded only modestly to a half-height version of this bush. (In the actual stimuli, only one bush appeared at a time.)

an object cannot be uniquely identified by cues like opposing motion in the two eyes, and perhaps there are no cells dedicated to detecting them. One might suppose that any cells responsive to moving images would serve this purpose — in the monkey, for example, cells in MT, or in the cat, cells in LS. However, the potent suppressive surrounds exhibited by many cells in these two areas (Von Grunau and Frost, 1983; Allman et al., 1985) could present a problem — they might prevent cells from responding to an individual image in a large optic flow field. While we do not know if this is the case in MT, in LS numerous cells do respond to individual objects in an optic flow field provided they are sufficiently large (Sherk et al., 1997). In a study with complex, 'naturalistic' stimuli, we found that cells commonly responded strongly to large objects, but weakly to half-height versions of these objects (compare the responses to the 'large dark bush' and the 'half-height dark bush' in Fig. 8). This outcome was somewhat surprising since the 'half-height' objects that we tested often filled most of a given cell's receptive field. Possibly these cells were sensitive to motion parallax — the difference in speed between images of nearby objects and distant objects as seen by a locomoting observer. This difference is generally largest for tall objects because they are often seen against a distant background that moves slowly (sometimes imperceptibly) on the retina. On the other hand, objects close to the ground give rise to weak motion parallax.

Foot placement

Detection of small objects or irregularities that require a walking or running observer to adjust his foot placement is a challenging problem. Although these objects are directly in the path of the observer, they are on the ground, well below eye level, and thus do not give rise to images that move in opposite direc-

Gibson, J.J. (1950) *The Perception of the Visual World*. Boston, Houghton-Mifflin.

Gibson, J.J. (1979) The *Ecological Approach to Visual Perception*. Boston, Houghton-Mifflin.

Gibson, A., Baker, J., Mower, G. and Glickstein, M. (1978) Corticopontine cells in area 18 of the cat. *J. Neurophysiol.*, 41: 484–495.

Graziano, M.S.A., Andersen, R.A. and Snowden, R.J. (1994) Tuning of MST neurons to spiral motions. *J. Neurosci.*, 14: 54–67.

Hollands, M.A., Marple-Horvat, D.E., Henkes, S. and Rowan, A.K. (1995) Human eye movements during visually guided stepping. *J. Motor Behav.*, 27: 155–163.

Hubel, D.H. and Wiesel, T.N. (1962) Receptive fields, binocular interaction and functional architecture in the cat' visual cortex. *J. Physiol.*, 160: 106–154.

Hubel, D.H. and Wiesel, T.N. (1965) Receptive fields and functional architecture in two nonstriate visual areas (18 and 19) of the cat. *J. Neurophysiol.*, 28: 229–289.

Kim, J.-N., Mulligan, K. and Sherk, H. (1997) Simulated optic flow and extrastriate cortex. I. Optic flow versus texture. *J. Neurophysiol.*, 77: 534–561.

Koenderink, J.J. (1986) Optic flow. *Vision Res.*, 26: 161–179.

Komatsu, H. and Wurtz, R.H. (1988) Relation of cortical areas MT and MST to pursuit eye movements. I. Localization and visual properties of neurons. *J. Neurophysiol.*, 60: 580–603.

Lagae, L., Maes, H., Raiguel, S., Xiao, D.-K. and Orban, G.A. (1994) Responses of macaque STS neurons to optic flow components: a comparison of areas MT and MST. *J. Neurophysiol.*, 71: 1597–1626.

Land, M.F. and Lee, D.N. (1994) Where we look when we steer. *Nature*, 369: 742–744.

Lappe, M., Bremmer, F., Pekel, M., Thiele, A. and Hoffmann, K.-P. (1996) Optic flow processing in monkey STS: a theoretical and experimental approach. *J. Neurosci.*, 16: 6265–6285.

Lappe, M., Pekel, M. and Hoffmann, K.-P. (1998) Optokinetic eye movements elicited by radial optic flow in the macaque monkey. *J. Neurophysiol.*, 79: 1461–1480.

Lee, D.N. (1976) A theory of visual control of braking based on information about time-to-collision. *Perception*, 5: 437–459.

Lee, D.N. (1994) An eye or ear for flying. In: M.N.O. Davies and P.R. Green (Eds.), *Perception and Motor Control in Birds*. Springer-Verlag, Berlin, pp. 270–291.

Lee, D.N. and Reddish, P.E. (1981) Plummeting gannets: a paradigm of ecological optics. *Nature*, 293: 293–294.

Miles, F.A. (1998) The neural processing of 3-D visual information: evidence from eye movements. *Eur. J. Neurosci.*, 10: 811–822.

Nace, K.L. and Britten, K.A. (1997) Microstimulation of macaque visual area MT during a heading discrimination task. *Soc. Neurosci. Abstr.*, 23: 458.

Orban, G.A., Lagae, L., Verri, A., Raiguel, S., Xiao, D., Maes, H. and Torre, V. (1992) First-order analysis of optical flow in monkey brain. *Proc. Natl. Acad. Sci. USA*, 89: 2595–2599.

Patla, A.E. and Vickers, J.N. (1997) Where and when do we look as we approach and step over an obstacle in the travel path? *NeuroReport*, 8: 3661–3665.

Poggio, G.F. and Fischer, B. (1977) Binocular interaction and depth sensitivity in the striate and prestriate cortex of the behaving monkey. *J. Neurophysiol.*, 40: 1392–1405.

Regan, D. and Beverley, K.I. (1982) How do we avoid confounding the direction we are looking and the direction we are going? *Science*, 215: 194–196.

Rieser, J.J., Ashmead, D.H., Talor, C.R. and Youngquist, G.A. (1990) Visual perception and the guidance of locomotion without vision to previously seen targets. *Perception*, 19: 675–689.

Saito, H.-A., Yukie, M., Tanaka, K., Hikosaka, K., Fukada, Y. and Iwai, E. (1986) Integration of direction signals of image motion in the superior temporal sulcus of the macaque monkey. *J. Neurosci.*, 6: 145–157.

Sherk, H. and Kim, J.-N. (1997) Neuronal responses to optic flow in extrastriate cortex: influence of receptive field surrounds. *Soc. Neurosci. Abstr.*, 23: 1126.

Sherk, H. and Mulligan, K.A. (1993) A reassessment of the lower visual field map in striate-recipient lateral suprasylvian cortex. *Vis. Neurosci.*, 10: 131–158.

Sherk, H., Mulligan, K. and Kim, J.-N. (1996) Optic flow during simulated turns: single unit responses in extrastriate cortex. *Soc. Neurosci. Abstr.*, 22: 1617.

Sherk, H., Mulligan, K. and Kim, J.-N. (1997) Neuronal responses in extrastriate cortex to objects in optic flow fields. *Vis. Neurosci.*, 14: 879–895.

Siegel, R.M. and Read, H.L. (1997) Analysis of optic flow in the monkey parietal area 7a. *Cereb. Cortex*, 7: 327–346.

Solomon, D. and Cohen, B. (1992) Stabilization of gaze during circular locomotion in light. I. Compensatory head and eye nystagmus in the running monkey. *J. Neurophysiol.*, 67: 1146–1157.

Steenhuis, R.E. and Goodale, M.A. (1988) The effects of time and distance on accuracy of target-directed locomotion: Does an accurate short-term memory for spatial locomotion exist? *J. Motor Behav.*, 20: 399–415.

Sun, H.-J. and Frost, B.J. (1998) Computation of different optical variables of looming objects in pigeon nucleus rotundus neurons. *Nat. Neurosci.*, 1: 296–303.

Tanaka, K. and Saito, H.-A. (1989) Analysis of motion of the visual field by direction, expansion/contraction, and rotation cells clustered in the dorsal part of the medial superior temporal area of the macaque monkey. *J. Neurophysiol.*, 62: 626–641.

Tanaka, K., Hikosaka, K., Saito, H., Yukie, M., Fukada, Y. and Iwai, E. (1986) Analysis of local and wide-field movements in the superior temporal visual areas of the macaque monkey. *J. Neurosci.*, 6: 134–144.

Thomson, J.A. (1983) Is continuous visual monitoring necessary in visually guided locomotion? *J. Exp. Psych. Hum. Percept. Perform.*, 9: 427–443.

Toyama, K. and Kozasa, T. (1982) Responses of Clare-Bishop neurones to three dimensional movement of a light stimulus. *Vision Res.*, 22: 571–574.

Toyama, K., Komatsu, Y. and Kozasa, T. (1986a) The responsiveness of Clare-Bishop neurons to motion cues for motion stereopsis. *Neurosci. Res.*, 4: 83–109.

Toyama, K., Fujii, K., Kasai, S. and Maeda, K. (1986b) The responsiveness of Clare-Bishop neurons to size cues for motion stereopsis. *Neurosci. Res.*, 4: 110–128.

Ungerleider, L.G. and Desimone, R. (1986) Cortical connections of visual area MT in the macaque. *J. Comp. Neurol.*, 248: 190–222.

Von Grunau, M. and Frost, B.J. (1983) Double-opponent process mechanism underlying RF-structure of directionally specific cells of cat lateral suprasylvian visual area. *Exp. Brain Res.*, 49: 84–92.

Wang, Y.-C. and Frost, B.J. (1992) Time to collision is signalled by neurons in the nucleus rotundus of pigeons. *Nature*, 356: 236–238.

Warren, W.H. and Hannon, D.J. (1988) Direction of self-motion is perceived from optical flow. *Nature*, 336: 162–163.

Warren, W.H., Morris, M.W. and Kalish, M. (1988) Perception of translational heading from optical flow. *J. Exp. Psych. Hum. Percept. Perform.*, 14: 646–660.

Zeki, S.M. (1974) Functional organization of a visual area in the posterior bank of the superior temporal sulcus of the rhesus monkey. *J. Physiol.*, 236: 549–573.

C. Casanova and M. Ptito (Eds.)
Progress in Brain Research, Vol. 134

CHAPTER 17

Behavioral cartography of visual functions in cat parietal cortex: areal and laminar dissociations

Stephen G. Lomber *

Laboratory for Visual Perception and Cognition, Department of Anatomy and Neurobiology, Boston University School of Medicine, 700 Albany Street, Boston, MA 02118, USA

Abstract: The purpose of this review is to: (1) compare and contrast the relative contributions that the four principle regions in cat extrastriate parietal cortex make to a battery of visual tasks which require motion, spatial, or attentional processing; and (2) examine the laminar parcellation of visual behaviors within one of these parietal regions which mediates multiple visual behaviors. We examined a battery of visual tasks presumed to be mediated by parietal cortex, including direction of motion, differential motion, and landmark discriminations, and visual orienting to moving stimuli. As a control, we also examined performance on form (pattern and object) recognition tasks mediated by the temporal processing stream. The four regions of parietal cortex we examined included the: middle suprasylvian (MS) gyrus (area 7), anterior middle suprasylvian (aMS) sulcus (AMLS, ALLS), posterior middle suprasylvian (pMS) sulcus (PMLS, PLLS), and the dorsal posterior suprasylvian (dPS) gyrus (area 21a). The contributions made to each of the six different behavioral tasks was examined before, during, and after reversible cooling deactivation of each cortical area. Deactivation of pMS sulcal cortex resulted in deficits on all four tasks that required motion, spatial or attentional processing. Deactivation of aMS sulcal cortex resulted in deficits on only tasks that required motion processing. Deactivation of neither aMS nor pMS sulcal cortex yielded any deficits on the form recognition tasks. In contrast, deactivation of dPS cortex only produced deficits on the form recognition tasks. This finding confirmed our early hypothesis that dPS cortex is a key component of the temporal, and not the parietal, processing stream. Regardless of the task, no deficits were identified on any of the six tasks during deactivation of the MS gyrus. We then more closely examined pMS sulcal cortex to determine if its multiple functions could be dissociated on a laminar level. We found that cooling deactivation of the superficial layers (I–III) of pMS sulcal cortex selectively and completely impaired performance on the direction of motion discrimination task, while leaving visual attention unimpaired. Additional deactivation of the deeper layers (IV–VI) resulted in impaired visual attention as assessed with visual orienting. These results show a functional bipartite division of labor between upper and lower cortical layers of pMS sulcal cortex. Therefore, spatial, motion and attentional functions can be localized within visuoparietal cortex on both an areal and laminar level.

Introduction

In cats, monkeys and humans, visual projections arising from primary visual cortex diverge into two functionally distinct processing pathways leading to visuoparietal and visuotemporal cortices (Ungerleider and Mishkin, 1982; Haxby et al., 1993; Payne, 1993; Ungerleider and Haxby, 1994). The visuoparietal pathway is essential for the processing of depth, motion and space (Mishkin et al., 1982; Mishkin and Ungerleider, 1982; Newsome and Paré, 1988; Kiefer et al., 1989; Newcombe and Ratcliffe, 1989; Pasternak et al., 1989; Krüger et al., 1993a; Zihl et al., 1991; Lomber et al., 1994, 1996a; Pasternak and Merigan, 1994; Milner and Goodale, 1995; Rudolph and Pasternak, 1996, 1999; Lomber and Payne, 2000a). The visuotemporal pathway is essen-

* Correspondence to: S.G. Lomber. Present address: Cerebral Systems Laboratory, School of Human Development, University of Texas at Dallas, P.O. Box 830688, Richardson, TX 75083-0688, USA. Tel.: +1-972-883-2235; Fax: +1-972-883-2491; E-mail: lomber@utdallas.edu

tial for pattern and object recognition (Gross, 1973; Sprague et al., 1977; Campbell, 1978; Gaffan et al., 1986; Damasio et al., 1989; Vaina, 1990; Milner and Goodale, 1995; Lomber et al., 1996a,b; Cornwell et al., 1998).

In the cat, the two principle targets of these two processing streams are middle suprasylvian (MS) cortex in visuoparietal cortex and ventral posterior suprasylvian (vPS) cortex in temporal cortex. The proposed routes of these two pathways have been previously described (Lomber et al., 1996a) and are illustrated in Fig. 1. MS cortex lies buried within the middle suprasylvian sulcus and much of vPS cortex continues onto the fusiform gyrus on the tentorial surface of the brain. Both MS and vPS have unique patterns of inputs from primary visual areas 17 and 18 and from the dorsal lateral geniculate nucleus (dLGN). MS cortex receives direct projections from areas 17 and 18 (Sherk, 1986; Grant and Shipp, 1991; MacNeil et al., 1996), whereas area 17 and 18 signals destined for vPS cortex are preprocessed in area 19 and/or dorsal posterior suprasylvian (dPS) cortex (Reinoso-Suárez, 1984; Symonds and Rosenquist, 1984). Transcortical efferent projections from MS cortex gain access to the limbic system via the posterior cingulate gyrus (pcg; Reinoso-Suárez, 1984; Olson and Musil, 1992) while efferents from vPS cortex project to entorhinal (er; Kuchiiwa et al., 1985; Witter and Groenewegen, 1986) cortex. From the thalamus, MS cortex receives input directly from the dLGN (Tong et al., 1982; Sherk, 1986; Lomber et al., 1995; Kawano, 1998), whereas dLGN inputs to vPS cortex are extremely weak (Raczkowski and Rosenquist, 1983) or non-existent (Cavada and Reinoso-Suárez, 1983).

In order to better understand the contributions that visuoparietal cortex in the cat makes to motion, spatial or attentional processing, this review compares and contrasts the relative contributions of four different regions within parietal cortex. We examined a battery of visual tasks, presumed to be mediated by parietal cortex, including direction of motion, differential motion, and landmark discriminations, and visual orienting to moving stimuli. The four regions we examined include: middle suprasylvian (MS) gyrus (area 7), anterior middle suprasylvian (aMS) sulcus (AMLS, ALLS), posterior middle suprasylvian (pMS) sulcus (PMLS, PLLS), and the dorsal posterior suprasylvian (dPS) gyrus (area 21a). In the first sections of the review, the areas studied and the reversible deactivation technique employed are detailed. Next, the four parietal tasks are examined in detail, followed by the results of two control form discrimination tasks. After considering the results of

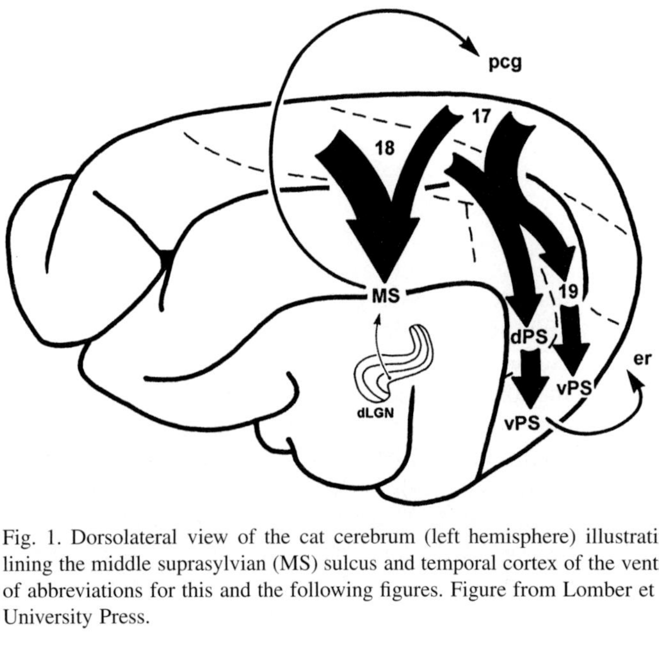

Fig. 1. Dorsolateral view of the cat cerebrum (left hemisphere) illustrating the major transcortical visual pathways to parietal cortex lining the middle suprasylvian (MS) sulcus and temporal cortex of the ventral-posterior suprasylvian (vPS) gyrus. Left is anterior. See list of abbreviations for this and the following figures. Figure from Lomber et al. (1996a) and reproduced with the permission of Cambridge University Press.

these studies in the context of other work, our results from a more detailed evaluation are considered in order to determine if the multiple functions mediated by pMS sulcal cortex can be dissociated on a laminar level.

Parietal cortical loci investigated

We used reversible cooling deactivation (Lomber et al., 1999) to examine the contributions that four regions of visuoparietal cortex made to motion, spatial, and attentional processing. The positions of these four loci, as well as how they relate to the retinotopic maps of other investigators, are described below.

(1) MS gyral cortex includes the entire central region of the middle suprasylvian gyrus and the lateral bank of the lateral sulcus (Fig. 2A). This deactivated region extended from approximately AP0 to A11 and included all of area 7 (Rosenquist, 1985) or area 7p (Olson and Lawler, 1987), depending upon nomenclature, and was slightly asymmetric in the medial direction.

(2) aMS sulcal cortex includes all of anterior middle suprasylvian and middle ectosylvian cortices that contribute to the medial and lateral banks of the aMS sulcus (Fig. 2B). The deactivated region abutting the aMS cryoloops extended from about A5 to A15, and corresponds to all of areas AMLS and ALLS and the anterior-most portion of areas PMLS and PLLS (Palmer et al., 1978).

(3) pMS sulcal cortex includes all of posterior middle suprasylvian and middle ectosylvian cortices that contribute to the medial and lateral banks of the pMS sulcus. The deactivated region extended from approximately coronal level P3 to A8. This region corresponds to all of areas PMLS and PLLS, dorsal-most DLS, the posterior-most portion of areas AMLS and ALLS (Palmer et al., 1978), and all of areas LS and PEV of Grant and Shipp (1991). The deactivation loci for both aMS and pMS sulcal cortex (Fig. 2B,C) appear to be smaller than those of the MS and dPS gyri (Fig. 2A,B). However, it should

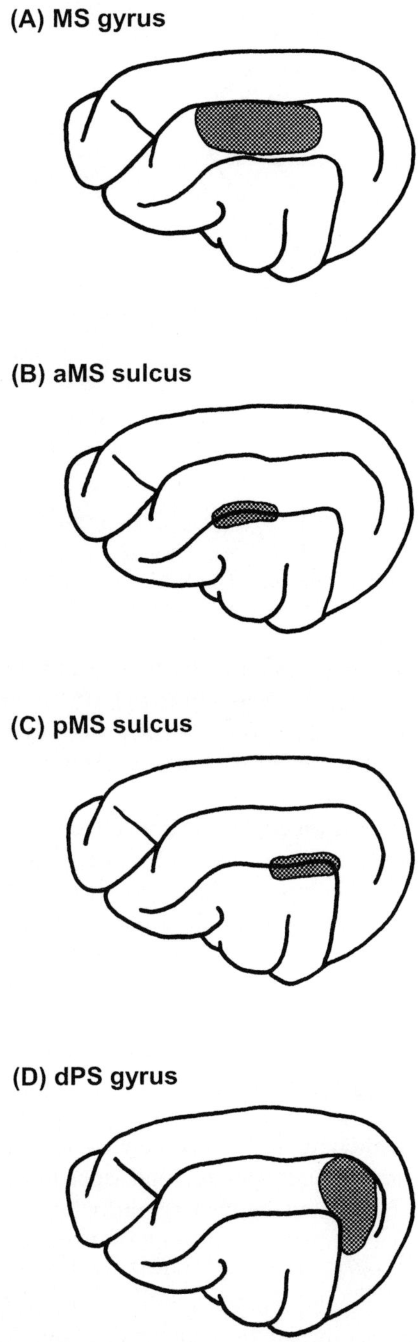

Fig. 2. Dorsolateral views of the cat cerebrum illustrating the positions of (A) MS gyral, (B) aMS sulcal, (C) pMS sulcal and (D) dPS gyral deactivation loci. Left is anterior and top is dorsal. These same illustrations are used as icons in subsequent figures. Note that the majority of aMS and pMS sulcal deactivations lie deep in the MS sulcus and are not visible on an exterior view of the cerebrum.

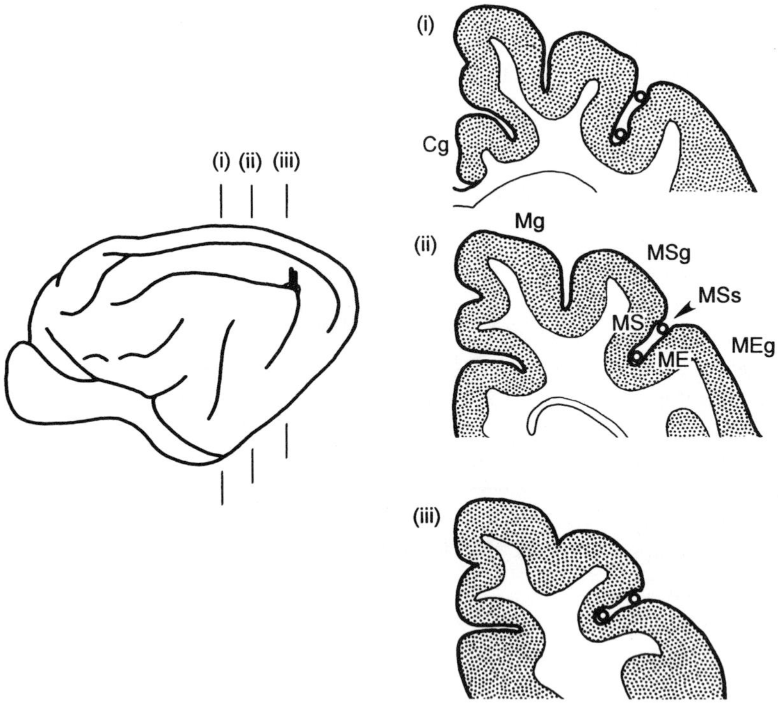

Fig. 3. Position of a cooling loop in the posterior middle suprasylvian sulcus (MSs). Left: Lateral view of the left hemisphere to show the site where the cooling tubes exited the sulcus and the A-P position of the three coronal sections (i–iii). Right) Coronal sections (i–iii) showing how the cooling loop was placed in the sulcus in contact with both the medial (MS) and lateral (ME) banks.

be noted that the vast majority of the deactivated sulcal cortices are hidden deep within the MS sulcus (Fig. 3). Therefore, if the cortical surface were to be flattened, the surface area of each deactivation locus would be very similar.

(4) dPS gyral cortex includes the dorsal half of the posterior suprasylvian gyrus and includes the entire posterior bend of the suprasylvian gyrus (Fig. 2D). The deactivated region includes all of retinotopically defined area 21a (Tusa and Palmer, 1980) and the central-vision representation of area 19 (Tusa et al., 1979).

Reversible cooling deactivation

The cooling method to reversibly deactivate neural tissue is an exciting, potent, and appropriate technique for examining cerebral contributions to behavior and has a number of highly beneficial and practical features (Lomber, 1999). (1) Limited regions of the cerebral cortex can be selectively and reversibly deactivated in a controlled and reproducible way. Baseline and experimental measures can be made within minutes of each other (Lomber et al., 1996a,b). (2) Repeated coolings over months or years produce stable, reversible deficits, with no evidence of attenuation, neural compensations or major variations (Lomber et al., 1994, 1999). (3) Repeated cooling induces neither local or distant degenerations that might compromise conclusions and do not induce types of neural compensations triggered by lesions. (4) Compared to traditional ablation studies, fewer animals are needed because sensitive within animal comparisons and double dissociations are possible, permitting large volumes of high quality data to be acquired from each animal (Lomber et al., 1996a). (5) Finally, as the major effect of cooling is to block synaptic transmission, activity in fibers of passage is not compromised (Jasper et al., 1970; Bénita and Condé, 1972).

We have verified that the surgical procedures to implant cryoloops, their presence in contact with the cerebrum, or their operation disrupts neither the normal structural nor functional integrity of cor-

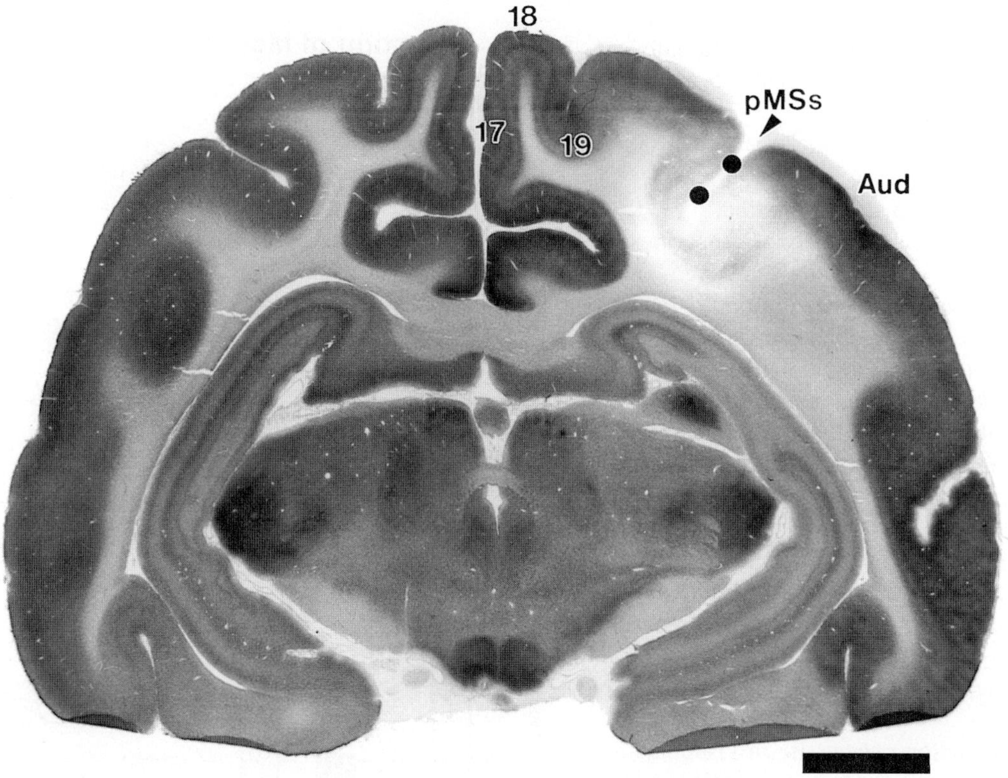

Fig. 4. 2-Deoxyglucose (2DG) autoradiogram of a coronal section showing diminished 2DG uptake in the posterior-middle suprasylvian sulcus (pMSs) adjacent to a pMS cryoloop (black dots) in the right hemisphere. Compare low 2DG uptake levels in pMS sulcal cortex of the right hemisphere with high levels in pMS sulcal cortex of the left hemisphere. High levels of 2DG uptake can also be identified in nearby areas 17, 18, 19 and auditory cortex (Aud). Note that only the right hemisphere loop was cooled at time of 2DG administration. Coronal section is approximately at A4. Scale bar: 5 mm.

tex (Lomber et al., 1999). In every instance, cell and myelin stains are rich, and the cyto- and myelo-architecture of the region are characteristic of the region investigated, with no signs of pathology, as might be revealed by a marked pale staining of neurons or gliosis or light staining of cytochrome oxidase (Lomber and Payne, 1996). However, the lack of any damage to the cortex means that it is not possible to use traditional histological techniques to determine the region that was deactivated. The most convenient and reliable way to estimate the extent of deactivated cortex is to administer radio-labeled 2-deoxyglucose (2DG) prior to sacrifice (Payne and Lomber, 1999). Since cooling silences evoked responses by neurons and depresses metabolic activity, little 2DG is taken up by the silenced neurons compared to regions at normal temperature and with normal levels of high activity. Consequently, the deactivated region is identified as a very pale region surrounded by dark gray, active tissue in autoradiograms (Payne and Lomber, 1999; Lomber and Payne, 2000a). An example of this from a pMS sulcal cryoloop deactivation is provided in Fig. 4. A region of very low 2DG uptake extends downwards from the lateral margin of the pMS sulcus (pMSs) to the fundus and upward to the medial margin and delimits the region of cortex silenced by the cooling (Fig. 4).

Contributions of individual parietal areas to motion, spatial and attentional processing

All of the studies described below were conducted using adult, intact cats under binocular viewing conditions. With the exception of the visual attention task, all pairs of cryoloops were bilaterally deactivated. For the visual attention task, data is presented during unilateral deactivation of the cryoloops.

Direction of motion

For the direction of motion discrimination, a two-choice Pennsylvania General Testing Apparatus (PGTA) was used and stimuli were displayed on 17 cm-diagonal black and white video monitors and were viewed through circular apertures (14.7° of visual angle in diameter). For more details, an explanation of the training procedures, and an illustration, see Fig. 2 of Lomber et al. (1996a). The stimuli consisted of a pair of identical, black, variously oriented, non-systematic angular shapes on a white background (Fig. 5, top) that moved at a constant velocity (13.6 deg/s from the decision line). The cats were trained to discriminate horizontal rightward motion, the designated positive (rewarded) direction, and upward and rightward movement of 45°, 30°, 15°, and 7.5°, the designated negative (unrewarded) directions.

Prior to the deactivation of any site in visuoparietal cortex, discrimination performance with a 30° angular difference was approximately 80%. However, deactivation of either aMS or pMS sulcal cortices significantly impaired performance, which dropped to chance levels (Fig. 5B,C). Similar results were obtained when the angular difference was decreased to 15° and 7.5°. However, no impairment was found with larger angular differences of 45° or 90° (Lomber et al., 1996a). Deactivation of other sites in visuoparietal cortex (MS or dPS gyri) did not result

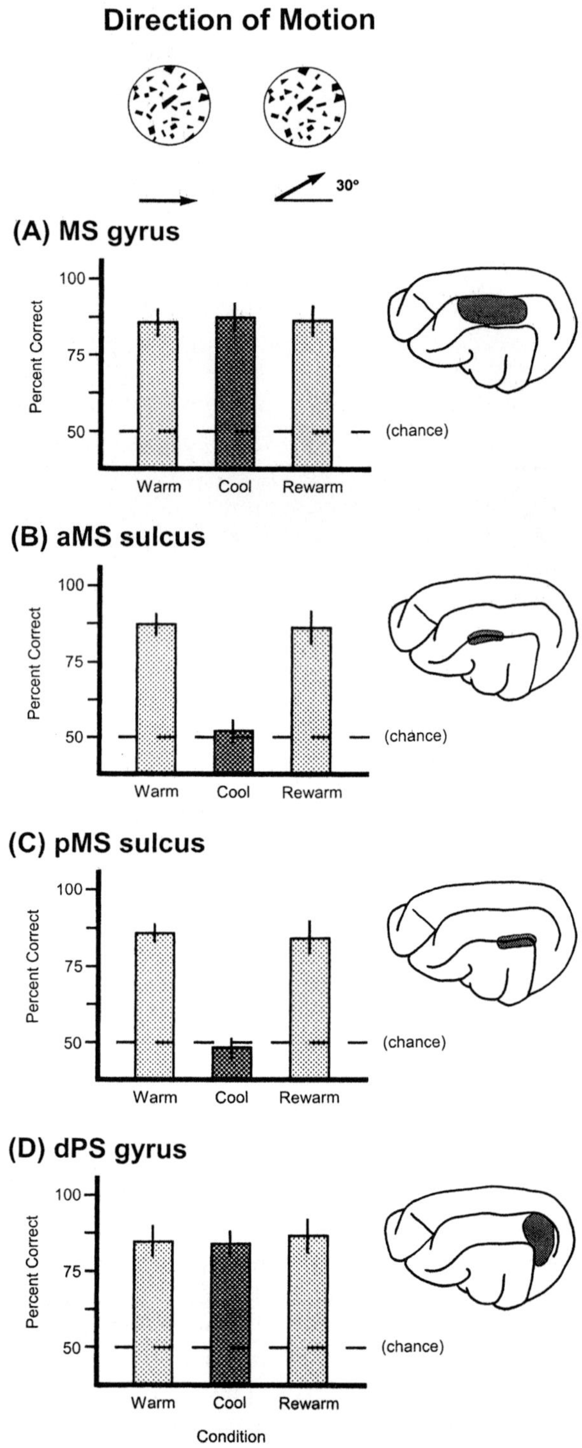

Fig. 5. Direction of motion task. The moving visual stimuli, viewed through circular apertures, are illustrated at top. Histograms of the mean (± 1 SE) percent correct responses while (A) MS gyral, (B) aMS sulcal, (C) pMS sulcal and (D) dPS gyral cortices are active (warm), deactivated (cool), and reactivated (rewarm). Data presented are when the animals discriminated between rightward (horizontal) movement and movement at and angular difference of 30° above horizontal. Dark stipple, cortical region was deactivated (cool); light stipple, cortex was uncooled (warm or rewarm). Chance performance = 50%. Note that there is no difference between performance before (warm) or after (rewarm) cooling deactivation of any parietal region.

in any significant changes in performance on the direction of motion discrimination task (Fig. 5A,D). Deactivation of sites in temporal cortex, such as vPS cortex, also did not have any affect on performance of the direction of motion task (Lomber et al., 1996a).

Differential motion

The stimulus for the differential motion discrimination consisted of an outline I or O partially obscured by a grid-like mask (Fig. 6, top) that were presented on black and white video monitors in a manner similar to the previous task. The grid, which partially masked the outline I and O patterns, oscillated up and down at a variable rate of 1–4 cycles/s. Performance was also examined with horizontal oscillations.

All cats tested could easily discriminate between the outline I or O behind the vertically moving grid with performance levels typically between 90 and 95%. However, performance fell to chance levels when aMS sulcal cortex was deactivated (Fig. 6B). An equivalently substantial decrease to chance levels of performance also occurred when pMS sulcal cortex was cooled (Fig. 6C; Lomber et al., 1994). Decreases in performance of a similar magnitude were also identical when either aMS or pMS sulcal cryoloops were cooled and the masking grid oscillated in the horizontal direction (Lomber et al., 1996a). Furthermore, other forms of masking, such as the black shapes used in the direction of motion task, also produced deficits when moved over the outline I and O shapes during deactivation of aMS and pMS cortices (Lomber et al., 1994). However, there was no change in performance when either MS or dPS gyral cortices were deactivated. Therefore, deactivation of either aMS or pMS sulcal, but not ad-

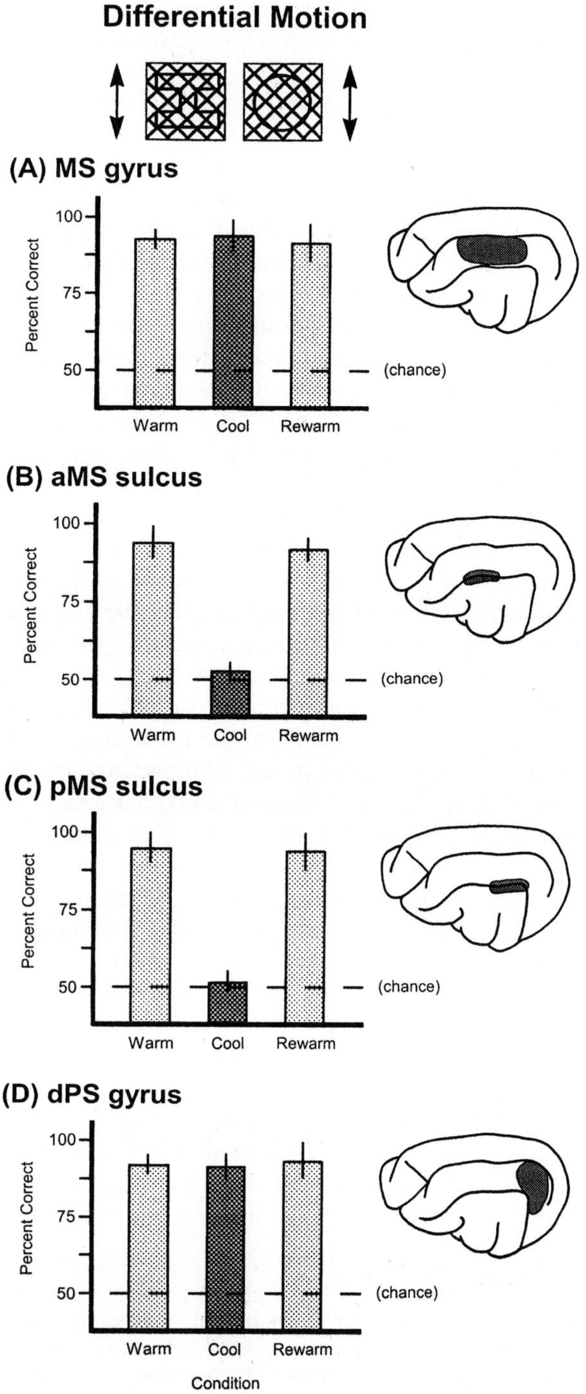

Fig. 6. Differential motion task. Top: Stationary, outline I and O stimuli viewed behind a vertically oscillating grid mask. Histograms of the mean (± 1 SE) percent correct responses while (A) MS gyral, (B) aMS sulcal, (C) pMS sulcal and (D) dPS gyral cortices are active (warm), deactivated (cool), and reactivated (rewarm). Data presented are when the animals discriminated outline I and O shapes from behind a vertically oscillating grid mask. Dark stipple, cortical region was deactivated (Cool); light stipple, cortex was uncooled (warm or rewarm).

jacent MS and dPS gyral, cortices resulted in deficits on both of the motion-related tasks examined.

Landmark discrimination

A modified PGTA was used for landmark discrimination training and testing (see Fig. 2 of Lomber et al., 1996a). In the modified testing apparatus, the center divider was removed to create one large open goal compartment with white walls. The landmark task we used is a variation of the landmark discrimination first described by Pohl (1973) and it was adapted for use with cats. Cats were presented with two wells, one on the left side of the apparatus and one on the right side (Fig. 7, top). One well contained a food reward that could not be seen by the cat. The location of the food was cued by the positioning of a black and white checkered box (6 cm wide × 8 cm high × 4 cm deep, with 2 cm checks) at one of six landmark locations between the food wells. Three left and three right, mirror-symmetric, positions were centered at 5, 14, or 23 cm from each reward compartment (Fig. 7, top). The cue was always presented on the same side of the center of the apparatus as the food reward. The location of the landmark was randomized across trials and the cat walked directly to the well containing the reward. A trial was scored as incorrect if the cat went to the unrewarded food compartment and a trial was not counted if the cat failed to make a choice.

Cooling deactivation and baseline performance are summarized in Fig. 7. The checkered landmark object was centered at the indicated distances in centimeters from the reward locus, and on each side of the midline. The lightly stippled bars represent composite performance during testing with all cortices warm, prior to *and* after each deactivation. The darkly stippled bars represent data collected during the cooling tests. Cats learned and performed this task at a high level of proficiency for all landmark positions (80–100% correct), although accuracy of reporting the location of the L23 and R23 positions, those farthest from the reward well and closest to the 30 cm midline, was somewhat lower than more proximal positions (Fig. 7, lightly stippled bars). Following cryoloop implantation, virtually identical performance levels were recorded prior to and after cortical deactivation.

During bilateral cooling of the MS gyral cortex loops, we found no deficits at any position of the landmark (Fig. 7A). Moreover, performance was indistinguishable from cooling deactivation of vPS gyral cortex (Lomber and Payne, 2000a), for which we did not anticipate any impairment on this task because of its contribution to the perception and recognition of forms and not spatial locations (Lomber et al., 1996a,b; Cornwell et al., 1998). In contrast, bilateral cooling of pMS sulcal cortex resulted in a profound impairment in reporting landmark position (Fig. 7C). For all six positions tested, performance dropped to chance levels during bilateral deactivation of pMS sulcal cortex, regardless of the proximity of the landmark to the reward locus. Finally, bilateral deactivation of dPS gyral cortex also had no influences on landmark discrimination performance. Therefore, pMS sulcal cortex function is critical for the reporting of visuospatial relations, as assessed with the landmark discrimination task.

Visual attention

A white semicircular arena was used to test the cat's ability to redirect its attention toward a visual stimulus introduced upwards through one of 13 openings in the floor of an arena and spaced around its circum-

Fig. 7. Landmark discrimination task. Task: Cats learned to discriminate whether a black and white checkered box (2 cm checks) was closer to a food reward locus on the left or the right side of the testing apparatus. Six landmark positions were used: three to the left of the midline (centered at 5, 14, or 23 cm from the reward locus) and three to the right of the midline in a mirror-symmetric configuration (top). Performance is expressed as a percent correct for each of the six different positions tested. The lightly shaded bars show normal, control data collected prior to and after cooling deactivation each day. As there was no difference between warm and rewarm performance levels, these two groups were combined and compared with the cooling deactivation state. The darkly shaded bars represent data collected during cooling deactivation. Hatched line represents chance performance (50% correct). Error bars are one standard error of the mean.

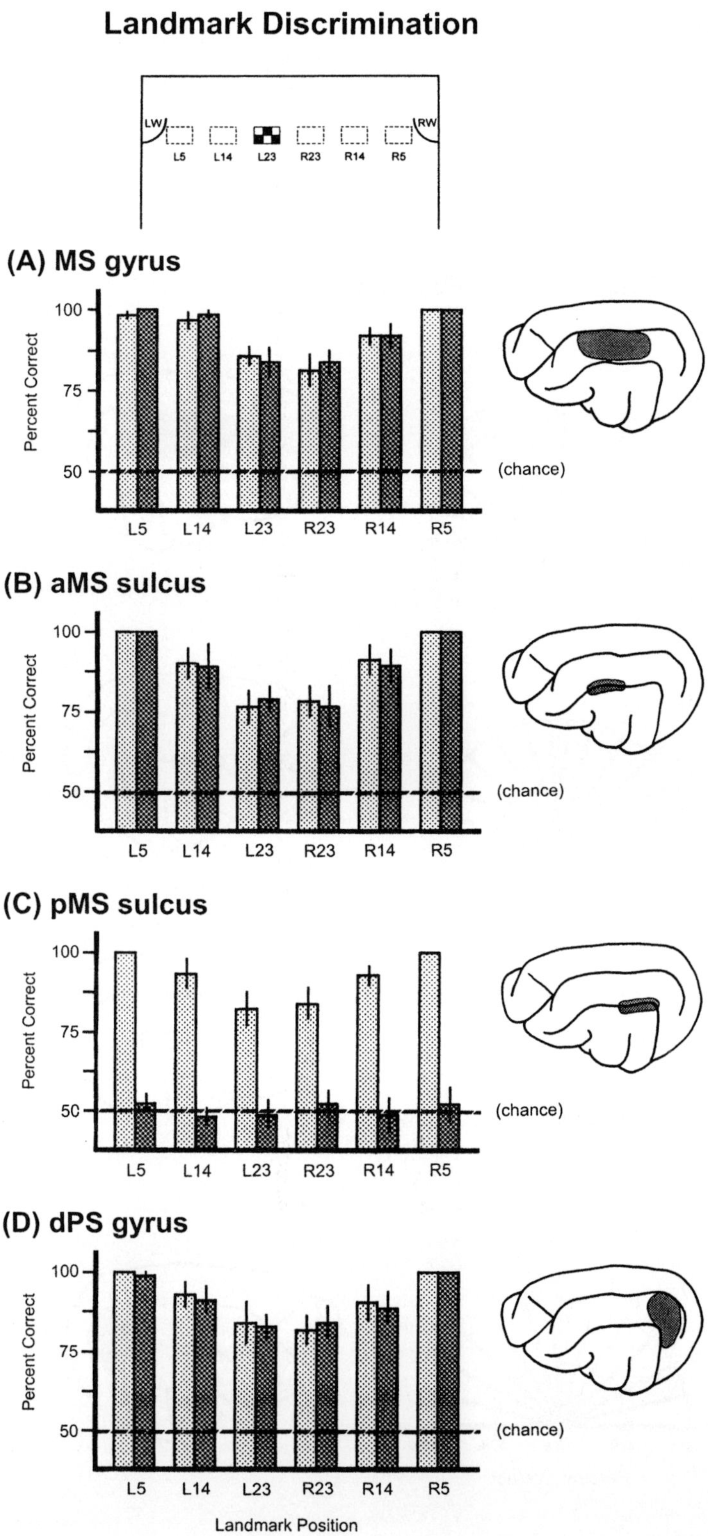
Landmark Discrimination
LW
RW
L5 L14 L23 R23 R14 R5
(A) MS gyrus
(B) aMS sulcus
(C) pMS sulcus
(D) dPS gyrus
Percent Correct
100
75
50
(chance)
L5 L14 L23 R23 R14 R5
Landmark Position

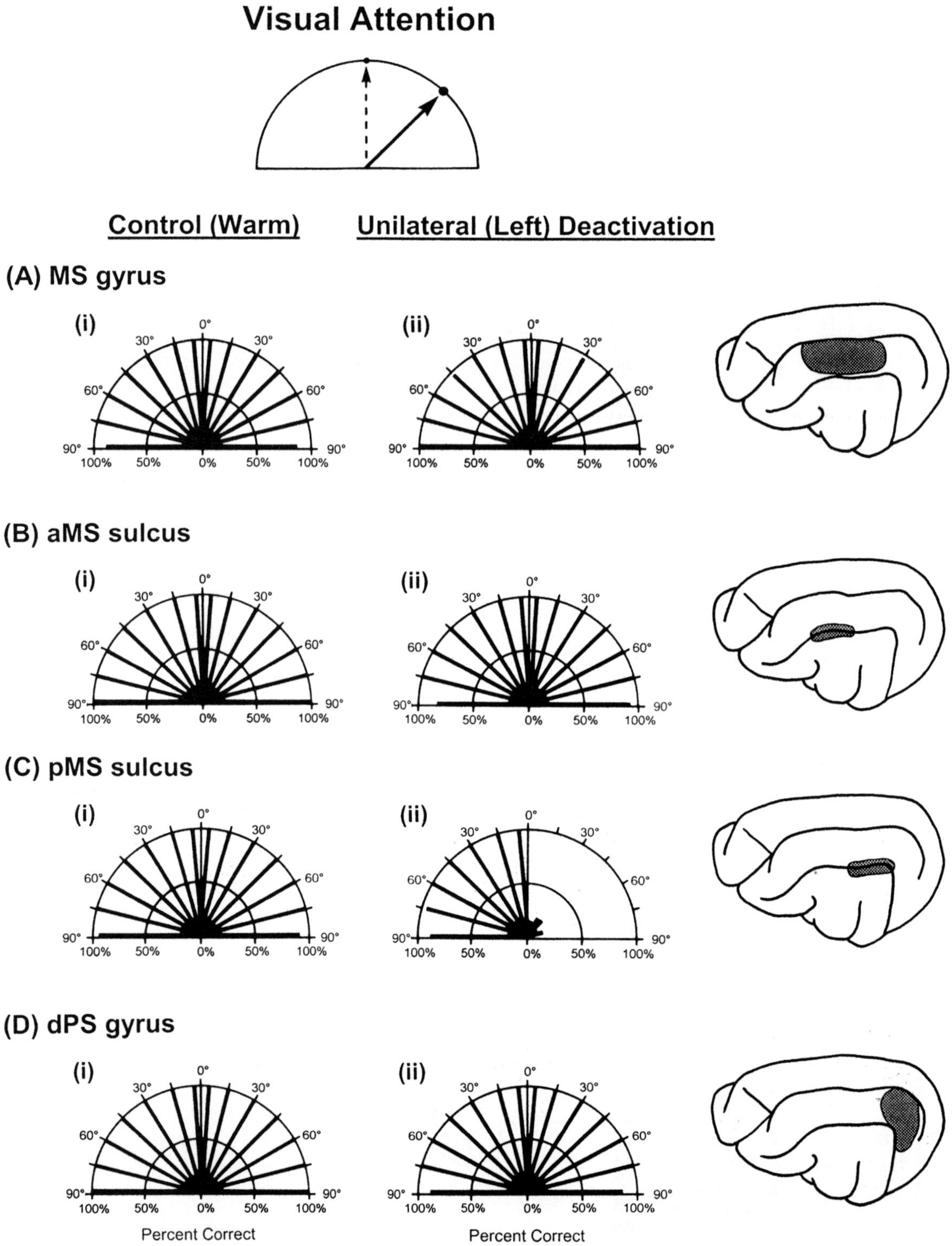
Visual Attention
Control (Warm)
Unilateral (Left) Deactivation
(A) MS gyrus
(i)
(ii)
(B) aMS sulcus
(i)
(ii)
(C) pMS sulcus
(i)
(ii)
(D) dPS gyrus
(i)
(ii)
0°
30°
60°
90°
100%
50%
0%
Percent Correct

ference at 15° intervals with respect to the arena's center. For more details and an illustration, see Fig. 2 of Lomber and Payne (1996). An initial target was introduced through the center opening to attract and hold the cat's attention (Fig. 8, top, small dot and dashed line). A second, higher incentive, stimulus was then introduced into the arena through the same or one of the peripheral openings. A strong and immediate redirection of the head and approach to the stimulus was scored as a positive response and the trial was scored as correct (Fig. 8, top, large dot and solid line). These testing procedures are similar to those of Sherman (1977).

Cats are able to learn to redirect their visual attention to a moving stimulus very quickly and accurately since the task is reflexive. Performance was at 100% for nearly all of the tested positions within the central 180° of the visual field (Fig. 8(i)). Typically, the only positions where performance was below 100% was at the right and left 90° positions. Furthermore, no change in visual orienting behavior was identified when MS gyral, aMS sulcal, or dPS gyral cortex was deactivated unilaterally (Fig. 8(ii) A–C). However, unilateral deactivation of pMS sulcal cortex resulted in a visual neglect of stimuli introduced into the contralateral visual field (Fig. 8C(ii); Lomber and Payne, 1996; Payne et al., 1996). This was a mirror-symmetric effect and resulted from unilateral deactivation of either left or right pMS sulcal cortex (Lomber and Payne, 1996). Interestingly, we have also identified that bilateral deactivation of pMS sulcal cortex restores visual attention into a previously neglected hemifield, thereby producing no effect during bilateral pMS sulcal cortex cooling (Lomber and Payne, 1996). In addition, no visual attention deficits have been identified during bilateral cooling of MS gyral, aMS sulcal, or dPS gyral cortices. Therefore, unilateral, but not bilateral, deactivation of pMS sulcal cortex has a profound influence on visual attention.

Fig. 8. Visual attention task. Task required the animal to redirect its attention from the centrally placed stimulus (small dot) to a stimulus moved into the visual periphery (large dot). (i) Control data collected prior to and after cooling deactivation. (ii) Data collected during unilateral cooling deactivation of the left cryoloop during binocular viewing conditions. Note that identical, mirror-symmetric data were obtained when the right cryoloop was deactivated. The two concentric semicircles represent 50 and 100% response levels and the length of each bold line corresponds to the percentage of responses at each location tested.

Contributions of individual parietal areas to form discriminations

Complex pattern discrimination

Complex patterns, comprised of outline I and O patterns partially obscured by a grid-like mask, were presented on video monitors in the PGTA and were identical to the stimuli used in the differential motion discrimination (Fig. 6, top). However, for this task, the overlaying mask remained stationary (Fig. 9, top). Interestingly, we had identified that cats performed better on this task when the overlaying mask was in motion (Fig. 6), compared to it being held stationary (Fig. 9). Typical performance was 10% better when the mask was in motion. We had previously found that this task is sensitive to temporal pathway deactivation, as cooling vPS gyral cortex profoundly impairs recall of these complex patterns (Lomber et al., 1996a,b).

Deactivation of dPS gyral cortex resulted in decreased performance on the complex pattern discrimination (Fig. 9D). Performance levels fell to approximately 74% correct and were significantly better than chance performance (Fig. 9D). Furthermore, similar deficits were also identified on a simpler pattern discrimination that lacked masking. In contrast, no deficits were identified on the complex pattern discrimination following deactivation of MS gyral, aMS sulcal, or pMS sulcal cortices (Fig. 9A–C). Therefore, only deactivation of the dPS gyrus resulted in a partial deficit on the complex pattern discrimination.

Object discrimination

Cats were tested on their ability to recall an object discrimination that consisted of solid-black I and O, 3-dimensional shapes. Deactivation of vPS gyral cortex reduces performance on this task to chance levels (Lomber et al., 1996a,b). However, deactivation of MS gyral, aMS sulcal or pMS sulcal cortices does not produce any deficit on this discrimination

(Fig. 10A–C). In contrast to this, but similar to the complex pattern discrimination (Fig. 9D), deactivation of dPS gyral cortex results in a partial deficit on the object discrimination which is above chance levels (Fig. 10D). Furthermore, similar results were also obtained during deactivation of dPS gyral cortex on junk objection discriminations. Therefore, deactivation of dPS gyral cortex produces partial deficits on both pattern and object discriminations.

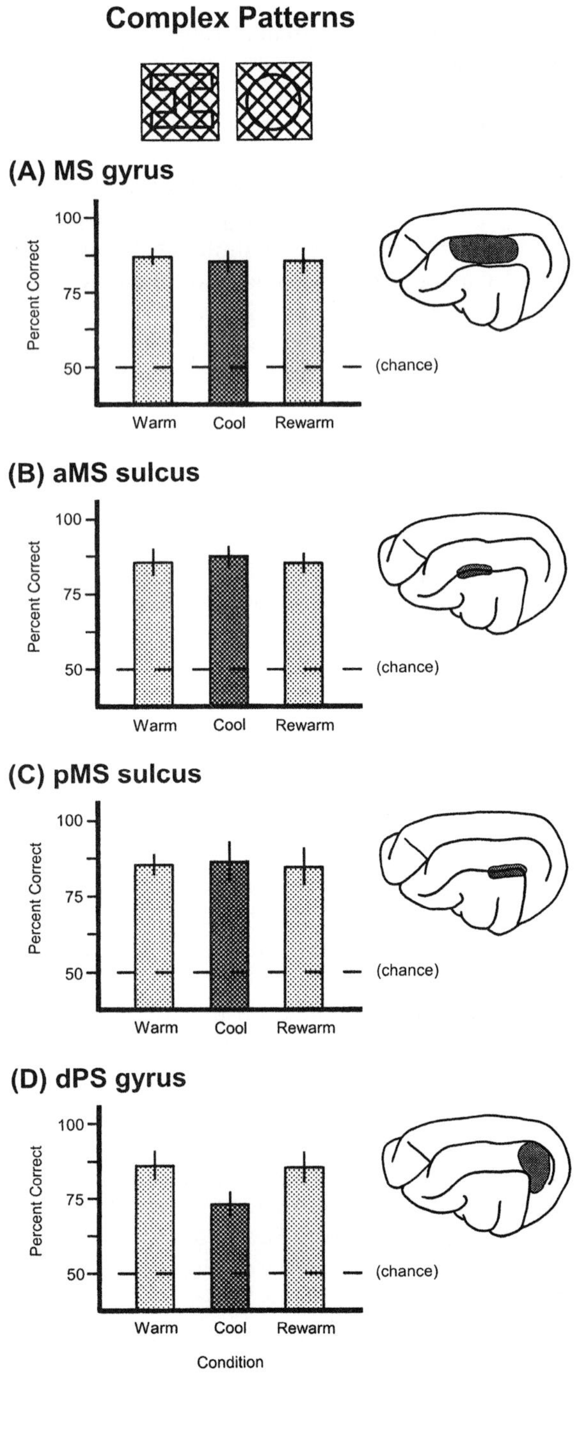

Fig. 9. Complex pattern discrimination task. Stimuli consisted of outline I and O shapes viewed behind a stationary grid mask (top). Histograms of the mean (± 1 SE) percent correct responses while (A) MS gyral, (B) aMS sulcal, (C) pMS sulcal and (D) dPS gyral cortices are active (warm), deactivated (cool), and reactivated (rewarm). Chance performance = 50%. Dark stipple, cortical region was deactivated (Cool); light stipple, cortex was uncooled (warm or rewarm).

Areal behavioral dissociations within visuoparietal cortex

In total, we have revealed that different motion, spatial and attentional tasks are mediated by individual regions within parietal cortex or some functions are shared between areas, such as motion processing in aMS and pMS sulcal cortices (see summary in Table 1). Furthermore, we have identified that numerous functions are mediated by pMS sulcal cortex. This will be the topic of the next section. dPS cortex does not mediate any of the functions typically associated with the parietal processing stream. In fact, deactivation of dPS cortex resulted in deficits on pattern and form discriminations mediated by the temporal processing stream. Therefore, these behavioral results confirm our earlier proposal that dPS is an important relay point in the temporal processing stream (Lomber et al., 1996a). Additional evidence for this is provided by electrophysiological studies which provide evidence that dPS cortex receives its principal excitatory input predominately from area 17 and that it is primarily involved in form analysis (Dreher et al., 1993, 1996), rather than the properties of motion analysis identified in pMS sulcal cortex (Dreher et al., 1996).

Unfortunately, no visual functions have yet been identified to be mediated by MS gyral cortex. It neither makes contributions to any of the motion, spatial or attentional tasks typical of visuoparietal cortex, nor the form discrimination tasks characteristic of visuotemporal cortex. Therefore, the next step in investigating visuoparietal cortex will be to examine the contributions that MS gyral cortex, as well as the other parietal regions, make to visuomotor control of actions, such as limb movements. There is substantial evidence that visuoparietal cortex makes significant contributions to the execution of visually directed movements (see Milner and Goodale, 1995).

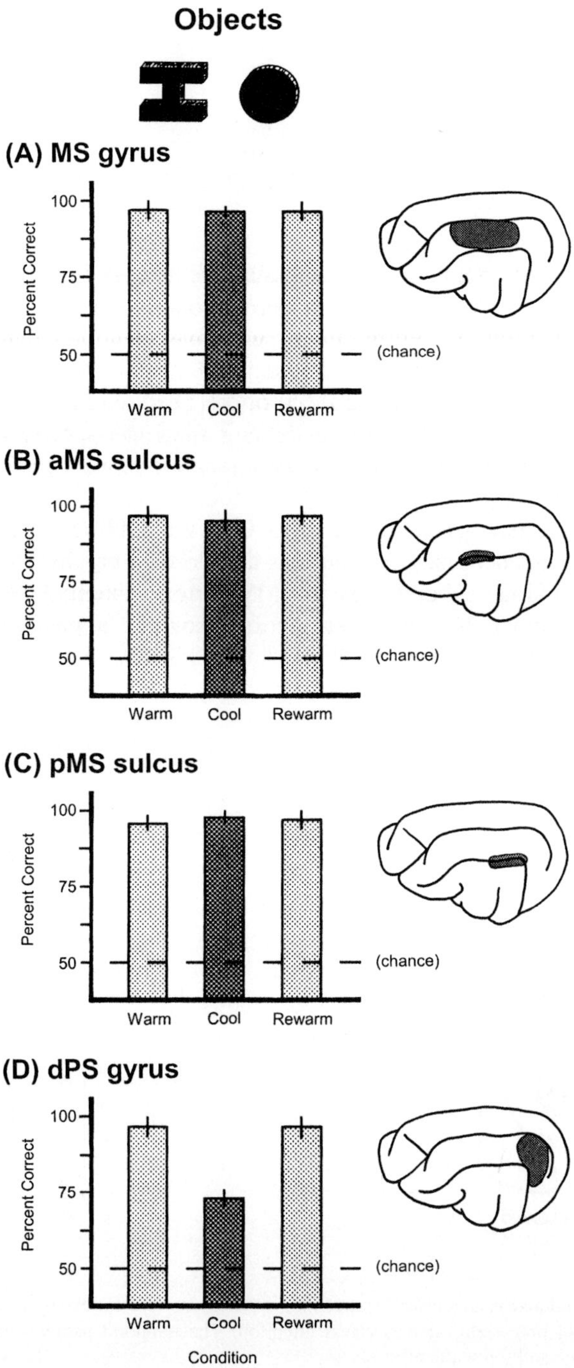

Fig. 10. Object discrimination task. Stimuli consisted of solid-black three-dimensional I and O shapes (top). Histograms of the mean (± 1 SE) percent correct responses while (A) MS gyral, (B) aMS sulcal, (C) pMS sulcal and (D) dPS gyral cortices are active (warm), deactivated (cool), and reactivated (rewarm). Chance performance = 50%. Dark stipple, cortical region was deactivated (Cool); light stipple, cortex was uncooled (warm or rewarm).

Fig. 11 summarizes the structure and function of the parietal and temporal processing streams through extrastriate visual cortex. Both pathways originate from primary visual areas 17 and 18. The parietal pathway is dominated by area 18 signals which project to MS sulcal cortex. In this pathway, MS sulcal cortex is implicated in motion and spatial processing as well as the direction of visual attention. The temporal pathway is dominated by area 17 signals which project to both dorsal posterior suprasylvian (dPS) cortex and area 19. In turn, these two areas then project to vPS gyral cortex. In this pathway, vPS gyral cortex is implicated in the learning and recognition of visual forms.

Multiple contributions to visual processing in pMS sulcal cortex

In the visual cortex, individual neurons have a unique signature-sensitivity for sets of stimulus parameters such as: size, line orientation, direction of movement, movement velocity, positional and movement disparity, contrast, spatial frequency, and so on. Moreover, populations of neurons with several signature-sensitivities in common are grouped in individual cortical layers and, on a larger scale, into cortical areas (for review see Payne, 1993) to produce unique laminar and cortical representations of the visual world. In classical terms, these representations are considered sensory, associational or motor, and the contiguity of these multiple representations in a single cerebral region is exemplified by pMS sulcal cortex, which

TABLE 1

Deficits on each of six visual tasks during reversible cooling deactivation of each cerebral region

Task	Cerebral region			
	MS gyrus	aMS sulcus	pMS sulcus	dPS gyrus
Direction of motion	–	Complete	Complete	–
Differential motion	–	Complete	Complete	–
Landmark discrimination	–	–	Complete	–
Visual attention	–	–	Complete	–
Complex patterns	–	–	–	Partial
Objects	–	–	–	Partial

(–) indicates that no deficit was identified.

contributes in many ways to both early and middle levels of visual processing and visually guided behavior. For example, temporary and permanent deactivation of pMS cortex depresses: (1) performance on a variety of tasks that require the processing of different directions of motion (Lomber et al., 1996b), differential motion (Kiefer et al., 1989; Lomber et al., 1994), different velocities of motion (Pasternak et al., 1989) and structure-from-motion (Rudolph and Pasternak, 1996); (2) the ability to detect and orient to a stimulus introduced into the contralateral visual field (Hardy and Stein, 1988; Lomber et al., 1996b; Payne et al., 1996); (3) proficient optokinetic nystagmus (Ventre, 1985; Tusa et al., 1989); (4) depth perception (Krüger et al., 1993a); (5) the ability to perform spatial discriminations (Lomber and Payne, 2000a); and (6) proficient visually guided locomotion (Sherk and Fowler, 2000). Together, these deficits span the spectrum from sensory, through associational, to motor contributions.

That accepted, we ask: Can we subfractionate the functional contributions and do they parallel the obvious subdivisions in pMS cortex anatomy? We believe that the next section provides a positive response to this question.

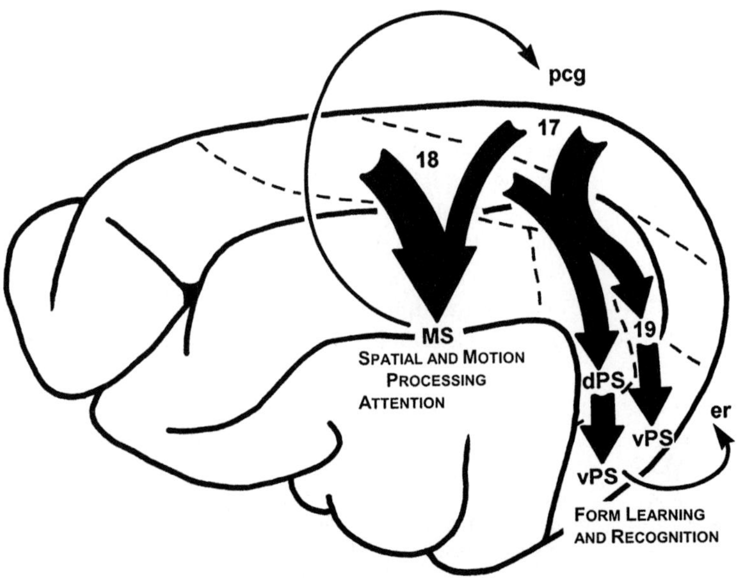

Fig. 11. Dorsolateral view of the cat cerebrum illustrating the visuoparietal and visuotemporal processing pathways across cat extrastriate visual cortex. The parietal pathway is implicated in motion and spatial processing and in visual attention. The temporal pathway is implicated in the learning and recognition of visual forms. Left is anterior and top is dorsal.

Laminar dissociations within pMS sulcal cortex

As we have demonstrated that pMS sulcal cortex makes multiple contributions to visual behavior, we next sought to determine if motion-processing and attentional machinery are dissociable in the laminar domain (Lomber and Payne, 2000b). Since disruption of normal function at the posterior end of parietal cortex in humans (Posner and Raichle, 1994; Rafal, 1994; Vaina and Cowey, 1996; Vaina et al., 1998), monkeys (Lynch and McLaren, 1989; Watson et al., 1994; Marcar et al., 1997) and cats (Pasternak et al., 1989; Lomber et al., 1994, 1996b; Payne et al., 1996) induces both motion and attentional deficits, we examined direction of motion discriminations and used visual orienting to assess visual attention in the cat. The approach was to apply lesser or greater levels of cooling to pMS sulcal cortex to deactivate the cortical thickness in a graded, yet consistent, way; the more-superficial layers alone or in combination with the deep layers (Lomber and Payne, 2000b).

With pMS sulcal cryoloop temperatures between 20 and 37ºC, cats are highly proficient at discriminating differences in movement direction of 30º of two identical non-systematic patterns moving at 6.4 deg/s (Fig. 5). Cooling to progressively lower temperatures (<20ºC) first initiated and then maximized an impairment in motion processing, which was reduced to a complete impairment, and chance levels of performance, at a cryoloop temperature of 8 ± 1ºC (Fig. 12(i)). Similar results were obtained with angular differences in motion direction of <30º. In contrast, performance on an easier 45º version of the task was completely unimpaired even when the pMS sulcal cryoloop was cooled to 3 ± 1ºC (Fig. 12, filled triangle). Presumably other regions of cortex are sufficient to maintain high performance when angular difference in direction is ≥45º (Lomber et al., 1996b).

A similar initiation, decline, and then complete blockade of visual attention is also effected by progressive cooling of the pMS sulcal cryoloop. However, the initiation temperature of the decline (<12ºC) and the final temperature of blockade (2–3ºC) was lower in all four cats examined than the respective initiation and blockade temperatures on the motion task. At the lowest temperatures used (2–3ºC) orienting into the ipsilateral hemifield was unimpaired (Fig. 12, filled circles).

The different temperatures for initiation and completion of blockade for the two tasks suggests that it is necessary to silence more neurons to block orienting performance than to block motion processing. Since 20ºC is the critical temperature below which neurons are silenced by blockade of synaptic transmission from afferent fibers (Jasper et al., 1970; Bénita and Condé, 1972; Lomber et al., 1999), we used arrays of microthermocouples to measure temperatures at more than 200 sites in two brains to ascertain the position of the 20ºC thermocline. A compilation of data from multiple tracks with the cryoloop sequentially cooled to two different temperatures (8 and 3ºC) are presented in Figs. 13 and 14. Cortex between the 20ºC thermocline and the cryoloop has temperatures of <20ºC and is deactivated by the cooling, whereas locations more distal from the cryoloop than the 20ºC thermocline have temperatures >20ºC and remain active.

It is readily apparent from Figs. 13 and 14 that the effect of reducing cryoloop temperature from 8 to 3ºC pushed the 20ºC thermocline from the middle cortical layers to the gray/white matter interface. In cross sectional terms, the linear area of cortex deactivated by lowering the temperature of the cryoloop in this way was increased by 138%, whereas estimates of lateral movement of the 20ºC thermocline on the cortical surface away from the cryoloop shows an increase in surface area of only 16%. Thus, the major effect of the additional cooling was to push the 20ºC thermocline across the deep layers of cortex with little lateral, surface movement.

The most parsimonious interpretation of the differences in extents of deactivations is that motion processing is critically dependent upon the superficial cortical layers and that the ability to redirect attention is critically dependent upon the deep layers. A critical component in acceptance of this interpretation is the recognition that deep layer neurons remain visually active when upper layer neurons are silenced. Control physiological measures made in other cats verify deep layer activity in the absence of upper layer activity, and confirm the results of others that deep layer neurons remain active in the absence of activity in the superficial layers (Schwark et al., 1986; Weyand et al., 1986, 1991; Ferster et al., 1996).

Another possible explanation of the results can also be considered. Several anatomical and electrophysiological studies suggest that the medial and lateral banks of the pMS sulcus have different anatomical connections and receptive field properties, respectively (Kawamura et al., 1978; Kawamura and Naito, 1980; Naito and Kawamura, 1982; Von Grünau et al., 1987). However, no behavioral evidence supports this possibility. For example, in all pMS cortex studies known to us that examined motion perception, all reports examined the medial bank or both banks, but never the lateral bank independently. Similarly, visual orienting studies have found similar deficits following lesions of either the medial or lateral banks (Hardy and Stein, 1988). Here, we have treated the medial and lateral banks collectively and not considered each bank individually. The possibility could therefore exist that the medial bank, for example, makes more of a contribution to motion sensitive tasks and the lateral bank is responsible for visual detection and orienting functions. However, even if this possibility were found to be true, this result would not weaken the significance of our laminar results. If the medial bank is found to be responsible for motion discriminations, then we would propose that it is the superficial layers of the medial bank which are responsible for contributions towards the successful completion of the motion tasks. Likewise, if visual orienting functions are localized to the lateral bank, we would propose that the deep

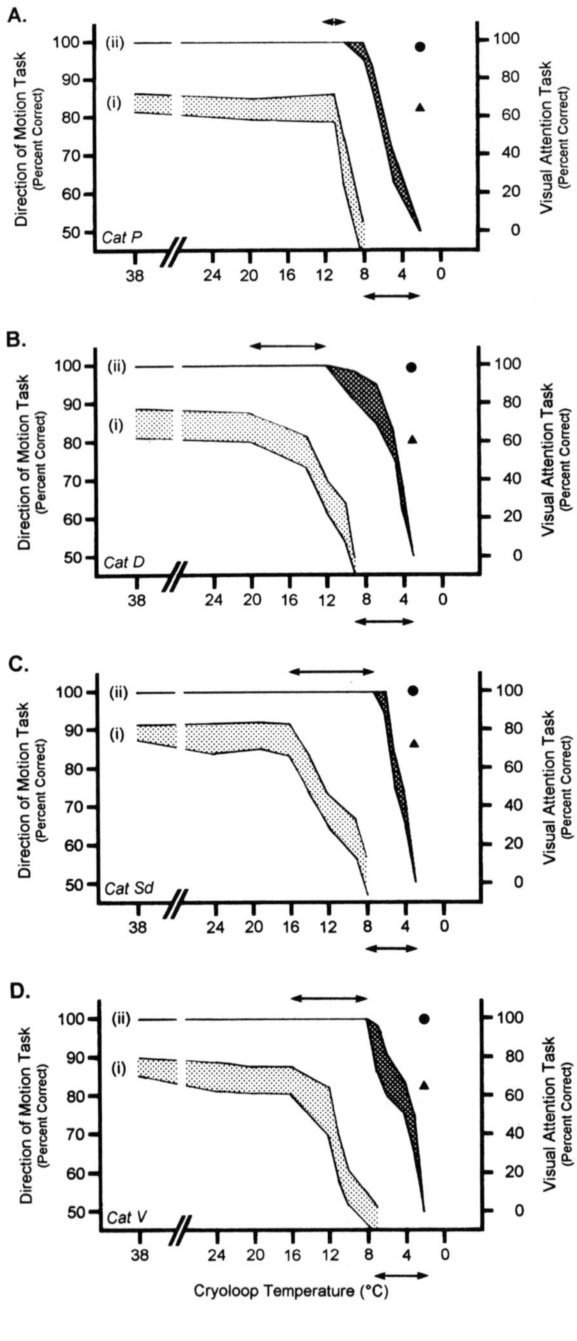

Fig. 12. Graphic representation of behavioral performance levels as a function of pMS cryoloop temperature for four cats. Each graph shows the mean ± 1 standard error performance for blocks of trials collected at different cryoloop temperatures (stipple). (i) Light stippling represents the range in performance on the 30° difference in direction of motion task. Filled triangle represents the mean performance on a 45° difference in direction of motion task when pMS sulcal cortex was fully deactivated. Note high performance on the 45° task when performance on the 30° task is reduced to chance. Slight differences in initiation temperature and slope of progressive deficits reflects slight differences in exact position of cryoloops, quality of contact between cryoloop and cortical surface, and vascular patterns (Lomber et al., 1999). (ii) Dark stippling represents the range of orienting performance on the visual attention task for stimuli introduced into the contracooled hemifield. Filled circle represents mean performance to stimuli introduced into the ipsicooled hemifield at 2 or 3°C. Upper arrows in each graph indicate differences in temperatures for initiation of impairments on the two tasks. Lower arrow indicates differences in temperature for complete blockade of both tasks.

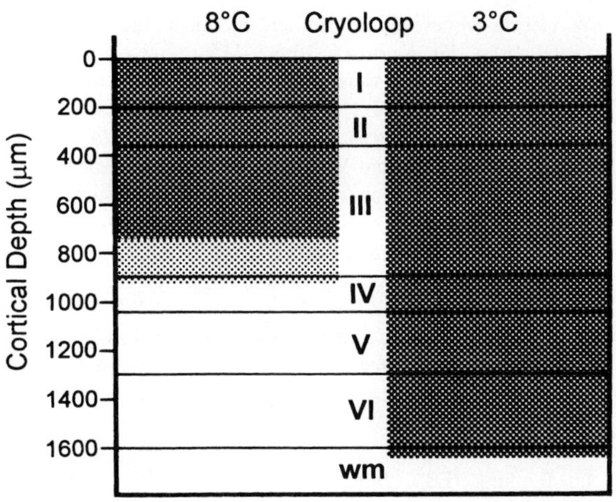

Fig. 13. Summary of deactivation depth when the cryoloop in the pMS sulcus was cooled to 8 and 3°C. Temperatures <20°C, where synaptic transmission is eliminated, are indicated by dark stipple. Temperature between 20 and 24°C, where synaptic activity is impaired, is indicated by light stipple. (From Lomber et al. (1999), reproduced with permission.)

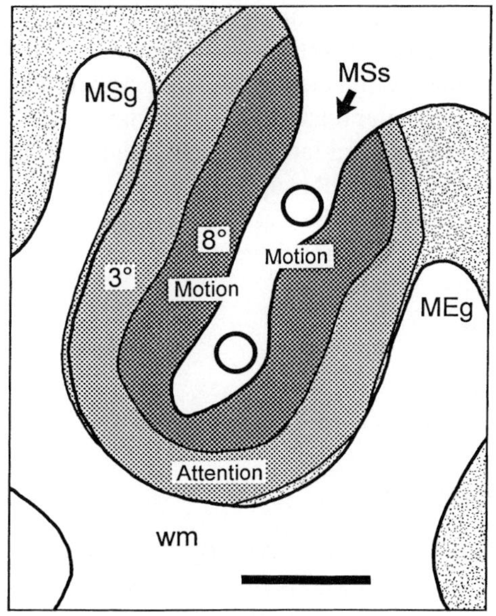

Fig. 14. Estimated position of the 20°C thermocline in the middle suprasylvian sulcus (MSs) during cooling of the loop to 8 and 3°C. With cooling to 8°C, the 20°C thermocline lay in the mid-depths of the cortex, whereas cooling to 3°C pushed the position of the 20°C to the vicinity of the gray/white matter (wm) junction. Dark stipple demarcates region of cortex with temperatures <20°C when the cryoloop was cooled to 8°C. Combined, the dark and light stipple zones demarcate the region of cortex <20°C when the cryoloop was cooled to 3°C. Circles show the position of the cooling loop in the sulcus. Outside diameter of cryoloop tubing is 0.63 mm. Impressions in the cortical surface indicate accurately the position of the cooling loops. Left is medial and scale bar = 2 mm.

layers of the lateral bank are responsible for contributions towards the successful completion of the detection and orienting task. Therefore, we do not consider the possibility that these functions may not be distributed across the entire sulcus, but instead be localized to a given bank, to undermine our conclusion that it is possible to localize functions to the superficial or deep layers of the cerebrum.

The massive effort invested in attempts over the previous one and a half centuries to localize functions to discrete regions of cerebral cortex have relied on ablation techniques to induce behavioral deficits and, more recently, on imaging techniques to localize discrete regions of activation. However, both approaches have limited their mapping exclusively to the two-dimensional sheet of cortex and have ignored the third dimension, depth. Our results confirm that a single cortical region can contribute to more than one visually guided behavior (Lomber et al., 1996b). They also show that motion processing is dominated by upper cortical layers, and that attentional mechanisms are dependent on deep cortical layers, thus, adding the long ignored third dimension to our view of the spatial organization of cerebral processing.

Abbreviations

Aud	auditory cortex
ALLS	anterolateral lateral suprasylvian
AMLS	anteromedial lateral suprasylvian
aMS	anterior middle suprasylvian
Cg	cingulate gyrus
dLGN	dorsal lateral geniculate nucleus
DLS	dorsal lateral suprasylvian
dPS	dorsal-posterior suprasylvian
er	entorhinal cortex
Mg	marginal gyrus
ME	middle ectosylvian
MEg	middle ectosylvian gyrus
MS	middle suprasylvian
MSg	middle suprasylvian gyrus
MSs	middle suprasylvian sulcus

pcg	posterior cingulated gyrus
PEV	posterior ectosylvian visual area
PGTA	Pennsylvania General Testing Apparatus
PLLS	posterolateral lateral suprasylvian
PMLS	posteromedial lateral suprasylvian
pMS	posterior middle suprasylvian
pMSs	posterior middle suprasylvian sulcus
vPS	ventral-posterior suprasylvian
wm	white matter
17	area 17
18	area 18
19	area 19
2DG	2-deoxyglucose

Acknowledgements

I am grateful to Professors Bert Payne, Paul Cornwell, and Jim Horel for their support and encouragement during these studies. I also wish to thank Margaret MacNeil, Helena Mariadason, Shana O'Marra, Greg Orpen, Rebbeca Huot, Christine Chizmar, Kevin Long, and Heather Foley for assistance with various portions of the experiments described in this review. Finally, I wish to thank Christian Casanova and Maurice Ptito for their gracious offer to participate in their symposium, *Vision: From Neurons to Cognition*, and this volume. This work was supported by the National Institute of Neurological Disorders and Stroke and the National Science Foundation.

References

Bénita, M. and Condé, H. (1972) Effects of local cooling upon conduction and synaptic transmission. *Brain Res.*, 36: 133–151.

Campbell Jr., A. (1978) Deficits in visual learning produced by posterior temporal lesions in cats. *J. Comp. Physiol. Psychol.*, 92: 45–57.

Cavada, C. and Reinoso-Suárez, F. (1983) Afferent connections of area 20 in the cat studied by means of the retrograde axonal transport of horseradish peroxidase. *Brain Res.*, 270: 319–324.

Cornwell, P., Nudo, R.J., Straussfogel, D., Lomber, S.G. and Payne, B.R. (1998) Dissociation of visual and auditory pattern discrimination functions within the cat's temporal cortex. *Behav. Neurosci.*, 112: 800–811.

Damasio, A.R., Tranel, D. and Damasio, H. (1989) Disorders of visual recognition. In: F. Boller and J. Grafman (Eds.), *Handbook of Neuropsychology*, Vol. 2. Elsevier, Amsterdam, pp. 317–332.

Dreher, B., Michalski, A., Ho, R.H.T., Lee, C.W.F. and Burke, W. (1993) Processing of form and motion in area 21a of cat visual cortex. *Vis. Neurosci.*, 10: 93–115.

Dreher, B., Wang, C., Turlejski, K.J., Djavadian, R.L. and Burke, W. (1996) Areas PMLS and 21a of cat visual cortex: two functionally distinct areas. *Cereb. Cortex*, 6: 585–699.

Ferster, D., Chung, S. and Wheat, H. (1996) Orientation selectivity of thalamic input to simple cells of cat visual cortex. *Nature*, 380: 249–252.

Gaffan, D., Harrison, S. and Gaffan, E.A. (1986) Visual identification following inferotemporal ablation in the monkey. *Q. J. Exp. Psychol. (B)*, 38: 5–30.

Grant, S. and Shipp, S. (1991) Visuotopic organization of the lateral suprasylvian area and of an adjacent area of the ectosylvian gyrus of cat cortex: a physiological and connectional study. *Vis. Neurosci.*, 6: 315–338.

Gross, C.G. (1973) Visual functions of inferotemporal cortex. In: R. Jung (Ed.), *Handbook of Sensory Physiology*, Vol. VII/3B, *Central Processing of Visual Information*, Part B. Springer-Verlag, Berlin, pp. 451–482.

Hardy, S.C. and Stein, B.E. (1988) Small lateral suprasylvian cortex lesions produce visual neglect and decreased visual activity in the superior colliculus. *J. Comp. Neurol.*, 273: 527–542.

Haxby, J.V., Grady, C.L., Horwitz, B., Salerno, J., Ungerleider, L.G., Mishkin, M. and Schapiro, M.B. (1993) Dissociation of object and spatial visual processing pathways in human extrastriate cortex. In: B. Gulyas, D. Ottoson and P.E. Roland (Eds.), *Functional Organisation of Human Visual Cortex*. Pergamon Press, Oxford, pp. 329–340.

Jasper, H.H., Shacter, D.G. and Montplaisir, J. (1970) The effect of local cooling upon spontaneous and evoked electrical activity of cerebral cortex. *Can. J. Physiol. Pharmacol.*, 48: 640–652.

Kawamura, K. and Naito, J. (1980) Corticocortical neurons projecting to the medial and lateral banks of the middle suprasylvian sulcus in the cat: an experimental study with the horseradish peroxidase method. *J. Comp. Neurol.*, 193: 1009–1022.

Kawamura, K., Konno, T. and Chiba, M. (1978) Cells of origin of corticopontine and corticotectal fibers in the medial and lateral banks of the middle suprasylvian sulcus of the cat. *Neurosci. Lett.*, 9: 129–135.

Kawano, J. (1998) Cortical projections of the parvocellular laminae C of the dorsal lateral geniculate nucleus of the cat: an anterograde wheat germ agglutinin conjugated to horseradish peroxidase study. *J. Comp. Neurol.*, 392: 439–457.

Kiefer, W., Krüger, K., Strauß, G. and Berlucchi, G. (1989) Considerable deficits in the detection performance of the cat after lesion of the suprasylvian visual cortex. *Exp. Brain Res.*, 75: 208–212.

Krüger, K., Kiefer, W. and Groh, A. (1993a) Lesion of the suprasylvian cortex impairs depth perception of cats. *NeuroReport*, 4: 883–886.

Krüger, K., Kiefer, W., Groh, A., Dinse, H.R. and von Seelen, W. (1993b) The role of the lateral suprasylvian visual cortex of the cat in object–background interactions: permanent deficits following lesions. *Exp. Brain Res.*, 97: 40–60.

Kuchiiwa, S., Kuchiiwa, T., Matsue, H. and Sukekawa, K. (1985) Efferent connections of area 20 in the cat: HRP–WGA and autoradiographic studies. *Exp. Brain Res.*, 60: 179–183.

Lomber, S.G. (1999) The advantages and limitations of permanent or reversible deactivation techniques in the assessment of neural function. *J. Neurosci. Methods*, 86: 109–117.

Lomber, S.G. and Payne, B.R. (1996) Removal of two halves restores the whole: reversal of visual hemineglect during bilateral cortical or collicular inactivation in the cat. *Vis. Neurosci.*, 13: 1143–1156.

Lomber, S.G. and Payne, B.R. (2000a) Contributions of cat posterior parietal cortex to visuospatial discrimination. *Vis. Neurosci.*, 17: 701–709.

Lomber, S.G. and Payne, B.R. (2000b) Translaminar differentiation of visually guided behaviors revealed by restricted cerebral cooling deactivation. *Cereb. Cortex*, 10: 1066–1077.

Lomber, S.G., Cornwell, P., Sun, J.-S., MacNeil, M.A. and Payne, B.R. (1994) Reversible inactivation of visual processing operations in middle suprasylvian cortex of the behaving cat. *Proc. Natl. Acad. Sci. USA*, 91: 2999–3003.

Lomber, S.G., MacNeil, M.A. and Payne, B.R. (1995) Amplification of thalamic projections to middle suprasylvian cortex following ablation of immature primary visual cortex in the cat. *Cereb. Cortex*, 5: 166–191.

Lomber, S.G., Payne, B.R., Cornwell, P. and Long, K.D. (1996a) Perceptual and cognitive visual functions of parietal and temporal cortices in the cat. *Cereb. Cortex*, 6: 673–695.

Lomber, S.G., Payne, B.R. and Cornwell, P. (1996b) Learning and recall of form discriminations during reversible cooling deactivation of ventral-posterior suprasylvian cortex in the cat. *Proc. Natl. Acad. Sci. USA*, 93: 1654–1658.

Lomber, S.G., Payne, B.R. and Horel, J.A. (1999) The cryoloop: an adaptable reversible cooling deactivation method for behavioral and electrophysiological assessment of neural function. *J. Neurosci. Methods*, 86: 179–194.

Long, K.D., Lomber, S.G. and Payne, B.R. (1996) Increased oxidative metabolism in middle suprasylvian cortex following removal of areas 17 and 18 from newborn cats. *Exp. Brain Res.*, 110: 335–346.

Lynch, J.C. and McLaren, J.W. (1989) Deficits of visual attention and saccadic eye movements after lesions of parieto-occipital cortex in monkeys. *J. Neurophysiol.*, 61: 74–90.

MacNeil, M.A., Lomber, S.G. and Payne, B.R. (1996) Rewiring of transcortical projections to middle suprasylvian cortex following early removal of cat areas 17 and 18. *Cereb. Cortex*, 6: 362–376.

Marcar, V.L., Zihl, J. and Cowey, A. (1997) Comparing the visual deficits of a motion blind patient with the visual deficits of monkeys with area MT removed. *Neuropsychologia*, 35: 1459–1465.

Milner, A.D. and Goodale, M.A. (1995) *The Visual Brain in Action*. Oxford University Press, Oxford, UK.

Mishkin, M. and Ungerleider, L.G. (1982) Contribution of striate inputs to the visuospatial functions of parieto-preoccipital cortex in monkeys. *Behav. Brain Res.*, 6: 57–77.

Mishkin, M., Lewis, M.E. and Ungerleider, L.G. (1982) Equivalence of parieto-preoccipital subareas for visuospatial ability in monkeys. *Behav. Brain Res.*, 6: 41–55.

Naito, J. and Kawamura, K. (1982) Thalamocortical neurons projecting to the areas surrounding the anterior and middle suprasylvian sulci in the cat. A horseradish peroxidase study. *Exp. Brain Res.*, 45: 59–70.

Newcombe, F. and Ratcliffe, G. (1989) Disorders in visuospatial analysis. In: F. Boller and J. Grafman (Eds.), *Handbook of Neuropsychology*, Vol. 2. Elsevier, Amsterdam, pp. 333–356.

Newsome, W.T. and Paré, E.B. (1988) A selective impairment of motion perception following lesions of the middle temporal visual area (MT). *J. Neurosci.*, 8: 2201–2211.

Olson, C.R. and Lawler, K. (1987) Cortical and subcortical afferent connections of a posterior division of feline area 7 (area 7p). *J. Comp. Neurol.*, 259: 13–30.

Olson, C.R. and Musil, S.Y. (1992) Topographic organization of cortical and subcortical projections to posterior cingulate cortex in the cat: evidence for somatic, ocular and complex subregions. *J. Comp. Neurol.*, 323: 1–24.

Palmer, L.A., Rosenquist, A.C. and Tusa, R.J. (1978) The retinotopic organization of lateral suprasylvian visual areas in the cat. *J. Comp. Neurol.*, 177: 237–256.

Pasternak, T. and Merigan, W.H. (1994) Motion perception following lesions of the superior temporal sulcus in the monkey. *Cereb. Cortex*, 4: 247–259.

Pasternak, T., Horn, K.M. and Maunsell, J.H.R. (1989) Deficits in speed discrimination following lesions of the lateral suprasylvian cortex in the cat. *Vis. Neurosci.*, 3: 365–375.

Payne, B.R. (1993) Evidence for visual cortical area homologs in cat and macaque monkey. *Cereb. Cortex*, 3: 1–25.

Payne, B.R. and Lomber, S.G. (1999) A method to assess the functional impact of cerebral connections on target populations of neurons. *J. Neurosci. Methods*, 86: 195–208.

Payne, B.R., Lomber, S.G., Geeraerts, S., van der Gucht, E. and Vandenbussche, E. (1996) Reversible visual hemineglect. *Proc. Natl. Acad. Sci. USA*, 93: 290–294.

Petrides, M. and Iverson, S.D. (1979) Restricted posterior parietal lesions in the rhesus monkey and performance on visuospatial tasks. *Brain Res.*, 161: 63–77.

Pohl, W. (1973) Dissociation of spatial discriminations deficits following frontal and parietal lesions in monkeys. *J. Comp. Physiol. Psychol.*, 82: 227–239.

Posner, M.I. and Raichle, M.E. (1994) *Images of Mind*. Freeman, New York.

Raczkowski, D. and Rosenquist, A.C. (1983) Connections of the multiple visual cortical areas with the lateral posterior-pulvinar complex and adjacent thalamic nuclei in the cat. *J. Neurosci.*, 3: 1912–1942.

Rafal, R.D. (1994) Neglect. *Curr. Biol.*, 4: 231–236.

Rauschecker, J.P., von Grünau, M.W. and Poulin, C. (1987) Centrifugal organization of direction preferences in the cat's lateral suprasylvian visual cortex and its relation to flow field processing. *J. Neurosci.*, 7: 943–958.

Reinoso-Suárez, F. (1961) *Topographischer Hirnatlas der Katz fur Experimentale Physiologische Untersuchungen*. [Topographical atlas of the cat brain for experimental-physiological research]. Merck, Darmstadt.

Reinoso-Suárez, F. (1984) Connectional patterns in parietotemporooccipital association cortex of the feline cerebral cortex. In: F. Reinoso-Suárez and C. Ajmone-Marsan (Eds.), *Cortical Integration*. Raven Press, New York, pp. 255–278.

Rosenquist, A.C. (1985) Connections of visual cortical areas in the cat. In: A. Peters and E.G. Jones (Eds.), *Cerebral Cortex*, Vol. 3, *Visual Cortex*. Plenum Press, New York, pp. 81–117.

Rudolph, K.K. and Pasternak, T. (1996) Lesions of cat lateral suprasylvian cortex affect the perception of complex motion. *Cereb. Cortex*, 8: 814–822.

Rudolph, K.K. and Pasternak, T. (1999) Transient and permanent deficits in motion perception after lesions of cortical areas MT and MST in the macaque monkey. *Cereb. Cortex*, 9: 90–100.

Schwark, H.D., Malpeli, J.G., Weyand, T.G. and Lee, C. (1986) Cat area 17: II. Response properties of infragranular layer neurons in the absence of supragranular layer activity. *J. Neurophysiol.*, 56: 1074–1087.

Sherk, H. (1986) Location and connections of visual cortical areas in the cat's suprasylvian sulcus. *J. Comp. Neurol.*, 247: 1–31.

Sherk, H. and Fowler, G.A. (2000) Visual guidance of locomotion after lesions of extrastriate cortex. *Soc. Neurosci. Abstr.*, 26: 2085.

Sherman, S.M. (1977) The effect of superior colliculus lesions upon the visual fields of cats with cortical ablations. *J. Comp. Neurol.*, 172: 211–230.

Spear, P.D. (1991) Functions of extrastriate visual cortex in non-primate species. In: A.G. Leventhal (Ed.), *Vision and Visual Dysfunction*, Vol. 4, *The Neural Basis of Visual Function*. Macmillan, Basingstoke, pp. 339–370.

Sprague, J.M., Levy, J., DiBerardino, A. and Berlucchi, G. (1977) Visual cortex areas mediating form discrimination in the cat. *J. Comp. Neurol.*, 172: 441–458.

Symonds, L.L. and Rosenquist, A.C. (1984) Corticocortical connections among visual areas in the cat. *J. Comp. Neurol.*, 229: 1–38.

Tong, L., Kalil, R.E. and Spear, P.D. (1982) Thalamic projections to visual areas of the middle suprasylvian sulcus in the cat. *J. Comp. Neurol.*, 212: 103–117.

Tusa, R.J. and Palmer, L.A. (1980) Retinotopic organization of areas 20 and 21 in the cat. *J. Comp. Neurol.*, 193: 147–164.

Tusa, R.J., Rosenquist, A.C. and Palmer, L.A. (1979) Retinotopic organization of areas 18 and 19 in the cat. *J. Comp. Neurol.*, 185: 657–678.

Tusa, R.J., Demer, J.L. and Herdman, S.J. (1989) Cortical areas involved in OKN and VOR in cats: cortical lesions. *J. Neurosci.*, 9: 1163–1178.

Ungerleider, L.G. and Haxby, J.V. (1994) 'What' and 'where' in the human brain. *Curr. Opin. Neurobiol.*, 4: 157–165.

Ungerleider, L.G. and Mishkin, M. (1982) Two cortical visual systems. In: D.J. Ingle, M.A. Goodale and R.J.W. Mansfield (Eds.), *Analysis of Visual Behavior*. MIT Press, Cambridge, MA, pp. 549–586.

Vaina, L.M. (1990) 'What' and 'where' in the human visual system: two hierarchies of visual modules. *Synthese*, 83: 49–91.

Vaina, L.M. and Cowey, A. (1996) Impairment of the perception of second order motion but not first order motion in a patient with unilateral focal brain damage. *Proc. R. Soc. Lond. B Biol. Sci.*, 263: 1225–1232.

Vaina, L.M., Makris, N., Kennedy, D. and Cowey, A. (1998) The selective impairment of the perception of first-order motion by unilateral cortical brain damage. *Vis. Neurosci.*, 15: 333–348.

Ventre, J. (1985) Cortical control of oculomotor functions. I. Optokinetic nystagmus. *Behav. Brain Res.*, 15: 211–226.

Von Grünau, M.W., Zumbroich, T.J. and Poulin, C. (1987) Visual receptive field properties in the posterior suprasylvian cortex of the cat: a comparison between the areas PMLS and PLLS. *Vision Res.*, 27: 343–356.

Watson, R.T., Valenstein, E., Day, A. and Heilman, K.M. (1994) Posterior neocortical systems subserving awareness and neglect. Neglect associated with superior temporal sulcus but not area 7 lesions. *Arch. Neurol.*, 51: 1014–1021.

Weyand, T.G., Malpeli, J.G., Lee, C. and Schwark, H.D. (1986) Cat Area 17. IV. Two types of corticotectal cells defined by controlling geniculate inputs. *J. Neurophysiol.*, 56: 1102–1108.

Weyand, T.G., Malpeli, J.G. and Lee, C. (1991) Area 18 corticotectal cells: response properties and identification of sustaining geniculate inputs. *J. Neurophysiol.*, 65: 1078–1088.

Witter, M.P. and Groenewegen, H.J. (1986) Connections of the parahippocampal cortex in the cat. III. Cortical and thalamic efferents. *J. Comp. Neurol.*, 252: 1–31.

Yamasaki, D.S. and Wurtz, R.H. (1991) Recovery of function after lesions in the superior temporal sulcus in the monkey. *J. Neurophysiol.*, 66: 651–673.

Zihl, J., von Cramon, D., Mai, N. and Schmid, C. (1991) Disturbance of movement vision after bilateral posterior brain damage. *Brain*, 114: 2235–2252.

C. Casanova and M. Ptito (Eds.)
Progress in Brain Research, Vol. 134

CHAPTER 18

Visual cortex organization in primates: theories of V3 and adjoining visual areas

Jon H. Kaas * and David C. Lyon

Department of Psychology, Vanderbilt University, Nashville, TN 37240, USA

Abstract: After years of experimentation and substantial progress, there is still only limited agreement on how visual cortex in primates is organized, and what features of this organization are variable or stable across lines of primate phylogeny. Only three visual areas, V1, V2, and MT, are widely recognized as common to all primates, although there are certainly more. Here we consider various concepts of how the cortex along the outer border of V2 is organized. An early proposal was that this region is occupied by a V3 that is as wide and as long as V2, and represents the visual hemifield as a mirror image of V2. We refer to this notion as the classical V3 or V3-C. Another proposal is that only the dorsal half of V3-C exists, the half representing the lower visual quadrant, and thus the representation is incomplete (V3-I) by half. A version of this proposal is that V3-I is discontinuous, extremely thin in places, and highly variable across individuals, much as a vestigial or degenerate structure might be (V3-IF-incomplete and fragmented). A fourth proposal is that there is no V3. Many results suggest that a series of visual areas border V2, none of which has the characteristics of V3. Alternatively, the possibility exists that primate taxa differ with regard to visual areas bordering V2. Currently, much of the supporting evidence for a classical V3 comes from fMRI studies in humans, much of the evidence for a series of bordering areas comes from New World Monkeys and prosimian galagos, and much of the evidence for a V3-I or V3-IF comes from macaque monkeys. Possibly all these interpretations of visual cortex organization are valid, but each for only one of the major groups of primate evolution. Here, we suggest that none of these interpretations is correct, and propose instead that a modified V3 (V3-M) exists in a similar form in all primates. This V3-M is smaller and thinner than V3-C, discontinuous in the middle, but with comparable dorsal and ventral halves representing the lower and upper visual hemifields, respectively. Because the evidence for V3-M is limited, and it stems in part from our ongoing but incomplete comparative studies of V1 connections in primates, this suggestion requires further experimental evaluation and it remains tentative.

Introduction

Nearly all current investigators agree with the premise that neocortex is divided into a number of areas of differing functional roles. Each area is thought to be interconnected with several others, usually neighbors, to form processing networks or systems with serial and parallel components, including feedforward, feedback, and lateral interconnections. Further components of this general agreement are that species vary in number of areas from few to many, that some basic areas are widely shared, and that closely related species are likely to share more areas (see Kaas, 1987).

While there is widespread agreement on the validity of this theoretical framework of brain function and organization, specific theories of how cortex is subdivided and interconnected have varied and continue to vary (see Kaas, 1995a, 1997b; Rosa, 1997). Since specific theories are highly valuable for interpreting and summarizing experimental and other observations, and they serve as guides for planning future research, it seems important to resolve the differ-

* Corresponding author: J.H. Kaas, Department of Psychology, 301 Wilson Hall, Vanderbilt University, 111 21st Avenue South, Nashville, TN 37203, USA.
Tel.: +1-615-322-6029; Fax: +1-615-343-8449;
E-mail: jon.kaas@vanderbilt.edu

ences in current theories and move toward a theory that best accounts for the accumulating observations.

Our review focuses on the organization of the more caudal visual cortex that is involved in the early stages of cortical processing. These visual regions have been the most intensively studied, and thus there are more relevant observations and interpretations of observations for comment and comparison. Our review also considers evidence and theories based on all major lines of primate evolution for several reasons. First, such comparative studies can more reliably guide theories of the organization of the human brain (Kaas, 1997a). We agree that it is natural to be especially interested in the organization of visual cortex in humans, and the use of non-invasive brain imaging techniques, such as fMRI, have already revealed much about the organization of visual cortex in humans (see Tootell et al., 1996). Yet, most of us recognize the limitations as well as the advantages of studies on humans, and believe that information and theories obtained and developed from other primates can be very useful in helping us understand the human brain. Thus, conclusions about the organization of visual cortex in other primates, especially macaque monkeys, are commonly considered, and they greatly influence interpretations of data from humans. The focus on results from macaque monkeys is reasonable, in that our closest relatives, the great apes, are as inaccessible as humans for many types of studies. However, any predictions based on macaques alone should be treated with caution, given the 30 or so million years of independent evolution (Kay et al., 1997) of Old World monkeys and hominids (apes and humans). We feel brain features that can be shown to be more widely distributed across primate taxa are more likely than variable features to be preserved in the human brain, and thus it is important to compare results across all studied primates (see Preuss and Kaas, 1999). Furthermore, proposed differences between primate species should be compatible with feasible courses of evolution, so that results and theories from one group of primates can be used to evaluate those from another group (see Kaas, 1997a). Of course, different primates also offer various advantages in experimentally addressing questions about brain organization. In particular, the small, relatively smooth brains of many New World monkeys expose more visual areas on the surface where they are more accessible for study. Conclusions based on species where more compelling data can be obtained can be seen as applicable to other species if less compelling and incomplete data are supportive.

Given these reasons for comparing primates, and our conclusion that the organization of much of visual cortex is poorly understood, let us start by considering three visual areas that seem to exist in all primates.

Areas no longer in contention: V1, V2, and MT

Most investigators now agree that most or all primates have V1, V2, and MT (Fig. 1). There is widespread agreement on their boundaries, retinotopic organizations, major connections, and architectonic features (see Kaas, 1997b). Yet, this was not always so.

V1 or primary visual cortex appears to exist in all but possibly a few blind or nearly blind subterranean mammals (Kaas, 1980). Architectonically, V1 is one of the most distinctive of cortical areas, and thus it was the first identified subdivision of neocortex (see Gross, 1997). Yet, in early architectonic studies, another retrosplenial field was once misidentified as primary visual cortex, and even Brodmann (1909) mistook the thinner medial part of V1 (area 17) for another field (area 18) in rodents. More recently, some investigators have wrongly concluded that the more differentiated V1 of cats and primates is not the same field as V1 in hedgehogs and rats (see Kaas, 1987).

The second visual area, V2, is also an area that likely exist in all mammals except those with a reduced visual system (see Catania et al., 1999). Yet, interpretations of the size, location, retinotopic organization, and even the existence of V2 have varied. Most notably, many investigators conclude that the lateral border of V1 in rats and several other rodents consists of a series of small areas rather than V2, while others consider the proposed areas as subdivisions of V2 (see, Kaas et al., 1988; Rosa and Krubitzer, 1999). Largely because a characteristic banding pattern exists in histological preparations of V2 of most primates (see Krubitzer and Kaas, 1989; Roe and Ts'o, 1997), there is now good agreement on the extent and location of V2 in these mammals.

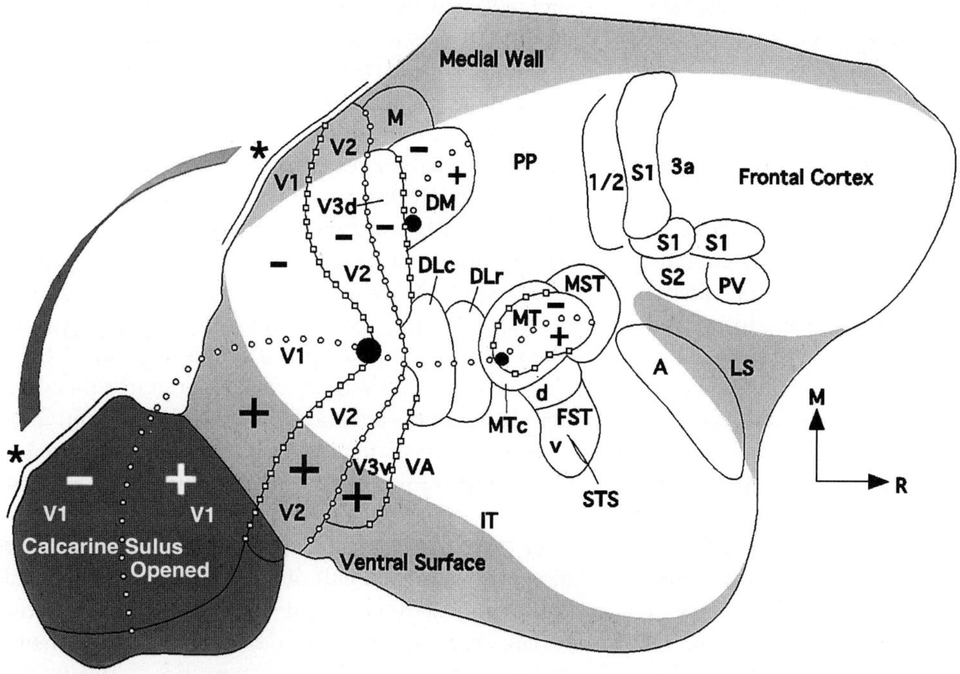

Fig. 1. Our current proposal for how visual cortex is subdivided into areas in primates shown on an unfolded view of neocortex in a New World monkey (marmoset). More established areas are outlined, others are indicated, while other proposed areas are not included. Outlined areas include primary visual cortex (V1), the second visual area (V2), dorsal and ventral V3 (V3d and V3v) as divisions of a redefined third visual area (V3), the dorsomedial area (DM), the middle temporal area (MT), the middle temporal crescent (MTc), the medial superior temporal area (MST), the dorsal and ventral divisions of the fundal area of the superior temporal sulcus (FSTd and FSTv), and caudal and rostral (DLc and DLr) divisions of the dorsolateral area (DL). Representations of the upper (+) and lower (−) visual quadrants are indicated for some of the visual areas. For some visual areas the zero horizontal (hollow circles) and the zero vertical (hollow squares) meridians are marked. Filled circles represent estimated location of foveal vision in DM and MT. The ventral anterior (VA), inferior temporal (IT), superior temporal 'sulcus' (STS) and posterior parietal (PP) visual regions are also indicated. For reference, the somatosensory areas, area 3b or primary somatosensory cortex (S1), the second somatosensory area (S2), the parietal ventral somatosensory area (PV), and the auditory core (A) are also outlined. LS, lateral sulcus. Shaded regions are parts of cortex that have been exposed by unfolding. Arrows indicate medial (M) and rostral (R) directions.

The middle temporal visual area, MT (also called the visual area of the superior temporal sulcus, the motion area, or V5), was first identified in owl monkeys as a densely myelinated oval of cortex with a systematic representation of the contralateral visual hemifield (Allman and Kaas, 1971). The approximate region of cortex was known to be responsive to visual stimuli (Woolsey et al., 1955), and to receive projections from V1 (Kuypers et al., 1965), but no MT-like area existed in early proposals of cortical organization based on architecture. Furthermore, while connections between V1 and MT are now recognized as retinotopically matched, various other concepts have been proposed. Initially, projections to the region were thought to be convergent, without a topographic pattern (Zeki, 1971) or convergent and to a larger ring-like area that circled V1 at a distance (Cragg, 1969). Another interpretation was that the V1 projection zones in the middle of the temporal lobes of owl monkeys and macaques were not to the same area (Zeki, 1980). The consensus opinion now is that MT exists as a densely myelinated V1 oval in the same relative position and with roughly topographic interconnections with V1 in all primates.

While V1 and V2 are areas that exist in most mammals, it is uncertain if MT exists in mammals other than primates. Since MT seems to be present in all primates, it is logical to assume that MT emerged with the first primates or even earlier. Because the Clare-Bishop region or area of cats has several of the features of MT in primates, including a representation of the visual hemifield, projections from V1, and a location displaced from the V1 border towards the upper temporal lobe, the Clare-Bishop area has often been considered to be a homologue of MT (e.g. Payne, 1993; Creutzfeldt, 1993). If the Clare-Bishop area and MT are homologous, one would expect to find an MT in many of the extant mammals that have descended from the common ancestors of cats and primates. Yet, there is little evidence for an MT-like area in other mammals. V1 projections to an oval of cortex lateral to V2 have been reported in several mammals including squirrels (Kaas et al., 1988) and tree shrews (Lyon et al., 1998). Admittedly, these regions of cortex resemble MT in having inputs from V1, in having a crude map of the visual hemifield, and perhaps in other ways, but they are located next to V2 rather than displaced into the temporal lobe. However, an MT-like area, slightly displaced from the V2 border, has been referred to as MT in megabats (Rosa, 1999). Possibly MT in primates and the Clare-Bishop region in cats both stem from an older area with V1 inputs that was independently displaced from the V2 border in lines of descent leading to these present-day mammals (Kaas, 1995b). Alternatively, MT and the Clare-Bishop region could be independent products of the evolution of complex visual systems with many cortical areas. Such issues of homology cannot be easily settled by studying cats and primates alone. A broader, cladistic approach is required (Harvey and Pagel, 1991).

Our purpose in mentioning all these various interpretations of visual cortex organization is not to devalue the serious efforts of previous researchers, but to emphasize how various interpretations typically are supportable, and that, with the accumulation of additional evidence, widespread agreements sometimes emerge. In the next section, we discuss views of how visual cortex along the outer border of V2 is organized, with the expectation that if we make differences in opinion more explicit, more research and progress toward a consensus view will occur.

Do primates have a V3?

With the evidence for a third visual area, V-III, in cats (see Hubel and Wiesel, 1965; we use the terms V-III in cats and V3 in primates to distinguish visual areas of the same name in the two taxonomic groups), it was logical to look for evidence for a V3 in primates. In cats, V-III has been described as a visual area along the complete length of the outer border of V2 with the width of V2 and a retinotopic organization that mirrors that of V2 (Tusa et al., 1979; Albus and Beckmann, 1980). V-III also receives retinotopically matched projections from V1 and V2. Indeed, early proposals of visual cortex organizations based on studies of V1 projections in macaque monkeys (Cragg, 1969; Zeki, 1969) included a V3 (then called 'area 19' or V-III) that had all of these characteristics of V-III of cats. We refer to this original depiction as the classical V3 or V3-C (Fig. 2A).

Since those early anatomical studies, evidence has accumulated to support several greatly modified concepts of V3. The modifications emerged in steps, with the most radical departure being the concept that only the dorsal half of V3 is V3, with the ventral half being another visual area, the ventroposterior visual area, VP (see Van Essen, 1985). We refer to this concept as V3-I because V3 is incomplete (representing only the lower visual quadrant) or, as previously noted (Kaas, 1996), improbable because it lacks an upper quadrant representation. Other modifications emerged so that a recent depiction is of a discontinuous remnant of dorsal V3 (Fig. 2B) that is as narrow as 1 mm in places, so limited in extent that it would not seem to be able to even represent all of the lower quadrant, and extremely variable in shape across individual macaque monkeys (Van Essen et al., 1986). This incomplete and fragmented V3 (V3-IF) is just a fraction of what one might expect for a visual area. The proposed variability in shape and extent across individuals, and the gross incompleteness of the representation suggest a visual area that is vestigial, one that has lost its functions and has been allowed to drift and degenerate without positive selection in evolution.

There were logical reasons for making this remarkable change in the proposed form of V3. First, the evidence for the classical V3 was based on assumptions about total projection patterns that were only partly known. Most of the accessible dorsal portion of V1 in macaque monkeys represents central and paracentral vision of the lower visual quadrant, and lesions and injections in this cortex did reveal projections to MT, dorsal V2, and cortex just outside

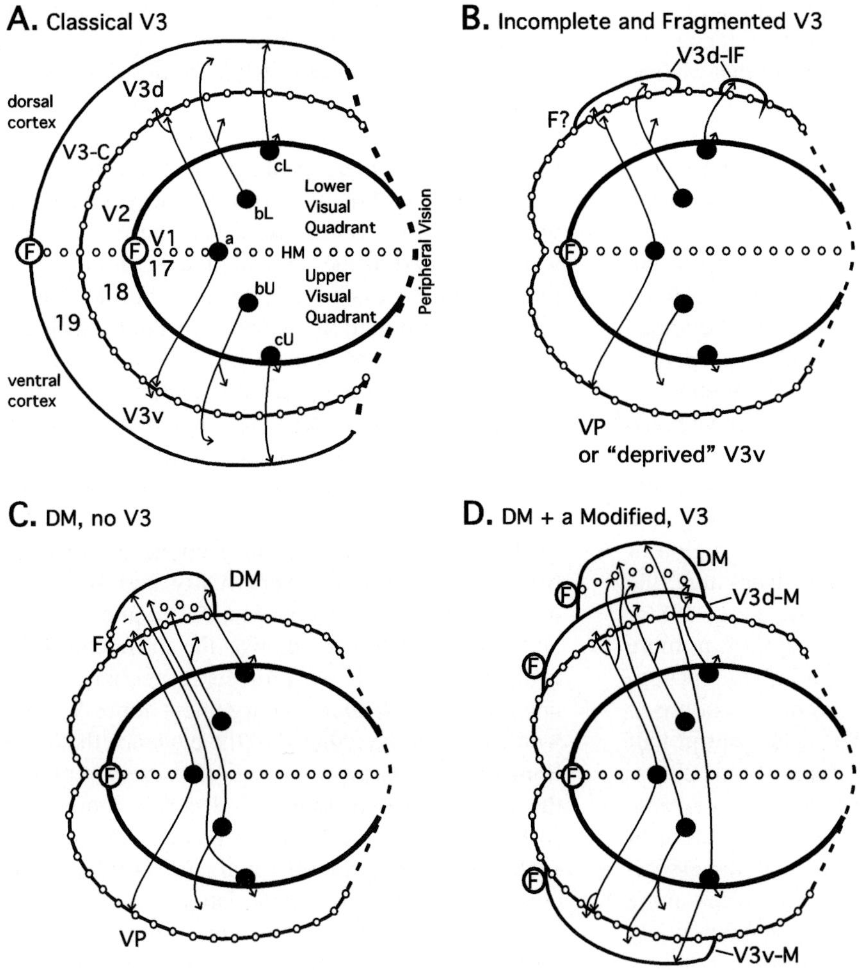

Fig. 2. Different concepts of V3 and visual cortex organization in primates. (A) In early and more classical or traditional views, V3 was seen as a third level of processing, equal in size and importance to V2. V2 and classical V3 (V3-C) were seen as successive ring-like areas around most of V1, with their common border formed by a representation of the horizontal meridian (HM; hollow circles), and the outer border of V3 by the vertical meridian. Both V2 and V3-C were thought to receive retinotopically congruent inputs from V1 in mirror reversal patterns. Thus, a region on the horizontal meridian in V1 (A) would project to the border regions of V2 and V3, both dorsally and ventrally due to the 'split' representation of the horizontal meridian. Locations centered in the representations of the lower (bL) and upper (bU) visual quadrants in V1 would project to the middle of dorsal or ventral V2 and V3, respectively. Finally, locations along the outer border of V1 would project locally to V2 and to the outer border of V3 (cL and cU). Note the representation of the fovea (F). (B) Subsequently, V3 was viewed as incomplete (V3-I), representing only the lower visual quadrant, or incomplete and fragmented (V3-IF), being separated into a larger part for more central lower field vision and a smaller part for more peripheral lower field vision. The former territory of ventral V3 was considered to be another visual area, the ventroposterior area (VP). According to this scheme, V1 would project in a retinotopic pattern to both dorsal and ventral V2, but only to dorsal V3. Alternatively, some theories retained a region of cortex for a ventral V3, but presumably this ventral V3 lacked V1 inputs and it differed from dorsal V3 in other ways. (C) Other investigators held that there was no V3. Projections from V1 to dorsomedial cortex along outer V2 were considered to be to a dorsomedial visual area (DM) rather than V3. Note that this theory predicts that all parts of V1 will project to the DM region, while the theory of an incomplete V3 (V3-I) predicts the existence of projections only from dorsal V1. (D) Our current proposal is that V3 exists as a complete representation that is nevertheless split into separate dorsal and ventral halves, each considerably smaller than the corresponding halves of classical V3 (V3-C). The dorsal half of this modified V3 (V3d-M) gets inputs from dorsal V1, while the ventral half (V3v-M) gets inputs from ventral V1. In addition, DM remains as a visual area with inputs from all parts of V1. In reduced size and location, this V3-M resembles the discontinuous and smaller V3 of Ungerleider and Desimone (1986) and Gattass et al. (1988).

the rostral border of dorsal V2. The terminations in cortex just rostral to dorsal V2 provided evidence for a V3, and it was reasonable to assume that ventral V1, representing the upper visual quadrant, would project to ventral V2 and cortex just rostral to ventral V2, providing missing evidence for a ventral V3. However, subsequent studies of V1 projections in macaques (e.g. Weller and Kaas, 1983; Van Essen et al., 1986) and other monkeys (e.g. Krubitzer and Kaas, 1993) failed to provide clear evidence for a ventral V3 (also see Newsome et al., 1986; Felleman et al., 1997). Furthermore, the response properties of neurons in the region of ventral V3 seemed to differ from those of dorsal V3 (Burkhalter and Van Essen, 1986; Burkhalter et al., 1986). Thus, there was no compelling evidence for a ventral V3, and the concept of V3 was modified by some of these investigators to exclude a ventral V3. The region of ventral V3 was assigned to another visual area, the ventroposterior area or VP (Newsome et al., 1986). However, others retained the concept of a more classical V3, with ventral and dorsal halves, but separated the halves in the region of central vision (see Ungerleider and Desimone, 1986). The ventral half of V3 would be 'deprived' of V1 input (Fig. 2B).

A further modification in the concept of V3 came from a careful analysis of the myeloarchitecture of the region (Van Essen et al., 1986). V3 was associated with a densely myelinated strip of cortex along the outer border of V2, and this strip appeared only dorsally, was narrow (1–3 mm in width), discontinuous, and variable. We refer to this as an incomplete, fragmented V3 or V3-IF (Fig. 2B). Further support for a discontinuous, narrow dorsal V3 came from a microelectrode mapping study of the region (Gattass et al., 1988). The concepts of V3-I and V3-IF differ so much from those of V-III in cats or V3-C in monkeys that one wonders if the designation 'V3' is more confusing than descriptive.

Arguments for a third major alternative were presented in the early microelectrode mapping studies of extrastriate cortex organization in owl monkeys by Allman and Kaas (e.g. Allman and Kaas, 1974, 1975, 1976). Although a cat-like classical V3 was expected at the time, no convincing evidence for such an area was found. Instead, the outer border of V2 seemed to be formed by a series of small visual areas. The proposal that V2 is bordered by a series of visual areas has been extended to include other primates (see Kaas, 1997b).

Originally, it appeared that V1 projections in New World monkeys were only to V2 and MT (Tigges et al., 1973; Spatz, 1977), but when more sensitive tracing methods were used, sparse projections to the approximate region of dorsal V3 were revealed as well (Lin et al., 1982). However, these projections were attributed to the dorsomedial visual area, DM, rather than to dorsal V3 (Fig. 2C). Further support for this interpretation of V1 projections followed, when a number of studies indicated that both V1 and V2 project in a topographic pattern to a zone of densely myelinated cortex just rostral to dorsal V2 in prosimian galagos, New World monkeys, and Old World monkeys (Krubitzer and Kaas, 1993; Stepniewska and Kaas, 1996; Beck and Kaas, 1998a,b, 1999). The evidence that projections originally attributed to dorsal V3 were really part of a more extensive pattern of V1 projections to another visual area, DM, seemed to remove the most compelling evidence for V3. If V1 projects to neither a ventral nor a dorsal V3, then the argument for a V3 at all would seem to be reduced to the evidence that cortex immediately rostral to dorsal V2 largely represents the lower visual quadrant, and cortex immediately rostral to ventral V2 largely represents the upper visual quadrant (e.g. Sereno et al., 1994, 1995; DeYoe et al., 1996). However, such data are open to the alternative interpretation of a series of bordering visual areas with largely matching or congruent retinotopic borders with V2 (see Sereno, 1998; Rosa, 1997).

Given these alternatives, some might be tempted to conclude that primate species differ in organization of extrastriate cortex along the outer border of V2 (e.g. Sereno, 1998). Current depictions of the retinotopic organization of human visual cortex as derived from fMRI studies typically contain a broad, classical V3 (e.g. Shipp et al., 1995) or a broad dorsal V3 and a broad ventral counterpart, a ventroposterior area with a retinotopy much like one would expect for the ventral half of classical V3 (e.g. Tootell et al., 1997). Much of the evidence for a series of visual areas bordering V2 comes from New World monkeys and prosimians, while arguments for a reduced, fragmented dorsal V3 stem only from results obtained from Old World monkeys. Possibly humans have a classical V3, macaques have an incomplete, fragmented V3, and other primates totally lack a V3. This conclusion would encompass most of the experimental observations, but it would require a very improbable evolutionary scenario.

A proposal for a modified V3 as an area common to primates

A fourth possibility for the interpretation of the organization of visual cortex immediately surrounding V2 is suggested by the results of our ongoing research on the connections of V1 in primates (Lyon and Kaas, 2001). While these studies are incomplete, and the evidence is limited, the results support an interpretation of the projection patterns of V1 to extrastriate cortex that may apply to all primates (Fig. 2D). Our proposal is based on the following observations and conclusions. First, considerable evidence now indicates that all parts of V1 project to DM, a visual area just rostral to the middle of dorsal V2 (see Beck and Kaas, 1999). The location of this projection zone appears to be similar in all studied primates. All of our recent results are consistent with the conclusion that DM is a target of V1 projections.

Second, dorsal V1 also projects, usually less densely, to a narrow strip of cortex we now locate between DM and V2, but was formerly included in either V2 or DM. Since the V1 projections to DM are immediately adjacent to those to V3d, it could be very difficult to distinguish the V3d terminations from DM terminations. However, the use of surface-view sections of flattened visual cortex convinced us that injections in dorsal V1 produced two distinct foci of terminations, one in cortex we now identify as V3d, and one in DM. We suggest that previous descriptions of projections from dorsal V1 to a dorsal V3 may have included terminations in DM, V3d, or even outer V2. Given the denser projections to DM, it seems likely that the more obvious DM terminations were most often detected and attributed to V3. While the full extent of V3d is not yet clear, it does appear from connection patterns and the architectonic features to be a narrow field that includes only part of the border of dorsal V2.

Third, as previously reported, ventral V1 also projects dorsally to DM, to complete the retinotopic representation in DM. However, our results indicate that ventral V1 also projects ventrally to a ventral V3 along the outer border of ventral V2. This proposed V3v exactly matches V3d in its narrow width and limited extent, but it represents the upper visual quadrant while V3d represents the lower visual quadrant. Although separated by a portion of dorsolateral cortex along the representation of central vision in V2, the two halves of V3 both get V1 inputs and they appear to be parts of the same visual area.

Our conclusion that ventral V1 projects to a ventral half of V3 is critically important for any firm acceptance of the concept of a V3 as an area common to primates. Yet our evidence is limited to results obtained from injections in New World monkeys and galagos (Lyon and Kaas, 2001) and thus our proposal should remain tentative. The lack of evidence for such a ventral projection in previous studies remains a concern, but there are several reasons why such projections may have been missed. Most importantly, the projections are sparse, and sparse projections are not always revealed. Injections in ventral V1 may have been small relative to those in dorsal V1 in order to avoid contamination of dorsal V1. Furthermore, the projections of the less accessible ventral half of V1 have been less often studied. In addition, even the projections to dorsal V3 may have been commonly missed, and the projections of dorsal V1 to DM may have been spuriously attributed to V3d. Finally, V3v and V3d are narrow, so that it would be difficult to distinguish terminations in V3 near the outer border of V2 from those in V2. Projections just beyond the outer border of V2 may have been assigned to V2. Thus, the evidence for V1 projections to either V3v or V3d has been questionable.

Our proposal of a redefined, narrow V3 raises the issue of how to interpret the evidence from previous studies of V3 connections, neuron response properties, and architecture. Clearly, we need ways of distinguishing conclusions that have been based solely on results from V3 and results contaminated by including parts of DM or other visual areas. A related question is how V3 functions in the visual system. This V3-M (Fig. 2D) is about half the width of V2 and fails to border central V2 and possibly the ends of V2. Thus, V3-M is significantly smaller than V2, and it receives less V1 input than V2, MT or DM. Obviously, this narrow, split V3-M cannot have the classically proposed role for V3 as the third major stage of visual processing, equal in importance to V2. Instead, we see V3 as one of several distribution targets of V1, with V2, MT and DM each receiving more of the output, and other areas receiving some of the V1 outputs (see Casagrande and Kaas, 1994). Furthermore, V3-M would contain compressed representations of the visual quadrants, and this would restrict some functions. In some sense, V3 may act as a transition zone between the retinotopy of V2 and the retinotopies of the ring of bordering areas. In marmosets, we have evidence that both dorsal and ventral portions of V3 get inputs from MT as well as V1 (Lyon and Kaas, 2001). The MT inputs suggest that V3 is functionally aligned with the dorsal stream of processing (Ungerleider and Mishkin, 1982) related to spatial aspects of vision.

The possibility that all primates have a V3, albeit not a classical V3, raises the possibility that V3 in primates and V-III in cats are homologous subdivisions of visual cortex, as often suggested (e.g. Albus and Beckmann, 1980; Rosenquist, 1985; Creutzfeldt, 1993; Payne, 1993). A cladistic analysis of the organization of visual cortex in studied mammals casts doubt on this attractive assumption. If carnivores and primates have inherited a V3 from a common ancestor, then members of sister orders of mammals should have a V3 as well. So far, there is little evidence that this is the case. For example, squirrels (Kaas et al., 1988) and other rodents (Rosa and Krubitzer, 1999), as well as tree shrews (Sesma et al., 1984; Lyon et al., 1998) do not appear to have a V3. Yet, new evidence may be forthcoming, and the interpretation of data on the organization of visual cortex is surprisingly difficult. Thus, the assumption of a homology between V-III of cats and V3 of primates is not supported by evidence for a V3 in sister orders of mammals. Yet, this possibility should remain open to further inquiry.

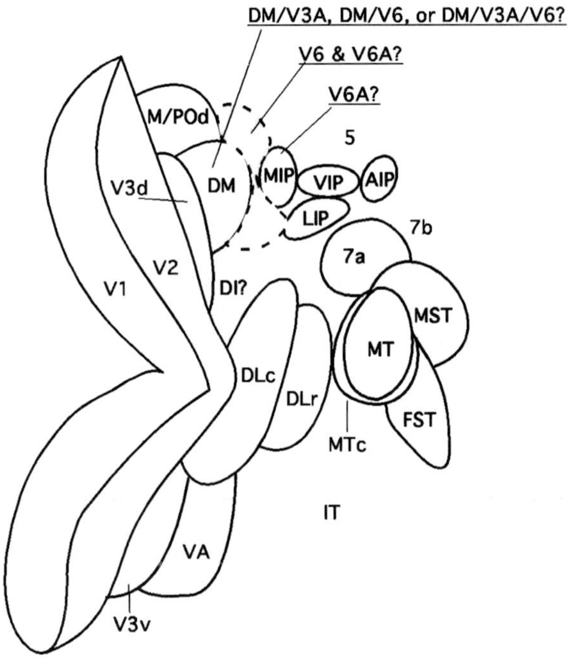

Fig. 3. Some unresolved issues of visual cortex organization. Borders for visual areas described in Fig. 1 (V1, V2, V3d, V3v, DM, M, DLc, DLr, VA, MT, MTc, MST, and FST) are shown on a diagram depicting proposed areas of visual cortex organization of Old World monkeys, based on previous diagrams (see Kaas, 1997b) and recent results from New World monkeys (Lyon and Kaas, 2001). Locations of area 7a and visual areas of the intraparietal sulcus, the medial intraparietal (MIP), ventral intraparietal (VIP), lateral intraparietal (LIP), and anterior intraparietal (AIP) areas, are based on other reports (see Rosa, 1997). The inclusion of a V3d displaces DM from the dorsal half of the V2 border (see Figs. 1 and 2D) and puts more of DM in a position very similar to area V3A of macaques and humans. The region rostral to DM bordered by a dashed line indicates the uncertainty as to where visual areas V6 and V6A (Galletti et al., 1995, 1999) fit within our current theory of primate visual cortex organization. It is possible that V6 may partially or completely overlap with DM and/or V3A. Furthermore, area V6A shows functional characteristics similar to those described for area MIP, namely visually guided reaching (Johnson et al., 1996). Other issues concern the similarity of visual areas M and POd (the surviving division of the parieto-occipital area) and whether these two regions actually represent the same cortical area. The dorsointermediate area (DI) is shown as a possible candidate for the region of visual cortex between DM and DL, but without any certainty of its borders. Inferior temporal visual cortex (IT), and somatosensory cortical areas 5 and 7b are shown for reference.

V3 and the revised status of DM

Our inclusion of a narrow dorsal V3 in our modified version of the organization of extrastriate cortex in primates is at the expense of the caudal part of DM and adjoining fields (Fig. 3). This DM remains as a possibly smaller visual area, somewhat displaced from the V2 border, but containing a complete representation of the contralateral visual hemifield and having inputs from all parts of V1 and V2. The way the visual field is represented in DM can be surmised from the input patterns (Krubitzer and Kaas,

1993; Beck and Kaas, 1998a,b, 1999; Lyon and Kaas, 2001) and from previous studies of retinotopy (Allman and Kaas, 1975; Krubitzer and Kaas, 1993; Rosa and Schmid, 1995). While the retinotopic organization of DM remains somewhat uncertain in detail, the representation of the lower visual quadrant is largely along the V3d border, and the representation of the upper visual quadrant is largely rostral and more lateral (Fig. 1). The representation of central vision may be more lateral than originally depicted (see Allman and Kaas, 1975), and peripheral vision is medial. The proposal that the representation of the upper visual quadrant is split in DM, with more central vision represented rostrocaudally and more peripheral vision caudomedially along the ventral border remains a possibility (Rosa and Schmid, 1995; Rosa, 1997) but further studies combining connectional, architectonic, and microelectrode mapping approaches would be useful. If the outer border of V3d represents the zero vertical meridian of the lower quadrant, as proposed, then we would expect adjoining parts of DM to match along the zero vertical meridian.

Our modified DM continues to occupy cortex assigned to other visual areas in other proposals, but exactly what other areas remains uncertain (Fig. 3). Clearly a modified DM would overlap with an outer portion of classical V3, but with little or none of the incomplete, narrow V3 of later proposals (Fig. 2). Much of DM may correspond to V3A (see Krubitzer and Kaas, 1993; Beck and Kaas, 1999). V3A was described as a visual area adjoining parts of the dorsal border of V3 in macaque monkeys (Zeki, 1978). Another possibility (see Rosa, 1997) is that DM overlaps partly or largely with another parietal-occipital visual area or PO (Colby et al., 1988). However, PO in macaques was originally thought to be the homologue of the medial visual area, M, first described in owl monkeys (Allman and Kaas, 1976). More recently a 'V6' has been described in the approximate location of DM in macaque monkeys (Galletti et al., 1995, 1999), and V6 may occupy much of the territory of DM. Other visual areas such as the posterior intra-parietal area, PIP, have been proposed for the region (Felleman and Van Essen, 1991). Thus, there is much uncertainty about how to divide this region into areas and how to name them.

This uncertainty stems in part from the difficulties in exploring cortex buried in the region where the lunate, intraparietal, and parieto-occipital sulci converge in macaque monkeys. Our initial studies focussed on marmoset monkeys where the region is exposed on the dorsolateral surface of the cerebral hemisphere, and none of these fissures exist. To the extent that visual cortex between New and Old World monkeys is subdivided into areas in a similar manner, it seems much more productive to determine the basic organization in such New World monkeys. Of course, a plan of organization developed from data on New World monkeys would need to be evaluated for applicability to Old World monkeys, but this could be done more reliably when highly specific hypotheses exist. For example, we propose that connection patterns with V1 and V2 can be used to reliably identify and delimit DM in macaques.

Of course it remains possible that the organization of extrastriate cortex will be found to differ significantly in New and Old World monkeys, even in the DM region. If this turns out to be the case, then humans and macaques may also differ and we should be very cautious about using results from macaque monkeys to model the organization of human visual cortex. However, much evidence supports the view that all primates share a number of visual areas. The evidence that all primates have a V1, V2, and MT is quite convincing. We would add V3-M, DM, DL and M to the list.

Acknowledgements

Research by the author was supported by NEI Grants EY-02686 (J.H.K.) and EY-07135 (D.C.L.). This paper was prepared while J.H.K. was a fellow at the Center for Advanced Study in the Behavioral Sciences at Stanford University. Financial support to the center was provided by the John D. and Catherine T. MacArthur Foundation. We thank N. Jain, C. Collins, and I. Stepniewska for helpful comments.

References

Albus, K. and Beckmann, R. (1980) Second and third visual area of the cat: interindividual variability in retinotopic arrangement and cortical location. *J. Physiol.*, 299: 276–297.

Allman, J.M. and Kaas, J.H. (1971) A representation of the

visual field in the posterior third of the middle temporal gyrus of the owl monkey (*Aotus trivirgatus*). *Brain Res.*, 31: 85–105.
Allman, J.M. and Kaas, J.H. (1974) A crescent-shaped cortical visual area surrounding the middle temporal (MT) in the owl monkey (*Aotus trivirgatus*). *Brain Res.*, 81: 199–213.
Allman, J.M. and Kaas, J.H. (1975) The dorsomedial cortical visual area: A third tier area in the occipital lobe of the owl monkey (*Aotus trivirgatus*). *Brain Res.*, 100: 473–487.
Allman, J.M. and Kaas, J.H. (1976) Representation of the visual field on the medial wall of occipital-parietal cortex in the owl monkey. *Science*, 191: 572–575.
Beck, P.D. and Kaas, J.H. (1998a) Cortical connections of the dorsomedial visual area in prosimian primates. *J. Comp. Neurol.*, 398: 162–178.
Beck, P.D. and Kaas, J.H. (1998b) Cortical connections of the dorsomedial visual area in New World owl monkeys (*Aotus trivirgatus*) and squirrel monkeys (*Saimiri sciureus*). *J. Comp. Neurol.*, 400: 18–34.
Beck, P.D. and Kaas, J.H. (1999) Cortical connections of the dorsomedial visual area in Old World macaque monkeys. *J. Comp. Neurol.*, 406: 487–502.
Brodmann, K. (1909) *Vergleichende Lokalisationslehre der Grosshirnrinde*. Leipzig, Barth.
Burkhalter, A. and Van Essen, D.C. (1986) Processing of color, form, and disparity information in visual areas VP and V2 of ventral extrastriate cortex in the macaque monkey. *J. Neurosci.*, 6: 2327–2351.
Burkhalter, A., Felleman, D.J., Newsome, W.T. and Van Essen, D.C. (1986) Anatomical and physiological asymmetries related to visual areas V3 and VP in macaque extrastriate cortex. *Vision Res.*, 26: 63–80.
Casagrande, V.A. and Kaas, J.H. (1994) The afferent, intrinsic, and efferent connections of primary visual cortex in primates. In: A. Peters and K. Rockland (Eds.), *Cerebral Cortex*, Vol. 10, *Primary Visual Cortex in Primates*. Plenum Press, New York, pp. 201–259.
Catania, K.C., Lyon, D.C., Mock, O.B. and Kaas, J.H. (1999) Cortical organization in shrews: evidence from five species. *J. Comp. Neurol.*, 410: 55–72.
Colby, C.L., Gattass, R., Olson, C.R. and Gross, C.G. (1988) Topographical organization of cortical afferents to extrastriate visual area PO in the macaque: a dual tracer study. *J. Comp. Neurol.*, 269: 392–413.
Cragg, B.G. (1969) The topography of the afferent projections in the circumstriate visual cortex of the monkey studied by the Nauta method. *Vision Res.*, 9: 733–747.
Creutzfeldt, O.D. (1993) *Cortex Cerebri* (English revision). Springer-Verlag, Berlin.
DeYoe, E.A., Carman, G.J., Bandettini, P., Glickman, S., Wieser, J. and Cox, R. (1996) Mapping striate and extrastriate visual areas in human cerebral cortex. *Proc. Natl. Acad. Sci. USA*, 93: 2382–2386.
Felleman, D.J. and Van Essen, D.C. (1991) Distributed hierarchical processing in primate cerebral cortex. *Cereb. Cortex*, 1: 1–47.
Felleman, D.J., Burkhalter, A. and Van Essen, D.C. (1997) Cortical connections of areas V3 and VP of macaque monkey extrastriate visual cortex. *J. Comp. Neurol.*, 379: 21–47.
Galletti, C., Battaglini, P.P. and Fattori, P. (1995) Eye position influence on the parieto-occipital area PO (V6) of the macaque monkey. *Eur. J. Neurosci.*, 8: 30–52.
Galletti, C., Fattori, P., Gamberini, M. and Kutz, D.F. (1999) The cortical visual area V6: brain location and visual topography. *Eur. J. Neurosci.*, 11: 3922–3936.
Gattass, R., Sousa, A.P.B. and Gross, C.G. (1988) Visuotopic organization and extent of V3 and V4 of the macaque. *J. Neurosci.*, 8: 1831–1845.
Gross, C.G. (1997) From Imhotep to Hubel and Wiesel: The story of visual cortex. In: K.S. Rockland, J.H. Kaas and A. Peters (Eds.), *Cerebral Cortex*, Vol. 12, *Extrastriate Cortex in Primates*. Plenum Press, New York, pp. 1–58.
Harvey, P.H. and Pagel, M.D. (1991) *The Comparative Method in Evolutionary Biology*. Oxford University Press, Oxford.
Hubel, D.H. and Wiesel, T.N. (1965) Receptive fields and functional architecture in two nonstriate visual areas (18 and 19) of the cat. *J. Neurophysiol.*, 28: 229–289.
Johnson, P.B., Ferraina, S., Bianchi, L. and Caminiti, R. (1996) Cortical networks for visual reaching: physiological and anatomical organization of frontal and parietal lobe of arm regions. *Cereb. Cortex*, 6: 102–119.
Kaas, J.H. (1980) A comparative survey of visual cortex organization in mammals. In: S.O.E. Ebbesson (Ed.), *Comparative Neurology of the Telencephalon*. New York, Plenum Press, pp. 483–502.
Kaas, J.H. (1987) The organization and evolution of neocortex. In: S.P. Wise (Ed.), *Higher Brain Functions*. John Wiley and Sons, New York, pp. 347–378.
Kaas, J.H. (1995a) Human visual cortex: progress and puzzles. *Curr. Biol.*, 5: 1126–1128.
Kaas, J.H. (1995b) The evolution of isocortex. *Brain Behav. Evol.*, 46: 187–196.
Kaas, J.H. (1996) Theories of visual cortex organization in primates: areas of a third level. In: M. Norita, T. Bando and B.E. Stein (Eds.), *Extrageniculostriate Mechanisms Underlying Visually-Guided Orientation and Behavior*. New York, Elsevier, pp. 213–221.
Kaas, J.H. (1997a) What comparative studies of neocortex tell us about the human brain. *Rev. Brasil. Biol.*, 56: 315–322.
Kaas, J.H. (1997b) Theories of visual cortex organization in primates. In: K.S. Rockland, J.H. Kaas and A. Peters (Eds.), *Cerebral Cortex*, Vol. 12, *Extrastriate Cortex in Primates*. Plenum Press, New York, pp. 91–125.
Kaas, J.H., Krubitzer, L.A. and Johanson, K.L. (1988) Cortical connections of areas 17 (V-I) and 18 (V-II) of squirrels. *J. Comp. Neurol.*, 281: 426–446.
Kay, R.F., Ross, C. and Williams, B.A. (1997) Anthropoid origins. *Science*, 275: 797–804.
Krubitzer, L.A. and Kaas, J.H. (1989) Cortical integration of parallel pathways in the visual system of primates. *Brain Res.*, 478: 161–165.
Krubitzer, L.A. and Kaas, J.H. (1993) The dorsomedial visual area of owl monkeys: connections, myeloarchitecture, and

homologies in other primates. *J. Comp. Neurol.*, 334: 497–528.

Kuypers, H.G.J.M., Szwarcbart, M.K., Mishkin, M. and Rosvold, H.E. (1965) Occipitotemporal corticocortical connections in the rhesus monkey. *Exp. Neurol.*, 11: 245–262.

Lin, C.S., Weller, R.E. and Kaas, J.H. (1982) Cortical connections of striate cortex in the owl monkey. *J. Comp. Neurol.*, 211: 165–176.

Lyon, D.C. and Kaas, J.H. (2001) Connectional and architectonic evidence for dorsal and ventral V3, and dorsomedial area in marmoset monkeys. *J. Neurosci.*, 21: 249–261.

Lyon, D., Jain, N. and Kaas, J.H. (1998) Cortical connections of striate and extrastriate visual areas in the tree shrew. *J. Comp. Neurol.*, 401: 109–128.

Newsome, W.T., Maunsell, J.H.R. and Van Essen, D.C. (1986) Ventral posterior visual area of the macaque: visual topography and areal boundaries. *J. Comp. Neurol.*, 252: 139–153.

Payne, B.R. (1993) Evidence for visual cortical area homologues in cat and macaque monkey. *Cereb. Cortex*, 3: 1–15.

Preuss, T.M. and Kaas, J.H. (1999) Human brain evolution. In: M.J. Zigmond, F.E. Bloom, S.C. Landis, J.L. Roberts and L.R. Squire (Eds.), *Fundamental Neuroscience*. Academic Press, San Diego.

Roe, A.W. and Ts'o, D.Y. (1997) The functional architecture of area V2 in the macaque monkey: physiology topography and connectivity. In: K.S. Rockland, J.H. Kaas and A. Peters (Eds.), *Cerebral Cortex: Extrastriate Cortex in Primates*, Vol. 12. Plenum Press, New York, pp. 259–333.

Rosa, M.G.P. (1997) Visuotopic organization of primate extrastriate cortex. In: K.S. Rockland, J.H. Kaas and A. Peters (Eds.), *Cerebral Cortex: Extrastriate Cortex in Primates*, Vol. 12. Plenum Press, New York, pp. 127–203.

Rosa, M.G.P. (1999) Topographic organization of extrastriate areas in the flying fox: implications for the evolution of mammalian visual cortex. *J. Comp. Neurol.*, 411: 503–523.

Rosa, M.G.P. and Schmid, L.M. (1995) Visual areas in the dorsal and medial extrastriate cortices of the marmoset. *J. Comp. Neurol.*, 359: 272–299.

Rosa, M.G.P. and Krubitzer, L.A. (1999) The evolution of visual cortex: Where is V2? *Trends Neurosci.*, 22: 242–248.

Rosenquist, A.C. (1985) Connections of visual cortical areas in the cat. In: A. Peters and E.G. Jones (Eds.), *Cerebral Cortex: Visual Cortex*, Vol. 3. Plenum Press, New York, pp. 81–155.

Sereno, M.I. (1998) Brain mapping in animals and humans. *Curr. Opin. Neurobiol.*, 8: 188–194.

Sereno, M.I., McDonald, C.T. and Allman, J.M. (1994) Analysis of retinotopic maps in extrastriate cortex. *Cereb. Cortex*, 4: 601–620.

Sereno, M.I., Dale, A.M., Reppas, J.B., Kwong, K.K., Belliveau, J.W., Brady, T.J., Rosen, B.R. and Tootell, R.R. (1995) Borders of multiple visual areas in humans revealed by functional magnetic resonance imaging. *Science*, 268: 889–893.

Sesma, M.A., Casagrande, V.A. and Kaas, J.H. (1984) Cortical connections of area 17 in tree shrews. *J. Comp. Neurol.*, 230: 337–351.

Shipp, S., Watson, J.D.G., Frackowiak, R.S.V. and Zeki, S. (1995) Retinotopic maps in human prestriate visual cortex: the demarcation of areas V2 and V3. *Neuroimage*, 2: 125–132.

Spatz, W.B. (1977) Topographically organized reciprocal connections between areas 17 and MT (visual area of superior temporal sulcus) in the marmoset *Callithrix jacchus*. *Exp. Brain Res.*, 27: 559–572.

Stepniewska, I. and Kaas, J.H. (1996) Topographic patterns of V2 cortical connections in macaque monkeys. *J. Comp. Neurol.*, 371: 129–152.

Tigges, J., Spatz, W.B. and Tigges, M. (1973) Reciprocal point-to-point connections between parastriate and striate cortex in the squirrel monkey (*Saimiri*). *J. Comp. Neurol.*, 148: 481–490.

Tootell, R.B.H., Dale, A.M., Sereno, M.I. and Malach, R. (1996) New images from human visual cortex. *Trends Neurosci.*, 19: 481–489.

Tootell, R.B.H., Mendola, J.D., Hadjikhani, N.K., Ledden, P.J., Liu, A.K., Reppas, J.B., Sereno, M.I. and Dale, A.M. (1997) Functional analysis of V3a and related areas in human visual cortex. *J. Neurosci.*, 17: 7060–7078.

Tusa, R.J., Rosenquist, A.C. and Palmer, L.A. (1979) Retinotopic organization of areas 18 and 19 in the cat. *J. Comp. Neurol.*, 185: 657–678.

Ungerleider, L.G. and Desimone, R. (1986) Projections to the superior temporal sulcus from central and peripheral field representations of V1 and V2. *J. Comp. Neurol.*, 248: 147–163.

Ungerleider, L.G. and Mishkin, M. (1982) The striate projection in the superior temporal sulcus of *Macaca mulata*: location and topographic organization. *J. Comp. Neurol.*, 188: 347–366.

Van Essen, D.C. (1985) Functional organization of primate visual cortex. In: A. Peters and E.G. Jones (Eds.), *Cerebral Cortex: Visual Cortex*, Vol. 3. Plenum Press, New York, pp. 259– 329.

Van Essen, D.C., Newsome, W.T., Maunsell, J.H.R. and Bixby, J.L. (1986) The projections from striate cortex (V1) to areas V2 and V3 in the macaque monkey: Asymmetries, areal boundaries, and patchy connections. *J. Comp. Neurol.*, 244: 451–480.

Weller, R.E. and Kaas, J.H. (1983) Retinotopic patterns of connections of area 17 with visual areas VII and MT in macaque monkeys. *J. Comp. Neurol.*, 220: 253–279.

Woolsey, C.N., Akert, K., Benjamin, R.M., Leibowitz, H. and Welker, W.I. (1955) Visual cortex in the marmoset. *Fed. Proc.*, 14: 166.

Zeki, S.M. (1969) Representations of central visual fields in prestriate cortex of monkey. *Brain Res.*, 14: 271–291.

Zeki, S.M. (1971) Convergent input from the striate cortex (area 17) to the cortex of the superior temporal sulcus in the rhesus monkey. *Brain Res.*, 28: 338–340.

Zeki, S.M. (1978) Uniformity and diversity of structure and function in rhesus monkey prestriate visual cortex. *J. Physiol.*, 277: 273–290.

Zeki, S.M. (1980) The response properties of cells in the middle temporal area (area MT) of owl monkey visual cortex. *Proc. R. Soc. Lond. B*, 207: 239–248.

C. Casanova and M. Ptito (Eds.)
Progress in Brain Research, Vol. 134

CHAPTER 19

From attentional gating in macaque primary visual cortex to dyslexia in humans

T.R. Vidyasagar *

Psychobiology Laboratory and Center for Visual Sciences, School of Psychology, Australian National University, Canberra, ACT 0200, Australia

Abstract: Selective attention is an important aspect of brain function that we need in coping with the immense and constant barrage of sensory information. One model of attention (Feature Integration Theory) that suggests an early selection of spatial locations of objects via an attentional spotlight would also solve the 'binding problem' (that is how do different attributes of each object get correctly bound together?). Our experiments have demonstrated modulation of specific locations of interest at the level of the primary visual cortex both in visual discrimination and memory tasks, where the actual locations of the targets was also important in being able to perform the task. It is suggested that the feedback mediating the modulation arises from the posterior parietal cortex, which would also be consistent with its known role in attentional control. In primates, the magnocellular (M) and parvocellular (P) pathways are the two major streams of inputs from the retina, carrying distinctly different types of information and they remain fairly segregated in their projections to the primary visual cortex and further into the extra-striate regions. The P inputs go mainly into the ventral (temporal) stream, while the dorsal (parietal) stream is dominated by M inputs. A theory of attentional gating is proposed here where the M dominated dorsal stream gates the P inputs into the ventral stream. This framework is used to provide a neural explanation of the processes involved in reading and in learning to read. This scheme also explains how a magnocellular deficit could cause the common reading impairment, dyslexia.

Introduction: role of attention in perception

The challenge facing a sensory system is not simply one of feature detection and pattern recognition, but also to select the bits of information that are relevant for the moment from the constant barrage of inputs flooding the sensory receptor surface. Apart from the task of choosing between sensory modalities (or in some cases integrating them appropriately), there is also the task of selecting the pertinent signals from the many inputs within any single modality. How do we manage to locate an object, such as a face in a crowd or that particular book among a number of cluttered papers and books on our desk, often in a surprisingly short time? How are we able to concentrate on the relevant locations and objects on the road and inside on the front panel while driving a car and even while talking to a passenger? This task does not get simplified as we begin to realize that the various stimulus attributes (color, form, movement, depth, etc.) are localized to a considerable degree in different neocortical areas (e.g. Livingstone and Hubel, 1988; Merigan and Maunsell, 1993; Van Essen et al., 1993; Zeki, 1993; Logothetis and Sheinberg, 1996). If, for example, color perception is localized in one area, form in another and spatial locations of objects in yet another cortical area, how do we correctly and effortlessly combine the correct location, form and color of each object? This is one of the many

* Correspondence to: T.R. Vidyasagar, Psychobiology Laboratory and Center for Visual Sciences, Division of Psychology, Australian National University, Canberra, ACT 0200, Australia. Tel.: +61-2-6249-2038; Fax: +61-2-6249-0499; E-mail: sagar@anu.edu.au

types of 'binding problems' in perception (Treisman, 1996, 1998). This task sounds particularly difficult when we consider the fact that the receptive fields of neurons in many of these specialized areas are quite large (Desimone and Ungerleider, 1989; Boussaoud et al., 1991) and may in most natural situations include a number of objects within them.

These fundamental problems in perception have been repeatedly recognized and many solutions have been offered. One of the most influential of these has been a model that has stressed the early selection of spatial locations for focal attention. This scheme, known as the 'Feature Integration Theory' (FIT), was put forward by Treisman and her colleagues (Treisman and Gelade, 1980; Treisman, 1988) and has since undergone some modifications (Wolfe et al., 1989; Wolfe, 1994; Vidyasagar, 1999). In its essence, the FIT argues that a top-down input selects a restricted region of an early visual area which has a good topographical representation, but not yet specialized for processing just one aspect (attribute) of the visual scene such as color, motion, disparity or form. The FIT was proposed on the basis of a series of delightfully simple experiments on visual search, where one looks for a unique target among a number of other distracting items (Treisman, 1988). It was found that the search tends to be serial when the target has no unique feature in comparison to other items (distracters) in the visual field, but is uniquely defined only by the *conjunction of two or more features*, each of which is shared by some of the other items too. The object that does have a *unique feature*, such as orientation or color, is seen in parallel or 'pre-attentively' and the search is 'flat', i.e. the time taken does not increase with the number of distracters.

Thus, detecting a single red vertical line among blue vertical lines or a single red vertical line among red horizontal lines is a 'parallel search' and is not dependent upon the number of distracting items. On the other hand, detecting a red vertical line among a field of red horizontal and blue vertical lines is a 'serial search', since the time taken increases with increasing number of distracters. Ostensibly, the visual system does a scan of the field until it sees the target it is looking for, if the presence of a single unique feature does not already lead to a 'pop-out'. Despite some notable exceptions (Nakayama and Silverman, 1986; McLeod et al., 1988), this general rule is followed in most experimental situations. The speed of such visual search has also been estimated to be between 13 and 44 ms per item (Wolfe et al., 2000).

Such an attentional spotlight acting at an early site in the visual pathway such as the primary visual cortex, solves a number of problems in one stroke:

(1) It helps in visual search where one needs to serially search through a number of items to detect the appropriate target (serial search à la Treisman).
(2) It reduces computational load for the brain, so that only information from a localized area of the visual field is available for detailed processing at any one instant.
(3) It provides a mechanism to home in on a focus of interest. This can aid other functions such as foveating and orienting towards the stimulus.
(4) It helps in binding the different attributes of an object together. Since at any one time only one object is processed by the different specialized cortical areas, those feature detectors activated by the object in these different areas can be easily bound together. The binding problem referred to above simply does not exist for any single moment.

Neural correlates of selective attention

With a huge psychophysical literature (reviewed in Treisman, 1998) favoring an attentional spotlight gating responses in some early visual area such as the striate cortex (V1) or the pre-striate area, V2, a number of electrophysiological studies have attempted to identify attentional effects in the responses of neurons at various levels of the visual pathway in the macaque. More recently fMRI and PET imaging studies in humans have also attempted to visualize cortical areas that might be specifically involved in attention. However, until 2 years ago, apart from a lone study by Motter (1993), most investigations had failed to see significant attentional effects in the primary visual cortex (Mohler and Wurtz, 1977; Moran and Desimone, 1985; Haenny and Schiller, 1988; Luck et al., 1997). On the other hand, many studies have identified attentional modulation in a number of extra-striate areas of the macaque, including area V4

(Moran and Desimone, 1985; Spitzer et al., 1988; Motter, 1993, 1994a,b), area V5/MT (Treue and Maunsell, 1996), inferotemporal cortex (Chelazzi et al., 1993), posterior parietal cortex (Lynch et al., 1977; Colby et al., 1993, 1996; Steinmetz and Constantinidis, 1995) and the prefrontal cortex (Lecas, 1995; Miller et al., 1996). For example, in a seminal study, Moran and Desimone (1985) found that area V4 neurons, when presented with two stimuli within their receptive fields, one an effective stimulus for the cell and the other an ineffective one, would respond to the effective stimulus only in those trials when the animal was paying attention to that stimulus. Motter (1993) did find some degree of modulation of visual responses in striate neurons in a paradigm that differed from the other studies in one significant way. He had introduced a situation where there were a number of competing items in the visual scene and the monkey needed to focus its attention in one particular area of the visual field for each trial to be able to perform the task. In the light of the human psychophysical studies and the context of an attentional spotlight mentioned earlier, it is conceivable that attentional modulation can be seen at the level of the primary visual cortex. However, such a modulation will be seen mainly in a situation where spatially selective attention is called into play to focus attention on one location at a time because of the clutter in the visual field due to a large number of distracters. This idea was specially exploited in a recent study in our laboratory and significant effects were demonstrated in the macaque striate cortex (Vidyasagar, 1998) which have been more marked than the earlier reports by Motter (1993).

Fig. 1 shows the paradigm which the monkeys learnt before they were used for electrophysiological recordings. Learning this rather complex paradigm involved a number of steps. First, the monkeys were trained on a simple fixation task. Here, they pressed a bar which brought a small fixation spot to appear on the monitor, which stayed for a variable period. As soon as this spot disappeared, the monkeys had to release the bar to obtain their fruit juice reward. After learning to fixate, the monkeys were trained on a visual discrimination task, where they had to covertly discriminate between a vertical and a horizontal grating at a particular part of the visual field while maintaining fixation. They were then trained to

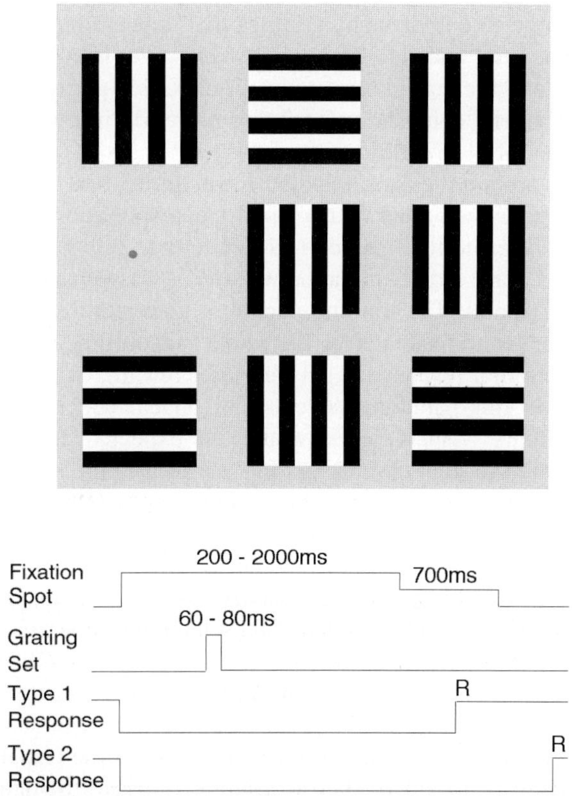

Fig. 1. Diagrammatic representation of the training paradigm. The upper panel shows the positions of the eight gratings relative to the fixation spot (not to scale). The grating patches (each $5 \times 5°$ or less; contrast 30%, 1–3 cycles/deg and average luminance 15 cd/m^2 on a background of 2.3 cd/m^2) usually occupied the centers of a virtual 3×3 grid, leaving out the middle left position for the fixation spot, the centers of the patches being 7–9° apart. In the lower panel, the uppermost trace represents the fixation spot, including the dimming period. The second trace refers to the grating set presented at a random interval after the onset of the fixation spot. In each trial, one of the gratings was cued by a small green spot (10–15 min arc) that appeared above it. The monkey had to direct its attention to the grating patch, which was so cued, and note the orientation of its lines. At the end of the fixation period, the fixation spot first dimmed for 700 ms before going off completely. If the cued grating was vertical, the monkey had to release the bar on dimming of the fixation spot to obtain a fruit juice reward (Type 1 response); for horizontal gratings, the bar had to be released on disappearance of the spot (Type 2). The reaction time allowed was a window of 200–650 ms. Both the duration of the fixation spot (200–2000 ms) and the interval before onset of the gratings (50–500 ms) were randomly varied to prevent animals using timing cues and to ensure that they maintained fixation throughout each trial. R denotes reward. (Figure reproduced from Vidyasagar, 1998.)

attend to one of many gratings that appeared simultaneously and discriminate it as vertical or horizontal (see figure legend for details). The fixation period for each trial could be up to 2 s or more, during which a set of (4–8) gratings were flashed for about 60–80 ms around the fixation point. In each trial, one of the gratings was cued with a small green spot above the grating and the monkey had to attend to this grating and make a discrimination whether it was vertical or horizontal. The training paradigm also required the monkey to fixate during the whole trial until he made the motor response to get fruit juice reward.

In this paradigm, a 'classical' visual cell in the primary visual cortex would be expected to respond to the flashed grating stimulus purely depending upon its stimulus requirements. Thus the fact whether the monkey had to pay attention to that particular grating or to another one on a particular trial would be of no consequence. On the other hand, in a situation where attentional selection of one grating at a particular location from among a number of gratings is essential for successful performance, a scheme such as Treisman's FIT that incorporates spatially focal attention at an early stage of the visual pathway would predict a different scenario. Striate cortical neurons would respond more vigorously for the appropriate stimulus in those trials where the monkey had to pay attention to that stimulus than in those trials where the monkey had to direct attention to a different location. Thus, for the same optimum stimulus flashed on the receptive field, the neuron's response would depend upon whether the monkey was paying attention to that location or to a different location. This is precisely what was seen in a subset of neurons in the primary visual cortex (Vidyasagar, 1998).

Fig. 2 shows the responses of six such neurons from macaque primary visual cortex. In the top row (A–C), responses are highly specific to the attentional state. There is a vigorous response to the stimulus for those trials in which attention is drawn to that location (top PSTHs or peristimulus time histograms). For other trials, where attention is drawn to a different location, but the receptive field is presented with the same stimulus as in the first situation, the response is very weak (bottom PSTHs in A–C). It is also noteworthy that the latencies of the responses of such attention-specific cells are generally longer than 70 ms. 'Classical' visual cells, on the other hand, which do not show any attentional modulation, have much shorter latencies (Maunsell and Gibson, 1992; Nowak et al., 1995). The longer latencies obtained here are consistent with the suggestion that such modulation is the result of a feedback that obviously requires a further lapse of time for the visual information to reach a higher area and then re-enter the primary visual cortex.

The three cells in the bottom row (D–F) are also modulated by attention, but in a somewhat different way. These cells show an early response, similar to the classical visual cells, but unaffected by whether the monkey is directing its attention to that spatial location or not. However, they also show a late response that is strongly influenced by attentional factors. In D, the early response continues into a sustained response that lasts well after the stimulus has disappeared. In E, the response is a very late one, occurring about 300 ms after stimulus onset. The cell in F responds to both stimulus onset and offset, but the attentional modulation is present only for the Off response. The latency of the early response of these cells is usually less than 70 ms. In general, these cells, which have been termed 'attention related cells' (Vidyasagar, 1998) show a vigorous early response (when measured during a window of 50–100 from stimulus onset) which is not dependent upon an attentional feedback, but show significant attentional modulation in the response component between 100 and 200 ms. Fig. 3 compares these responses in these temporal windows for six cells from a larger set of similar striate cortical cells that were recorded.

Whether these two types of cells that show attentional modulation in the macaque striate cortex — the attention specific and the attention related — form two separate categories or are two ends of a continuum is probably too early to say. In any case, together with the classical visual neurons, these cells could form the neuronal substrate in the striate cortex that enable early attentional selection. One can visualize how, in the specific training paradigm we used, the classical visual cells process and relay the first wave of signals from the retinogeniculate stream to higher areas. As the feedback from one or more of these higher areas re-enter the striate cortex to facilitate the spatial location of interest, the activity

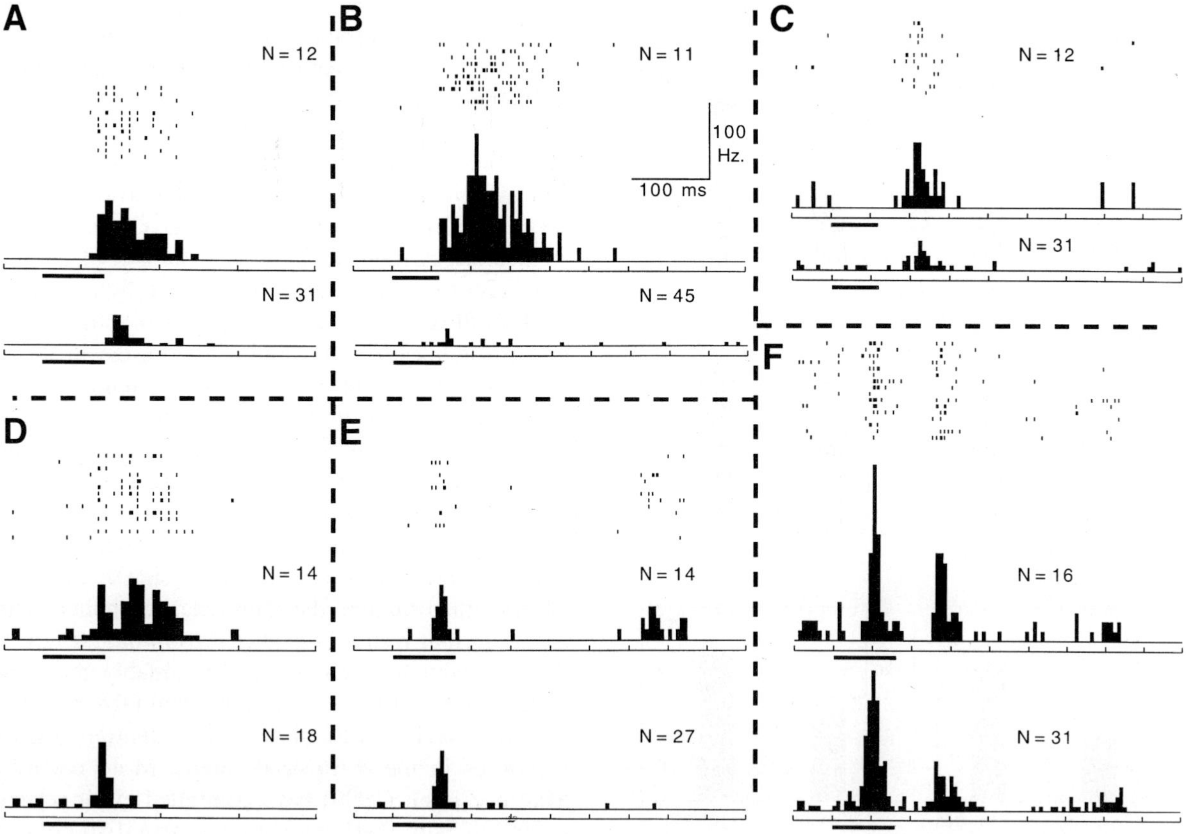

Fig. 2. Responses of three attention specific or AS (A–C) and three attention related or AR (D–F) cells. For each cell, responses to either the vertical or horizontal grating presentations are shown (whichever was the better stimulus) when the monkey had to direct its attention to it (top PSTH) and the PSTH representing responses to the same grating when he had to direct its attention to another grating among the set (lower PSTH). Number of trials (*N*) for each PSTH is shown and the raster display shows the occurrence of spikes for each trial for the top PSTHs. The scale is in spikes/s, so that the amplitude of the histograms can be directly compared. (Figure reproduced from Vidyasagar, 1998.)

in the area of interest would be maintained in the continued activity of the attention-related cells and finally these and the attention specific cells would be sending their signals to the extra-striate areas for processing the relevant stimulus attributes. In this scheme, once the feedback reaches back to the striate cortex, the major topographic source of the striate input to extra-striate areas will be the area of interest spotlighted by the feedback. It appears from the results shown above that the attentional gating of striate neurons is clearly operational by about 100 ms after stimulus onset.

It has been established that in primates, the magnocellular (M) and parvocellular (P) divisions of the retinogeniculostriate pathway carry distinctly different types of information (e.g. Hicks et al., 1983) and they remain fairly segregated in their cortical terminations and in their further projections into the extra-striate areas (e.g. Livingstone and Hubel, 1988; Merigan and Maunsell, 1993). Barring some restricted cross-talk between the two streams (Ferrera et al., 1992, 1994), the magnocellular pathway dominates the visual inputs into a dorsal parietal stream, namely to area V5/MT and then on to the posterior parietal cortex and the parvocellular stream mainly projects into a ventral temporal stream of brain regions, namely into area V4 and thence on to the inferotemporal cortex. It is broadly acknowl-

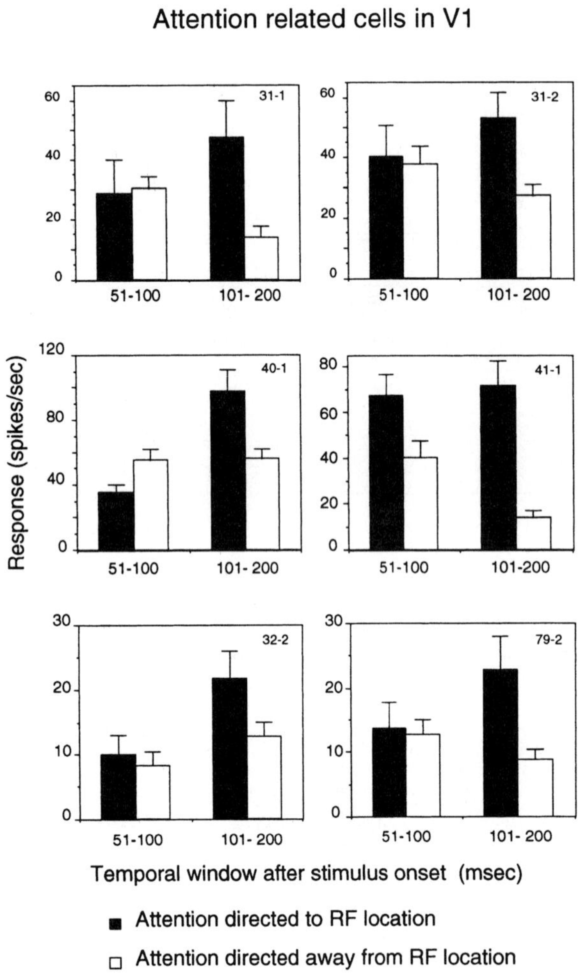

Fig. 3. Mean response rates of six AR cells (with SE) showing no significant influence of attention between 51 and 100 ms after stimulus onset, but a significant modulation in the 101–200 ms window depending upon attention. (Figure reproduced from Vidyasagar, 1998.)

edged that the dorsal stream deals with movement, disparity and spatial position of objects in the visual scene, whereas the ventral stream deals with the pattern itself, namely, form, color, etc. (e.g. Livingstone and Hubel, 1988; Schiller and Logothetis, 1990; Merigan and Maunsell, 1993; Logothetis and Sheinberg, 1996). It is possible that in the behavioral paradigm we used, the early wave of activity is mediated by the faster conducting magnocellular pathway, essentially fast tracking the input necessary for the attentional feedback. This is particularly plausible in view of the role that the posterior parietal cortex plays in attentional control (see later sections) and the fact that the main visual input into this region is magno-dominated.

The timing of the attentional modulation seen in the above study (Vidyasagar, 1998) is consistent with the latencies of typical attention related events observed in the human visual system. There are two studies (Heinze et al., 1994; Martinez et al., 1999) that have provided data on this question. Heinze et al. (1994) combined event-related potentials with positron emission tomography to localize in space and time visual inputs related to focal attention. They found that inputs from attended locations lead to enhanced processing at 80–130 ms after stimulus onset in the fusiform gyrus, an area which is probably the human analogue of macaque V4 (McKeefry and Zeki, 1997). While the localization to area V4 may itself just indicate the specific processing demands of the task, the timing of the attentional component is in the range that would be expected from the latency of the V1 effects seen in our data. Presumably, the modulation of V1 responses by attentional factors would roughly overlap with the earliest attention related responses in the extra-striate areas. More recently, Martinez et al. (1999) have combined event related potentials with fMRI to study the neural sources of attention related events and their time courses. They found that the early sensory events in the striate cortex, i.e. up to 50–55 ms after stimulus onset was not modulated by attention. They also found that the earliest attentional signals found in extra-striate areas were around 70–75 ms. Therefore they postulate that the attentional modulation found in the striate cortex in fMRI images is a re-entrant signal after this latency, i.e. after 75 ms. These time courses closely match our own results mentioned above (Vidyasagar, 1998).

Attentional feedback to primary visual cortex in a memory task

We have recently trained monkeys in a memory task, where both their behavior and electrophysiology indicate that the primary visual cortex is involved in the task more than as a relay station or as just an area of basic feature detectors (Chelvanayagam et al., 1999; Vidyasagar et al., 1999). Our results suggest that in these tasks significant feedback modulation and even some longer term plastic changes can be demonstrated in the striate cortex. The monkeys were trained on a delayed match to sample (DMS) task, where they had to remember both the orientation (vertical or horizontal) and the visual field location of a briefly presented grating and match them to those of a grating flashed a second or so later. While the monkeys took about 8 months from the very beginning to fully learn this task and reach a performance score of over 90%, it was possible to test a few hypotheses during this period of learning. In particular, two ideas were rigorously tested at the stage where each monkey had learnt to perform a DMS task in one retinal location only. They had learnt to match the orientation of the second grating to that of the first, but both gratings were being presented at the same retinal location. So at this stage, the DMS task was to do only with the pattern, but not the retinal location. Since the monkeys were trained to maintain fixation on a fixation spot during the trails, we could test whether the learning transferred from one retinal location to the other. Since the areas that are classically associated with learning and memory, such as hippocampus, parahippocampus, amygdala and the inferotemporal cortex (e.g. Ungerleider and Mishkin, 1982; Squire, 1986; Miyashita, 1988; Fuster, 1990) code retinal location poorly and have rather large receptive fields (Desimone and Ungerleider, 1989; Boussaoud et al., 1991), one would expect that the learning of the DMS task in our situation would readily transfer from one retinal location to another. However, to our surprise, it did not (Chelvanayagam et al., 1999; Pigarev et al., 2001). In fact, the learning was highly retinal position specific, so that even small displacements of 2°, which meant that the new position still overlapped with the old one over 3°, was sufficient to significantly reduce performance. It took many thousands of trials to relearn the task at the new location, though ultimately faster than in the original location. This indicates that at least some component of the learning in our DMS task was occurring at an early visual area such as area V1 which has a fairly fine grain topographical representation.

The other idea that we tested was to see whether at an early stage of learning the DMS task, when the monkey had not learnt to generalize for stimuli of different sizes, he would display size constancy. Since there is evidence that size constancy occurs at an early extra-striate area (Ungerleider et al., 1977), though not at the level of the primary visual cortex (Blakemore et al., 1972), one would expect according to the prevailing ideas of brain regions involved in memory functions (e.g. Ungerleider and Mishkin, 1982; Squire, 1986; Miyashita, 1988; Fuster, 1990), that the site of learning a DMS memory task would be beyond the site of site constancy. Therefore, changing the viewing distance, but not the absolute size should not make a difference to the degree of performance. This was not the case (Vidyasagar et al., 1999; Pigarev et al., 2001). The learning was specific to the retinal size. Changing either the absolute size or the distance of the stimuli markedly affected the performance. However, once the monkey had learnt the full DMS task (i.e. at the end of 8 months when he had learnt the DMS task for both pattern and position), he could transfer the learning easily to other sizes, whether retinal or absolute. Thus these two behavioral experiments strongly suggest that an early visual area such as V1 is involved in at least some component of learning our DMS task.

Consistent with these behavioral studies, single unit responses recorded during the performance of the DMS task showed very significant modulation of the activity of primary visual cortical neurons (Vidyasagar et al., 2000; Vidyasagar and Pigarev, in preparation). This was evident in a number of cells in the striate cortex in two different ways, as shown diagrammatically in Fig. 4. The figure represents trials where matching grating stimuli (either both vertical or both horizontal) were presented at the receptive field position of the neuron under study. The top trace represents responses in the DMS task, where the monkey was actively paying attention to the grating stimuli. The bottom trace represents one of those trials from another block of trials, where exactly similar stimuli were applied to the receptive field location and elsewhere, but the monkey was not working for reward in a DMS task; he simply had to maintain his fixation on the fixation spot and respond by releasing the bar as soon as the fixation spot disappeared. Therefore, in this passive situation, the monkey's attention was on the fixation spot and the gratings had to be ignored. A classical visual neuron that is not under any modulation due

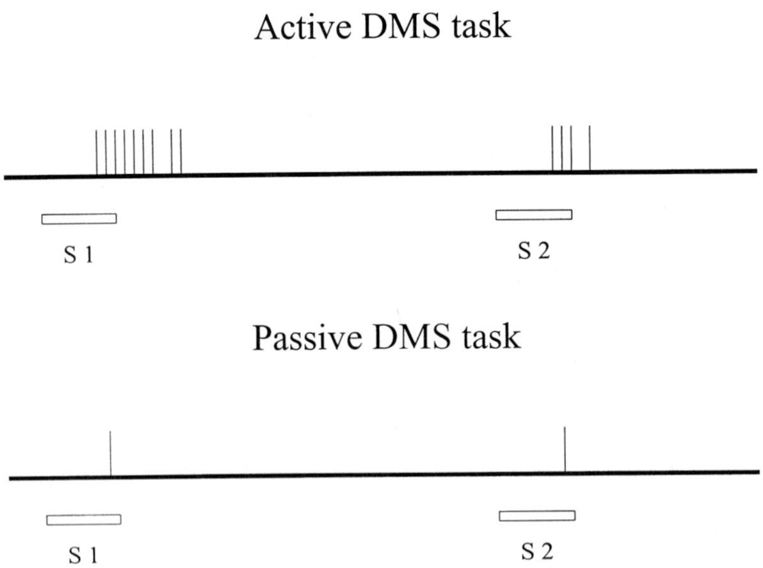

Fig. 4. A diagrammatic representation of responses in a macaque striate cortical neuron in a delayed match to sample memory task (top panel). In this 'active' version, one grating (S1) was flashed at one position around the fixation spot and after a delay a second grating (S2) was flashed in the same position or at a different position. The monkey had to remember both the grating orientation and the position of S1 and match them with S2. The top panel represents a typical response for the match trials of the cell for the orientation that gave the better response. In many cells, there was a significant difference between the responses for S1 and S2, even though the stimuli were identical and appeared at exactly the same position. In some cells, the S1 response was greater and in other cells, the S2 response was bigger. The bottom panel represents the typical response of the same cell to exactly the same stimuli as in the top panel, but in a 'passive' task, where the monkey was simply performing a fixation task, where he had to wait until the fixation spot disappeared to release the bar and obtain reward ignoring the gratings. The cell's response in this passive task was much poorer than in the active one.

to feedback influences would be expected to give the same response for all four stimuli, i.e. for both S1 and S2 in both the active and passive cases. However, the cells showed modulatory influences in two ways:

(1) The responses often were much more vigorous in the active DMS task, where the monkey's attention was on the grating stimuli, compared to the responses in the passive task, where the attention was focussed on the fixation spot. It should be noted that the grating stimuli are exactly the same in the two situations. The only cue for the monkey that the task is a fixation task rather than a DMS task is that the fixation spot was tinged slightly red.

(2) The responses for the two visual stimuli in the active DMS task were not the same, even though the two stimuli in these match trials were identical. In some cells, the response was greater for the first grating stimulus (as shown in Fig. 4) and in others, the response was significantly greater for the second grating.

These experiments constitute the first results that show very significant modulatory influences acting on the primary visual cortex related to attention and memory. They are surprising in the context of classical views on neural sites of memory functions, which have localized them exclusively in higher brain areas. However, our physiological results are very consistent with our own behavioral observations mentioned earlier.

Except the study by Motter (1993), previous neurophysiological attempts (Mohler and Wurtz, 1977; Luck et al., 1997; Haenny and Schiller, 1988) at showing attentional effects in V1 have faltered, largely because of the difference in the experimental design. In Motter's and our studies (Motter, 1993; Vidyasagar, 1998), the crucial factor was the use of a number of distracters in the visual field. As explained earlier and elsewhere (Vidyasagar, 1999), any sort of attentional spotlighting of restricted areas of area V1 would be necessary only if there are a number of competing items in the visual field. If there are only one or a small number of objects, there is no need for focal facilitation in the striate cortex. Despite the large sizes of the receptive fields of the ventral stream structures that process the visual information for object recognition, they will not be confounded in the absence of a clutter of objects in the scene. This point has been appreciated recently also in human fMRI and EEG studies that have confirmed such attentional modulation of neuronal activity in the primary visual cortex (Brefczynski and DeYoe, 1999; Gandhi et al., 1999; Martinez et al., 1999; Somers et al., 1999; Gilbert et al., 2000).

Source of the attentional feedback

What is the likely source of the feedback that might modulate striate cortical responses for spatially focussed attention? This neocortical region might have a role not only in facilitating visual responses at the topographical region of interest, but also in enabling visual search by providing a mechanism to sweep an attentional spotlight across the visual field. There is a wealth of indirect evidence that suggests that the ultimate source of such a feedback is probably the posterior parietal cortex. Single unit studies from macaques have indicated that neurons here could be involved in spatial mapping and could initiate neuronal outputs for directing voluntary spatial attention (e.g. Mountcastle et al., 1975; Bushnell et al., 1981; Duhamel et al., 1992; Andersen et al., 1993; Colby et al., 1993; Andersen, 1995; Steinmetz and Constantinidis, 1995). There is also a large clinical literature linking visual neglect where there is a spatial deficit in one half of the visual field, to parietal lobe dysfunction (for review, Heilman and Valenstein, 1985; Robertson, 1998).

Studies using positron emission tomography (Corbetta et al., 1995) and event-related functional magnetic resonance imaging, or ER-fMRI (Corbetta et al., 2000) have identified the posterior parietal cortex as being preferentially activated in visuo-spatial attention tasks. In fact, Corbetta et al. (2000) have also been able to visualize two different regions in the parietal cortex that may be associated with two different ways of attending to visual stimuli based on their spatial locations. They found that when attention is voluntarily maintained at a cued location of the visual field, the only brain area that showed sustained activation was the intraparietal sulcus. On the other hand, when attention was drawn by a cue to a previously unattended location, they found that it was the temporoparietal junction that was preferentially activated. Therefore reorienting visual attention to an unattended location seems to be anatomically localized to a different region of the parietal cortex from the region that controls maintenance of attention on a location of interest. It would appear that in the paradigms we have used in the awake monkey experiments mentioned above, both these parietal regions would be involved. Other ER-fMRI studies (Wojciulik and Kanwisher, 1999; Downar et al., 2000) also suggest that the parietal areas are preferentially activated by attention-drawing stimuli in a number of different tasks and in all of the three sensory modalities, visual, auditory and tactile.

There are also further indications from clinical studies that processes that wield an attentional spotlight might be associated with the parietal cortex. In patients with unilateral visual neglect due to parietal lesions, there is a marked difference in their performance between a preattentive, parallel (feature) search and an attentive, serial (conjunction) search. The patients perform poorly in searching for conjunction of features, which presumably involves an attentional feedback to an early visual area, but do well in a feature search (Eglin et al., 1989; Humpherys and Riddoch, 1993). Finally, there was a remarkable patient with parietal damage described by Friedman-Hills et al. (1995), who seemed to have lost the ability to bind different stimulus attributes of objects correctly. According to Treisman's Feature Integration theory, such binding problems would accompany any inability to employ an attentional spotlight to perform visual search.

A neural model of attentional gating

Assuming from these studies that the attentional feedback for striate modulation arises from the parietal cortex and that such attentional focussing is a constant process necessary to deal with the richness of information in the sensory environment, I have formulated a neural theory of attention that has implications for normal perception as well as for pathologies such as dyslexia and attention deficit disorders (Vidyasagar, 1999). The theory draws particularly upon the following major electrophysiological and psychophysical findings:

(1) In primates, there are two major afferent pathways from the primary visual cortex (Livingstone and Hubel, 1988; Merigan and Maunsell, 1993), a dorsal, parietal and a ventral, temporal stream.
(2) Despite some limited cross-talk (Ferrera et al., 1992, 1994), most of the parvocellular information goes into the ventral stream and the dorsal stream receives mainly magnocellular signals (Livingstone and Hubel, 1988).
(3) The striate cortex receives significant feedback inputs from higher cortical areas (Motter, 1993; Salin and Bullier, 1996; Vidyasagar, 1998; Hupe et al., 1998).
(4) The visually responsive neurons in the inferotemporal cortex, presumably involved in object recognition, usually have large receptive fields and display position invariance (Desimone and Ungerleider, 1989; Boussaoud et al., 1991).
(5) When there are a large number of distracting items in the visual field, one can show significant attentional modulation of striate cortical responses to appropriate visual stimuli (Motter, 1993; Vidyasagar, 1998).
(6) The parietal cortex plays a critical role in accessing spatial information for the purpose of focal attention (e.g. Robertson, 1998).
(7) Visual search for a unique feature is pre-attentive and parallel, whereas conjunction searches are mostly serial (Treisman, 1988).
(8) Some conjunction searches are more flat than would be predicted by the FIT. In these situations, one of the features is usually an attribute that can be processed by the magnocellular stream (Vidyasagar, 1999).

The crux of the theory is that the posterior parietal cortex uses the spatial information it receives through the magnocellular signals to gate the information going into the temporal stream via an (attentional) feedback to the striate cortex or to anyone of the regions further down the stream into the temporal cortex (Vidyasagar, 1999). Since the ventral pathway has large receptive fields, which is a necessary requirement for achieving position invariance in object recognition, the problem arises of how the different attributes of each object (color, shape, size, etc.) can be correctly bound together. However this ceases to be a problem, if a dorsal stream area which retains precise spatial information were to spotlight one location of the visual field at a time. Since all the attributes of any one object have inevitably the same local sign, these will be automatically bound together by the time at which they get processed in relation to other objects each of which will be processed at a different point in time. It is not quite essential that the gating always needs to operate at an early level such as the striate cortex. If there are only a very limited number of objects in the visual field, the object recognition by the networks of neurons in the inferotemporal cortex can be carried out without being confounded by the binding problem. As we go along the ventral stream from the striate cortex, there is a progressive increase in receptive field size. The typical receptive fields in areas V1, V4, TEO and TE are of the order of 0.2°, 3°, 6° and 25°, respectively (Desimone and Ungerleider, 1989; Boussaoud et al., 1991). Therefore, the target area of the spotlight need not always be as early a station as the striate cortex, but it would be efficient to direct it to the cortical level that is just sufficient to perform the task depending upon the density of objects in the scene. This point was exploited in the electrophysiological experiments (Motter, 1993; Vidyasagar, 1998) that have indeed found significant attentional modulation in the striate cortex when using a large number of visual items. More recent human studies that have also successfully shown attentional effects in the primary visual cortex have used a similar paradigm (Brefczynski and DeYoe, 1999; Martinez et al., 1999), namely discriminations on targets embedded in a cluttered visual scene. The scaling of the attentional spotlight depending upon task demands was also suggested by a recent fMRI study (Kastner et al., 1998), where a progression of increasing lateral suppression from V2 to V4 to TEO under focal attentional control was demonstrated.

The above line of argument also means that for those attributes that are processed by the dorsal stream which does retain spatial information, searches need not be serial. Furthermore, in cases where at least one of the features in a conjunction search is an attribute that can be processed by the dorsal stream, the searches would be more flat than expected by the classical FIT of Treisman (1988), a point discussed at length by Vidyasagar (1999). This is indeed the case as shown by a number of exceptions (Wolfe et al., 1989) to the rule à la Treisman (1988) that search for feature conjunctions are serial.

There is already a large literature linking parietal cortical damage to attentional impairments (reviewed in Heilman and Valenstein, 1985). However, the present proposal that signals entering the ventral stream are gated by an attentional spotlight originating in a dorsal stream structure such as the posterior parietal cortex, has potentially a number of further clinical implications. Most notably, a disruption of dorsal stream functions could in principle also affect functions that are primarily the preserve of the ventral cortical stream. This will be particularly true if each target of interest is surrounded by a number of distracting items. As described earlier, a cluttered visual scene would confound the temporal neocortical modules concerned with object recognition, unless helped by a process of attentional searchlight that lets through only signals from one visual location at a time. This means that a purely magnocellular deficit can lead to an impairment in parvocellular functions if the target is embedded in a visual field full of distracters. If the target is surrounded by very few items, there would be no deficit noticeable in the parvo-mediated functions.

Visual attention and dyslexia

One commonplace application of this theory that has been recently suggested is to the uniquely human function of reading and to its impairment, usually known as dyslexia (Vidyasagar, 1999). Given the dichotomy of functions claimed for the parvo- and magnocellular pathways, it would be expected that the fine pattern vision and object recognition essential for reading is a parvocellular mediated function processed in the ventral stream. Nevertheless, there are a number of papers that have linked the reading deficits in developmental dyslexia with a specific magnocellular pathway impairment (Lovegrove et al., 1980, 1986, 1990; Breitmeyer, 1980, 1993; Livingstone et al., 1991; Lovegrove, 1993; Cornelissen et al., 1995, 1998; Borsting et al., 1996; Stein and Walsh, 1997; but see also Skottun, 1997, 2000). Breitmeyer (1980) attempted to solve this paradox by the following theory: During reading, the eyes make saccades from one point in the line to another, fixating at each point for about 250 ms and taking in approximately about 7 letters at each fixation. Breitmeyer suggested that during each saccade, there is a suppression on the parvocellular neurons by the magnocellular neurons that get activated by the movement of visual stimuli. Such suppression, he claimed, helps to keep the packets of parvo-mediated information that are processed during the series of fixations separate from each other. When the magno pathway is impaired, this no longer happens, so that the two packets of information supposedly merge into each other causing the typical reading difficulty.

While this may seem to be a reasonable framework for explaining how a magno deficit could lead to a reading problem, it has been pointed out (Vidyasagar, 1999) that this model cannot be true for a number of reasons:

(1) Burr et al. (1994) have shown that the suppression elicited during saccades is all within the magnocellular system and parvocellular mediated functions are unaffected during saccades.
(2) According to the Breitmeyer theory, since the two consecutive packets of parvo-information get superimposed, one should expect a dyslexic to confuse a particular letter with the letter removed by one fixation length, say the eighth letter. However, this is not the case in reality. Dyslexics usually confuse adjacent letters.
(3) The Breitmeyer theory still leaves another question unanswered: During the fixation period itself, how does the packet of 7 or so letters get appropriately processed, retaining the spatial order of the letters, when the receptive fields of neurons in area V4 and the inferotemporal cortex are quite large in comparison to the size of the letters.

This leaves us with the conundrum that a magnocellular deficit has been identified in dyslexics, but whose specific reading impairment is with functions that are probably mediated by the parvocellular pathways. However, under the framework of attentional gating proposed earlier, parvocellular functions could indeed be affected by a magnocellular deficit if the task is one which requires extensive attentional spotlighting. It is not too speculative to suggest that reading would be impossible without the aid of the dorsal stream in spotlighting one or a small number of letters at a time. Given the large size of the receptive fields of temporal neocortical neurons, it would not be possible to ascertain the spatial sequence of the recognized letters unless they are processed one at a time. The spotlighting of consecutive letters (or up to two letters at a time in the case of faster readers?) would permit the sequential processing of the letters by the ventral stream.

However, the problem with such attentional gating of letters in a reading material is that voluntary switching of attention is a very slow process (Wolfe et al., 2000), requiring many hundreds of milliseconds to change the focus of attention. On the other hand, serial visual search can proceed at a rate of 13–44 ms per item (Wolfe et al., 2000) and this inherently involuntary process is a random one and has no 'memory' (Horowitz and Wolfe, 1998). This means that visual search does not keep track of locations that have been inspected. Such random direction of the attentional focus is generally a functionally useful strategy to avoid the immense computational load of keeping track of the search history. One major reason why learning to read is such a difficult process taking years may be because the usually random visual search mechanisms have to be trained to perform spatially sequential spotlighting. In modern civilization, reading may well be the most challenging task for the attentional resources of the dorsal stream and thus any deficit in the magnocellular system or posterior parietal cortical functions is likely to lead to reading difficulties. This may be the reason for the consistent finding of magnocellular deficits in dyslexics and also for the frequent association of dyslexia with parietal cortical damage.

One of the predictions of this theory would be that dyslexics should show significantly reduced performance in visual search, particularly for conjunction searches that presumably employ an attentional spotlight. This was tested in our laboratory recently (Vidyasagar and Pammer, 1999) by comparing the

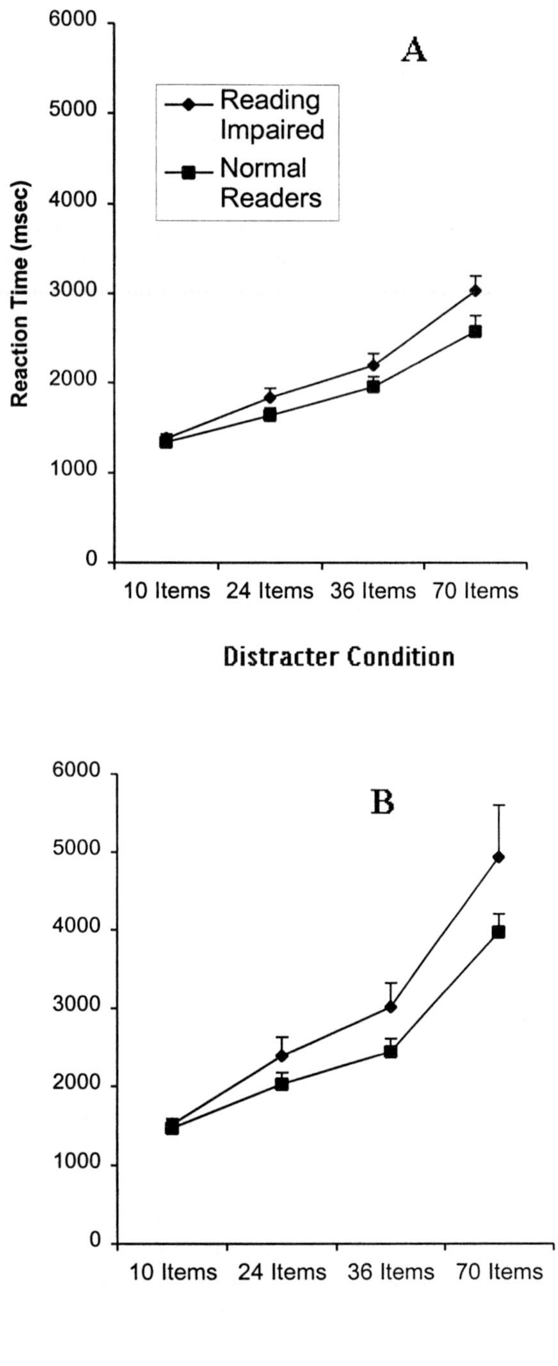

Fig. 5. Reaction time scores for both the normal and impaired reading groups over the different distracter conditions. There was an increasing difference between the groups when the target was present (upper graph), although a significant difference was obtained only when the distracter condition displayed the largest number of background items. There was no significant difference between reading groups when the target was absent (lower graph), even though all the means were higher for dyslexics. Vertical lines represent standard errors of the means. (Figure reproduced from Vidyasagar and Pammer, 1999.)

performance of reading impaired children and normal readers in parallel and serial search tasks. In parallel searches, there was no significant difference between the two groups. However, as predicted, in serial search, as the number of distracters in the visual display was increased, the reading impaired group showed longer reaction times to see the target than the control group (Fig. 5). More recently, we have used a more rigorous paradigm than reaction times to test the idea (Buchholz, Pammer and Vidyasagar, submitted). We designed a paradigm of visual search where as the number of distracters increased, the time of exposure increased at a rate of about 30 ms per item. This meant that the curve of percentage correct against target size for the serial search should be nearly a straight line parallel to the abscissa. This was indeed the case for normal readers, but for the reading impaired children, performance was not only coming down with target size, but the whole curve was shifted down. This meant that dyslexic children require greater time per item for visual search. These experiments show that mechanisms necessary for covert attention are impaired in dyslexia. With such an impairment, it is reasonable to postulate that an attentional deficit is the critical pathophysiological mechanism underlying the reading difficulties seen in dyslexics. There have been other recent studies that have also supported such a view (Facoetti et al., 2000; Facoetti and Molteni, 2001). One of these studies also specifically implicates a disorder of the right posterior parietal cortex and its role in attention in leading to a reading disability (Facoetti and Molteni, 2001).

Summary

For two decades, human psychophysical studies had indicated that attentionhelps in early selection of the incoming sensory information. While previous attempts had failed to show neuronal correlates of such attentional modulation at the level of the primary visual cortex, recent electrophysiological studies in macaques have clearly demonstrated such feedback influences on the striate cortex. These have been followed up by brain imaging studies in humans which are consistent with such early modulation of the visual input. The success of these studies in demonstrating this was largely due to the fact that the serial visual search task they used involved discriminating the target among a number of other distracting items. The model proposed in this paper suggests that such attentional feedback originates in the posterior parietal cortex, which receives its visual information largely though the magnocellular inputs. The scheme explains how purely magnocellular pathway impairments could lead to deficits when testing parvocellular functions, since the magno-mediated attentional feedback would be essential in organizing the spatial information entering the ventral stream via the parvocellular pathway. One application of this idea discussed at length in this paper is how a magnocellular impairment could underlie the reading impairment seen in developmental dyslexia.

It would be interesting to investigate whether attentional problems seen in other conditions such as attentional deficit disorder (ADD) and schizophrenia may be related to a dysfunction in the magnocellular pathway or in the parietal structures involved in the attentional feedback.

Acknowledgements

The work was supported by a Project Grant from the National Health and Medical Research Council of Australia. The experiments on visual attention were done with the help of Ms. Melinda Irving and Mrs. Eva Henry, those on memory functions in the macaque were done in collaboration with Dr. Ivan Pigarev, Dr. David Chelvanayagam and Ms. Jean Cappello and the experiments on dyslexia were done with Dr. Kristen Pammer and Ms. Judy Buchholz.

References

Andersen, R.A. (1995) Encoding of intention and spatial location in the posterior parietal cortex. *Cereb. Cortex*, 5: 457–469.

Andersen, R.A., Snyder, L.H., Li, C.S. and Stricanne, B. (1993) Coordinate transformations in the representation of spatial information. *Curr. Opin. Neurobiol.*, 3: 171–176.

Blakemore, C., Garner, E.T. and Sweet, J.A. (1972) The site of size constancy. *Perception*, 1: 111–119.

Borsting, E., Ridder, W.H., Dubeck, K., Kelley, C., Matsui, L. and Motoyama, J. (1996) The presence of a magnocellular defect depends on the type of dyslexia. *Vision Res.*, 36: 1047–1053.

Boussaoud, D., Desimone, R. and Ungerleider, J.G. (1991) Visual topography of area TEO in the macaque. *J. Comp. Neurol.*, 306: 554–575.

Brefczynski, J.A. and DeYoe, E.A. (1999) A physiological correlate of the 'spotlight' of visual attention. *Nat. Neurosci.*, 2: 370–374.

Breitmeyer, B.G. (1980) Unmasking visual masking: a look at the 'why' behind the veil of the 'how'. *Psychol. Rev.*, 87: 52–69.

Breitmeyer, B.G. (1993) The roles of sustained (P) and transient (M) channels in reading and reading disability. In: S.F. Wright and R. Groner (Eds.), *Facets of Dyslexia and its Remediation*. Elsevier, Amsterdam, pp. 13–31.

Burr, D.C., Morrone, M.C. and Ross, J. (1994) Selective suppression of the magnocellular visual pathway during saccadic eye movements. *Nature*, 371: 503–511.

Bushnell, M.C., Goldberg, M.E. and Robinson, D.L. (1981) Behavioral enhancement of visual responses in monkey cerebral cortex. I. Modulation in posterior parietal cortex related to selective visual attention. *J. Neurophysiol.*, 46: 755–772.

Chelazzi, L., Miller, E.K., Duncan, J. and Desimone, R.J. (1993) A neural basis for visual search in inferior temporal cortex. *Nature*, 363: 345.

Chelvanayagam, D.K., Pigarev, I., Cappello, J.Y. and Vidyasagar, T.R. (1999) Evidence for learning in striate cortex: Performance in a delayed match to sample memory task is retinal position specific. *Proc. Aust. Neurosci. Soc.*, 10: 201.

Colby, C.L., Duhamel, J.R. and Goldberg, M.E. (1993) The analysis of visual space by the lateral intraparietal area of the monkey: the role of extraretinal signals. *Prog. Brain Res.*, 95: 307–316.

Colby, C.L., Duhamel, J.R. and Goldberg, M.E. (1996) Visual, presaccadic, and cognitive activation of single neurons in monkey lateral intraparietal area. *J. Neurophysiol.*, 76: 2841–2852.

Corbetta, M., Shulman, G.L., Miezin, F.M. and Petersen, S.E. (1995) Superior parietal cortex activation during spatial attention shifts and visual feature conjunction. *Science*, 270: 802–805.

Corbetta, M., Kincade, J.M., Ollinger, J.M., McAvoy, M.P. and Shulman, G.L. (2000) Voluntary orienting is dissociated from target detection in human posterior parietal cortex. *Nat. Neurosci.*, 3: 292–297.

Cornelissen, P., Richardson, A., Mason, A., Fowler, S. and Stein, J. (1995) Contrast sensitivity and coherent motion detection measured at photopic luminance levels in dyslexics and controls. *Vision Res.*, 35: 1483–1494.

Cornelissen, P.L., Hansen, P.C., Hutton, J.L., Evangelinou, V. and Stein, J.F. (1998) Magnocellular visual function and children's single word reading. *Vision Res.*, 38: 471–482.

Desimone, R. and Ungerleider, L.G. (1989) Neural mechanisms of visual processing in monkeys. In: F. Boller and J. Grafman (Eds.), *Neuropsychology*, Vol. 2. Elsevier, New York, pp. 267–299.

Downar, J., Crawley, A.P., Mikulis, D.J. and Davis, K.D. (2000) A multimodal cortical network for the detection of changes in the sensory environment. *Nat. Neurosci.*, 3: 277–283.

Duhamel, J., Colby, C.L. and Goldberg, M.E. (1992) The updating of the representation of visual space in parietal cortex by intended eye movements. *Science*, 255: 90–92.

Eglin, M., Roberstson, L.C. and Knight, R.T. (1989) Visual search performance in the neglect syndrome. *J. Cogn. Neurosci.*, 4: 372–381.

Facoetti, A. and Molteni, M. (2001) The gradient of visual attention in developmental dyslexia. *Neuropsychologia*, 39: 352–357.

Facoetti, A., Paganoni, P. and Lorusso, M.L. (2000) The spatial distribution of visual attention in developmental dyslexia. *Exp. Brain Res.*, 132: 531–538.

Ferrera, V.P., Nealey, T.A. and Maunsell, J.H. (1992) Mixed parvocellular and magnocellular geniculate signals in visual area V4. *Nature*, 358: 756–761.

Ferrera, V.P., Nealey, T.A. and Maunsell, J.H. (1994) Responses in macaque visual area V4 following inactivation of the parvocellular and magnocellular LGN pathways. *J. Neurosci.*, 14: 2080–2088.

Friedman-Hills, S.R., Robertson, L.C. and Treisman, A. (1995) Parietal contributions to visual feature binding: evidence from a patient with bilateral lesions. *Nature*, 269: 853.

Fuster, J.M. (1990) Inferotemporal units in selective visual attention and short-term memory. *J. Neurophysiol.*, 64: 681–697.

Gandhi, S.P., Heeger, D.J. and Boynton, G.M. (1999) Spatial attention affects brain activity in human primary visual cortex. *Proc. Natl. Acad. Sci. USA*, 96: 3314–3319.

Gilbert, C., Ito, M., Kapadia, M. and Westheimer, G. (2000) Interactions between attention, context and learning in primary visual cortex. *Vision Res.*, 40: 1217–1226.

Haenny, P.E. and Schiller, P.H. (1988) State dependent activity in monkey visual cortex. 1. Single cell activity in V1 and V4 on visual tasks. *Exp. Brain Res.*, 69: 225–244.

Heilman, K.M. and Valenstein, E. (1985) *Clinical Neurophysiology*. Oxford University Press, New York.

Heinze, H.J., Mangun, G.R., Burchert, W., Hinrichs, H., Scholz, M., Munte, T.F., Gos, A., Scherg, M., Johannes, S. and Hundeshagen, H. et al. (1994) Combined spatial and temporal imaging of brain activity during visual selective attention in humans. *Nature*, 372: 543–546.

Hicks, T.P., Lee, B.B. and Vidyasagar, T.R. (1983) The responses of cells in macaque lateral geniculate nucleus to sinusoidal gratings. *J. Physiol.*, 337: 183–200.

Horowitz, T.S. and Wolfe, J.M. (1998) Visual search has no memory. *Nature*, 394: 575.

Humpherys, G.W. and Riddoch, M.J. (1993) Interactive attentional system in unilateral visual neglect. In: I.H. Robertson and J.C. Marshall (Eds.), *Unilateral Neglect: Clinical and Experimental Studies*. Lawrence Erlbaum, Hillsale, NJ, pp. 139–168.

Hupe, J.M., James, A.C., Payne, B.R., Lomber, S.G., Girard, P. and Bullier, J. (1998) Cortical feedback improves discrimination between figure and background by V1, V2 and V3 neurons. *Nature*, 394: 784–787.

Kastner, S., De Weerd, P., Desimone, R. and Ungerleider, L.G. (1998) Mechanisms of directed attention in the human extrastriate cortex as revealed by functional MRI. *Science*, 282: 108–111.

Lecas, J.C. (1995) Prefrontal neurones sensitive to increased visual attention in the monkey. *NeuroReport*, 7: 305–309.

Livingstone, M. and Hubel, D.H. (1988) Segregation of form, color, movement and depth: anatomy, physiology and perception. *Science*, 240: 740–749.

Livingstone, M.S., Rosen, G.D., Drislane, F.W. and Galaburda, A.M. (1991) Physiological and anatomical evidence for a magnocellular defect in developmental dyslexia. *Proc. Natl. Acad. Sci. USA*, 88: 7943–7947.

Logothetis, N.K. and Sheinberg, D.L. (1996) Visual object recognition. *Annu. Rev. Neurosci.*, 19: 577–621.

Lovegrove, W. (1993) Do dyslexics have a visual deficit? In: S.F. Wright and R. Groner (Ed.), *Facets of Dyslexia and its Remediation*. Elsevier, Amsterdam.

Lovegrove, W.J., Bowling, A., Badcock, D. and Blackwood, M. (1980) Specific reading disability: differences in contrast sensitivity as a function of spatial frequency. *Science*, 210: 439–440.

Lovegrove, W., Martin, F. and Slaghuis, W. (1986) A theoretical and experimental case for a visual deficit in specific reading disability. *Cogn. Neuropsychol.*, 3: 225–267.

Lovegrove, W.J., Garzia, R.P. and Nicholson, S.B. (1990) Experimental evidence for a transient system deficit in specific reading disability. *Am. Optom. Assoc. J.*, 61: 137–146.

Luck, S.J., Chelazzi, L., Hillard, S.A. and Desimone, R. (1997) Neural mechanisms of spatial selective attention in area V1, V2 and V4 of macaque visual cortex. *J. Neurophysiol.*, 77: 24–42.

Lynch, J.C., Mountcastle, V.B., Talbot, W.H. and Yin, T.C.T. (1977) Parietal lobe mechanisms for directed visual attention. *J. Neurophysiol.*, 40: 362–389.

Martinez, A., Anllo-Vento, L., Serono, M.I., Frank, L.R., Buxton, R.B., Dubowitz, D.J., Wong, E.C., Hinrichs, H.J. and Hillard, S.A. (1999) Involvement of striate and extrastriate cortical areas in spatial attention. *Nat. Neurosci.*, 2: 364–369.

Maunsell, J.H. and Gibson, J.R. (1992) Visual response latencies in striate cortex of the macaque monkey. *J. Neurophysiol.*, 68: 1332–1344.

McKeefry, D.J. and Zeki, S. (1997) The position and topography of the human color center as revealed by functional magnetic resonance imaging. *Brain*, 120: 2229–2242.

McLeod, P., Driver, J. and Crisp, J. (1988) Visual search for a conjunction of movement and form is parallel. *Nature*, 332: 154–155.

Merigan, W.H. and Maunsell, J.H.R. (1993) How parallel are the primate visual pathways?. *Annu. Rev. Neurosci.*, 16: 369–402.

Miller, E.K., Erickson, C.A. and Desimone, R. (1996) Neural mechanisms of visual working memory in prefrontal cortex of the macaque. *J. Neurosci.*, 16: 5154–5167.

Miyashita, Y. (1988) Neuronal correlate of visual associative long-term memory in the primate temporal cortex. *Nature*, 335: 817–820.

Mohler, C.W. and Wurtz, R.H. (1977) Role of striate cortex and superior colliculus in visual guidance of saccadic eye movements in monkeys. *J. Neurophysiol.*, 40: 74–94.

Moran, J. and Desimone, R. (1985) Selective attention gates visual processing in the extrastriate cortex. *Science*, 229: 782–784.

Motter, B.C. (1993) Focal attention produces spatially selective processing in visual cortical areas V1, V2 and V4 in the presence of competing stimuli. *J. Neurophysiol.*, 70: 909–919.

Motter, B.C. (1994a) Neural correlates of attentive selection for color or luminance in extrastriate area V4. *J. Neurosci.*, 14: 2178–2189.

Motter, B.C. (1994b) Neural correlates of feature selective memory and pop-out in extrastriate area V4. *J. Neurosci.*, 14: 2190–2199.

Mountcastle, V.B., Lynch, J.C., Georgopoulos, A., Sazskata, H. and Acuna, C. (1975) Posterior parietal association cortex of the monkey: command function for operations within extrapersonal space. *J. Neurophysiol.*, 38: 871–908.

Nakayama, K. and Silverman, G.H. (1986) Serial and parallel processing of visual feature conjunctions. *Nature*, 320: 264–265.

Nowak, L.G., Munk, M.H., Girard, P. and Bullier, J. (1995) Visual latencies in areas V1 and V2 of the macaque monkey. *Vis. Neurosci.*, 12: 371–384.

Pigarev, I., Chelvanayagam, D.K. Cappello, J. and Vidyasagar, T.R. (2001) Primary visual cortex and memory: Retinal position specificity and lack of size constancy at early stages of learning a visual memory task in the macaque. *Exp. Brain Res.*, in press.

Robertson, L.C. (1998) Visuospatial attention and parietal function: their role in object perception. In: R. Parasuraman (Ed.), *The Attentive Brain*. MIT Press, Cambridge, pp. 255–278.

Salin, P. and Bullier, J. (1996) Corticocortical connections in the visual system: structure and function. *Physiol. Rev.*, 75: 107–154.

Schiller, P.H. and Logothetis, N.K. (1990) The color-opponent and broad-band channels of the primate visual system. *Trends Neurosci.*, 13: 392–398.

Skottun, B.C. (1997) Some remarks on the magnocellular deficit theory of dyslexia. *Vision Res.*, 37: 965–966.

Skottun, B.C. (2000) The magnocellular deficit theory of dyslexia: the evidence from contrast sensitivity. *Vision Res.*, 40: 111–127.

Somers, D.C., Dale, A.M., Seiffert, A.E. and Tootell, R.B.H. (1999) Functional MRI reveals spatially specific attentional modulation in human primary visual cortex. *Proc. Natl. Acad. Sci. USA*, 96: 1663–1668.

Spitzer, H., Desimone, R. and Moran, J. (1988) Increased attention enhances both behavioral and neuronal performance. *Science*, 240: 338–340.

Squire, L.R. (1986) Mechanisms of memory. *Science*, 232: 1612–1619.

Stein, J. and Walsh, V. (1997) To see but not to read; the magnocellular theory of dyslexia. *Trends Neurosci.*, 20: 147–152.

Steinmetz, M.A. and Constantinidis, C. (1995) Neurophysiological evidence for a role of posterior parietal cortex in redirecting visual attention. *Cereb. Cortex*, 5: 448–456.

Tootell, R.B., Hadjikhani, N., Hall, E.K., Marrett, S., Vanduffel,

W., Vaughan, J.T. and Dale, A.M. (1998) The retinotopy of visual spatial attention. *Neuron*, 6: 1409–1422.

Treisman, A. (1988) Features and objects: the fourteenth Bartlett memorial lecture. *Q. J. Exp. Psychol.*, 40A: 201–237.

Treisman, A. (1996) The binding problem. *Curr. Opin. Neurobiol.*, 6: 171–178.

Treisman, A. (1998) Feature binding, attention and object perception. *Philos. Trans. R. Soc. Lond. B. Biol. Sci.*, 353: 1295–1306.

Treisman, A.M. and Gelade, G. (1980) A feature integration theory of attention. *Cogn. Psychol.*, 12: 97–136.

Treue, S. and Maunsell, J.H.R. (1996) Attentional modulation of visual motion processing in cortical areas MT and MST. *Nature*, 382: 539–541.

Ungerleider, L.G. and Mishkin, M. (1982) Two cortical visual systems. In: D.J. Ingle, M.A. Goodale and R.J.W. Mansfield (Eds.), *Analysis of Visual Behavior*. MIT Press, Cambridge, MA, pp. 549–586.

Ungerleider, L.G., Ganz, L. and Pribram, K.H. (1977) Size constancy in rhesus monkeys: effects of pulvinar, prestriate and inferotemporal lesions. *Exp. Brain Res.*, 27: 251–269.

Van Essen, D.C., Olshausen, B., Gallant, J., Press, W., Anderson, C., Drury, H., Carman, G. and Felleman, D. (1993) Anatomical, physiological and computational aspects of hierarchical processing in the macaque visual cortex. In: B. Albowitz, K. Albus, U. Kuhnt, H.C. Nothdurft and P. Wahle (Eds.), *Structural and Functional Organization of the Neocortex*. Springer-Verlag, Berlin, pp. 317–329.

Vidyasagar, T.R. (1998) Gating of neuronal responses in macaque primary visual cortex by an attentional spotlight. *NeuroReport*, 9: 1947–1952.

Vidyasagar, T.R. (1999) A neuronal model of attentional spotlight: parietal guiding the temporal. *Brain Res. Rev.*, 30: 66–76.

Vidyasagar, T.R. and Pammer, K. (1999) Impaired visual search in dyslexia relates to the role of the magnocellular pathway in attention. *NeuroReport*, 10: 1283–1287.

Vidyasagar, T.R., Pigarev, I., Chelvanayagam, D.K. and Cappello, J.Y. (1999) Monkeys do not show size constancy at the earlier stages of learning a delayed match to sample memory task. *Proc. Aust. Neurosci. Soc.*, 10: 200.

Vidyasagar, T.R., Pigarev, I., Cappello, J.Y. and Chelvanayagam, D.K. (2000) Mnemonic components modulate responses of macaque striate cortical neurones in a delayed match to sample memory task. *Proc. Aust. Neurosci. Soc.*, 11: 57.

Wojciulik, E. and Kanwisher, N. (1999) The generality of parietal involvement in visual attention. *Neuron*, 23: 747–764.

Wolfe, J.M. (1994) Guided search 2.0: a revised model of visual search. *Psychonomic Bull. Rev.*, 1: 202–238.

Wolfe, J.M., Cave, K.R. and Franzel, S.L. (1989) Guided search: an alternative to the feature integration model for visual search. *J. Exp. Psychol. Hum. Percept. Perform.*, 15: 419–433.

Wolfe, J.M., Alvaerz, G.A. and Horowitz, T.S. (2000) Attention is fast but volition is slow. *Nature*, 406: 691.

Zeki, S. (1993) *A Vision of the Brain*. Blackwell Scientific, Oxford.

C. Casanova and M. Ptito (Eds.)
Progress in Brain Research, Vol. 134

CHAPTER 20

Different spaces and different times for perception and action

Melvyn A. Goodale *

Departments of Psychology and Physiology, University of Western Ontario, London, ON N6A 5C2, Canada

Abstract: Separate, but interacting, visual systems have evolved in the primate brain for the perception of objects on the one hand and the control of actions directed at those objects on the other. This 'duplex' account of high-level vision suggests that 'reconstructive' approaches and 'purposive–animate–behaviorist' approaches need not be seen as mutually exclusive, but as complementary in their emphases on different aspects of visual function. Indeed, the limitations of one system are the strengths of the other. Perception (which is mediated by the ventral stream of visual projections in primate cortex) delivers a rich and detailed representation of the world, but does not compute the detailed metrics of the scene with respect to the observer. In contrast, the action system (which depends heavily on dorsal-stream projections) delivers accurate metrical information about an object in the required egocentric coordinates for action, but these computations are fleeting and are for the most part limited to the particular goal object that has been selected. Both systems work together in the production of purposive behavior — one system selects the goal object from the visual array, the other carries out the required metrical computations for the goal-directed action.

Introduction

It seems self-evident that perception is a necessary antecedent to action. Most of us take for granted, for example, that we need to *see* an object before we can pick it up. But the truth is that perception [1] and action are not that tightly coupled. Even though seeing an object enables us to select it as a target for action, the programming and control of the action itself makes use of visual information that is not gleaned from what we think we see. Indeed, contrary to what our phenomenology tells us, evidence from a broad range of studies on both neurological patients and normal observers suggests that the processes mediating the visual control of goal-directed actions are quite independent from those mediating the conscious perception of objects. In this chapter, I will explore some recent work from our own laboratory that has contributed to this idea, particularly work showing dissociations between *vision for perception* and *vision for action* in the normal observer. But first some background.

* Correspondence to: M.A. Goodale, Department of Psychology, University of Western Ontario, London, ON N6A 5C2, Canada. Tel.: +1-519-661-2070; Fax: +1-519-661-3961; E-mail: mgoodale@julian.uwo.ca

[1] In this chapter, I use the term 'perception', not in the broad sense of *any* processing of sensory input, but in the more restricted sense of assigning meaning and significance to external objects and events. This usage, which is most common in philosophical and psychological writings, often (though not always) carries experiential connotations, and tends to be identified with one's phenomenological experience of the world.

Two visual systems in the primate cerebral cortex

Traditional accounts of vision, from Helmholtz to Marr, have assumed that the function of vision is to construct an internal model of the external world, which then serves as a perceptual foundation for all visually driven thought and action. Even though recent versions of such accounts have postulated that there are separate 'modules' for the processing of different visual features such as motion, color, texture, and form, there is still an implicit assumption that in the end vision delivers some sort of unified representation of the external world (for a discussion of this issue, see Goodale and Humphrey, 1998).

The idea of a single 'general purpose' visual system has begun to be challenged however. In 1992, David Milner and I proposed, on the basis of evidence derived from work with both humans and monkeys, that the neural mechanisms mediating conscious visual perception are functionally and anatomically distinct from those mediating the visual control of actions (Goodale and Milner, 1992). We went on to suggest that the distinction between vision for perception and vision for action can be mapped onto two streams of visual processing in the brain, which were first identified in the cerebral cortex of the monkey: the so-called *ventral stream* projecting from primary visual cortex to inferotemporal cortex and the so-called *dorsal stream* projecting from primary visual cortex to posterior parietal cortex (Ungerleider and Mishkin, 1982). The major projections and cortical targets for these two streams are illustrated in Fig. 1. Although one must always be cautious when drawing homologies between monkey and human neuroanatomy (Crick and Jones, 1993), recent neuroimaging work suggests that the visual projections from the primary visual cortex to the temporal and parietal lobes in the human brain may involve a separation into ventral and dorsal streams similar to that seen in the macaque brain (for review, see Tootell et al., 1996).

David Milner and I have argued that the ventral stream plays the major role in constructing the perceptual representation of the visual world and the objects within it, while the dorsal stream mediates the visual control of actions directed at those objects (for a more detailed discussion, see Goodale and Milner, 1992; Milner and Goodale, 1995; Goodale and Humphrey, 1998). In other words, processing within the ventral stream allows us to recognize an object, such as a banana in a bowl of fruit, while processing within the dorsal stream provides critical information about the location, orientation, size, and shape of that banana so that we can reach out and pick it up. Note that this is not the distinction between what and where (object vision and spatial vision) that was originally put forward by Ungerleider and Mishkin in 1982. In our scheme, the structural and spatial attributes of the goal object are being processed by both streams, but for different purposes. In the case of the ventral stream, information about a broad range of object parameters is being transformed for perceptual purposes; in the case of the dorsal stream, some of these same object parameters are being transformed for the control of actions. This is not to say that the distribution of subcortical visual inputs does not differ between the two streams, but rather that the main difference lies in the nature of the transformations that each stream performs on those two sets of inputs. Of course, as I will discuss in more detail later, the two streams are not hermetically sealed from one another. Indeed, they work together in controlling our behavior as we live our complex lives — but they play separate and complementary roles in the production of adaptive behavior.

The metrics and timing of perception and action

Vision for action and vision for perception differ both with respect to the metrics and frames of reference that each system uses and with respect to the time scale over which each system operates. To be able to grasp and/or manipulate an object, for example, it is essential to 'compute' the absolute[2] size of the object and its orientation and position with respect to the observer. This information is critical to the formation of the anticipatory posture of the hand and fingers as they are moved towards the object (Jeannerod, 1988). Moreover, the programming and control of such an action require that the metrical information about the location and disposition of the object be computed in *egocentric* frames of reference — in other words, in frames of reference that take into account the location and disposition of the object with respect to the effector that is to be used to perform the action. Although the position of a goal object appears to be computed initially in

[2] The term 'absolute' is used here to refer to the actual size of an object. An object's absolute size, unlike its relative size, does not vary with respect to other objects in the scene.

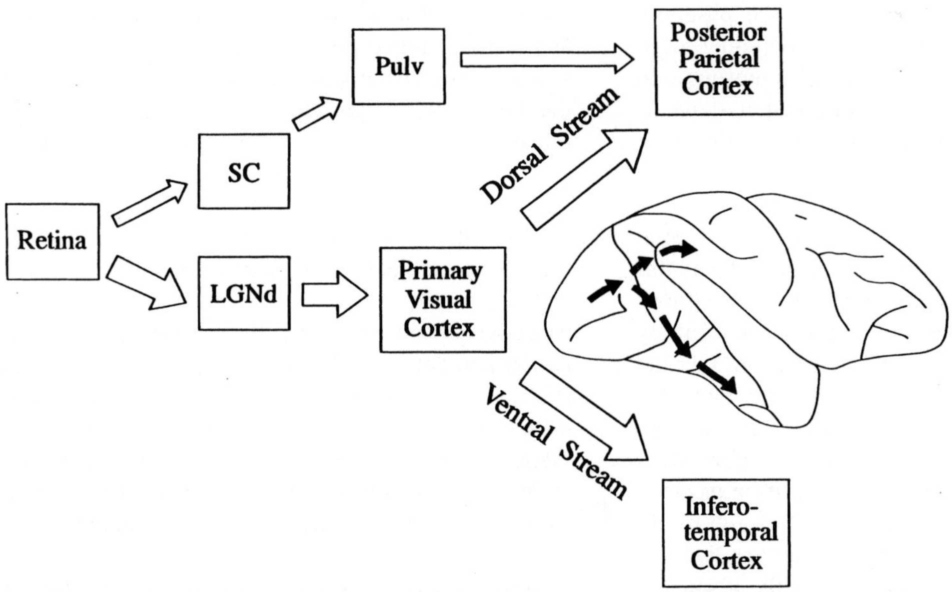

Fig. 1. The major routes whereby retinal input reaches the dorsal and ventral streams. The diagram of the macaque brain (right hemisphere) on the right of the figure shows the approximate routes of the cortico-cortical projections from the primary visual cortex to the posterior parietal and the inferotemporal cortex, respectively. LGNd, lateral geniculate nucleus, pars dorsalis; Pulv, pulvinar; SC, superior colliculus.

oculocentric coordinates (Batista et al., 1999), eventually this information must be transformed within frames of reference that reflect the position of the goal with respect to effectors being used to perform the planned action, such as the arm, hand, and fingers, for example, in the case of an object-directed grasping movement.

The time at which these computations are performed is also critical. Observers and goal objects rarely stay in a static relationship with one another and, as a consequence, the egocentric coordinates of a target object can often change dramatically from moment to moment. It makes sense, therefore, that the required coordinates for action be computed immediately before the movements are initiated and it makes little sense that these coordinates (or the resulting motor programs) be stored for more than a few milliseconds before executing that action. Indeed, there is evidence that the motor program begins to change or decay almost immediately if it is not used — in less than 800 ms for saccades (Gnadt et al., 1991) and in less than 2 s for manual aiming movements and grasping (Elliot and Madalena, 1987; Goodale et al., 1994). Thus, actions directed to remembered objects (objects that were present in the visual array, but are no longer there after a delay) look quite different from actions directed to objects that remain visible (Bridgeman et al., 1997; Hu et al., 1999). In short, visual information about the goal object for an intended action must be computed in 'real time'.

The situation is quite different for conscious perception, both in terms of the spatial frame of reference used to construct the percept and the time frame over which that percept (or some version of it) can be accessed. Vision for perception appears not to rely on computations about the absolute size of objects or their egocentric locations — a fact that explains why we have no difficulty watching television, a medium in which there are no absolute metrics at all. Instead of using absolute metrics and egocentric frames of reference, our perceptual system computes the size, location, shape, and orientation of an object primarily in relation to other objects and surfaces in the scene. In other words, the metric of conscious perception is inherently relative. Of course, conscious perception is primarily concerned with the identity and meaning of objects — not their absolute size or their precise location with respect to the observer. The main function of perception is to render what appears to be a detailed and 'faithful' representation of the world. This representation, which depends on memory as well as direct visual input (Rensink et al., 1997), allows us to think about the world, communicate with others, and plan various courses of action. In other words, it provides a perceptual foundation for cognitive operations. Encoding an object in a scene-based frame of reference (sometimes called an *allocentric* frame of reference, particularly with respect to the object's spatial location) permits a perceptual representation of the object that preserves the relations between the object parts and its surroundings without requiring precise information about absolute size of the object or its exact position with respect to the observer. Indeed, if our perceptual machinery attempted to deliver the real size and distance of all the objects in the visual array, the computational load on the system would be astronomical.

Perception also operates over a much longer time scale than that used in the control of action. We can recognize objects we have seen minutes, hours, days — or even years before. In fact, the time scale for visual perception is several orders of magnitude larger than the time scale for the visual control of action in real time. When objects (and scenes) are coded in allocentric frames of reference, it is much easier to preserve their identity over relative long periods of time. In other words, we can recognize objects that we have seen before, even though the position of those objects with respect to our body might have changed considerably since the last time we saw them.

Several lines of evidence provide support for the idea that vision for action uses egocentric frames of reference, whereas vision for perception uses allocentric frames of reference. For example, Wong and Mack (1981) carried out an experiment in which subjects fixated a small target that was presented within a surrounding frame in an otherwise dark room. After a 500-ms blank period, the frame and target re-appeared, but the frame was displaced a few degrees to the left or right. The target itself stayed at the same location as before. Nevertheless, subjects consciously perceived the target as having moved in a direction opposite to that of the actual displacement of the frame, instead of perceiving the frame as having changed position. This illusory perception was sustained even when, after the blanking period, the target was displaced in the same direction as the frame, but by only one third of the distance. In this case, the perceived and actual changes of target position were in opposite directions. Yet despite the presence of this strong illusory displacement of the target, subjects consistently directed their saccades towards the true location of the target (i.e. its retinocentric location). Similar dissociations between perception and action have been observed in studies using aiming movements. Bridgeman et al. (1981), for example, found that even though a fixed visual target surrounded by a moving frame appeared to drift in a direction opposite to that of the frame, subjects persisted in pointing to the veridical location of the target. In short, conscious perception of the location of a visual stimulus is computed in allocentric frames of reference, whereas visuomotor output to the same target is computed in egocentric frames of reference.

As I mentioned earlier, just as the frames of reference mediating the conscious perception of *object location* differ from those underlying the visual control of actions directed at that object, so do the metrics underlying the conscious perception of *object size*. In our daily life, we rarely make judgements of the absolute size of an object, but instead make judgements based on the relative size of objects in the visual scene. These relative judgements can be quite subtle and precise — and we are capable of making fine discriminations between the dimensions of different objects in a scene. There is no need to compute the real size of the objects, a much more complex computation, unless — as will become clear later — we plan to act up the object.

These relative judgements of object size are also obligatory. We cannot stop ourselves from comparing the sizes of different objects. Such comparisons are automatic and effortless — a fact that explains why many optical illusions involving judgements of size continue to work even when we know full well that what we are looking at is just an illusion. A prototypical example of such an illusion is the Ebbinghaus Illusion (or Titchener Circles Illusion) in which two target circles of equal size, each surrounded by a circular array of either smaller or larger

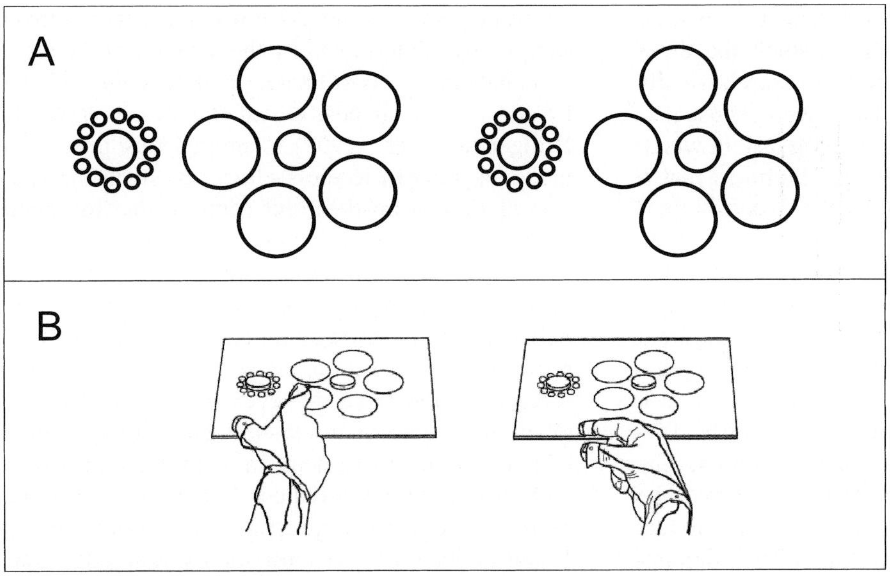

Fig. 2. The 'Ebbinghaus' illusion. (A) In the standard version of the illusion, the target circles in the center of the two arrays appear to be different in size even though they are physically identical is shown in the left-hand figure. For most people, the circle in the annulus of smaller circles appears to be larger than the circle in the annulus of larger circles. The right-hand figure shows a version of the illusion in which the target circle in the array of larger circles has been made physically larger than the other target circle. The two target circles should now appear to be perceptually equivalent in size. (B) An illustration of the two tasks performed by each subject using a three-dimensional version of the Ebbinghaus illusion. Light emitting diodes were attached to the finger, thumb and wrist to allow for optoelectronic tracking. The grasping task is illustrated on the left. In this illustration, the subject's hand is pictured in-flight on the way to the target disk. The right-hand drawing illustrates the manual estimation task. The heel of the subject's hand rested on the table and the subjects opened their thumb and index finger by an amount that matched the perceived size of the target disk. (Adapted with permission from Goodale and Humphrey, 1998.)

circles, are presented side by side (see Fig. 2A). Subjects typically report that the target circle surrounded by the array of smaller circles appears larger than the one surrounded by the array of larger circles, presumably because of the difference in the contrast in size between the target circles and the surrounding circles. In another version of the illusion, also shown in Fig. 2A, the target circles can be made to appear identical in size by increasing the actual size of the target circle surrounded by the larger circles. What is striking about these illusions and many other size-contrast illusions is that even when the trick is explained to the subjects and the true size of the targets circles is demonstrated, they continue to experience these illusions.

Although perceptual judgements are clearly affected by these manipulations of the stimulus array, there is good reason to believe that the calibration of size-dependent motor outputs, such as grip aperture during grasping, would not be. Instead, the visuomotor transformations that mediate the grasp might be expected to use metrical computations that are centered on the target itself without taking into account the size and location of surrounding objects in the scene. The production of successful and reliable actions demands computations that are refractory to the kinds of pictorial cues that drive our perception of familiar illusions. After all, an accidental conjunction of object features that created an illusion in a natural scene could lead to disastrous consequences if the programming of an action was sensitive to that illusion. To reiterate, to grasp an object efficiently, we must compute its real size.

The insensitivity of grasp to size-contrast illusions was recently demonstrated in two experiments that used a three-dimensional version of the Ebbinghaus illusion in which two thin 'poker-chip' disks were arranged as pairs on a standard annular circle display (Aglioti et al., 1995; Haffenden and Goodale, 1998). Trials in which the two disks appeared perceptually identical but were physically different in size were randomly alternated with trials in which the disks appeared perceptually different but were physically identical. Even though subjects showed robust perceptual illusions — even in a matching task in which they opened their index finger and thumb to match the perceived diameter of one of the disks — their grip aperture was correlated with the real size of the disk when they reached out to pick it up. In other words, as their hand moved toward the target object, it was scaled in flight for the real not the apparent size of target. The dissociation between perceptual judgements and the calibration of grasping is not limited to the Ebbinghaus Illusion. The vertical—-horizontal illusion is one in which a vertical line that bisects a horizontal line appears longer than the horizontal line even though both lines are in fact the same length. Vishton and Cutting (1995) demonstrated, however, that subjects do not show this bias when they reach out and 'grasp' the vertical line. Using a three-dimensional version of the same illusion, Servos et al. (2000) showed that subjects scale their grasp to the real size of the target object, even though they perceive it to be longer than it really is. The relative insensitivity of reaching and grasping to pictorial illusions has also been demonstrated for the Müller–Lyer illusion (Gentilucci et al., 1996) and the Ponzo illusion (Brenner and Smeets, 1996; Jackson and Shaw, 2000). Creem et al. (1998) have even used a large-scale Müller–Lyer illusion to demonstrate that locomotor accuracy can escape the illusion even though subjects report that the line with outward pointing arrows is longer than the one with inward pointing arrows.

But skilled motor actions are not always immune to the influences of conscious perception. There is evidence, for example, that conscious perception of an object position *can* affect motor performance. This reliance on allocentric information about position is typically seen, however, in situations where the actions are not initiated immediately, but only after a delay. In the Wong and Mack (1981) experiment described earlier, for example, saccades made to a remembered visual target were made to the consciously perceived target position rather than to the true location where it had appeared. In other words, the trajectory of the memory-driven saccade was determined by the location of the target with respect to the frame, whereas the trajectory of the target-driven saccade was determined by the location of the target in oculocentric co-ordinates, and was not affected by the change in position of the frame. Recently, Bridgeman et al. (1997) examined this interaction using an induced Roelofs effect, in which the position of a target inside an off-center frame appears to be biased in the direction opposite that of the frame. The same effect appeared in manual pointing — but only when the movement was executed after a 4-s delay between viewing the target and initiating the movement. In real time, the pointing movement was directed at the target — even in visual open loop when the target was not visible during the execution of the pointing movement. In a similar vein, Creem and Proffitt (1998) studied verbal judgments and motor adjustments of geographical slant perception. When subjects viewed a hill, their verbal judgements of the incline of the hill were greatly overestimated compared to their motor adjustments. Yet after a delay, when the hill was no longer visible, their motor adjustments were similar to their exaggerated verbal judgements. Creem and Proffitt argued that actions after a delay are guided by an explicit stored representation of visual information. Thus, if motor actions are driven by stored representations that are derived from conscious perception of object location, then they will use the same allocentric frames of reference as the original perception.

If actions initiated after a delay use allocentric rather than egocentric frames of reference to localize the goal, then by the same token one might expect that the size-scaling of a delayed action, such as grasping, would use relative rather than absolute metrics. In other words, one might expect that the scaling of grip aperture would move into relative metrics if a delay is interposed between viewing the goal object and initiating the grasp — since now the subject would have to rely on a stored percept of the object rather than on some version of normal on-line visuomotor computations. Although earlier studies have shown that the kinematics of grasping after a delay are certainly different from the kinematics of normal grasping, these studies did not examine the metrics used to scale the two different kinds of grasping movements (Goodale et al., 1994; Hu et al., 1999). In a recent experiment, however, Yaoping Hu and I compared the metrics used to scale grasping movements directed at objects in real time with the metrics used to scale similar movements initiated to the same objects but after a 5-s delay (Hu and Goodale, 2000).

Absolute versus relative metrics in grasping: experiments in a virtual workspace

To carry out this kind of experiment, we had to devise a method of presenting objects where we had complete control over the visual appearance of the goal objects and other objects in the workspace. It is almost impossible to equate the appearance of real three-dimensional objects so that they differ in only one dimension such as size or orientation. More often than not there are small differences in the visual appearance of the objects' surfaces, perhaps a finger smudge or a nick in the paint, which can be used by a subject to tell one object from another. We had to have objects that were as identical from trial to trial as those used by visual psychophysicists. To do this we developed a virtual workbench, illustrated in Fig. 3, in which a high-resolution monitor was positioned directly above a first-surface mirror. When subjects viewed the reflected image of the monitor screen through stereo goggles, they saw a virtual three-dimensional object below the surface of the mirror. A real object identical in size to the virtual object was positioned by means of a robot arm at the corresponding location below the mirror. Thus, when subjects reached out to pick up the virtual object, they ended up grasping the real object under the mirror. This arrangement ensured that the subject experienced haptic feedback that corresponded to the visual information from the virtual image. The movements of the hand and fingers were tracked using conventional opto-electronic recording, in which small infra-red light-emitting diodes attached to the index finger, thumb, and wrist were tracked at 100 Hz by two infra-red sensitive cameras.

In our first experiment, undergraduate students were required to make an explicit comparison between the sizes of two virtual objects before picking up one of them. In one condition, subjects were asked to pick up the larger one of two objects, in the other condition, they were asked to pick up the smaller one. In fact, as Fig. 4 shows, in both conditions, they were picking up the same target objects, each of which had been paired with a corresponding smaller or larger object. One group of subjects were required to pick up the target object (the larger or

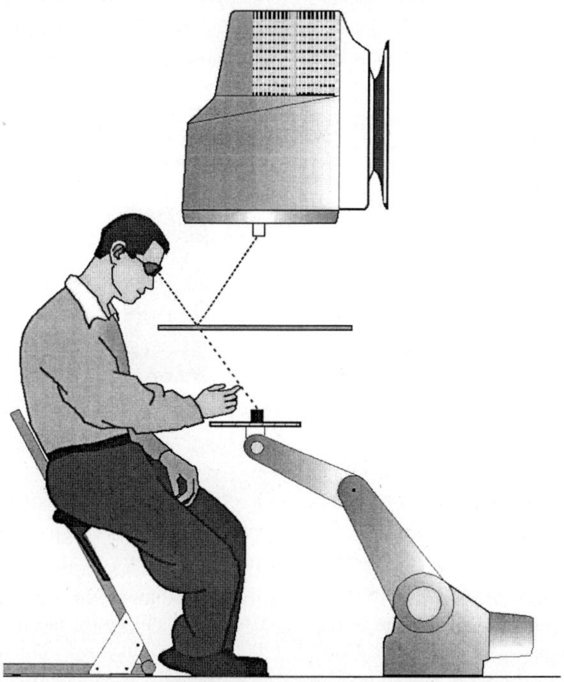

Fig. 3. Simple illustration of the virtual workbench showing the relationship between the virtual and real objects. (Adapted with permission from Hu and Goodale, 2000.)

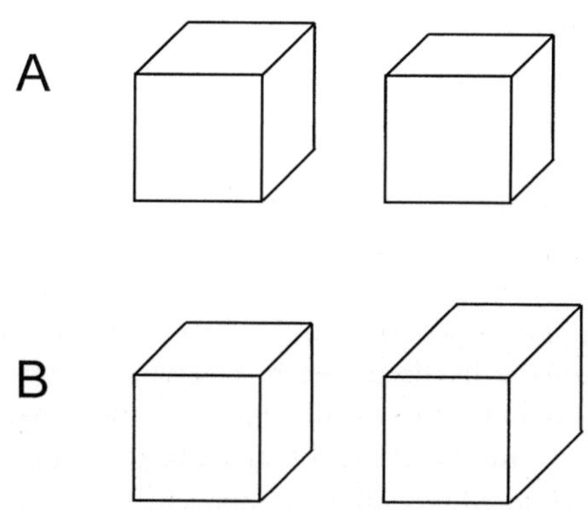

Fig. 4. The 3-dimensional virtual objects used in the 'virtual workbench' experiments carried out by Hu and Goodale (2000). Subjects were instructed to grasp the larger object in display A and the smaller object in display B. In fact, these two objects were identical in size. (Adapted with permission from Hu and Goodale, 2000.)

the smaller one) as soon as the two objects came into view. A second group of subjects were required to pick up the target object after a 5-s delay during which the two objects were no longer in view. In both cases, the actual grasping movement was made in 'visual open loop' and neither the objects nor the moving hand was visible during the hand movement. We had to run the study in open loop to avoid subjects having the potentially unsettling experience of reaching towards a visible object without seeing their hand. These open loop grasping movements feel quite 'normal' and in fact, such movements are only slightly different from grasping movements made in closed loop, where the subject can see their hand and the object throughout the movement (Jakobson and Goodale, 1991).

We anticipated that those subjects who grasped the target object immediately in 'real time' would not be influenced by the difference in size between the target object and its companion. In other words, we predicted that maximum grip aperture, a kinematic parameter that has been shown to be highly correlated with object size (Jeannerod, 1988; Jakobson and Goodale, 1991), would not be influenced by this relative size information. The reason for this prediction is clear. Although the subjects' choice of target object (the smaller one or the larger one) would be mediated by the conscious perception of the entire visual array, the grasping movement itself would be programmed on the basis of the actual size of the target object — not its relative size with respect to the other object. In other words, we expected that the scaling of maximum grip aperture, which is achieved well before contact with the target object, would reflect the absolute size of that object rather than its relative size with respect to the smaller or larger object with which it had been paired. In the case of the delayed grasping movements, however, we expected that the maximum grip aperture would now be influenced by the relative difference in size between the two objects. In this case, any real-time visuomotor program that might have been formed would have decayed over the 5-s delay period, and the grasp instead would have to be programmed on the basis of stored information about object size. We expected that this stored information would have been formed on the basis of earlier perceptual processing of the visual array, and thus would have incorporated the relative size of the two objects. In other words, we expected that after a delay, subjects would open their fingers wider for a target object paired with a smaller object than they would for the same object when it was paired with a larger object.

What did we find? As predicted, the scaling of the grasping movements produced by subjects who reached out immediately to pick up the target object was not affected by the presence of another larger or smaller object — even though the subjects had been asked to make an explicit comparison between the size of the two objects in the array. As the difference score in Fig. 5 illustrates, maximum grip aperture was the same for a given target object whether that object was accompanied by a larger object or by a smaller one. It is also important to note that subjects were still scaling for the real width of the different target objects that were presented. In other words, the larger the target object, the wider they opened their hand.

The picture was quite different for the subjects who reached out to pick up the object after a 5-s delay. In their case, maximum grip aperture was larger when the target object was accompanied by

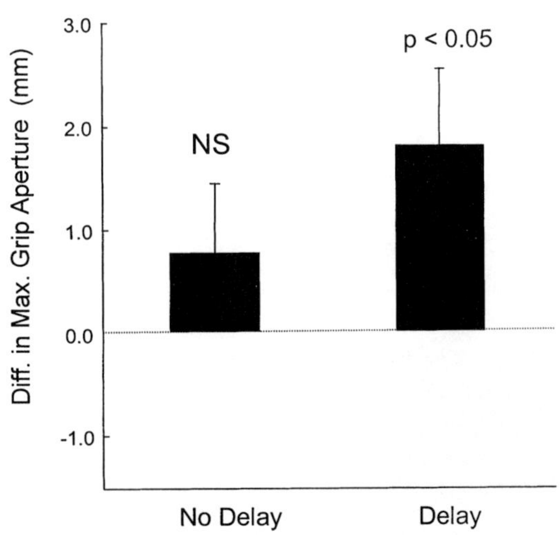

Fig. 5. Mean values of the difference in maximum grip aperture between grasping the 'larger' and 'smaller' objects in the first experiment by Hu and Goodale (2000). In fact, the target object was the same size in both cases; it was simply accompanied by a larger object in one case and a smaller object in the other. (Error bars represent the standard error of the mean difference.) (Adapted with permission from Hu and Goodale, 2000.)

a smaller object than when it was accompanied by a larger object. Overall, as the difference score in Fig. 5 shows, subjects opened their fingers significantly wider when they were required to pick up the larger of the two objects than when they were required to pick up the smaller one, even though the target object was in fact the same one in both conditions. Of course, superimposed on this relative size effect was the effect of the real width of the target object: the wider the target object, the wider they opened their hand.

The fact that grip scaling becomes sensitive to the relative size of an object after a delay, I believe, reflects a shift in motor programming from absolute to relative metrics. Even a delay as short as 5 s forces the subject to rely, not on the real-time visuomotor transformations that would normally be used to program an object-directed grasping movement, but on stored perceptual memories of the target object and the array in which it was embedded. Because conscious perception uses relative metrics, the relative size of the two objects in the array stored in memory can influence the scaling of the grasp when the object is no longer in view.

But perhaps we were biasing the subjects to use relative information. After all, the subjects had been asked to make an explicit comparison between the sizes of the two objects in the array. Perhaps these instructions primed subjects to store the relative size of the two objects in memory. Alternatively the very language, 'larger' or 'smaller', could have led to the use of a larger or smaller grasp when subjects were working 'off-line' after a delay, and were recalling what it was they had seen 5 s earlier.

To eliminate these possibilities, we carried out a second experiment in which subjects were not required to make a size discrimination. In this experiment, one of the objects was marked with a red dot and subjects were simply instructed to pick up the marked object. Over a series of randomized trials, the object marked with a red dot was paired with a smaller object, a larger object, or an object of the same size. We found that subjects who picked up the marked object in 'real time' were not affected by the presence of another larger or smaller object. As Fig. 6 illustrates, maximum grip aperture was the same for a given target object whether that object was larger or the smaller of the two objects in the array. Just as was the case in Experiment 1, however, the subjects' grip aperture was sensitive to the actual width of the target object. As expected, the picture was quite different for the subjects who reached out to pick up the marked object after a 5-s delay. As can be seen in the difference scores summarized in Fig. 6, subjects opened their fingers significantly wider when the marked object was the larger of the two objects than when it was the smaller one — even though the marked object was the same size in both kinds of trials. Again, as was the case in the first experiment, an effect of the real width of the object was superimposed on the relative size effect: the wider the target object, the wider the subjects opened their hand.

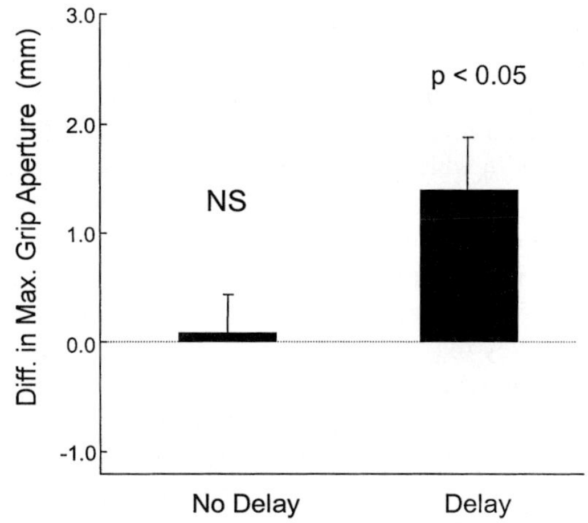

Fig. 6. Mean values of the difference in maximum grip aperture in the second experiment by Hu and Goodale (2000) between grasping the marked objects accompanied by a larger object and grasping the marked objects accompanied by a smaller object. (Error bars represent the standard error of the mean difference.) (Adapted with permission from Hu and Goodale, 2000.)

The results of this second experiment showed that the shift from an absolute to a relative metric for grip scaling during the delay period is not dependent on some sort of instructional or verbal mediation. Instead, it appears that stored perceptual memories of the objects that are used to program the delayed response are indeed organized in relative metrics.

If the relative metrics displayed in the scaling of the grip aperture after a delay truly reflect the invocation of stored percepts, then subjects should show relative scaling of their conscious judgements of object size in this situation — and this relative scaling should occur even when subjects make these judgements in real time. To demonstrate that this was indeed the case, Yaoping Hu and I conducted a third experiment in which subjects were requested to make estimate the size of target objects in the same two-object array that we had used in the second experiment. In other words, subjects were asked to judge the size of the virtual object that was marked with a red dot. They made these estimates of size by opening their thumb and index finger a matching amount while keeping their hand on the start platform of the apparatus. The dimension they were asked to estimate was the width of the object, the same dimension across which subjects in the two earlier experiments had grasped the object. Once subjects had given their manual estimate, they too were required to reach out and pick up the object — thus ensuring that they had the same haptic feedback about object size as the subjects in the grasping experiments.

As the difference scores depicted in Fig. 7 illustrate, the conscious estimates of the width of the marked object were influenced by the other object in scene, no matter whether subjects gave the estimates immediately or after a 5-s delay. In both delay and no-delay conditions, subjects opened their fingers significantly wider when the marked object was the larger of the two objects than when it was the smaller one — even though the marked object was the same size in both kinds of trials. Again, superimposed on this relative size effect was the effect of the real width of the object: in all conditions, the wider the target object, the wider the subjects opened their fingers in manual estimations. The results of this experiment show that even in real time our conscious perception is influenced by the relative size of objects in the visual scene. Moreover the order of magnitude of the difference in estimation that we observed in this experiment was similar to that seen in grip scaling after a delay.

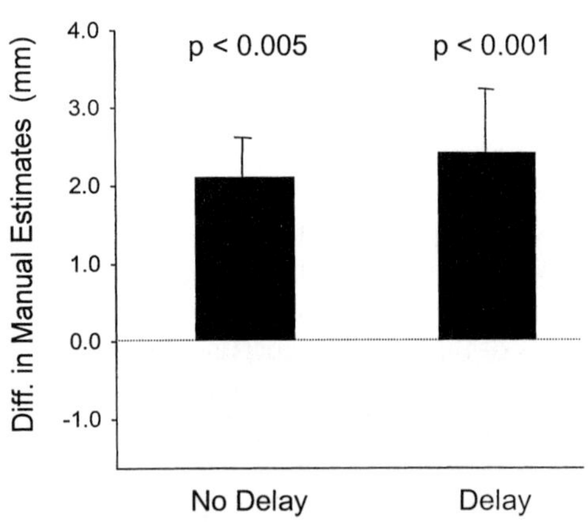

Fig. 7. Mean values of the difference in perceptual estimates in the third experiment by Hu and Goodale (2000) between estimating the width of the marked objects accompanied by a larger object and estimating the width of the marked objects accompanied by a smaller object. (Error bars represent the standard error of the mean difference.) (Adapted with permission from Hu and Goodale, 2000.)

Taken together, the results of the three experiments that Yaoping Hu and I carried out provide convincing evidence for a dissociation between the metrics used by the visual mechanisms mediating perception and those used by the visual mechanisms mediating the control of action. The fact that grip scaling was insensitive to the contrast in size between the two objects in the scene parallels the findings of studies discussed earlier where pictorial illusions that fool our perception of object size were shown not to affect the real-time scaling of object-directed actions (Aglioti et al., 1995; Vishton and Cutting, 1995; Brenner and Smeets, 1996; Gentilucci et al., 1996; Haffenden and Goodale, 1998; Jackson and Shaw, 2000). Interestingly, a recent report by Westwood et al. (2000) provides evidence that the Müller–Lyer illusion can affect grip scaling if a short delay in introduced between viewing the display and grasping an object placed on the display. In real time, of course, grip scaling remains refractory to the illusion.

It is important to note that the stimulus array that Yaoping Hu and I used was not so much a contrived illusion, as it was an example of a situation in our daily life when we are confronted with two or more possible goal objects. Yet even though there were only two objects in the array, subjects' perception of one object's size was influenced by the presence of the other, while their real-time grip scaling was not.

Delayed visuomotor responses in neurological patients

The demonstration of a shift from on-line visuomotor metrics to stored perceptual metrics may help explain some otherwise puzzling observations in neurological patients. Consider, for example, the patient D.F., a young woman who developed visual form agnosia as a result of anoxia from carbon monoxide poisoning (Milner et al., 1991). Even though D.F. is unable to indicate the size, shape, and orientation of an object, either verbally or manually, she shows normal preshaping and rotation of her hand when reaching out to grasp it (Goodale and Milner, 1992). Although one must always be cautious when interpreting neuroimaging data from patients with brain damage that resulted from anoxia, MRI scans taken a year after her accident are consistent with the suggestion that the human homologue of the ventral stream in D.F. is compromised while the dorsal pathway to the posterior parietal cortex is relatively spared. Despite the fact that D.F. shows accurate scaling of grasp aperture in real time, all evidence of such scaling vanished when she was required to initiate her hand movements following a 2-s delay after viewing the object (Goodale et al., 1994). Now there was no correlation at all between the size of the object and the aperture of her grasp in flight. Presumably, D.F. — unlike the normal subjects in the present experiment — could not use a visual memory of the objects that were presented earlier to program her delayed grasping movements, because D.F. did not perceive those objects in the first place.

A converse example is the patient A.T., who suffered damage to the visuomotor systems in her dorsal stream and is unable to scale her grasp for unfamiliar 'neutral' targets, whose size and shape have to computed directly on-line. Surprisingly, when presented with familiar objects of the same size, A.T. showed much better scaling (Jeannerod et al., 1994), probably because she was able to invoke stored perceptual memories of those objects and use those memories to program her actions. It would be interesting in this context to see what would happen if A.T. were asked to delay her grasping to neutral objects. One might expect to see an improvement in grip scaling with delay since now she would be forced to rely on perceptual memories of what she had just seen rather than on the more 'automatic' visuomotor computations that are clearly not working properly. Although no evidence has been published to support this prediction, David Milner and his colleagues have recently shown a paradoxical improvement in A.T.'s performance on a pointing task when she was asked to delay her response for 5 s after the visual target had disappeared (Milner et al., 1999). Intact subjects, of course, typically get worse when a delay is introduced. As the authors themselves comment "when an immediate response was required, A.T.'s damaged visuomotor system caused her to make large errors; but when a delay was required, a different, more flexible, visuospatial coding system — presumably relatively intact in her brain — came into play, resulting in much more accurate responses. The data are consistent with a dual processing theory whereby motor responses made directly to visual stimuli are guided by a dedicated system in the superior parietal and premotor cortices, while responses to remembered stimuli depend on perceptual processing and may thus crucially involve processing within the temporal neocortex." (p. 2225).

The effect of other objects on target-directed grasping

The fact that normal grasping movements are scaled for the real and the not the relative size of the goal object does not mean that the visuomotor system completely ignores other objects that might be present in the workspace. The most obvious way that other objects can influence the shaping of a grasping movement is by blocking access to the goal. In short, other objects can act as obstacles. In programming the grasping movement, the visuomotor system must certainly take into account the position of potential obstacles so that collision with them can be avoided (for review, see Tresilian, 1998).

This means that under certain conditions the presence of objects in the vicinity of a target object could have effects not only on the perception of the target but also on the actions directed at the target. But the range over which these effects are likely to operate is going to be different for perception and action — with objects at some distance from the target having a greater effect on perception than on action. Indeed, unless the objects are potential obstacles for a target-directed action, they are likely to have no effect at all on the constituent movements of the action once the goal for the action has been selected. In the study that Yaoping Hu and I carried out, for example, the companion object, which was located to the left or right of the target object in the virtual array, was not close enough (or in the right position) to interfere with the grasping movement. As a consequence, the visuomotor system did not have to take the flanking object into account when programming the grasping movement directed at the target. But the presence of the companion object, as we saw, did affect the perceptual judgments of object size — by providing a contrast against which the size judgments could be implicitly compared.

There are some displays, however, in which the elements in the array can have dual effects on the scaling of grasp and perceptual estimates of size. One such display is the Ebbinghaus illusion described earlier, in which two target circles, each surrounded by a circular array of either smaller or larger circles, are presented side by side (see Fig. 2). Although in the Aglioti et al. (1995) and Haffenden and Goodale (1998) studies there was a clear dissociation between the effects of the illusion on perceptual judgments and the scaling of the grasp, there appeared to be a small effect of the illusion on grasping, particularly in the condition where the two target circles were the same physical size. In the Aglioti et al. study, the effect reached significance but was significantly smaller than the perceptual effect. In the Haffenden and Goodale study, the effect on grasp was not significant. As small as the effect was, it needed to be explained. At the time, we suggested that the small effect reflected the fact that the control of skilled movements is not completely isolated from perceptual information. It is self-evident, after all, that the perceived function of an object will influence the nature of the grasp that we adopt when we pick up that object. There is some possibility, therefore, that perceptual analysis of the scene could affect grip scaling to some degree, even though that effect would undoubtedly be much smaller than the effect on the subjects' conscious judgements of size. Although this explanation appeared to be quite parsimonious, there was evidence in the Haffenden and Goodale study that could provide an alternative account — one that is more consistent with the idea outlined above that the objects surrounding a target are treated as potential obstacles by the visuomotor system.

In the Haffenden and Goodale (1998) study, we included a control condition designed to test whether

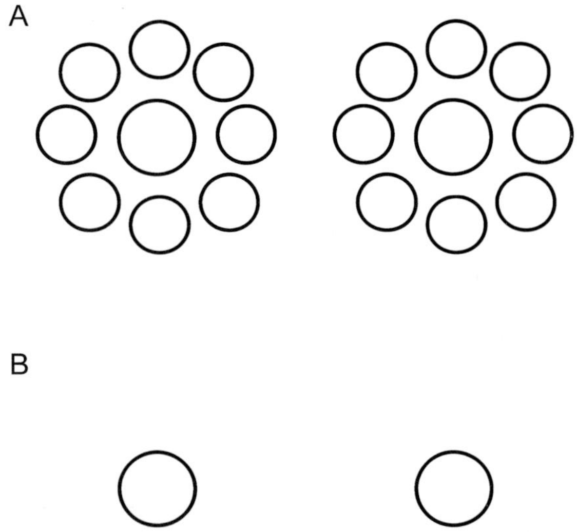

Fig. 8. The two control displays used by Haffenden and Goodale (1998) to examine the effects of surrounding elements on the control of visually guided prehension. (A) The equal-annuli display in which the perceptual effect of the surrounding elements on the two target disks was equivalent. (B) The 'control' display in which the target disks were presented without surrounding elements. (Adapted with permission from Haffenden and Goodale, 2000.)

or not the simple presence of flanking stimuli (i.e. the surrounding annulus) would affect the scaling of the grasp independent of any illusory effect. To do this, we created two displays: one in which the two targets were presented on their own, and another in which the two targets were surrounded by identical annuli made up of circles that were slightly smaller than the target disks (see Fig. 8). Because the two annuli were identical in the one display, any perceptual influence of the annuli would have to be the same on both disks in that display. Nevertheless, a size-contrast effect was produced on the perceptual judgements such that the disks surrounded by annuli were estimated to be larger than the same disks presented on their own. Quite the opposite effect, however, occurred in grasping. When subjects reached out to pick up one of the target disks on trials in which the two disks were surrounded by control annuli, their grip aperture was not as large as it was on trials when the disks were presented without surrounding annuli. To compare the differential effects of the displays on grip scaling and on manual estimations of size, difference scores were calculated in which

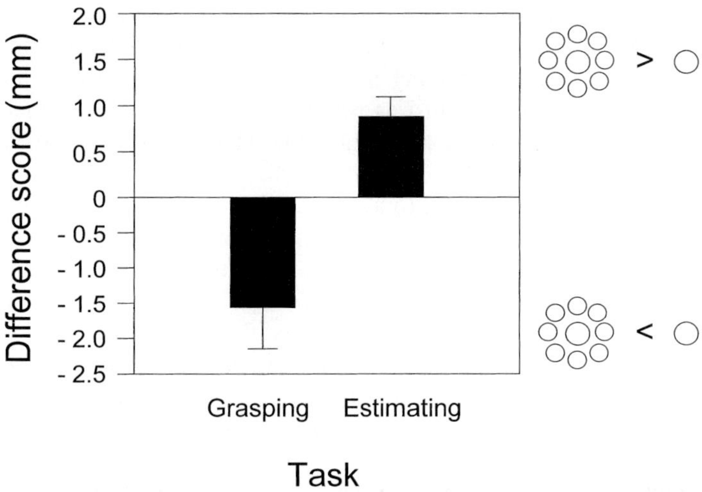

Fig. 9. The differing effects of the control displays on grip scaling and perceptual judgments of size. The bars represent the mean difference scores (the response to the targets presented on the equal annuli display minus the response to targets presented without surrounding annuli) for grasp and manual estimates. (Adapted with permission from Haffenden and Goodale, 2000.)

the average response to the targets presented without annuli was subtracted from the average response to the targets surrounded by the control annuli. For grip scaling, the difference score was negative, and for manual estimations the difference score was positive (see Fig. 9). Both these scores differed significantly from zero and from each other.

Why did the presence of the annuli have opposite effects on grasp and perceptual judgements? It is easy to see why there was an effect on perception. There was a size-contrast effect: the target disks were noticeably smaller than the circles that made up the surrounding annuli. The effect of the surrounding annuli on grip aperture, however, cannot be explained as a perceptual influence on grip scaling since the presence of the annuli made the grip smaller rather than larger. Instead, in line with the argument made earlier, it looks as though the surrounding annuli might have been treated as obstacles to be avoided. This situation is similar to that faced when reaching into a hole; the hand must open wide enough to encompass the target object, but not so wide that it cannot fit into the hole. When faced with a target object surrounded by potential obstacles, the visuomotor system must ensure that the opening of the hand is 'pared down' to avoid collision with those obstacles. For these reasons, the hand would be expected not to open as wide when the target disks were surrounded by the annuli as it would when the disks were presented on their own.

Of course, the circles in the annuli of the Ebbinghaus display are not really obstacles. They are, after all, only line drawings. Nevertheless, visuomotor systems depend on rapid and reliable computations for which edges, even two-dimensional edges, could form part of the input for programming and controlling the movement. The main function of the visuomotor control mediating the grasp is to get the hand safely to the target and the fingers on stable grasp points. In the real world, sharp edges signal the presence of potential obstacles or targets. Thus, the most efficient strategy would be to take into account any visual contours around the target that could potentially interfere with the execution of the grasp.

Although this 'ecological' account of the effects of obstacles on grip scaling is speculative, it does help explain why, in the Haffenden and Goodale (1998) control experiment just described, the effects of the surrounding annulus on perceived size and grip scaling were in the opposite directions. Such an account, however, need not always predict opposite effects on perception and action. In fact, there may be circumstances under which the effect of pictorial illusion on perception might coincide with the effect of the non-target stimuli on visuomotor programming. Take the case of the small effect of the Ebbinghaus display on grasp in the Aglioti et al. (1995) study that we described earlier. In that study, subjects opened their hand slightly wider for the target disk surrounded by an annulus of small circles than they did for the same disk surrounded by the annulus of large circles. Although this was interpreted as a small effect of perception on grasp, it can also be explained by the ecological account described above. When the target disk was surrounded by the annulus made up of large circles, the situation was similar to that of the control annuli. In other words, the target was flanked on all sides by circles, with a finger-width gap between the target and the surrounding circles. Thus one might expect that the opening of the hand would be scaled down to fit inside the annulus and grasp the target. This effect is in the same direction as the perceptual effect of the large-circle annulus; when the target disk was presented in the annulus comprised of large circles it appears to be smaller than it actually is. In contrast to this, when the target was surrounded by the small circle annulus, there was essentially no gap between the target and surrounding stimuli, thus in this case making it impossible to fit the hand between the annuli and target disk. In fact, here it is possible that subjects might actually open their hand slightly wider as if to grasp the entire display.

So far all of this is essentially a post hoc argument. Recently, however, Angela Haffenden and I tested this idea in two separate experiments. In the first experiment (Haffenden and Goodale, 2000), we systematically varied the location of potential 'obstacles' with respect to the target by manipulating the orientation of flanking elements in the classic 'assimilation' or 'attraction' illusion. In this illusion, the edges of the target are thought to be perceptually drawn towards the edge of the nearby flanking elements (for review see Rock, 1995). Thus, the closer the flanking elements, the stronger the attraction, and consequently the larger the perceived size of the target. We reasoned that varying the orientation of flanking elements around a target object in this illusion would have no effect on perceptual judgements of target size, but would have an effect on grasp depending on whether or not the elements were adjacent to the contact points for the grasp (see Fig. 10). Thus, two flanking objects that were oriented horizontally, one close to the far edge and one close to the near edge of the target, could potentially interfere with a grasping movement directed at the near and far edges. Just as was the case with the Ebbinghaus control display used in the Haffenden and Goodale (1998) study, subjects might 'pare down' the opening of their hand to avoid 'collision' with the horizontal flankers. The same flanking objects oriented vertically and placed to the left and right of the same target should not interfere with the grasp, at least not in the same way, since they would not be close to the contact points for the grasp. But, to reiterate, there is no a priori reason to expect that perceptual judgements of size would be affected by this manipulation.

The results of the experiment were straightforward. There was a large effect of the flanking elements on the manual estimates of target size: the closer the flanking elements, the larger the estimates of target size. But importantly, this effect was independent of the orientation of the flanking elements. In other words, the effect on perception was the same whether the flanking elements were oriented horizontally or whether they were oriented vertically — and this was true for all distances between the flanking elements and the target. In contrast to the clear effect of the flanking elements on the perception of target size, there was no overall effect of the flanking elements on grip scaling. Nevertheless, close examination of grip aperture on those trials where there was a 'finger-sized gap' between the target and the flanking elements revealed a small but consistent effect of flanker orientation on grip aperture, such that the grip aperture was smaller for horizontally oriented flankers than for vertically oriented flankers. In other words, there was a small reduction in grip aperture when flankers were placed adjacent to contact points for the grasp. The magnitude of this effect corresponded nicely with the effects on grip aperture observed in the earlier Ebbinghaus experiments.

In our second experiment (Haffenden et al., 2001), we decided to test more directly the possible independence of the effects of the Ebbinghaus display on grasp and on perceptual judgments. We did this by manipulating the size of the gap between the annulus and the target disk. Three different displays, each consisting of a single target disk surrounded by an annulus, were used. These displays are illustrated

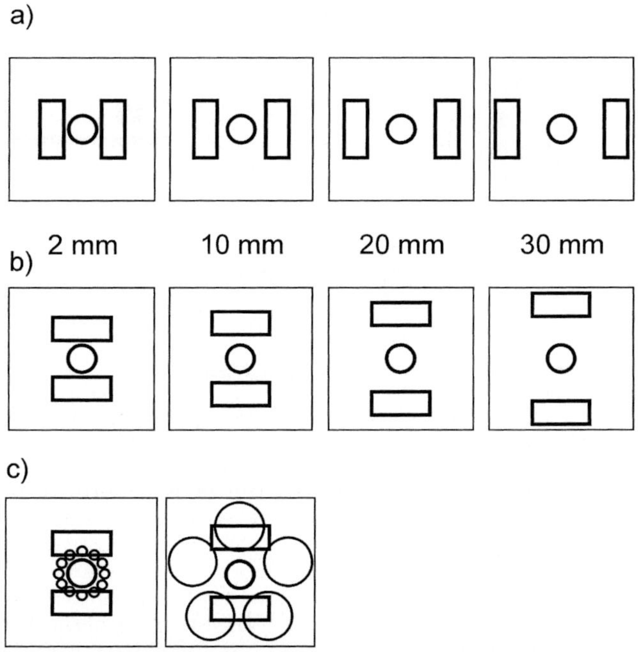

Fig. 10. The displays used in the flanking element study. The plastic target disks were centered between two-dimensional flanking rectangles that were placed at four different distances from the target in two different orientations: (a) vertically oriented flanking elements placed beside the left and right edges of the target; or (b) horizontally oriented flanking elements placed next to the near and far edges of the target. Subjects were instructed to grasp the disks at the near and far edges. (c) A schematic diagram illustrating how the flanking rectangle displays were designed to emulate the target–annulus distances of the Ebbinghaus display used in previous studies. The display in which the flanking rectangles were 3 mm away from the mean of the two sizes of target disks matched the distance in the small circle annulus. The display in which the flanking rectangles were 11 mm away from the mean of the two sizes of target disks matched the distance in the large circle annulus. (Adapted with permission from Haffenden and Goodale, 2000.)

in Fig. 11. Two of the displays consisted of the conventional small-circle and large-circle annuli that we and others had employed earlier. The remaining display consisted of a small-circle annulus in which the gap between the annulus and the target disk was the same size as the gap between the annulus and target in the large-circle display, a gap that was big enough for the fingers to fit into. In other words, two displays had annular circles of the same size but different gap sizes, and two displays had annular circles of different sizes but the same 'finger-sized' gap between the annulus and the target. When subjects were asked to judge the size of the target disks, they judged the disks that were surrounded by large-circle annuli as being much smaller than identical targets surrounded by either of the two annuli of small circles. The difference in the size of the gap between the annulus and the target in the two small-circle displays had only a small effect on size judgments. Quite the opposite pattern was observed for grip aperture. Now the size of the gap mattered a great deal. Subjects 'pared' down their grasp when picking up the target disk when there was a finger-sized gap between the annulus and the target, independent of whether the annulus was made up of large circles or small circles. They opened their hand wider for the target surrounded by a small-circle annulus that had only a narrow gap between the annulus and the target. The differential effects of these displays on manual estimates of target size and grip scaling are illustrated in Fig. 12. As this figure indicates, perceptual judgements of target size were affected most by the size of the surrounding circles, while grip scaling was affected most by the size of the gap between the target and the surrounding circles.

The results of all these experiments make it clear that pictorial displays can have quite independent and opposite effects on perception and action. As

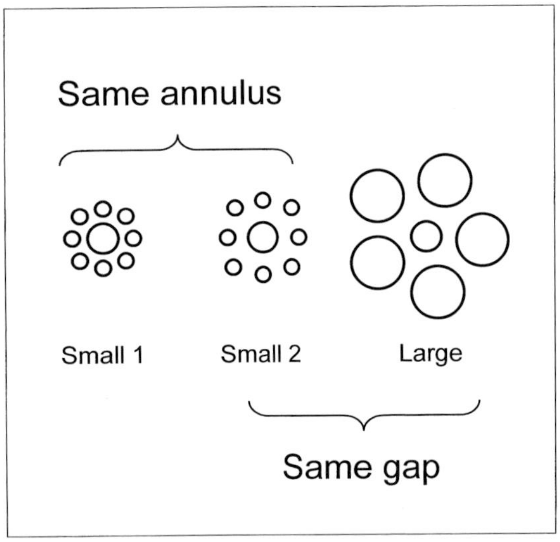

Fig. 11. The three displays used in the last experiment by Haffenden and Goodale. 'Small 1' and 'Small 2' had the same small-circle annuli but different sized gaps between the annuli and the target disk. 'Small 2' and 'Large' had different annuli but the same finger-sized gap between the annuli and the target disk. (Adapted with permission from Haffenden et al., 2001.)

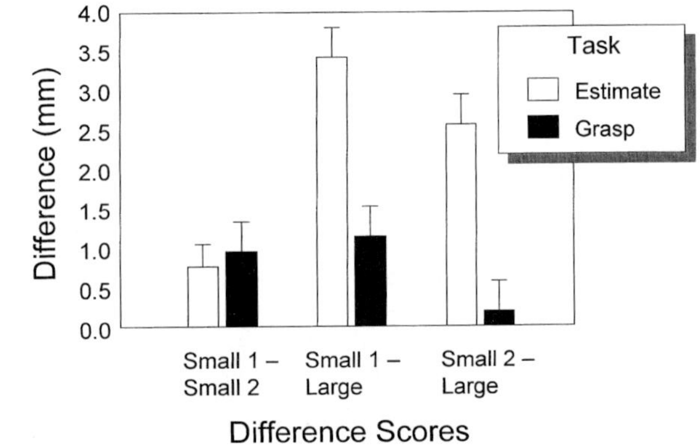

Fig. 12. Graph illustrating the mean differences between the manual estimates and grip aperture for each of the possible comparisons between the three displays. Note that for manual estimates, the smallest difference was obtained between the two displays in which the circles in the annuli were the same size (both small) but the gaps were different sizes, whereas for grip aperture, the smallest difference was obtained between the displays in which the circles in the annuli were different sizes but the gaps were the same size. (Adapted with permission from Haffenden et al., 2001.)

I pointed out earlier, however, the direction of the effect of the flanking elements on grip scaling can sometimes coincide with the direction of the predicted perceptual effect. For example, in a particular display, both grip aperture and manual estimates could be reduced by the presence of flanking objects — albeit for quite different reasons. Indeed, it is possible that previous experiments reporting significant effects of illusory displays on grip scaling did not adequately account for this possibility, and confused the treatment of flanking elements as obstacles with the effects of the illusion on perceived size. This may have been the case in a recent study employing the Ebbinghaus Illusion (Franz et al., 2000). Franz et al. presented subjects with half of the Ebbinghaus illusion on each trial, that is, a single target surrounded by either the large or the small circle annulus. In doing so, they attempted to equate the attentional demands of the perceptual task with the demands of the grasping task. As they clearly show, the magnitude of the perceptual effect is greatly reduced by this single annulus presentation method, as compared to the perceptual effect produced by presenting two targets simultaneously, one surrounded by large circles and the other by small circles. This reduced perceptual effect resulting from the single annulus presentations was similar in magnitude to that seen in the grasp, leading the authors to conclude that the same internal representation of target size was used for both perceptual judgments and the programming of the grasp. This is a strong conclusion, particularly since the authors did not control for the differences in distance between the targets and edge of the circles making up the two different sized annuli. Nor did they include a grasping condition in which the target disk was presented on its own. Their conclusion rests entirely on the fact that the effect on perceptual judgments and the effect on grasp are in the same direction and of similar magnitude. But as the experiments discussed above demonstrate, pictorial elements can have independent effects on perception and action. The direction of these independent effects can sometimes coincide by virtue of the layout of the display that is used to test them. Only by careful design can the two effects be pulled apart.

Coincidental perceptual and visuomotor effects may also help to account for the effects of other illusory displays on grip scaling. For example, take the recent observation by Daprati and Gentilucci (1997) that the illusion has a small but significant effect on grip scaling. The authors raised the possibility that the open-wing elements could have acted as obstacles to the grasping hand, but in the end decided that this could not be the case since only the shaft of the Müller–Lyer display was a three-dimensional object; the wings of each configuration were two-dimensional figures. Our experiments, however, suggest that such two-dimensional elements can be treated as obstacles by the visuomotor system and can generate effects on pre-contact grip scaling that are quite separate from the effects the display might have on perceptual judgements. In the Daprati and Gentilucci experiment, the predicted 'obstacle' effect of the wings on grasp coincided with the established (and much larger) perceptual effect of the wings. Only with a different arrangement of the display would it be possible to disentangle the small effects of two-dimensional 'obstacles' from any putative perceptual effects on grasp scaling.

In summary, it seems clear that two-dimensional displays, such as those used to create size-contrast illusions, can influence grasping in ways that are quite separate from the influence of these displays on perception. This observation opens up the possibility of designing displays that reveal even more about how the different movements that constitute a grasp are programmed and controlled. It also suggests that patients, such as D.F., who show intact visuomotor control despite profound deficits in perception, should continue to be sensitive to the presence of potential obstacles when reaching out to grasp goal objects. In fact, recent experiments by Rob McIntosh and colleagues (personal communication) show that this is the precisely the case, suggesting that her intact dorsal action stream takes into account the position of potential obstacles when programming a grasping movement.

Biological tele-assistance

Throughout this chapter, I have emphasized the distinction between vision for perception and vision for action — two decidedly different visual systems within the primate brain. It is important to remember, however, that the two systems evolved together and play complementary roles in the control of behavior. In some ways, the limitations of one system are the strengths of the other. Perception (which is mediated by the ventral stream of visual projections in primate cortex) delivers a rich and detailed representation of the world, but does not compute the detailed metrics of the scene with respect to the observer. In contrast, the action system (which depends heavily on dorsal stream projections) delivers accurate metrical information about an object in the required egocentric coordinates for action, but these computations are fleeting and are for the most part limited to the particular goal object that has been selected.

A useful analogy for understanding the different contributions of the dorsal action stream and the ventral perception stream to visually guided behavior can be found in robotic engineering. That analogy is *tele-assistance* (Pook and Ballard, 1996), one of the general schemes that have been devised whereby human operators can control robots working in hostile environments, such as a deep mine shaft or the surface of another planet. In tele-assistance, a human operator identifies the goal, such as interesting geological specimen on the surface of Mars, and then uses a symbolic language to communicate with a semi-autonomous robot that actually picks up the rock that has been identified or 'flagged' by the human operator. The semi-autonomous robot uses its on-board rangefinders and other devices to compute the location and disposition of the rock with respect to itself and its end-effectors.

Tele-assistance is much more flexible than a completely autonomous robot. Autonomous robots are very useful in certain environments such as an automobile assembly line, where the tasks that the robot has to perform are highly constrained and well-specified. But even though autonomous robots can carry out highly precise operations, they can do this only in the working environment for which they have been designed. Such robots could not cope with events that their programmers had not anticipated. Imagine the difficulty, for example, of programming an autonomous robot so that it could deal with everything it might encounter on the surface of Mars.

At present, the only way to make sure that the robot does the right thing in a novel environment is to have a human operator somewhere in the loop. One way to do this is to have the human operator control the movements of the robot in a one-to-one fashion, where the movements or instructions of the human operator (the master) are simply reproduced by the robot (the slave). For instance an operator in a nuclear plant might move a joystick, which in turn directly controls the movements of a robot arm in a radioactive laboratory. Such tele-operation, as this method of control is sometimes called, cannot cope well with sudden changes in scale (on the video monitor) or with a significant delay between the communicated action and feedback from that action. But tele-assistance can.

In tele-assistance, the human operator does not have to worry about the real metrics of the workspace or the timing of the movements made by the robot; instead, the human operator has the job of identifying a goal and specifying an action on that goal in general terms. Once this information is communicated to the semi-autonomous robot, the robot can use its on-board range finders and other sensing devices to work out the required movements for achieving the specified goal. In short, tele-assistance combines the flexibility of tele-operation with the precision of autonomous robotic control.

The division of labor between the two visual systems in the primate brain corresponds nicely to this engineering principle. The perceptual–cognitive system in the ventral stream, like the human operator in tele-assistance, identifies different objects in the scene — using a representational system that is rich in detail but not metrically precise. When a particular goal object has been flagged, dedicated visuomotor networks in the dorsal stream, in conjunction with output systems elsewhere in the brain (located in premotor cortex, basal ganglia, and brainstem) are activated to perform the desired motor act. In other words, the action systems in the dorsal stream, with their precise egocentric coding of the location, size, orientation, and shape of the goal object, are like the robotic component of tele-assistance. Both systems have to work together in the production of purposive behavior — one system to select the goal object from the visual array, the other to carry out the required metrical computations for the goal-directed action. In short, the existence of separate, but interacting, visual systems for perception and action is a clear case in which biology has once again anticipated an elegant solution to a difficult problem in engineering science.

References

Aglioti, S., DeSouza, J.F.X. and Goodale, M.A. (1995) Size-contrast illusions deceive the eye but not the hand. *Curr. Biol.*, 5: 679–685.

Batista, A.P., Buneo, C.A., Snyder, L.H. and Andersen, R.A. (1999) Reach plans in eye-centered coordinates. *Science*, 285: 257–260.

Brenner, E. and Smeets, J.B.J. (1996) Size illusion influences how we lift but not how we grasp an object. *Exp. Brain Res.*, 111: 473–476.

Bridgeman, B., Kirch, M. and Sperling, A. (1981) Segregation of cognitive and motor aspects of visual function using induced motion. *Percept. Psychophys.*, 29: 336–342.

Bridgeman, B., Peery, S. and Anand, S. (1997) Interaction of cognitive and sensorimotor maps of visual space. *Percept. Psychophys.*, 59: 456–469.

Creem, S.H. and Proffitt, D.R. (1998) Two memories for geographical slant: separation and interdependence of action and awareness. *Psychon. Bull. Rev.*, 5: 22–36.

Creem, S.H., Wraga, M. and Proffitt, D.R. (1998) Perception-action dissociation in a large-scale Müller–Lyer figure. *Invest. Ophthalmol. Vis. Sci.*, 39: 1095.

Crick, F. and Jones, E. (1993) Backwardness of human neuroanatomy. *Nature*, 361: 109–110.

Daprati, E. and Gentilucci, M. (1997) Grasping an illusion. *Neuropsychologia*, 35: 1577–1582.

Elliot, D. and Madalena, J. (1987) The influence of premovement visual information on manual aiming. *Q. J. Exp. Psychol.*, 39A: 541–559.

Franz, V.H., Gegenfurtner, K.R., Bülthoff, H.H. and Fahle, M. (2000) Grasping visual illusions: no evidence for a dissociation between perception and action. *Psychol. Sci.*, 11: 20–25.

Gentilucci, M., Chieffi, S., Daprati, E., Saetti, M.C. and Toni, I. (1996) Visual illusion and action. *Neuropsychologia*, 34: 369–376.

Gnadt, J.W., Bracewell, R.M. and Andersen, R.A. (1991) Sensorimotor transformations during eye movements to remembered targets. *Vision Res.*, 31: 693–715.

Goodale, M.A. and Milner, A.D. (1992) Separate visual pathways for perception and action. *Trends Neurosci.*, 15: 20–25.

Goodale, M.A. and Humphrey, G.K. (1998) The objects of action and perception. *Cognition*, 67: 179–205.

Goodale, M.A., Jakobson, L.S. and Keillor, J.M. (1994) Differences in the visual control of pantomimed and natural grasping movements. *Neuropsychologia*, 32: 1159-1178.

Haffenden, A.M. and Goodale, M.A. (1998) The effect of pictorial illusion on prehension and perception. *J. Cogn. Neurosci.*, 10: 122–136.

Haffenden, A.M. and Goodale, M.A. (2000) Independent effects of pictorial displays on perception and action. *Vision Res.*, 40: 1597–1607.

Haffenden, A.M., Schiff, K.C. and Goodale, M.A. (2001) The dissociation between perception and action in the Ebbinghaus illusion: nonillusory effects of pictorial cues on grasp. *Curr. Biol.*, 11: 177–181.

Hu, Y. and Goodale, M.A. (2000) Grasping after a delay shifts size-scaling from absolute to relative metrics. *J. Cogn. Neurosci.*, 12: 856–868.

Hu, Y., Eagleson, R. and Goodale, M.A. (1999) The effects of delay on the kinematics of grasping. *Exp. Brain Res.*, 126: 109–116.

Jackson, S.R. and Shaw, A. (2000) The Ponzo illusion affects grip-force but not grip-aperture scaling during prehension movements. *J. Exp. Psychol. Hum. Percept. Perform.*, 26: 418–423.

Jakobson, L.S. and Goodale, M.A. (1991) Factors affecting higher-order movement planning: a kinematic analysis of human prehension. *Exp. Brain Res.*, 86: 199–208.

Jeannerod, M. (1988) *The Neural and Behavioural Organization of Goal-Directed Movements*. Oxford University Press, Oxford, pp. 1–283.

Jeannerod, M., Decety, J. and Michel, F. (1994) Impairment of grasping movements following a bilateral posterior parietal lesion. *Neuropsychologia*, 32: 329–380.

Milner, A.D. and Goodale, M.A. (1995) *The Visual Brain in Action*. Oxford University Press, Oxford, pp. 1–248.

Milner, A.D., Perrett, D.I., Johnston, R.S., Benson, P.J., Jordan, T.R., Heeley, D.W., Bettucci, D., Mortara, F., Mutani, R., Terazzi, E. and Davidson, D.L.W. (1991) Perception and action in 'visual form agnosia'. *Brain*, 114: 405–428.

Milner, A.D., Paulignan, Y., Dijkerman, H.C., Michel, F. and Jeannerod, M. (1999) A paradoxical improvement of misreaching in optic ataxia: new evidence for two separate neural systems for visual localization. *Proc. R. Soc. Lond. B Biol. Sci.*, 266: 2225–2229.

Pook, P.K. and Ballard, D.H. (1996) Deictic human/robot interaction. *Robot. Auton. Syst.*, 18: 259–269.

Rensink, R.A., O'Regan, J.K. and Clark, J.J. (1997) To see or not to see: the need for attention to perceive changes in scenes. *Psychol. Sci.*, 8: 368–373.

Rock, I. (1995) *Perception*. Scientific American Library, New York, pp. 1–243.

Servos, P., Carnahan, H. and Fedwick, J. (2000) The visuomotor system resists the horizontal–vertical illusion. *J. Motor Behav.*, 32: 400–404.

Tootell, R.B., Dale, A.M., Sereno, M.I. and Malach, R. (1996) New images from human visual cortex. *Trends Neurosci.*, 19: 481–489.

Tresilian, J.R. (1998) Attention in action or obstruction of movement? A kinematic analysis of avoidance behavior in prehension. *Exp. Brain Res.*, 120: 352–368.

Ungerleider, L.G. and Mishkin, M. (1982) Two cortical visual systems. In: D.J. Ingle, M.A. Goodale and R.J.W. Mansfield (Eds.), *Analysis of Visual Behavior*. MIT Press, Cambridge, MA, pp. 549–586.

Vishton, P.M. and Cutting, J.E. (1995) Veridical size perception for action: reaching vs. estimating. *Invest. Ophthalmol. Vis. Sci.*, 36: 358.

Westwood, D.A., Chapman, C.D. and Roy, E.A. (2000) Pantomimed actions may be controlled by the ventral visual stream. *Exp. Brain Res.*, 130: 545–548.

Wong, E. and Mack, A. (1981) Saccadic programming and perceived location. *Acta Psychol.*, 48: 123–131.

C. Casanova and M. Ptito (Eds.)
Progress in Brain Research, Vol. 134

CHAPTER 21

Asymmetrical masking between radial and parallel motion flow in transparent displays

Marta Iordanova * and Michael W. von Grünau

Department of Psychology, Concordia University, 7141 Sherbrooke Street West, Montreal, PQ, H4B 1R6 Canada

Abstract: Human spatial behavior remains surprisingly accurate and stable, despite the complexities of the concurrent retinal image flow. How does visual motion analysis contribute to behavioral stability? To approach this question, we rely on current knowledge about heading perception and coherent motion extraction from animated random dot displays. This chapter presents psychophysical evidence for an asymmetry in the global visual decomposition of the retinal motion flow. We examined the ability of human observers to identify the radial and the parallel flow component in displays where the two motions were transparently superimposed. Whereas sensitivity to the radial motion remained unaffected by the presence of parallel flow, sensitivity to the latter was greatly degraded in the presence of radial flow. This imbalance was observed within the first 200 ms of motion exposure, prior to the perception of heading (430 ms; Hooge et al. (1999) *Exp. Brain Res.*, 129: 615–628). Although such an asymmetrical masking is well suited to minimize heading errors, whether it really contributes to the extraction of behavioral direction remains an open question.

Introduction

Despite profound differences in their visual systems, all animals are very sensitive to visual motion. Virtually all neurons in the mammalian visual cortex are triggered by motion stimulation, and a large portion of the cortical surface is dedicated to motion processing (Nakayama, 1994). Such redundancy in the neural representation of visual motion is consistent with its important behavioral functions. It is well known, for example, that visual motion controls directly the flight and the landing behavior of flying insects (Srinivasan and Zhang, 2000). In primates and humans, visual motion controls oculomotor pursuit (Ilg, 1997) and induces postural sway (Lee and Aronson, 1974; Stoffregen et al., 1987). Furthermore, large-scale motion creates ego-displacement illusions in passive observers (Brandt et al., 1973) and modulates perceived ego-speed during walking (Rieser et al., 1995). These observations suggest that motion input, which normally works together with the vestibular and kinesthetic senses, can strongly influence and even override the latter.

Despite the obvious biological importance of visual motion, it is still unclear how global motion analysis contributes to different aspects of human spatial orientation and behavior, such as the control of heading during walking and driving, postural stability, or obstacle avoidance. Ever since James J. Gibson drew attention to these issues (Gibson, 1954), they have stirred lively debates. Apart from other considerations, the study of visually guided behaviors in higher vertebrates is especially challenging due to anatomical complications. Whereas insects have immobile eyes, the human retina is placed on top of a series of mobile supports (e.g. the hips, the torso, the head and the eye), which can all rotate relative to one another (Van den Berg, 2000). All these ego-motions introduce retinal image motion.

* Corresponding author: M. Iordanova, Department of Psychology, Concordia University, 7141 Sherbrooke Street West, Montreal, PQ, H4B 1R6 Canada.
Tel.: +1-514-848-2212; Fax: +1-514-848-4545;
E-mail: martai@vax2.concordia.ca

Retinal motion during self-motion

The retinas of the active observer receive complex dynamic stimulation. Many local image motions occur together and their global organization changes rapidly over time. Some of these motions are continuous, others erratic, some are spatially confined, whereas others merge into larger coherent patterns. Typically, motions of limited spatial extent reflect the movement of objects independent of the observer. Object motions, however, may also extend over larger areas of the visual field. This occurs, for example, when groups of small objects move together (e.g. flock of birds or a snowstorm) or when a textured surface slides before the observer (e.g. a train passing by). Self-motion adds a new level of complexity as object motions occur within the context of large-scale self-induced motions which affect the image as a whole. For example, the entire projection expands during forward locomotion, contracts while stepping backwards, rotates during head tilts and shifts during movements of the eyes. It is thus common that during self-motion different global patterns of flow share the same image space.

In particular, we will focus on two different large-scale patterns of retinal flow produced by two common self-motions — forward or backward egomotion along a linear track and horizontal oculomotor pursuit. For simplicity, we will not consider additional retinal motions produced by displacement of the torso and the head.

Radial motion flow

Advancing forward through a rigid three-dimensional world creates a radial pattern of retinal motion flow in which all local motions are directed away from a motionless point in the image. This special point is known as the focus of outflow, the focus of expansion or, more generally, as the focus of motion. Similarly, backward egomotion results in radial contraction with all local motions directed towards the focus of inflow. As long as the gaze remains fixed on an object along the direction of heading, the radial motion flow is symmetrical and is centered at the fovea.

Normally, the radial motion flow contains a gradient of speeds. Local speed varies as a function of the distance between objects and the observer and thus depends on the spatial layout of the environment through which one is moving. Local speed would be slowest for the central images of far objects in the direction of heading and fastest for the peripheral images of close objects which sweep on each side as the observer passes them by. A typical, expanding pattern of radial motion flow is represented in Fig. 3c. Each arrow represents the local velocity vector at a particular point of the image. The arrow's direction represents the local direction of motion, whereas the arrow's length indicates the local motion speed.

Parallel motion flow

By parallel flow we mean global one-directional motion in which all local motions have the same orientation and speed (see Fig. 3a). The impression is of sliding motion along the frontoparallel plane. Pure parallel retinal motion flow is produced by the image of the background when the eyes of a stationary observer pursue a target of interest. Rightward rotation of the eye, for example, transposes the entire retinal image leftwards. The local speed of this parallel flow depends entirely on the rotation speed of the eye — thus all image points move with the same speed, regardless of spatial layout. Parallel retinal motion may also reflect the movement of a textured surface independent of the observer. Such retinal motions, however, are normally offset by optokinetic nystagmus and they rarely affect the entire field of view except under very special conditions (e.g. optokinetic drum stimulation).

Parallel and radial motion flow combined

Of course, pure radial or parallel image motion occur very rarely. During ego-motion, the gaze normally strays away from the direction of heading as one explores points of interest or follows the movement of an object. Consider the motion flow on the retinas of a soccer player who runs across the field while keeping his eyes on the ball. In this, and many other natural situations the retinal motion flow is a combination of at least two self-motion components — radial flow due to ego-motion and parallel flow due to oculomotor pursuit. The extraction of heading direction from such compound retinal motion flow is of special interest for the present discussion (see below). To avoid ambiguity, we will use the term 'retinal flow' to indicate the overall pattern of motion on the retinal surface, be it radial, parallel or a combination of the two. We will avoid the term 'optic flow' because of its exclusive association with the radial structure of the retinal flow during forward egomotion (Gibson, 1954; Van den Berg, 2000).

Heading perception from retinal motion flow

In the 1950s, James Gibson noted that the global pattern of motion flow on the retinas of a moving observer contains regularities which carry useful information about the direction and speed of the self-motion. In particular, Gibson made three strong assertions about the nature of this information and the way in which it is being used (Gibson, 1950, p. 123).

First, Gibson suggested that behavioral direction is completely specified by the radial motion flow. More specifically, he pointed out that the focus of expansion, defined by the radial structure of the motion flow, provides a 'point of aim' that allows the observer to "see where he is going" — that is, to identify the direction of heading. Second, Gibson acknowledged that a pursuit eye movement complicates the radial flow because it adds a constant to the motion of each point in the image. He claimed, however, that despite such addition, the pattern of radial motion is still implicitly present and will still indicate heading direction whether or not the eye is rotating. Finally, Gibson advanced the general notion that the optic flow (i.e. the radial flow) is the basis for the visual control of all aspects of human locomotion.

In the 1970s, it became possible to formally test some of Gibson's intuitions with large-scale simulations of the retinal motion flow. Typically, these simulation's mimic the retinal input for an eye that moves through an environment without recognizable features (randomly scattered dots). This may be a frontoparallel surface, a ground plane or a three-dimensional cloud of dots. Prolonged viewing of these motion fields induces the impression of self-movement with respect to a rigid environment. The perception of heading direction, which precedes the onset of vection has been extensively studied in psychophysical experiments.

Results are consistent with Gibson's first hypothesis: it appears that the visual system can accurately extract the direction of heading from pure radial expansion over a range of conditions relevant to normal locomotion (see Warren, 1998 and Van den Berg, 2000 for recent reviews). In such displays, heading direction can be discriminated from a reference target with a just noticeable difference of 1–2° (Warren et al., 1988). This level of accuracy is sustained despite drastic changes in scene layout (Warren et al., 1991) and despite large amounts of directional noise, suggesting that heading perception relies on pooled local motion signals across the entire flow field, rather than on the focus of expansion, or on other local feature of the display (Warren et al., 1991). The importance of spatial pooling is reinforced by the fact that reducing dot lifetime to two frames eliminates acceleration and trajectory information, yet heading accuracy remains very high (i.e. 1.1°; Warren et al., 1991).

Addressing Gibson's second hypothesis, however, has produced mixed results. The visual estimation of heading during eye movements has turned out to be problematic. In this case the radial motion flow is 'contaminated' by concurrent parallel flow.

The need to decompose the retinal motion flow

As mentioned earlier, when the gaze deviates from the direction of heading, a constant amount of parallel motion is being added to each point of the radial motion flow. Most importantly, such a compound field is asymmetrical and the focus of outflow on the retina does not correspond any more to the direction of heading. For example, if the motion pattern on the screen simulates central approach towards an extended wall, an eye rotation will shift the focus of outflow on the retina away from the center of the screen, that is, away from the actual direction of heading. The shift will be in the eye-movement direction. This happens because only one dot from the flow will move with the eye and will be stabilized on the retina, whereas all other dots (including the old focus of outflow) will be displaced in the opposite direction. Thus a new retinal focus of outflow is formed which confounds the true focus of heading. If the simulated scene is not a wall, the effect of an eye movement is similar: although there may be no clear retinal focus of expansion there may be an apparent focus of 'best fit' derived from all local motions in the retinal flow (Van den Berg, 2000). How do human observers distinguish the direction in which they are looking from the direction in which they are heading? This is a central question in the heading literature which is known as 'the rotation problem'.

It appears that human observers are able to resolve the rotation problem, as long as the parallel flow on the retina is produced by an actual shift of the gaze. With real pursuit eye movements made while viewing radial motion flow, heading errors are invariably small, ranging only between 2° and 4°. All studies addressing this question agree on this estimate (see Van den Berg, 2000 for a review). In support of Gibson's second hypothesis, it seems that observers can somehow discount the eye-movement-related parallel flow, while their heading perception relies primarily on the radial flow component. The nature of this 'recovery', however, is controversial.

Evidence for and against visual decomposition

Real eye movements are accompanied by non-visual signals of vestibular or motor (efference copy) origin, which could account for the presence of parallel image flow, thus offsetting its contribution to heading perception. It is also possible, however, to separate the parallel and the radial motion flow by strictly visual mechanisms. Is there evidence that such visual decomposition takes place?

Warren and Hannon (1988, 1990) compared perceived heading during a smooth pursuit eye movement with perceived heading from simulations of the same retinal flow presented to the stationary eye. Whereas with real eye movements both extraretinal and visual decomposition may be at work, heading extraction in simulated displays must rely on visual decomposition alone. Results indicated that heading accuracy was not reduced in the absence of the extraretinal signal, as long as the simulated scene was three-dimensional (i.e. a cloud or a ground plane). This suggested that in depth-rich environments visual decomposition alone is sufficient to support accurate heading perception. This was not true, however, when observers judged their heading towards a wall. With simulated eye movements, large errors were observed, whereas accuracy remained high when the eyes were actually moving. The heading biases in the absence of an extraretinal signal were, as expected, in the direction of the parallel flow. In other words, observers saw themselves as heading towards the retinal focus.

It must be noted, however, that in the above experiments the speeds of eye rotation (both simulated and real) were rather slow (up to 1.5 deg/s). Results with faster parallel flow are more variable. Some researchers, have reported biases of 15° or more for cloud environments at simulated eye rotation of 5 deg/s (Royden et al., 1992, 1994; Banks et al., 1996). One must be aware of the difficulties in comparing results from different laboratories. Apart from discrepancies in simulated environments, and response measures (pointing vs. discrimination) it is also likely that observers approach the heading task differently (Van den Berg, 2000). Whereas some subjects may attempt to extract heading direction from the global pattern of motion and independent of retinal focus (i.e. heading observers), others may not be making such an effort (i.e. retinal focus observers). A careful meta-analysis of the existing literature indicates that the data range from supporting pure visual decomposition to no visual decomposition (Van den Berg, 2000).

Taken together, the above investigations suggest that a visual decomposition of the retinal motion flow contributes to heading accuracy in the presence of eye movements. This visual mechanism, however, has certain limitations — it is optimal only at slow parallel motion speeds, high ratios of radial to parallel motion speed and at low levels of motion noise. This range corresponds to most common situations such as walking or running while pursuing a relatively distant target in a well-defined three-dimensional environment. An extraretinal compensation becomes essential under more challenging or ambiguous circumstances. In addition, individual observers may use strategies favoring one mechanism over the other. The next section describes a stimulus in which the visual compensation is perceptually explicit.

Visual compensation in a motion flow illusion

As mentioned above, the independent movement of objects can also complicate the retinal flow. Heading accuracy, however, remains high even if half of the dots in a radial flow field undergo incoherent motion or remain stationary (Van den Berg, 1992). A consistent perceptual bias occurs, however, if the distracting dots take part in a coherent parallel motion. This bias is illusory and results from the interaction between parallel and radial flow in the absence of an extraretinal signal.

Duffy and Wurtz (1993) created a transparent motion display, in which radial and parallel motion are not vectorially added to one another, but are independently superimposed. This was done by dividing all dots in the flow field into two equally sized sets. Radial motion was assigned to the dots in one set and parallel motion to those in the other (see Fig. 2). It is important to note, that physically, the radial and the parallel motion signals are equally prominent because they are carried by the same number of local elements. With unlimited viewing, both types of flow are clearly visible under these transparent conditions. Furthermore, the overlap preserves the original symmetrical structure of the radial flow and physically, the focus of outflow remains centered on the display. Yet perceptually, observers vividly experience an illusory shift of the focus of expansion in the direction of the concurrent parallel flow.

The transparent flow field described above does not correspond to any natural situation. Whereas the radial flow component simulates forward egomotion, the interpretation of the parallel flow is ambiguous. On the one hand, it is possible that the visual system attributes the parallel flow to an independent lateral translation of an extended frontoparallel surface at some distance in front of the observer. The illusory shift of the center of the radial flow can be explained as follows: parallel motion to the right, for example, induces motion to the left in other moving or stationary objects; this leftward induced motion is added to every dot of the radial flow, resulting in a rightward shift of the focus of outflow (Meese et al., 1995). This is equivalent to subtracting the original rightward parallel flow from every point of the symmetrical radial motion flow (Pack and Mingolla, 1998). Duffy and Wurtz (1993) proposed another related account of the illusion. They suggested that the visual system attributes the parallel component to the execution of an eye movement and attempts to compensate for it. For example, if there is rightward parallel motion, the assumption is that the eye must have rotated to the left. As discussed earlier, an actual leftward eye rotation would have displaced the radial focus to the left, whereas in fact, the stimulus remains centered on the retina. The goal of a visual compensation mechanism is to counteract the presumed leftward retinal shift by subtracting the rightward parallel flow from the overall radial motion flow. Were there a real eye movement to the left, the subtraction would center the representation of the radial flow by resetting it back to the right. Since in reality, the eye remains stationary, and the radial flow remains centered on the retina, this rightward correction is actually perceived.

The above analysis illustrates that to recover egomotion direction, the visual compensation mechanism needs to subtract any parallel flow from the representation of the overall motion flow. This is regardless of whether the overall radial pattern is distorted and requires correction (simulated eye movements) or is symmetrical and centered on the retina (illusion in transparent displays). It thus appears, that the visual system treats the parallel retinal flow component in a similar way, regardless of its origin. Such a strategy would be adequate, because both surface motion and eye movement induced parallel flow may potentially bias the extraction of behavioral direction. Background parallel flow biases judgments of straight-ahead egocentric direction (Howard, 1982, pp. 302–304; Karnath, 1996) as well as performance on spatial tasks such as line-bisection (Pizzamiglio et al., 1990; Vallar et al., 1997). Similar to the motion flow illusion, the biases are in the direction of the parallel flow (i.e. erroneous correction in the absence of retinal shift), or in the direction of the slow tracking phase of the corresponding nystagmus (i.e. inability to correct for the retinal shift). Neurological patients with damage to the posterior parietal cortex exhibit large errors on these tasks, suggesting a faulty visual compensation. By contrast, for healthy observers these errors are consistent but small, indicating an adequate visual compensation. The magnitude of the illusory shift, for example, varies between 0.3° and 1.2° for each degree per second increment in parallel motion speed.

Few authors have taken advantage of the opportunity to study the properties of the visual compensation with the transparent flow stimulus. The magnitude of the illusory shift can be used to estimate the strength of the visual compensation mechanism over a range of stimulus parameters (Pack and Mingolla, 1998; Grigo and Lappe, 1998). This approach has revealed some of the important limitations of a purely visual compensation, which are consistent with the conclusions from the heading literature.

The speed limits of visual compensation

Similar to the actual retinal focus shift when radial and parallel motion are vectorially added, the magnitude of the illusory shift depends on the ratio of radial to parallel motion speed. The bias increases with increase in the speed of the parallel flow and decreases with increasing radial motion speed (Duffy and Wurtz, 1993). Pack and Mingolla (1998) estimated the gain of the visual compensation by measuring the magnitude of the illusory shift over a range of parallel motion speeds, while radial speed was constant. A monotonic increase in the shift with parallel motion speed will indicate a gain of 1, or perfect visual compensation. This is what is needed to offset the linear displacement of the retinal focus in flow fields simulating eye movements where parallel and radial motion are vectorially combined. Results revealed an adequate but imperfect visual compensation for slow parallel motion speeds and no visual compensation at fast speeds (Pack and Mingolla, 1998; see their Fig. 5). Also, the degree of visual compensation varied between observers. These results are in striking agreement with the accuracy data for human heading perception for simulated eye movements (Van den Berg, 2000). The less than perfect compensation gain was attributed to the speed limits of local center–surround mechanisms responding to relative motion which are known to exist in the medial temporal area (MT) (Tanaka et al., 1986). On the other hand, the adequate gain at slow parallel speeds and its dependence on the areal extent of the parallel field argued for the involvement of a global process.

Visual stabilization depends on relative depth

Another line of evidence indicates that visual stabilization is also dependent on the perceived depth order in the motion flow. Using the transparent flow stimulus, Grigo and Lappe (1998) presented the parallel flow at different stereoscopic depth planes relative to the radial flow. They found that the illusory shift occurs only if the parallel motion is defined by uncrossed disparity and appears behind the radial flow. The interaction between radial and parallel flow is reduced if the two sets of dots are separated in depth, and is almost completely abolished if the parallel flow is presented in front of the radial flow. This is consistent with both the eye movement compensation and the induced motion accounts. An eye movement interpretation of the parallel flow requires that the simulated depth arrangement is compatible with natural experience. When forward self-motion and eye rotation occur together, the ratio of radial to parallel motion component is large in the foreground and small in the background. Thus points in the scene that take part primarily in a fast radial motion should be near, whereas points of the slower parallel flow should be far away. Similarly, classical induced motion is greatly diminished if the inducer appears in the foreground, in front of the test motion (Grigo and Lappe, 1998).

The dependence of the illusion on relative depth suggests that the visual stabilization mechanism requires the involvement of global, large-scale levels of motion analysis, where disparity and eye-movement information converge and modulate the responses of motion selective neurons. Whereas disparity-dependent motion signals have been identified in both the MT and in the dorsal portions of the medial superior temporal area (MSTd) of the primate cortex (Roy and Wurtz, 1990; Bradley et al., 1995), eye-movement-specific activity occurs only at the level of MST and beyond (Ilg, 1997; Kawano et al., 2000).

Addressing the visual compensation mechanism

So far, the visual compensation mechanism has been addressed by manipulating the parameters of the parallel flow component and measuring changes in the magnitude of the illusion. Instead, we focused our attention on the phenomenal transparency of the stimulus which allows a different psychophysical approach.

According to the preceding review, a motion based visual compensation involves decomposition of the retinal motion flow and subtraction of the parallel component. In the transparent displays introduced by Duffy and Wurtz (1993) the flow field is already 'decomposed' in that the parallel and the radial component are defined independently and perceptually explicit. Yet, the signals contributing to these representations must interact to produce an illusory distortion of the radial motion pattern. This allows exploration of the subtractive process in its own right. The concept of 'decomposition' implies that at some level of processing the parallel and the radial component of the retinal motion flow generate sufficiently distinct neural representations. The subtractive process can be conceptualized as selective modulation of the parallel and the radial motion signals. The goal of this modulation would be to remove the parallel motion signal from the final, behaviorally relevant representation of the flow field.

To address the subtractive process, we investigated how the perception of each flow component is affected by the presence of the other component. Specifically, we measured the sensitivity to each flow component in the transparent presence of the other. This allowed us to assess the relative signal strength of the radial and the parallel motion flow as they are being concurrently processed. It must be emphasized that we assume a positive correlation between the strength of the neural signal and psychophysical sensitivity. In other words, the stronger signal is expected to gain faster and more complete perceptual access. In the next section, we discuss some relevant processing considerations.

Motion processing of radial and parallel flow

The perception of global patterns of motion requires pooling of local motion signals over large areas of the visual field. There are many ways in which spatial pooling may be carried out and this appears to depend on the stimulation that enters the system, as well as on the perceptual task (Zohary et al., 1996). Motion transparency illustrates clearly the sophisticated, selective nature of this integration: the initial local measurements are not simply combined, but they are also segregated into distinct but spatially superimposed perceptual representations (Braddick, 1997). This segregation could be mediated by cooperative and competitive interactions between or within the receptive fields of neurons within the same or different areas, or between global neural representations at different stages along the motion pathway. Thus the nature of the segregation process in transparency depends on whether the motions to be segregated are processed along the same or different channels. This brings us to an important question: are parallel and radial patterns of motion processed along the same channel or along distinct and specialized channels?

Despite intensive efforts, the above question remains unresolved. On the one hand, it has been shown that speed discrimination thresholds are the same for radial and parallel flow (Sekuler, 1992; Clifford et al., 1999), and that both motions exhibit similar and extensive spatial summation (Burr et al., 1998). In line with the above, neurons with large receptive fields in MSTd have been found to respond selectively not only to radial flow but also to large-scale parallel motion flow (Duffy and Wurtz, 1991). This has led some authors to suggest that the integration of both motions proceeds in a common manner and involves similar areas along the motion pathway (Sekuler, 1992).

By contrast, other results suggest that the integration of radial motion flow is carried out by a specialized channel. Regan and Beverley (1978) showed that adaptation to the global looming motion of several elements decreases sensitivity to each element's motion in a way that cannot be accounted for by local adaptation alone. Similarly, Bex et al. (1999) showed that radial motion produces a stronger motion aftereffect (MAE) than parallel motion, when the MAE was measured in local regions of the global configuration. Also, radial flow is perceived as being faster than parallel flow of the same physical speed, suggesting the involvement of a specialized mechanism integrating local speed information along radial directions (Bex and Makous, 1997; Clifford et al., 1999). In addition, several studies report consistently higher sensitivity for radial motion than for parallel motion in random dot kinematograms (Freeman and Harris, 1992).

Only few experiments have examined the perception of different motion flow patterns in transparent displays and some of the results are conflicting. If the parallel and the radial motion are processed by separate channels, they are not expected to interfere with each other's visibility. If, on the other hand, parallel and radial flow are processed by the same channel they may compete with one another for perceptual representation and may interfere with one another in a reciprocal manner. Psychophysically, however, it may be hard to distinguish the lack of interference from reciprocal interference. To claim no interference, for example, it must be shown that the identification of the target motion is as good in the presence of the secondary transparent motion, as it is in the presence of the same amount of directional noise. In addition, there are other considerations. For instance, the fact that with unlimited viewing, transparently overlapping motion patterns remain readily visible could be taken as face evidence for simultaneous and independent processing. De Bruyn and Orban (1993), however, have seriously challenged the validity of such an assumption. They demonstrated that the segregation of the component motions in transparent displays depends on viewing time, as well as on whether observers know beforehand the identity of the target motion. To illustrate the importance of these factors, consider the following discrepancy. De Bruyn and Orban (1993) showed that for very short exposure times and without prior knowledge about the motion patterns, observers identify rotation much better than radiation, although these motions were equally identifiable when embedded in directional noise. By contrast, Freeman and Harris (1992) reported lack of interference between superimposed radial and rotary motion and argued for processing independence. Freeman and Harris, however, informed their subjects about the target motion, used much longer exposure times and varied motion amplitude and not motion direction. Interestingly, De Bruyn and Orban (1993) found that when observers knew the identity of the irrelevant motion, superimposed parallel flow was effectively filtered from radial or rotary motion, whereas these same complex motions could not be filtered from the parallel flow. These authors refrained from interpreting this asymmetry and attributed it to methodological factors (e.g. differential effect of their backward mask).

Overall, the existing evidence suggests that the processing of the coherent components of the retinal motion flow is not carried out by parallel, and completely separate channels. Yet some degree of specialization seems to exist. This is consistent with the recently established consensus that neuronal responses to complex patterns of motion at the level of MSTd are less specialized than previously believed. There seems to be a continuum of response selectivities, with many neurons responding to more than one flow component (Duffy and Wurtz, 1991; Lappe, 1997). In fact, as a result of their compound selectivity to both parallel and radial flow, MSTd neurons respond systematically to shifts of the focus of motion (Duffy and Wurtz, 1995a). Little is known, however, about the interactions between these flow field components and this issue deserves special consideration.

The next section is an overview of our recent psychophysical experiments in which we used a replication of the original transparent flow stimulus introduced by Duffy and Wurtz (1993). Although we did not measure the magnitude of the illusory shift, it was experienced by all our observers. Our goal was to examine in detail the complementary masking between parallel and radial motion flow and to relate it to parameters known to influence the illusion. It was of interest whether one motion will be prioritized over the other, as the findings of De Bruyn and Orban (1993) suggest. In particular, we examined whether the parallel/radial motion interaction is speed dependent and whether it is influenced by the presence of acceleration in the pattern of radial flow. We also explored the spatial extent of this interaction by limiting dot lifetime and by confining the component motions to non-overlapping segments of the display.

Sensitivity to transparently superimposed parallel and radial motion flow

Motion stimulation

The transparent motion stimulus was rear-projected on a translucent screen and occupied almost the entire visual field (see Fig. 1 for details). To avoid inhomogeneities in motion sensitivity and to discourage judgments based on individual dot motions, stimulation was not presented within a small area around fixation (diameter 5°). As explained earlier, the flow field consisted of two superimposed sets of dots, with half of the dots participating in the radial flow, and the other half defining the parallel flow (see Fig. 2 for details). Despite their overlap, both flow

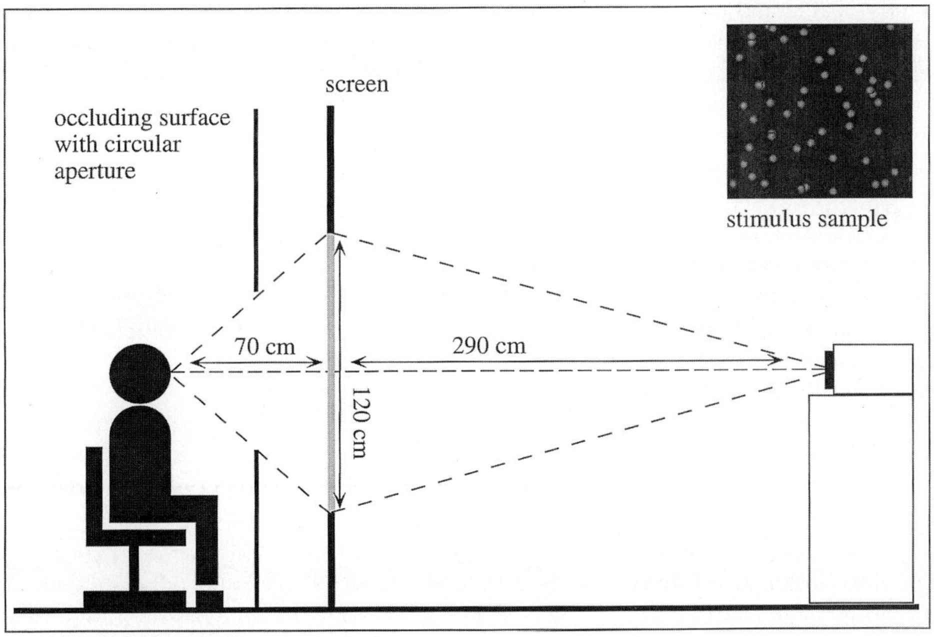

Fig. 1. Viewing arrangement for the rear projection of the motion flow. Observers viewed the screen through a circular aperture. Stimulation extended over a large circular area of the visual field (diameter: 100° of visual angle) and was centered at fixation. Observers were trained to keep their gaze on the fixation point. Head position was straight ahead and stabilized with a head/chin rest. The inset (top right) shows a sample of the random dot field presented to the observers. The field contained 400 bright Gaussian dots (0.3°) presented on a dark background (Michelson contrast = 0.20). During animation, a specialized algorithm kept dot density constant across all regions of the display.

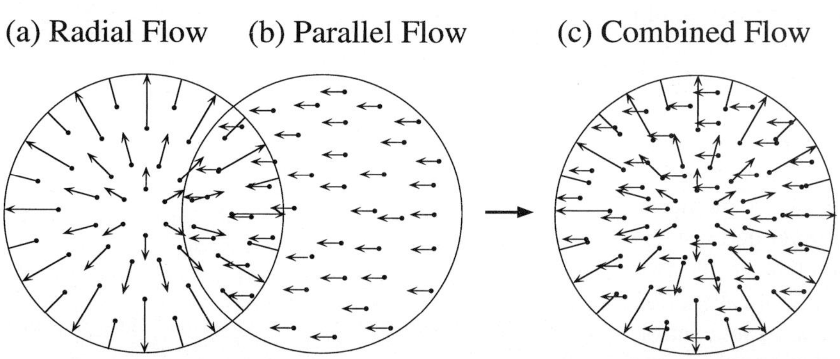

Fig. 2. Combining parallel and radial flow in transparent displays. Arrows represent local motion vectors. Half of the dots (200) defined the radial flow and the other half (200) moved horizontally, defining the parallel flow. The two sets of dots were superimposed over the same display area. Dots in the two sets were identical except for their motion assignment. Depending on the experimental condition, observers judged the global direction of motion of either component of the transparent displays while the other component acted as a mask. Parallel motion speed was constant across the display and was 9 deg/s for all the experiments. In the radial flow, dot speed increased as a function of eccentricity (illustrated by arrow length). Such motion flow creates the impression of movement in depth with respect to a three-dimensional cloud of dots even though there were no other depth cues such as changes in size and density. We refer to this radial flow as three-dimensional and accelerating. Note: in some of the experiments, we kept the speed of the radial dots constant across the display (not illustrated). We sometimes refer to this radial flow as two-dimensional or 'flat'.

components were transparently visible and uniquely defined by the pattern of motion in the two sets of dots. Besides motion, there were no other cues to help one distinguish between the parallel and the radial flow.

The masking paradigm

Before each trial, observers fixated a central mark. When ready, they pressed a key to initiate the exposure to the transparent motion flow. To prevent eye movements, stimulation was brief (typically, 200 ms) and had a gradual onset and offset. No fixation point was present during the exposure to motion but observers were trained not to blink and to keep their gaze steady. Observers were asked to indicate the global direction of the designated motion flow while ignoring any other motions that may be concurrently present. The task was a two-alternative forced choice. For example, if the observer judged the direction of the parallel flow component, he or she indicated whether it was to the left, or to the right, regardless of the nature of the accompanying mask.

To measure sensitivity to each flow component (the test motion) in the presence of the other (the masking motion), the coherence of the test motion was systematically degraded. Thresholds are defined as the percentage of coherently moving dots supporting 82% correct directional judgments (Weibull fit). Each threshold is based on 80–100 repetitions of six coherence levels (0, 20, 40, 60, 80 and 100%). We evaluated direction-specific masking by comparing the test motion threshold obtained with a fully coherent mask (100%) to the one obtained with a fully incoherent mask (0%, see Fig. 3). It should be noted that the orientation and the magnitude of the local motion vectors remained the same in the two masking conditions — it was only the local motion direction that was manipulated. Thus the control, jittering mask was identical in all respects to the motion mask but lacked the coherent motion. Sensitivity to parallel flow was measured in the presence of a radial mask — either radial flow (Fig. 3c) or radial jitter (Fig. 3d). Conversely, sensitivity to radial flow was measured in the presence of a parallel mask — either parallel flow (Fig. 3a) or parallel jitter (Fig. 3b). In some of the experiments, we also measured sensitivity to the test motion in the presence of a stationary mask, to evaluate baseline differences in parallel and radial motion sensitivity.

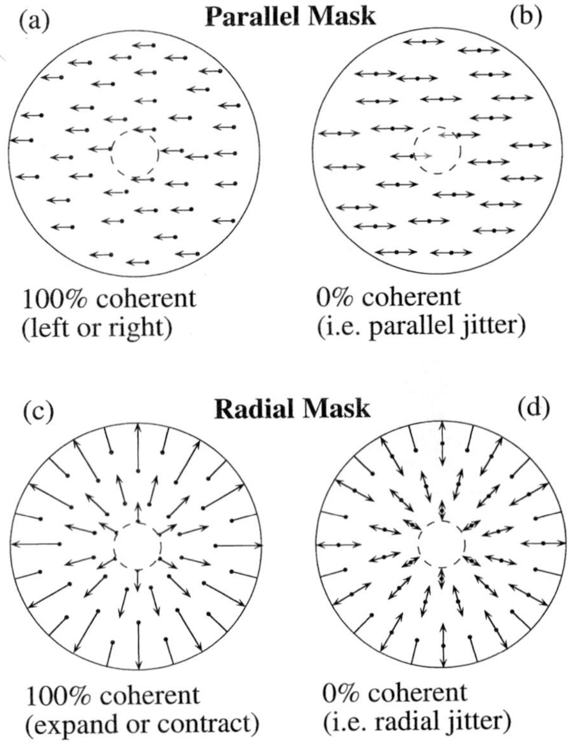

Fig. 3. Masking conditions. When observers judged the lateral global direction of motion (parallel test), the radial flow acted as a mask. When observers judged the global radial direction of motion (radial test), the parallel flow acted as a mask. The masking flow was fully coherent (100%) or incoherent (0%). In the fully coherent conditions (a,c), for the duration of its lifetime, each dot moved consistently in the same direction along the corresponding motion trajectory (e.g. to the left for leftward parallel flow; centrifugally, for expanding radial flow). In the zero coherence conditions (b,d), the motion of each dot reversed direction randomly on a frame-by-frame basis while the speed and the global direction structure of the flow were preserved. This created the impression of parallel motion jitter (b) or radial motion jitter (d). Test motion thresholds obtained with the jitter mask were used as a baseline to evaluate the influence of the corresponding coherent motion mask. To determine thresholds, the motion coherence of the test flow was varied by assigning 'jitter' and consistent direction of motion to different proportions of dots.

Overview of the experiments

Initially, we explored the nature of the complementary masking between the radial and parallel motion flow and its dependence on exposure duration. Similar to the original transparent displays (Duffy and Wurtz, 1993), the radial flow was accelerating with eccentricity from 0 to 70 deg/s. The speed of the parallel motion was fixed at 9 deg/s for all experiments. To encourage global motion discrimination judgments, each test motion dot had a limited lifetime — moved continuously for 91 ms (7 frames) and was then redrawn at a new random location, consistent with the density control algorithm. To optimize interference, masking dots had infinite lifetime (moved continuously throughout the entire exposure).

With this stimulus, we confirmed the observation of De Bruyn and Orban (1993) that the radial and the parallel component of the transparent flow field interact in an asymmetrical manner (Iordanova and von Grünau, 1999). Whereas the radial mask elevated discrimination thresholds for the parallel motion flow, radial thresholds were little affected by the parallel motion mask (Fig. 4). The suppression of the parallel motion flow was strong and direction specific — on average, parallel motion thresholds were twice as high in the presence of radial flow than in the presence of radial jitter (Fig. 5). Furthermore,

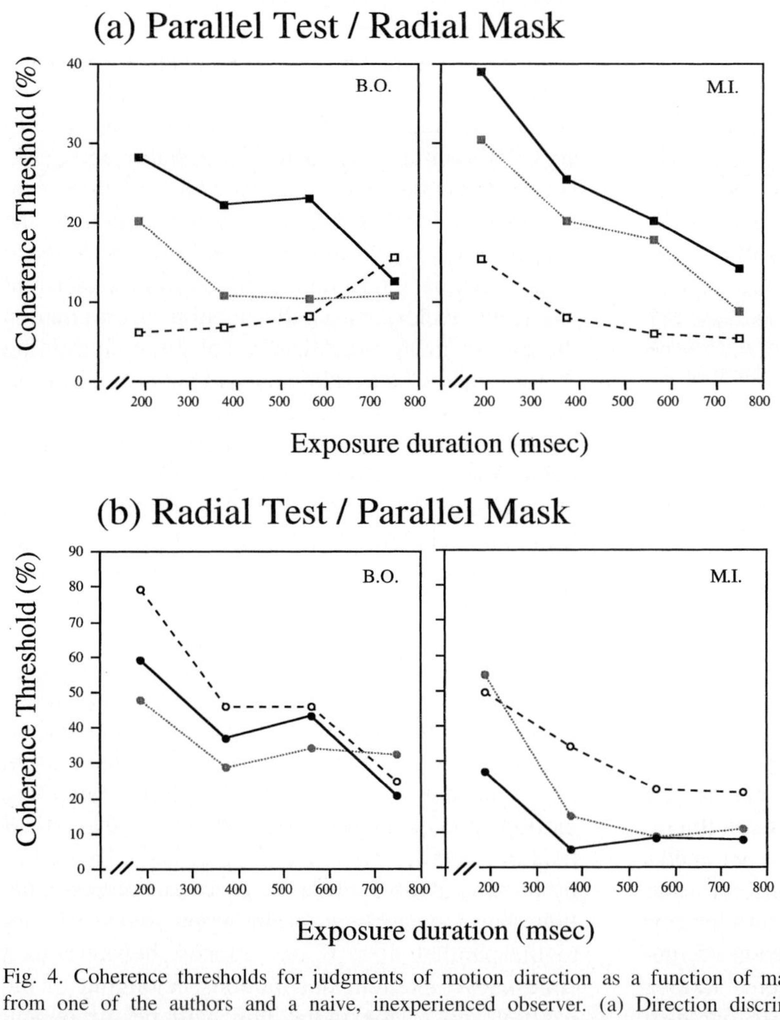

Fig. 4. Coherence thresholds for judgments of motion direction as a function of mask type and exposure duration. Individual data from one of the authors and a naive, inexperienced observer. (a) Direction discrimination thresholds (left/right) for horizontally oriented frontoparallel flow masked by radial jitter (– –□– –) or by radial flow (—■—, expansion; ···■···, contraction). (b) Direction discrimination thresholds (expand/contract) for radial flow masked by parallel jitter (– –○– –) or by parallel flow (—●—, rightward; ···●···, leftward).

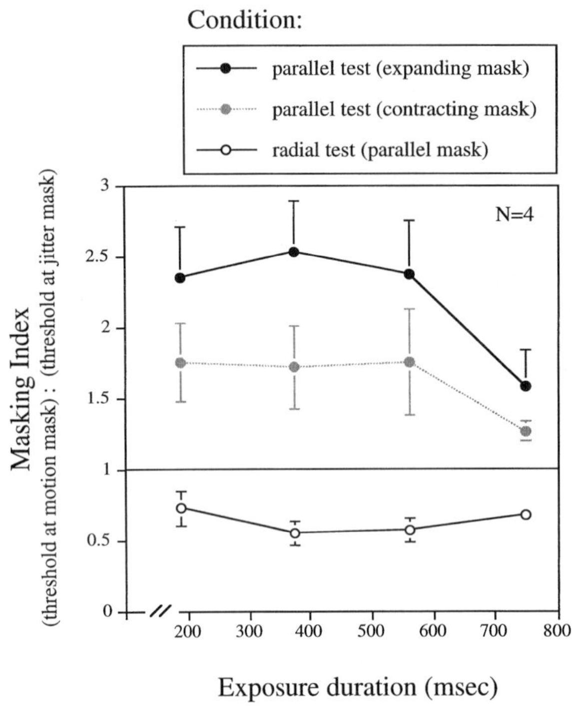

Fig. 5. Complementary masking between transparently superimposed radial and parallel flow at four exposure durations (187, 374, 561 and 748 ms). The masking index summarizes individual data and indicates the factor by which coherence thresholds for each type of flow changed in the presence of the other type of flow, relative to thresholds obtained with the jitter mask. Ratios larger than 1 indicate threshold elevation (masking), values smaller than 1 indicate threshold reduction (i.e. 'unmasking'), a value of 1 indicates no threshold change. Averaged masking indices from four observers (one author and three naive).

the selective suppression of the parallel motion flow developed fast and was optimal only at short exposure durations (i.e. 187 and 300 ms). In addition, the masking influence of expanding radial flow was stronger than that of the contracting radial flow.

Of course, the above asymmetry could be at least partially due to the speed difference between the radial and the parallel flow. The radial flow contained a gradient of local speeds with predominance of faster peripheral speeds. Most importantly, the acceleration in the radial flow produced the impression of motion in depth, rather than two-dimensional motion towards or away from a central point. In our next experiment, we removed the speed gradient from the radial flow and matched its local speed to that of the parallel flow (i.e. 9 deg/s). We also measured thresholds to radial and parallel motion in the presence of a stationary mask, to examine whether there are any a priori differences in the sensitivity to the two motion components. Given the short latency of the asymmetric masking, we limited the exposure duration to 200 ms which minimized eye-tracking concerns.

A clear asymmetric masking effect was observed again, even after removing the speed difference between the parallel and the radial flow (see Fig. 6). Whereas sensitivity to the parallel flow was very susceptible to dynamic masking, sensitivity to the radial motion flow remained superior and robust to interference. On average, observers reliably discriminated the direction of the radial flow when only 10–15% of the radial dots were coherently moving. This level of performance was maintained regardless of the masking condition (i.e. dynamic or stationary). By contrast, compared to a stationary mask, both radial jitter and coherent radial motion were detrimental for the direction discrimination of the parallel flow, suggesting a general susceptibility to local dynamic interference. In addition, a coherent radial mask elevated parallel motion discrimination thresholds much more than radial jitter, confirming the presence of an additional and substantial masking effect which is specific to the radial motion flow. To summarize, it appears that accelerating and 'flat' radial flow are equally effective in masking the parallel motion flow. Removing the velocity gradient from the radial flow, however, had one important consequence — expansion lost its masking advantage over contraction and there was even a trend in the opposite direction.

In the above experiments, the long lifetime of individual dots provided abundant trajectory information. It is thus possible that observers based their judgments on the relative motion in a limited portion of the display, instead of on the global pattern of motion. For example, if one attends to the left of fixation, parallel motion will be effectively masked by horizontal dot motion which is part of the radial flow. This may account for the suppressed sensitivity to the parallel flow. If one attends, however, to a zone above fixation, dot motions belonging to the parallel and to the radial flow will be orthogonal to each other. Although it is unlikely that subjects chose a strategy that is detrimental to their perfor-

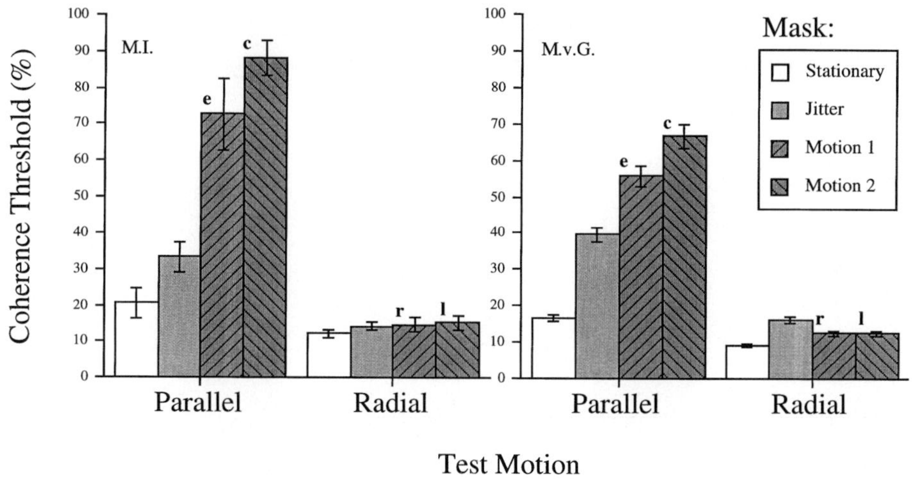

Fig. 6. Motion coherence thresholds for the two types of test motion under four masking conditions. To ease the comparison, parallel and radial motion thresholds are plotted side by side for each observer. Mask symbols should read as follows. For parallel test motion: (1) dots comprising the stationary mask did not undergo any displacement; (2) the jitter mask consisted of radial jitter; and (3) motion masks were radial expansion (e) and radial contraction (c). For radial test motion: (1) dots comprising the stationary mask did not undergo any displacement; (2) the jitter mask consisted of parallel jitter; and (3) motion masks were rightward (r) or leftward parallel motion (l). Thresholds obtained in each condition are averaged over five blocks of trials for each one of the authors. Error bars reflect individual threshold fluctuations over five testing sessions. Masking dots had an infinite lifetime, test motion dots had a lifetime of 7 frames (91 ms). The local speed of masking and test dots was the same (9 deg/s). The radial flow was 'flat' since speed was held constant across the display.

mance, in principle, judgments of the parallel flow could rely on individual dot motions. To examine whether the asymmetric masking depends on trajectory information we reduced dot lifetime in a systematic manner, applying the same lifetime to all stimulus dots regardless of whether they belonged to the test or to the mask (see Fig. 7 for details). In this context, the shortest lifetime at which thresholds could be obtained was four frames, or 52 ms at a screen refresh rate of 75 Hz. It was also observed that at the shortest lifetime, displays had a shimmering appearance and the perception of transparency was greatly diminished. In such displays the extraction of global motion direction requires integration of local motions over space since integration over time is limited. Nevertheless, results indicate that the asymmetrical masking was present at the shortest lifetime duration and was essentially independent of dot lifetime, despite the absolute threshold reduction with increase in lifetime duration (Fig. 7). Overall, there was substantial elevation of parallel motion thresholds in the two dynamic masking conditions, and especially when the radial mask was coherent (top curve, Fig. 7a). By contrast, radial motion thresholds remained uniformly low (Fig. 7b). Most importantly, even at this shortest lifetime duration, the suppression of parallel flow sensitivity was strong and direction-specific, whereas no direction-specific effects were observed for the radial motion flow. Thus it appears, that the asymmetric interaction between parallel and radial motion flow is mediated by a global mechanism which integrates local motion signals over space.

In another experiment, we examined the spatial extent over which the radial flow suppresses sensitivity to the parallel flow. We addressed this question by confining the two flow components to adjacent but non-overlapping equally sized segments (see Fig. 8 for details). In these displays, there was no spatial overlap between the local motions carrying the radial and the parallel flow. We manipulated the spatial extent of the segments by varying their number from 16 to two (i.e. the fewer the segments, the larger they are). It was of interest to find out at which point the extent of the segments would exceed the spatial limits of the suppression. In these experiments, we measured only parallel motion thresholds. Consistent with our previous findings for accelerating radial

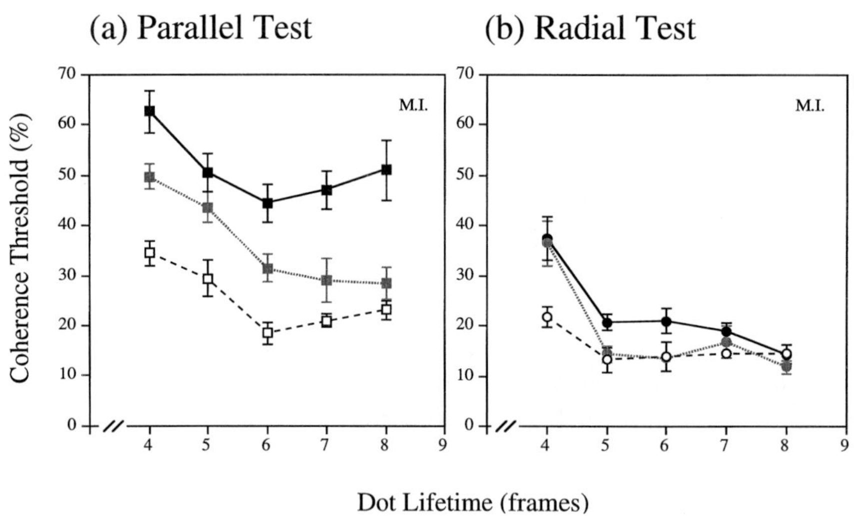

Fig. 7. Direction discrimination thresholds for parallel (a) and radial (b) flow as a function of mask type and lifetime duration. Masking and test motion dots had the same lifetime and speed (9 deg/s). Radial dot speed was constant across the display. Exposure duration was 180 ms. Thresholds obtained in each condition are averaged over five blocks of trials for one of the authors. Error bars indicate individual threshold fluctuations over five measurements. (a) Parallel motion thresholds (squares) were obtained with the following masks: stationary (– –□– –); radial jitter (· · ·■· · ·); coherent radial flow (—■—; data for expanding and contracting masks are collapsed). (b) Radial motion thresholds (circles) were obtained in the following masking conditions: stationary (– –○– –); parallel jitter (· · · ● · · ·) and coherent parallel flow (—●—; data for rightward and leftward masks are collapsed).

flow, we found much stronger masking effects for expansion than for contraction (Fig. 9). On average, contraction elevated parallel motion thresholds by 50%, compared to the radial jitter baseline. The magnitude of this effect remained constant, regardless of whether the flow components were transparently overlapping (0°) or segmented, and regardless of the segments' extent. By contrast, expansion produced twice as much threshold elevation which weakened only for segments exceeding 45°. The expansion advantage was still present when the two flow components were confined to separate quadrants of the display (90°). These results emphasize the global nature of the interaction between parallel and radial motion flow in our displays. Furthermore, it appears that the mechanisms encoding radial expansion show

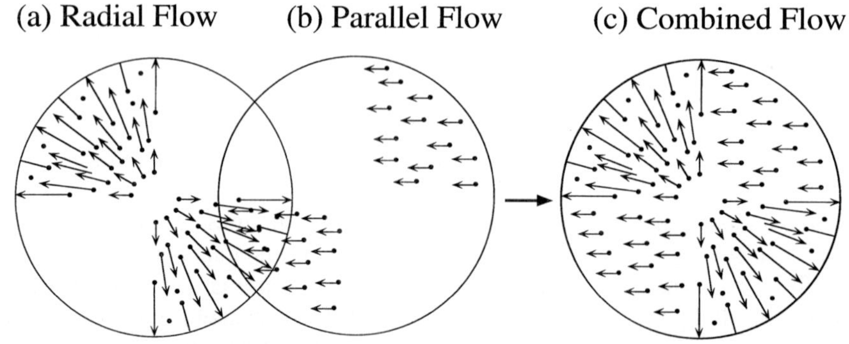

Fig. 8. Combining radial and parallel flow in segmented displays. As in the transparent displays, there was a total of 400 dots, with 200 defining the radial flow and the other 200 assigned to the parallel flow (dot density was the same as in the transparent displays and was held constant across the display). Each set of dots was distributed evenly and confined to alternating and non-overlapping segments. Thus the radial and the parallel flow were projected together over different portions of the visual field. The curtailment of the display into four segments (90° each) is illustrated above.

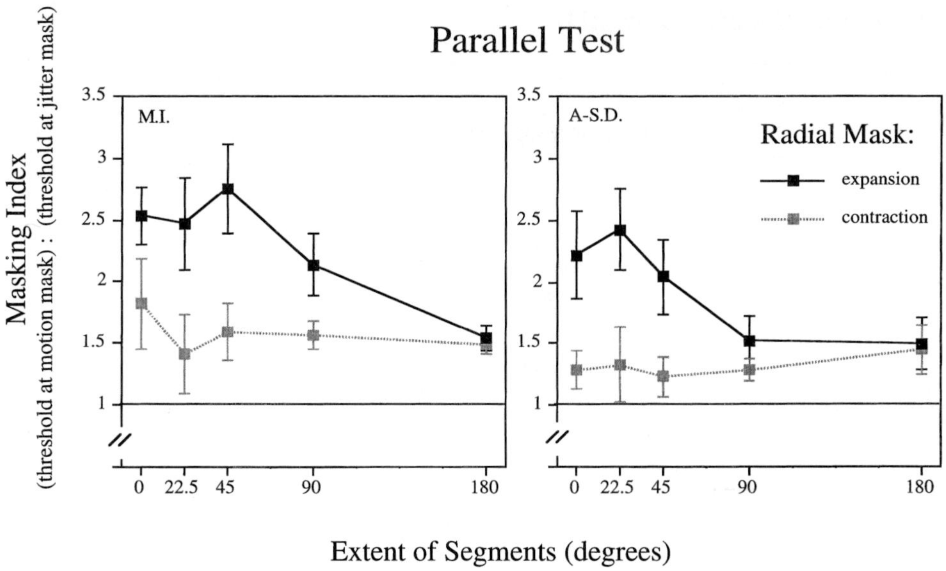

Fig. 9. Masking of parallel flow by concurrent radial flow in progressively segmented displays. The masking index indicates parallel threshold elevation due to radial flow beyond that due to local radial jitter (see legend to Fig. 5 for details). Results for expanding (—■—) and contracting (· · ·■· · ·) masks are plotted separately for two observers (one author and one naive). We varied the number and the spatial extent of the segments in the following graded manner: 0 segments (0° each) corresponded to our standard transparent stimulus with complete spatial overlap; 16 segments (22.5° each); 8 segments (45° each); 4 segments (90° each, see Fig. 8) and 2 segments (180° each). The absolute position and the motion content of the segments were swapped from trial to trial to avoid repeated exposure to one type of motion an attentional narrowing to a particular region of the visual field. The radial flow in this experiment was accelerating with eccentricity (0–70 deg/s). Dot lifetime was 7 frames for the parallel test motion and infinite for the radial mask.

more extensive spatial summation, than those encoding radial contraction (Iordanova and von Grünau, 2000).

As previously noted, increasing the speed of the radial flow reduces the magnitude of the illusory shift of the focus of expansion, observed in our displays. If the suppression of parallel motion flow contributes to visual compensation, it is expected to show positive dependence on radial motion speed. To test our hypothesis, we examined the dependence of the parallel motion suppression on radial motion speed. This was done for 'flat' (Fig. 10a) and accelerating radial flow (Fig. 10b; Del Vecchio et al., 2000). Consistent with our expectations, for both types of radial flow, the magnitude of the suppression increased with radial motion speed. In the absence of acceleration, sensitivity to parallel flow declined at the same rate as a function of speed, regardless of whether the radial flow was expanding or contracting (Figs. 10a and 11). For accelerating radial flow, however, the magnitude of the suppression was speed dependent only if the masking flow was expanding (Figs. 10b and 11). This pattern of results is consistent with the idea that the visual suppression of parallel motion flow is well suited to support behavioral stability during forward locomotion. It is natural to expect that the gain of the visual compensation mechanism will be superior during forward ego-motion than during backward ego-motion. The subsequent sections highlight the most important aspects of our results and provide a framework for their interpretation.

Processing advantage for radial motion flow

According to our results, the radial motion appears to generate a very robust neural signal, which is extremely resistant to interference, whereas the perception of parallel flow is greatly degraded. This confirms the initial report by De Bruyn and Orban (1993). In addition, the dominance of the radial signal does not seem to depend on the presence of acceleration in the radial flow, and is not limited to conditions in which the radial motion was

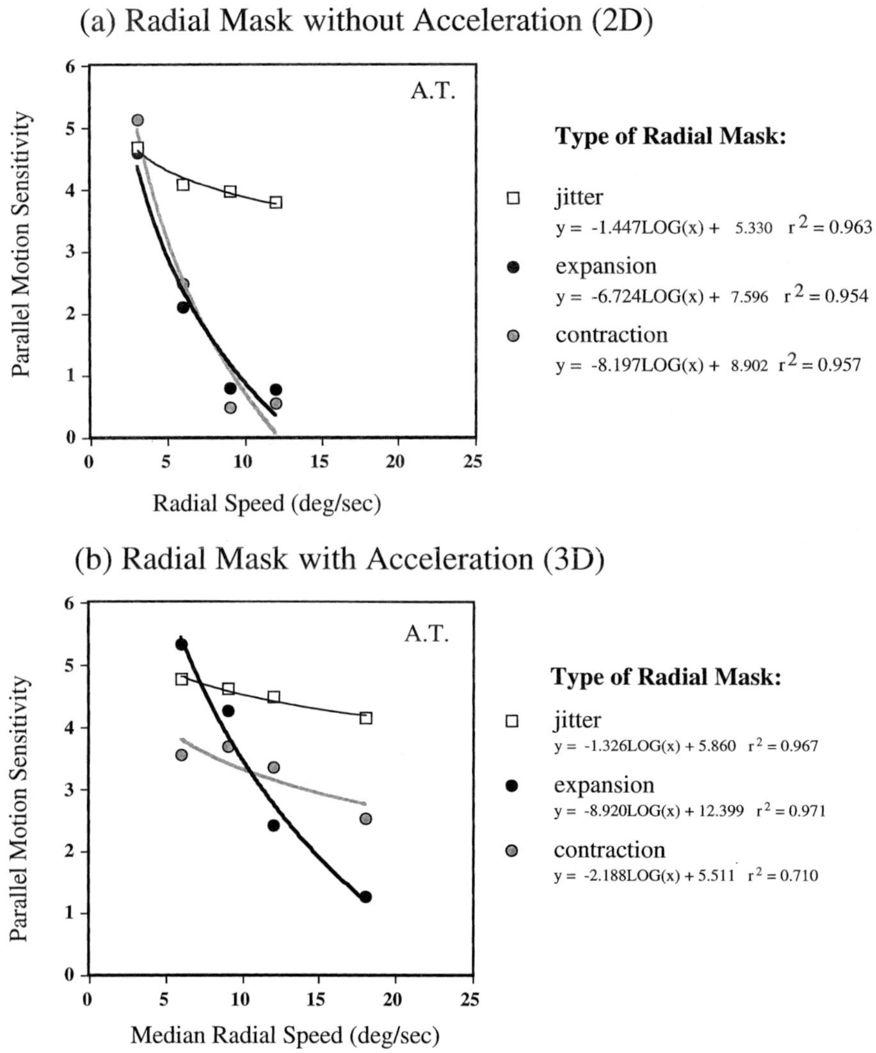

Fig. 10. Parallel motion sensitivity as a function of the overall speed and the speed profile of the radial flow. Representative data from one naive, inexperienced observer. Three other observers produced very similar results (not presented due to space limitations, summarized in Fig. 11). Sensitivity is defined as 1/(coherence threshold). (a) Parallel flow sensitivity (y-axis) was measured in the context of a radial mask in which dot speed remained constant across eccentricity. For this observer, absolute radial speed values (x-axis) were 3, 6, 9 and 12 deg/s (parallel motion thresholds reached a ceiling at higher mask speeds). A logarithmic function with a negative slope accounted well for the decline in parallel motion sensitivity in each of the three radial masking conditions (see legend, equations and r^2). (b) Parallel flow sensitivity measured in the context of a radial mask in which dot speed accelerated exponentially with eccentricity. The median radial speed (x-axis) was used as an index of overall speed and was defined as the speed of a dot located midway between fixation and the edge of the display (i.e. at 25° eccentricity). The effective values of median speeds for this observer were 6, 9, 12 and 18 deg/s (parallel motion thresholds saturated at higher mask speeds). It should be noted that a median speed of 6 deg/s represents a wide range of absolute radial speeds — i.e. from 0 deg/s at fixation to 24 deg/s at the extremes of the display. Again, a logarithmic fit was appropriate for the sensitivity data obtained in each of the three radial masking conditions (see legend, equations and r^2).

faster. It appears, that the perceptual dominance of the radial flow depends primarily on the directional structure of the radial flow. Thus our results support the special status of radial motion and suggest a strong cooperative interaction among radially oriented local motion detectors, selective for centrifugal

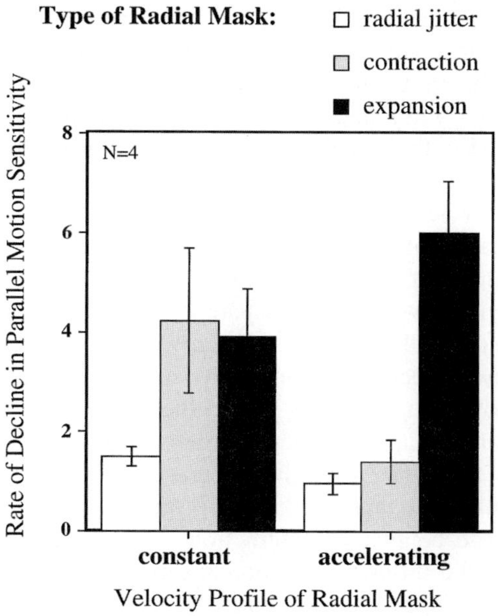

Fig. 11. The rate of decline in parallel motion sensitivity with increase in radial motion speed is represented by the absolute value of the slope of the logarithmic functions fitted through the individual data (see equations, Fig. 10). The average slopes obtained from four observers are plotted on the y-axis together with the associated standard error. The rate of decline in parallel motion sensitivity is plotted for both constant speed and accelerating radial masks (x-axis) for each of the three masking conditions (radial jitter, contraction and expansion).

or centripetal directions of motion. This strong cooperativity overrides local interference and this may be reinforced at many levels of the motion hierarchy, including by large-scale detectors in MSTd (Smith et al., 1994). Thus it appears that the parallel motion signals are treated as noise or may be partially assimilated by the stronger radial integration process. By contrast, the cooperative links between one-directional local motion detectors appear to be weak, hence irrelevant local motions disrupt easily the spatial integration of the parallel motion flow. If these 'irrelevant' motions are organized in a radial flow, the disruption is even more dramatic.

It should also be noted that during the motion discrimination task observers directed all their attention to only one flow component (parallel or radial). Parallel motion sensitivity was substantially degraded despite this selection effort. In a separate pilot experiment, we asked observers to make directional judgments with respect to both flow components. When attention was split in this way and both components were fully coherent, both radial and parallel motion were equally identifiable even at very brief exposures (150–300 ms). Thus it appears that attention has unequal influence over the integration of the parallel and the radial motion flow — it can boost sensitivity to the radial flow, but has no access to the neural representation of the parallel flow. This reinforces the idea that the motion processing system is designed to favor the efficient extraction of the radial flow and may employ relatively specialized and 'pre-wired' mechanisms to carry out this task. Also, the unequal attentional access suggests that the activation of global levels in the motion pathway is essential for the integration of radial motion, whereas the integration of parallel flow depends primarily on local mechanisms.

Suppression of parallel motion flow

It is also possible that the perception of the parallel flow was actively suppressed and not simply overridden by the stronger radial signal. Direction-specific suppression appears to play an important role in transparent motion perception where local signals may compete with each other while contributing to distinct but spatially overlapping motion percepts. Quian and Andersen (1994) found that MT neuronal responses were suppressed when confronted with parallel transparent motion in which the preferred motion component was coupled with motion of the opposite or an orthogonal direction. The suppression was enhanced by local pairings of the component dot motions, which abolished transparency (Quian et al., 1994). This effect operated on a very small spatial scale (0.4°) and was not observed in V1 neuronal responses. There are also psychophysical reports of reciprocal direction-specific suppression between the component motions in transparent displays (Mather and Moulden, 1983; Snowden, 1989). The interpretation of these reports, however, has been challenged on methodological grounds (Edwards and Nishida, 1999). Whereas the physiological suppression correlates with the perception of transparency, it does not seem to transfer directly into selective suppression of visibility. In a masking paradigm very similar to ours, Edwards and Nishida (1999) found no evidence for direction-specific suppression between superimposed parallel motion streams. Sensitivity to each flow component was the same in the transparent presence of an orthogonal or opponent parallel motion or the same amount of directional noise. This is consistent with Quian and Andersen's ideas that the primary purpose of the local directional suppression in MT is to reduce noise within the same motion channel, by separating 'true' motion signals from uncorrelated noise. A local mechanism of this sort is not sufficient to explain our results.

Our report of asymmetrical masking between parallel and radial motion flow contrasts sharply with the above findings. The direction-specific suppression of parallel motion flow appears to involve interactions at a more global spatial scale. This is supported by the fact that the suppression persists in the absence of local motion overlap between the two flow components and is little affected by reducing the lifetime of the local motion signals. Furthermore, we observed that the effect is dependent on the global perception of depth from motion in the scene, in the absence of changes in disparity. Thus it is possible that a higher level, three-dimensional representation of the radial flow exerts an active influence over the spatial integration of the parallel motion flow.

The role of motion in depth

The presence of acceleration in the radial motion flow creates a secondary motion signal of changing distance between the observer and a three-dimensional cloud of dots. Our exposure times were too short for the development of vection, but there was a clear sense of relative motion in depth. In this situation, we observed striking differences between the masking effects of expanding and contracting radial flow. The destructive influence of expansion was much stronger, operated across larger portions of the visual field and was speed dependent, whereas contraction exerted a constant and much smaller amount of suppression.

This difference is consistent with the distribution of response selectivities in the primate area MSTd, which is biased in favor of expansion (Geesaman and Andersen, 1996). Consequently, expansion is expected to generate a stronger neural response in MSTd than contraction. The presence of acceleration in the radial flow modulates MSTd neuronal responses (Duffy and Wurtz, 1995b) and may be essential for the psychophysical expression of the neuronal anisotropy at this level.

Another account, based on the three-dimensional interpretation of the scene, would be consistent with the findings of Grigo and Lappe (1998) that the interaction between the transparently superimposed radial and parallel flow depends on whether the parallel flow is perceived 'in front' or 'behind' the radial flow. Our observers shared the impression of change in the apparent depth order of the parallel and the radial flow. In the context of expansion, the parallel flow appeared more distant and slower than in the context of contraction. This is consistent with the difference in scanning patterns during exposure to motion simulations of forward and backward ego-motion (Niemann et al., 1999). Slow and less frequent eye movements occur during forward ego-motion as the gaze explores distant points in the scene. By contrast, backing up requires active scanning of objects in the vicinity the observer. There are obvious ecological reasons why visual compensation during forward locomotion should be more efficient. This issue, however, requires further exploration.

Conclusions

The psychophysical work described in this chapter provides further evidence for a purely visual compensation for the image motion produced by oculomotor pursuit: there is an asymmetrical interaction between the radial and the parallel component of the retinal motion flow which preserves the integrity of the former and minimizes the influence of the latter. Although we can only speculate about the nature of this interaction, it seems to operate on a large spatial scale and takes into account the depth information carried by the motion flow. In addition, the suppression of the parallel flow is optimal under the same conditions which support heading accuracy in the presence of simulated eye movements (e.g. high ratios of radial to parallel speeds, depth quality in the motion flow). Therefore, it is likely that the visual processes we describe contribute to the maintenance of stable and accurate behavioral direction.

Acknowledgements

This work was supported by FCAR and NSERC research grants to Michael von Grünau. Special thanks to Peter April for his programming and technical support (www.vpixx.com).

References

Banks, M.S., Ehrlich, S.M., Backus, B.T. and Crowell, J.A. (1996) Estimating heading during real and simulated eye movements. *Vision Res.*, 36: 431–443.

Bex, P.J. and Makous, W. (1997) Radial motion looks faster. *Vision Res.*, 37: 3399–3405.

Bex, P.J., Metha, A.B. and Makous, W. (1999) Enhanced motion aftereffect for complex motions. *Vision Res.*, 39: 2229–2238.

Braddick, O. (1997) Local and global representations of velocity: transparency, opponency, and global direction perception. *Perception*, 26: 995–1010.

Bradley, T., Quian, N. and Andersen, R. (1995) Integration of motion and stereopsis in middle temporal cortical area of macaques. *Nature*, 373: 609–611.

Brandt, Th., Dichgans, J. and Koenig, E. (1973) Differential effects of central versus peripheral vision on egocentric and exocentric motion perception. *Exp. Brain Res.*, 16: 476–491.

Burr, D.C., Morrone, M.C. and Vaina, L.M. (1998) Large receptive fields for optic flow detection in humans. *Vision Res.*, 38: 1731–1743.

Clifford, C.W.G., Beardsley, S.A. and Vaina, L.M. (1999) The perception and discrimination of speed in complex motion. *Vision Res.*, 39: 2213–2227.

De Bruyn, B. and Orban, G.A. (1993) Segregation of spatially superimposed optic flow components. *J. Exp. Psychol. Hum. Percept. Perform.*, 19: 1014–1027.

Del Vecchio, A., Iordanova, M. and von Grünau, M.W. (2000) Depth from radial motion enhances suppression of frontoparallel motion in superimposed flow fields. *Invest. Ophthalmol. Vis. Sci.*, 41: S717.

Duffy, C.J. and Wurtz, R.H. (1991) Sensitivity of MST neurons to optic flow stimuli. I. A continuum of response selectivities to large-field stimuli. *J. Neurophysiol.*, 65: 1329–1345.

Duffy, C.J. and Wurtz, R.H. (1993) An illusory transformation of optic flow fields. *Vision Res.*, 33: 1481–1490.

Duffy, C.J. and Wurtz, R.H. (1995a) Response of monkey MST neurons to optic flow stimuli with shifted centers of motion. *J. Neurosci.*, 15: 5192–5208.

Duffy, C.J. and Wurtz, R.H. (1995b) Medial superior temporal area neurons respond to speed patterns of optic flow. *J. Neurosci.*, 17: 2839–2851.

Edwards, M. and Nishida, S. (1999) Global-motion detection with transparent-motion signals. *Vision Res.*, 39: 2239-2249.

Freeman, T.C. and Harris, M.G. (1992) Human sensitivity to expanding and rotating motion: Effects of complementary masking and directional structure. *Vision Res.*, 327: 81–87.

Geesaman, B.J. and Andersen, R.A. (1996) The analysis of complex motion patterns by form/cue invariant MSTd neurons. *J. Neurosci.*, 16: 4716–4732.

Gibson, J.J. (1950) *The Perception of the Visual World.* Hougton Mifflin, Boston.

Gibson, J.J. (1954) The visual perception of objective motion and subjective movement. *Psychol. Rev.*, 61: 304–314.

Grigo, A. and Lappe, M. (1998) Interaction of stereo vision and optic flow processing revealed by an illusory stimulus. *Vision Res.*, 38: 281–290.

Hooge, I.Th.C., Beintema, J.A. and van den Berg, A.V. (1999) Visual search of heading direction. *Exp. Brain Res.*, 129: 615–628.

Howard, I.P. (1982) *Human Visual Orientation.* John Wiley and Sons, Chichester.

Ilg, U.J. (1997) Slow eye movements. *Prog. Neurobiol.*, 53: 293–329.

Iordanova, M. and von Grünau, M.W. (1999) Sensitivity to planar and radial motion in superimposed flow fields. *Invest. Ophthalmol. Vis. Sci.*, 40: S424.

Iordanova, M. and von Grünau, M.W. (2000) Suppression of frontoparallel motion by radial flow shows spatial spreading. *Invest. Ophthalmol. Vis. Sci.*, 41: S720.

Karnath, H.O. (1996) Optokinetic stimulation influences the disturbed perception of body orientation in spatial neglect. *J. Neurol. Neurosurg. Psychiatry*, 60: 217–220.

Kawano, K., Inoue, Y., Takemura, A., Kodaka, Y. and Miles, F.A. (2000) The role of MST neurons during ocular tracking in 3D space. In: M. Lappe (Ed.), *Neuronal Processing of Optic Flow, International Review of Neurobiology*, Vol. 44. Academic Press, San Diego, pp. 49–63.

Lappe, M. (1997) Analysis of self-motion by parietal neurons. In: P. Thier and H.O. Karnath (Eds.), *Parietal Lobe Contributions to Orientation in 3D Space.* Springer-Verlag, New York, pp. 597–618.

Lee, D.N. and Aronson, E. (1974) Visual proprioceptive control of standing in human infants. *Percept. Psychophys.*, 15: 529–532.

Mather, G. and Moulden, B. (1983) Thresholds for movement detection: two directions are less detectable than one. *Q. J. Exp. Psychol. A*, 35A: 513–518.

Meese, T.S., Smith, V. and Harris, M.G. (1995) Induced motion may account for the illusory transformation of optic flow fields found by Duffy and Wurtz. *Vision Res.*, 35: 981–984.

Nakayama, K. (1994) James J. Gibson — an appreciation. *Psychol. Rev.*, 101: 329–335.

Niemann, T., Lappe, M., Büscher, A. and Hoffman, K.-P. (1999) Ocular responses to radial optic flow and single accelerated targets in humans. *Vision Res.*, 39: 1359–1371.

Pack, C. and Mingolla, E. (1998) Global induced motion and visual stability in an optic flow illusion. *Vision Res.*, 38: 3083–3093.

Pizzamiglio, L., Frasca, R., Guariglia, C., Incoccia, C. and Antonucci, G. (1990) Effect of optokinetic stimulation in patients with visual neglect. *Cortex*, 26: 535–540.

Quian, N. and Andersen, R.A. (1994) Transparent motion perception as detection of unbalanced motion signals. II. Physiology. *J. Neurosci.*, 14: 7367–7380.

Quian, N., Andersen, R.A. and Adelson, E.H. (1994) Transparent motion perception as detection of unbalanced motion signals. I. Psychophysics. *J. Neurosci.*, 14: 7357–7366.

Regan, D. and Beverley, K.I. (1978) Looming detectors in the human visual pathway. *Vision Res.*, 18: 415–421.

Rieser, J.J., Pick Jr., H.L., Ashmead, D.H. and Garing, A.E. (1995) Calibration of human locomotion and models of perceptual-motor organization. *J. Exp. Psychol. Hum. Percept. Perform.*, 21: 480–497.

Roy, J.P. and Wurtz, R.H. (1990) The role of disparity-sensitive cortical neurons in signaling the direction of self-motion. *Nature*, 348: 160–162.

Royden, C.S., Banks, M.S. and Crowell, J.A. (1992) The perception of heading during eye movements. *Nature*, 360: 583–585.

Royden, C.S., Crowell, J.A. and Banks, M.S. (1994) Estimating heading during eye movements. *Vision Res.*, 34: 3197–3214.

Sekuler, A.B. (1992) Simple-pooling of unidirectional motion predicts speed discrimination for looming stimuli. *Vision Res.*, 32: 2277–2288.

Smith, A.T., Snowden, R.J. and Milne, A.B. (1994) Is global motion really based on spatial integration of local motion signals? *Vision Res.*, 34: 2425–2430.

Snowden, R.J. (1989) Motions in orthogonal directions are mutually suppressive. *J. Opt. Soc. Am. A Opt. Image Sci. Vis.*, 6: 1096–1101.

Srinivasan, M.V. and Zhang, S. (2000) Visual navigation in flying insects. In: M. Lappe (Ed.), *Neuronal Processing of Optic Flow, International Review of Neurobiology*, Vol. 44. Academic Press, San Diego, pp. 67–92.

Stoffregen, T.A., Schmuckler, M.A. and Gibson, E.J. (1987) Use of central and peripheral optic flow in stance and locomotion in young walkers. *Perception*, 16: 113–119.

Tanaka, K., Hikosaka, K., Saito, H., Yukie, M., Fukada, Y. and Iwai, E. (1986) Analysis of local and wide-field movements in the superior temporal visual areas of the macaque monkey. *J. Neurosci.*, 6: 134–144.

Vallar, G., Guariglia, C. and Rusconi, M.L. (1997) Modulation of the neglect syndrome by sensory stimulation. In: P. Thier and H.O. Karnath (Eds.), *Parietal Lobe Contributions to Orientation in 3D Space*. Springer-Verlag, New York, pp. 555–578.

Van den Berg, A.V. (1992) Robustness of perception of heading from optic flow. *Vision Res.*, 32: 1285–1296.

Van den Berg, A.V. (2000) Human ego-motion perception. In: M. Lappe (Ed.), *Neuronal Processing of Optic Flow, International Review of Neurobiology*, Vol. 44. Academic Press, San Diego, pp. 3–25.

Warren, H.W. Jr. (1998) The state of flow. In: T. Watanabe (Ed.), *High-level Motion Processing: Computational, Neurobiological, and Psychophysical Perspectives*. MIT Press, Cambridge, pp. 315–358.

Warren Jr., H.W. and Hannon, D.J. (1988) Direction of self-motion is perceived from optical flow. *Nature*, 336: 162–163.

Warren Jr., H.W. and Hannon, D.J. (1990) Eye movements and optical flow. *J. Opt. Soc. Am. A Opt. Image Sci. Vis.*, A7: 160–169.

Warren Jr., H.W., Morris, M.W. and Kalish, M. (1988) Perception of translational heading from optic flow. *J. Exp. Psychol. Hum. Percept. Perform.*, 14: 646–660.

Warren Jr., H.W., Blackwell, A.W., Kurtz, K.J., Hatsopolous, N.G. and Kalish, M.L. (1991) On the sufficiency of the velocity field for perception of heading. *Biol. Cybern.*, 65: 311–320.

Zohary, E., Scase, M.O. and Braddick, O.J. (1996) Integration across directions in dynamic random dot displays: Vector summation or winner take all? *Vision Res.*, 36: 2321–2331.

C. Casanova and M. Ptito (Eds.)
Progress in Brain Research, Vol. 134

CHAPTER 22

Speculations on the neural basis of islands of blindsight

Robert Fendrich *, C. Mark Wessinger and Michael S. Gazzaniga

Center for Cognitive Neuroscience, Dartmouth College, Hanover, NH 03755-3547, USA

Abstract: Blindsight, residual visual function in the absence of conscious awareness, can sometimes be found within the scotomas of patients with lesions to primary visual cortex. However, cases in which blindsight is distributed across large regions of a scotoma are extremely rare. In contrast, blindsight is relatively frequent within small islands of residual visual function. We review the evidence for the existence of these islands. We argue that blindsight is likely to depend on vestiges of geniculostriate function, and that in humans the secondary retinotectal pathway has little functional utility in the absence of geniculostriate support. To account for the frequency of blindsight within residual islands of function, we speculate that patients may be unaware of such islands precisely because they are *islands*, which are isolated from the integrated network of neural activity that represents visual space. The relationship of blindsight to the hemispatial neglect is considered in this context.

Blindsight

In 1973, Pöppel, Held and Frost reported a correlation between the distance of flashed stimuli and the amplitude of saccades directed towards those stimuli, when the stimuli were presented within the scotomas of four partially hemianopic patients. This ability was present although the patients claimed they had no conscious awareness of the saccadic targets. The localization abilities documented by this report are limited and erratic; the observed correlation is very weak in three of the four subjects, and in every subject the increase in amplitude with increasing target distance reverses at one or more target positions. Nevertheless, this report triggered a wave of research in the ensuing years which has argued that a wide variety of visual abilities can sometimes be found in visual field regions that are phenomenally blind. These include the ability to detect stimulus presentations with forced choice procedures (e.g. Fendrich et al., 1992; Kentridge et al., 1997; Wessinger et al., 1997; Azzopardi and Cowey, 1998), localize stimuli with saccadic eye movements (Weiskrantz et al., 1974; Zihl and von Cramon, 1980; Weiskrantz, 1986; Blyth et al., 1987; Barbur et al., 1988) and manual pointing responses (Bridgeman and Staggs, 1982; Weiskrantz, 1986; Blyth et al., 1987; Corbetta et al., 1990), detect flashing and moving stimuli (Barbur et al., 1980; Blyth et al., 1986), perform discriminations based on wavelength (Stoerig and Cowey, 1989, 1992) or pattern (Torjussen, 1978; Weiskrantz, 1986, 1987; Marcel, 1998), and extract semantic (Marcel, 1983, 1998) and (most recently) affective information from blind field stimuli (Morris et al., 1999). In the last case, recognition of an angry facial expression was required so detailed form perception is also implied. In addition, both facilitory and inhibitory interactions between blind and seeing field stimuli have been reported. In some subjects, reaction times to stimulus presentations in a subject's seeing hemifield can be reduced by simultaneous presentations in the blind hemifield (Marzi et al., 1986; Corbetta et al., 1990). On the other hand, saccadic reaction times to seeing field stimuli can be increased by simultaneous presentations in the blind hemifield (Rafal et al., 1990). Larry Weiskrantz coined the general term

* Corresponding author: R. Fendrich, Center for Cognitive Neuroscience, Dartmouth College, Hanover, NH 03755-3547, USA. Tel.: +1-802-646-1190; Fax: +1-802-646-1181; E-mail: robert.fendrich@dartmouth.edu

'blindsight' to describe such "residual visual abilities within a field defect in the absence of acknowledged awareness" (Weiskrantz et al., 1974).

Blindsight seemed to open a doorway for investigations of consciousness. Since the loss of phenomenal vision appeared to be a consequence of an interruption of the primary visual pathway, it seemed reasonable to attribute the residual function to a secondary pathway. By determining what neural structures were not accessed by this secondary pathway, the neural systems mediating consciousness might be identified. Moreover, to the extent that patients with blindsight can exhibit behaviors that are normally guided by visual awareness, blindsight provides a means of evaluating the specific contribution of awareness to these behaviors (see Marzi, 1999, and Guzeldere et al., 2000, for discussions of these points).

Secondary pathways

One viable secondary system was already known: the 'retino-tectal' pathway going from the retina to extrastriate cortex via the superior colliculus and pulvinar (Schneider, 1969). In monkeys, substantial visual function remains after the ablation of V1. (e.g. Humphrey, 1974; Weiskrantz et al., 1977; Mohler and Wurtz, 1977; Pasik and Pasik, 1982). Moreover, some recent investigations have argued that the tectal based visual function in monkeys may be akin to human blindsight insofar as its occurs in monkeys who behave as if they have lost phenomenal vision (Moore et al., 1995; Cowey and Stoerig, 1995, 1997). At least part (and conceivably all) of this residual function appears to be mediated by the retino-tectal system. Following striate lesions, monkeys are still able to saccade to visual targets, but additional lesions to the superior colliculus abolish this residual capacity (Mohler and Wurtz, 1977). Following total hemispherectomy in infancy, the ipsilateral dLGN in monkeys degenerates almost completely, but there is residual function in the 'blind' hemifield coupled with almost complete preservation of the ipsilesional superior colliculus (Ptito et al., 1996). In addition, motion sensitive cortical area MT remains responsive in monkeys following striate ablations, but this sensitivity is lost when the SC is also removed (Rodman et al., 1990). Other secondary pathways have also been proposed as playing a role in blindsight; most notably a sparse direct geniculo-extrastriate projection (Cowey et al., 1989; see Cowey and Stoerig, 1991 for a review). In humans, neuroimaging and MEG data have provided indications of a non-striate pathway capable of activating motion-sensitive areas of extrastriate cortex (Barbur et al., 1993; Zeki et al., 1996; Holliday et al., 1997; Stoerig et al., 1998).

Alternative explanations

Almost from the start, however, there have been calls for caution regarding the interpretation of blindsight in terms of secondary pathways: In 1983, Campion et al. argued in detail for alternative accounts of the phenomenon. One alternative is that the residual vision may be due in part or full to surviving vestiges of the primary visual pathway (Campion et al., 1983; Fendrich et al., 1992; Wessinger et al., 1997; Schaerli et al., 1999). This was a possibility Pöppel et al. (1973) had, in fact, acknowledged. Another possibility is that scattered light accounts for much of the residual function. Campion et al. (1983) demonstrate that such scatter can mediate localization capabilities of the sort found in blindsight patients. This is shown both in hemianopic subjects and in normal subjects using stimulus presentations to the natural blindspot. Recently, Faubert et al. (1999) have argued that reports of residual sensitivity in the blind field of some hemispherectomy patients can generally be explained by lambertian intraocular scatter (although see Bittar et al., 1999).

Giving credence to such alternative explanations, blindsight did not turn out to be a frequent phenomenon, as one might expect if it was mediated by a secondary system. Blindsight, in fact, is a phenomenon which is only evident in a small number of individuals. In many patients with lesions that are restricted to V1, no residual vision can be found. Holtzman (1984), for example, tested a patient who had a surgical ablation of striate cortex to treat an AVM, and found no hint of surviving localization abilities. Marzi et al. (1986) found evidence of blindsight in only four of 20 patients, and consistent evidence of blindsight in only one of those patients. However, calls for caution have failed to sway many blindsight investigators; in recent years, a substantial number of studies have been carried out in a single individual (GY) in whom the phenomenon can be readily demonstrated.

Islands of blindsight

In the late 1980s, we began to investigate the relationship of blindsight to cortical sparing in patients with focal striate lesions (full reports of these investigations can be found in Fendrich et al., 1992 and Wessinger et al., 1997). We reasoned that if residual abilities in cortically blind field regions were the result of cortical sparing, it would sometimes be the case that irregularities in the pattern of cortical damage would result in a patchy distribution of the residual abilities. We attempted to observe such a patchy distribution by performing very dense perimetry on hemianopic patients. Blindsight cannot be detected with standard perimetry because this perimetry depends upon a subject's phenomenal awareness of stimulus presentations, so we employed an interval two-alternative forced-choice method. We also used a Purkinje image eyetracker to retinally stabilize our stimuli, insuring the accurate placement of our perimetric targets irrespective of subject eye motions.

Subject CLT

Our first subject was CLT, a 54-year-old man who became hemianopic following a stroke in 1987. CLT's clinical visual field, assessed by standard Humphreys perimetry, is shown in Fig. 1 (clinical perimetry).

CLT proved to be a wonderful subject who was willing to work in a seemingly interminable series of testing sessions. We tested 68 locations in the central 15 × 24° of CLT's hemianopic field. On each trial, tones defined two successive 600-ms intervals. During one of the intervals, a dark 1° diameter circle was flashed three times against a light background. At the end of the second interval, the subject indicated with a keypress the interval in which the flashes had occurred. He also called out a number between one and five to indicate his confidence, with one designating a total guess. We took his confidence reports to be an indication of his conscious awareness of the stimulus presentations.

As indicated, our goal was to look for a patchy distribution of residual visual function. What we found was a single isolated retinal island with preserved detection, completely surrounded by a region that was totally blind (see Fig. 1, stabilized I2AFC field). In this single spot, CLT could report the interval containing the test stimulus with an accuracy of about 65%. This 65% is reliable: it achieves statistical significance even with a Bonferroni correction for 68 test locations. However, CLT's confidence for stimuli presented in this region only measured 1.05, which did not differ from his confidence in surrounding completely blind regions. This meant that CLT's detection abilities within the island were occurring in the absence of any awareness on his part, and therefore met the definition of blindsight.

In subsequent testing, we micromapped the boundaries of this island and found it was in fact not much larger than 1° (see Fig. 1, micromapping). We also investigated the extent of the visual abilities present within CLT's island. This yielded a result which was surprising given the results of previous blindsight investigations: CLT appeared to have no information about the location of the island. In one experiment, we flashed targets within CLT's island or at the corresponding location in his blind lower left visual field. Since he could not see these targets, he was instructed to guess the flash location and initiate his saccade in response to an audible signal. When stimuli were presented in the island, the distribution of upward and downward saccades was identical to the distribution obtained when targets were presented at the lower field location. CLT also could not detect drifting gratings covering the island any better than stationary gratings. However, CLT did appear to have some shape discrimination abilities within the island. When asked to distinguish between a square and diamond, he could do this better than chance if their borders fell within the island, but could not distinguish between a larger square and diamond with borders falling outside the island. Wavelength discrimination was also possible within the island: CLT could discriminate between isoluminant red and green stimuli if they were presented in the island, but not outside the island.

Additional subjects

The fact that we found an island of residual function in the *first* patient we tested suggested that such

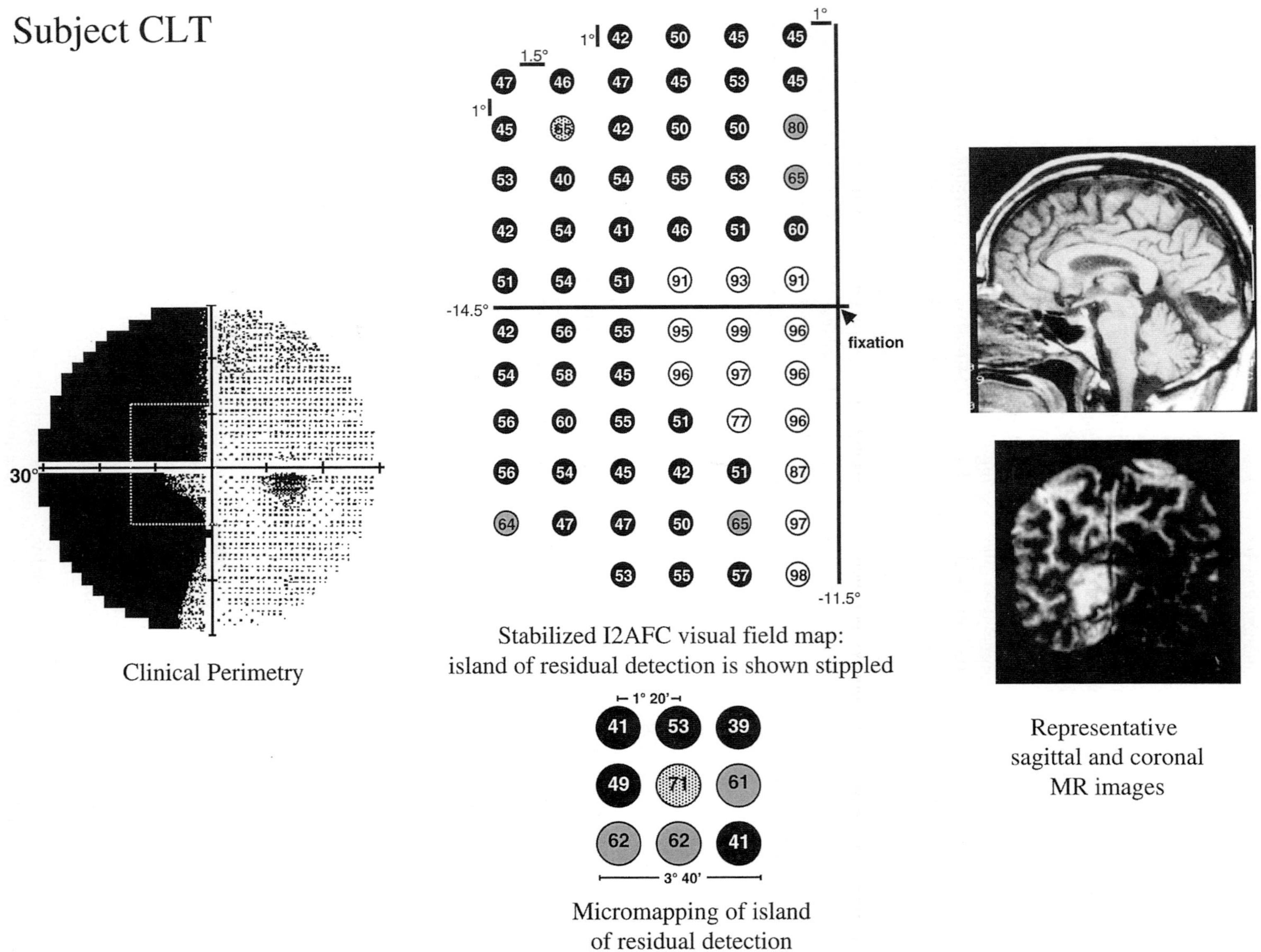

Fig. 1. MR images of CLT's lesion, his clinically assessed visual field, and the fields we obtained with I2AFC testing. The upper MR image is T1 weighted, so the lesioned area is dark. The lower MR image is T2 weighted, so the lesioned area is bright. In the clinical field, the dotted rectangle in the blind field marks the region where we tested. Values given in the I2AFC field are percent correct performance, based on 36–276 trials. The value for the island is based on 166 trials. Values in the micromaps of the islands are based on 66 trials.

islands were probably not rare, but testing with additional patients was clearly necessary. We undertook this testing program, using a grid of contiguous 3.3 degree squares in an effort to improve the efficiency of our mapping procedure. Testing was carried out on six additional patients, two with scotomas due to surgical resections, three with scotomas due to stroke. and one with an occipital cyst probably due to a perinatal stroke. The surgical patients and one of the stroke patients showed no sign of any residual vision in our I2AFC detection task or a saccadic localization task. Of the three remaining stroke patients, one showed a probable island but withdrew from the study before this could be confirmed, and each of the other two showed two definite islands.

Fig. 2 shows a standard Humphreys perimetric field from patient FN, who had a stroke when he was 50, six years before we initially tested him.

Stabilized I2AFC testing indicated FN has two islands of preserved detection, one in his upper visual field close to a zone of macular sparing, and the second is in his lower visual field displaced outward about 10° from that zone (see Fig. 2, stabilized I2AFC field). For both islands, FN's confidence values were close to 1 and did not differ from those obtained in surrounding blind regions. FN therefore exhibits blindsight. Fig. 2 also shows the results of our micromapping of both of FN's islands, which was carried out using a set of five contiguous 1.3 degree squares. This microperimetry revealed that FN's lower island consists or an oblique oval with spared visual function which subtends about $1 \times 2°$. However, in the upper island, micromapping provided no indication of residual function at any location. When we got this result, we rechecked using our larger 3° stimuli and the island was still there. This outcome suggests that in FN's upper field island, preserved detection depends on the spatial summation of attenuated signals from a relatively large retinal area.

Subsequent testing showed a pattern of surviving abilities quite different from that obtained in CLT. FN showed no indication of preserved wavelength or shape discrimination, either within or outside his islands. However, he was able to direct saccades toward stimuli presented within both his islands, but not to stimuli presented at blind control locations. FN was also able to discriminate moving from static stimuli in both his islands, but not in control locations.

Patient, JC has a huge porencephalic occipital cyst (see Fig. 3, MR images), probably due to a perinatal. stroke, and is densely hemianopic in her right visual field (see Fig. 3, clinical field). One amazing thing about JC is that she reached the age of 35 before anyone became aware of her pathology. A seizure in 1974 led to a CT scan which revealed the cyst. Like FN, JC has two islands with preserved detection and no apparent awareness of the residual vision within her islands (Fig. 3, stabilized I2AFC field). Her confidence values for reports of stimuli presented to the islands are close to 1. Stimulation of JC's upper islands influences the direction of her saccades, but not stimulation in blind upper field control locations. This is also the case for stimulation in the lower island, but also, notably, in two lower field control locations where she had no detection abilities. Microperimetry (see Fig. 3, micromapping) shows JC's islands subtend only about 1°, but suggests the upper island could be a peninsula attached to an irregular band of visual sparing which runs along her retinal vertical meridian. When we first found indications of islands in JC, we had only seen the sagittal and horizontal MRIs, and it was a mystery where the islands might be coming from. Coronal MRIs, shown in Fig. 4, provide an answer.

Despite the massive cyst, a small region of preserved convoluted cortex can be seen at JC's occipital pole. We believe this cortex is the likely substrate for her residual left field visual abilities.

Finally, we note that recent testing with a new hemianopic patient has resulted in the discovery of another probable island (Wessinger et al., 1999). Patient WS is a 62-year-old man who is densely hemianopic in RVF due to 1996 left hemisphere bleed. CT scans show a large area of lesioned tissue affecting WS's left occipital, temporal and parietal and occipital lobes. Testing has revealed a likely island of detection 10° out and just above the horizontal meridian, where WS's detection accuracy is about 70%. However, WS reports no phenomenal awareness of stimuli presented to this location.

Implications

Our success in finding islands in a small patient group appears to confirm that such islands are commonplace, if one looks for them with appropriate

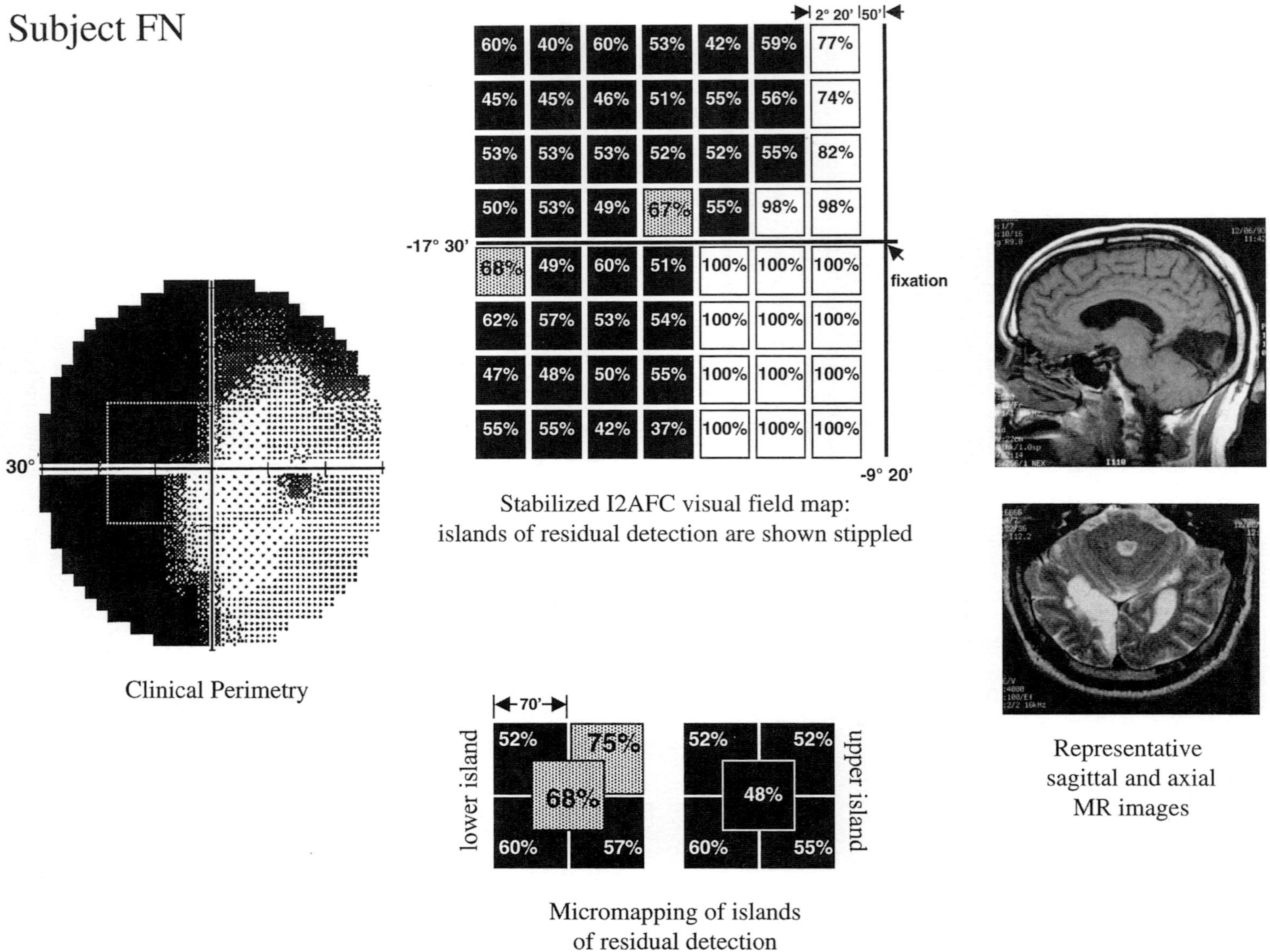

Fig. 2. MR images of FN's lesion, his clinically assessed visual field, and the fields we obtained with I2AFC testing. The general format is the same as in Fig. 1. The percent correct performance value for the upper field island is based on 192 trials. The value for the lower island is based on 90 trials. Micromapping values are based on 60–66 trials.

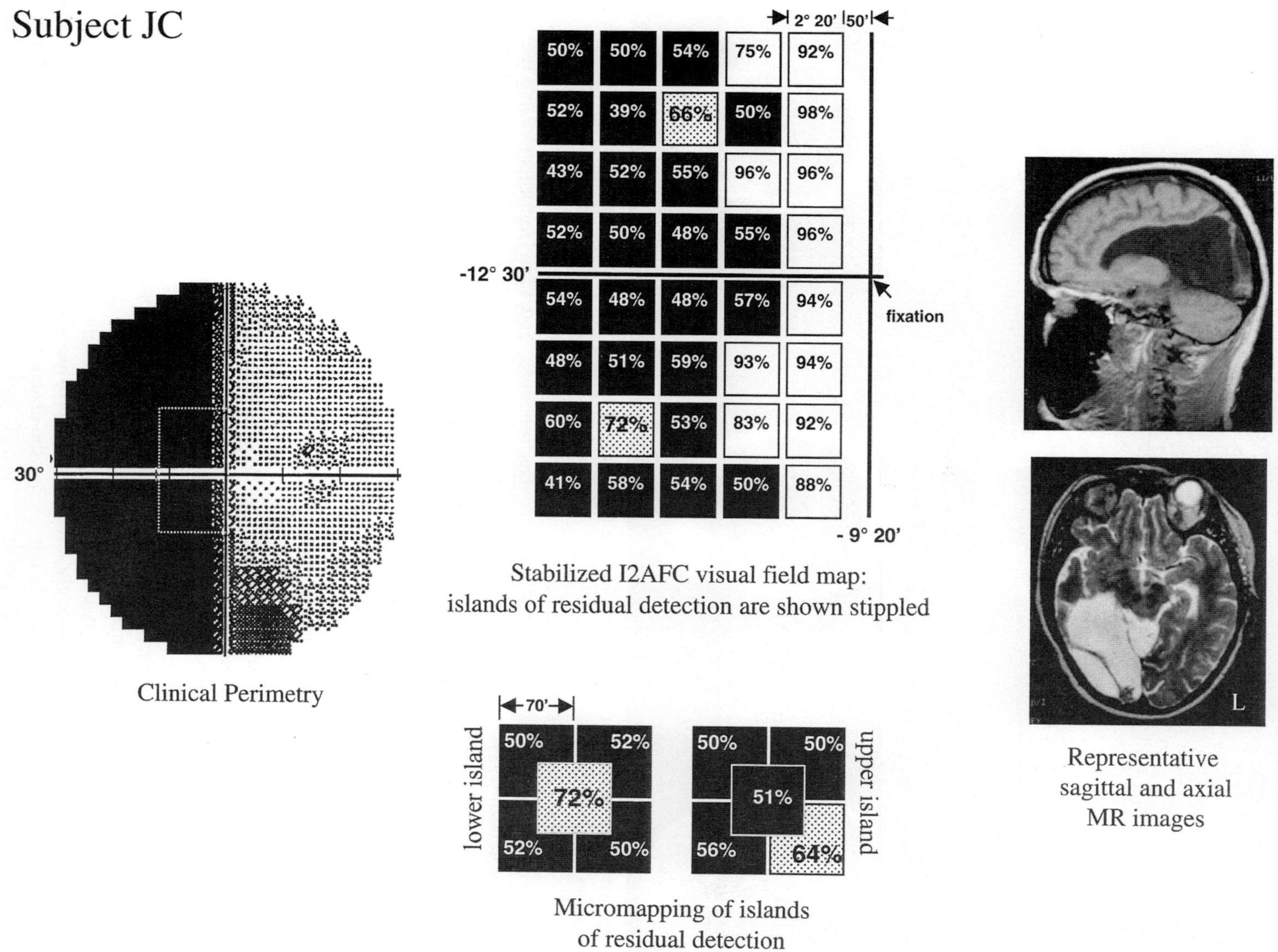

Fig. 3. MR images of JC's porencephalic cyst, her clinically assessed visual field, and the fields we obtained with I2AFC testing. The general format is the same as in Fig. 1. The percent correct performance value for the upper field island is based on 122 trials. The value for the lower island is based on 108 trials. Micromapping values are based 70 trials in the upper island and 66 trials in the lower island.

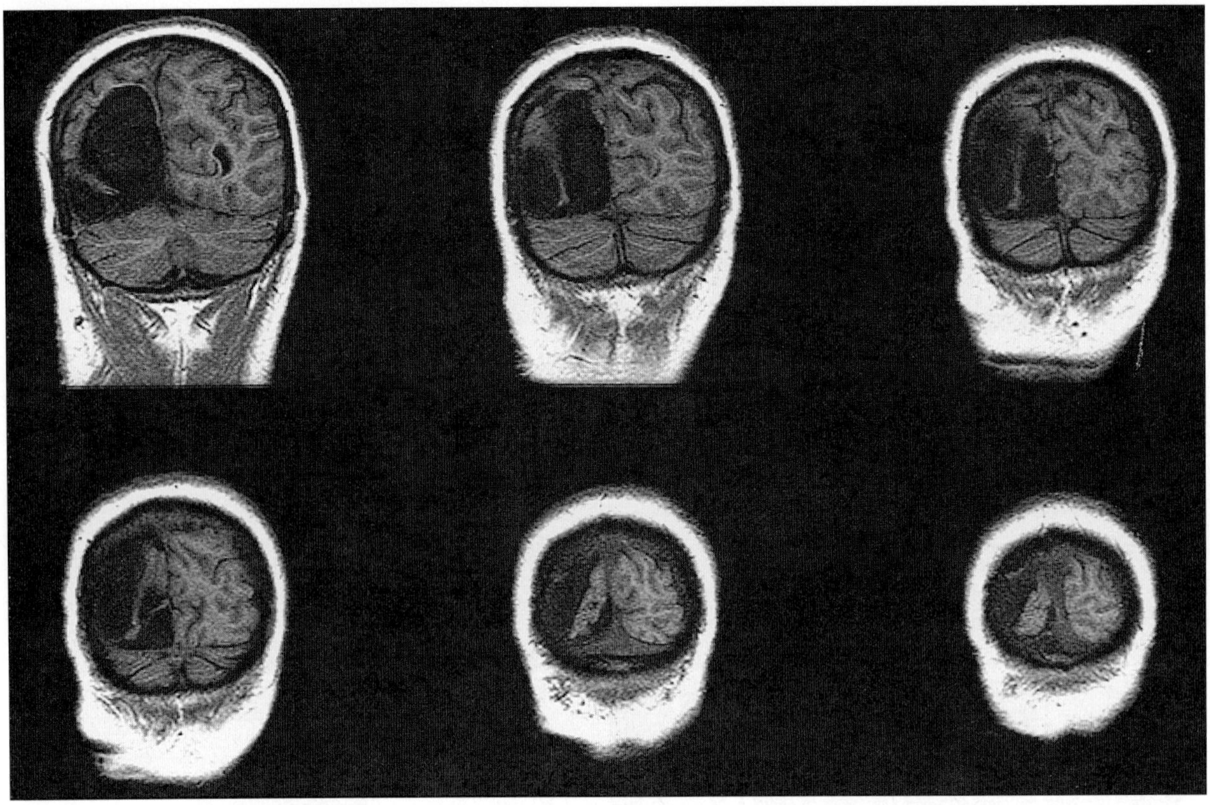

Fig. 4. Coronal MR images for subject JC. Despite the huge fluid filled cavity in the right posterior of her brain, there is a small region of convoluted cortex at her occipital pole.

methods. We continue to believe that the best way to account for these islands is to posit corresponding patches of surviving tissue which can reside within lesioned cortical areas. The variability we observed in patterns of preserved abilities supports this argument. Even within a single individual, preserved visual functions can apparently dissociate, with some present at one retinal location and not another. The pattern of preserved abilities in each patient may reflect a patchy sparing in extrastriate regions. However, the small and well defined nature of many of the islands suggests that access to spared extrastriate regions is generally mediated by islands in V1.

Since we find blindsight in these islands, our research does not support the premise that blindsight is specific to the case where visual functions are mediated by a secondary system. Whether residual vision in humans can ever be due exclusively to the operation of a secondary system remains, in our view, uncertain. Certainly, the retino-tectal system has functions, and visual information may be able reach cortical and other structures via this and other non-striate visual streams. However, it may also be that few if any visual functions can normally be realized without some geniculostriate support. An experiment we are currently conducting is worth mentioning in this regard.

The ventriloquism effect in hemianopic subjects

Rationale

In the monkey, the superior temporal polysensory area continues to be visually responsive following striate ablations, but this responsiveness vanishes when the SC is also removed (Gross, 1991). We therefore thought that visual–auditory interactions might provide a marker for tectopulvinar function in the absence of V1. In particular, we thought that visual capture of auditory location (the 'ventriloquism effect'; see Welch and Warren, 1986 for a review) might provide a marker for such function. This seemed especially likely to be the case if eye movements were used to index auditory localization. The colliculus plays a major role in the initiation and control of saccadic eye motions, and appears to be the motor output nexus where the spatial maps for the various modalities are brought into final alignment (for reviews see Stein and Meredith, 1993; Sparks and Groh, 1995).

Method

To evaluate this idea, we constructed an apparatus which consists of a row of five speakers separated by 10º, with a red light emitting diode (LED) mounted just above each speaker. LED flashes and speaker 'clicks' can be initiated singly or in any combination under computer control. In the experimental task, the LED at the left or right end of the row served as a fixation point, and the room was darkened so subjects could not see the speakers. On each trial, subjects were asked to saccade to a click from one of the speakers. The speaker producing the click was either 20º or 30º from the fixation point. However, subjects did not know that the speakers 10º and 40º from the fixation point were not being used. When a click was presented, an LED in the same position or 10º to the left or right of it was also flashed. Subjects were specifically informed that the LED might not be spatially aligned with the click, and they should not use the LED to judge the click position. Nevertheless, based on the literature (Bermant and Welch, 1976; Warren, 1979), we expected the flash would produce a ventriloquism effect, causing the heard location of the click to shift towards the flash when the two locations were not identical. The critical question was if this capture effect would also occur when the flashes were presented in the blind field of hemianopic subjects, who could not consciously see the flashes due to lesions in the primary visual pathway. Eye motions were monitored and stored with an Iscan video eye tracking system.

Results

We initially tested four neurologically normal observers. A robust ventriloquism effect was observed, as illustrated in Fig. 5A,B. When the click and flash were presented at the same horizontal location, the mean endpoint of saccades to the click was at 19.2º if the click was located at 20º and 27.7º if the click was located at 30º. When the flash was offset 10º from the click location, saccades to the click were shifted by an mean of 5.45º towards the flash when the click was at 20º, and by 5.00º when the click was at 30º.

Two hemianopic subjects have now been tested, CLT who is blind in his LVF due to a right hemisphere stroke (see Fig. 1) and WS who is blind in his RVF due to a LH bleed. Both these patients are completely blind in their hemianopic fields at the positions where our LEDs were placed. Combined results for the two patients are presented in Fig. 5C,D.

Patient CT showed a robust ventriloquism effect in his seeing RVF. With the click position at 20º, LED placements at 10º, 20º, and 30º resulted in mean saccadic endpoints of 10.5º, 23.6º, and 29.7º, respectively. With the click position at 30º, LED placements at 20º, 30º, and 40º resulted in mean saccadic endpoints at 26.6º, 33.8º, and 39.4º, respectively. However, he showed no sign of any ventriloquism effect in his blind LVF: when the click was at 20º saccadic endpoints at were 15.5º, 17.6º, and 15.4º, and when the click was at 30º saccadic endpoints were at 24.5º, 25.3º, and 23.0º.

The same outcome was obtained with patient WS. Although his saccades were generally hypometric in his seeing LVF, a ventriloquism effect is evident. With the click position at 20º, LED placements at 10º, 20º, and 30º resulted in mean saccadic endpoints of 5.8º, 14,4º, and 25.4º, respectively. With the click position at 30º, LED placements at 20º, 30º, and 40º resulted in mean saccadic endpoints at 15.5º, 26.0º, and 36.1º, respectively. No ventriloquism effect was found in his blind RVF: when the click was at 20º, saccadic endpoints for the three LED positions were 25.6º, 27.9º, and 27.2º. When the click was at 30º, saccadic endpoints were at 33.8º, 32.3º, and 31.6º.

Results to date therefore do not support the premise that the tectopulvinar system can support visual capture in the absence of phenomenal awareness. These results must be regarded as preliminary. Additional testing is needed, and it is possible that the sought for auditory–visual interaction will be

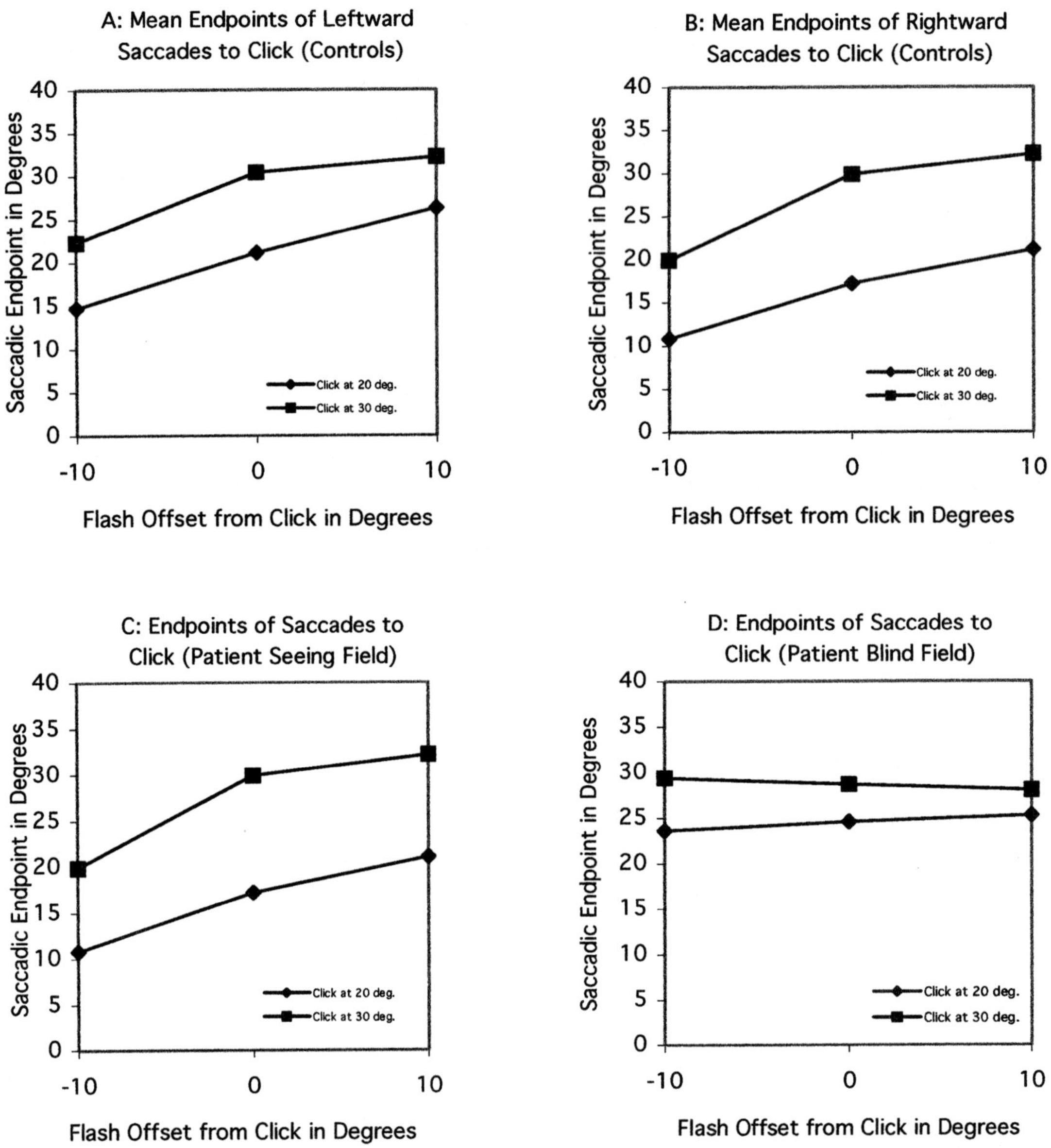

Fig. 5. Results of the testing for the ventriloquism effect. Control subject data show the mean results for four subjects; patient data shows the means for two hemianopic subjects. The click was randomly presented 20° or 30° from the fixation point, to the left or right in different trial blocks. A −10 on the abscissa indicates the flash was 10° closer to the fixation point than the click, while a +10 indicates the flash was 10° farther from the fixation point. A strong ventriloquism effect is evident for the controls and in the seeing field of the patients, but is absent in the blind field of the patients. Each patient data point is based on 12 saccades from CLT and 18 saccades from WS.

found in other hemianopic patients. However, from the limited data that has been gathered, it does not seem likely that this interaction will prove to be a routine indicator of surviving tectopulvinar function. Here, then, is another case in which monkey anatomy and physiology suggests that a visual process might survive without geniculostriate support, but in humans this does not occur.

Islands of blindsight: speculations on their neural basis

If blindsight is not restricted to cases where visual functions are mediated by a secondary pathway, what are the conditions that produce it? One possibility is that blindsight occurs whenever sensory signals are almost lost in noise. It is commonplace for normal subjects in psychophysical testing procedures to perform above chance with just liminal stimuli when they have little or no confidence in the accuracy of their judgments. Specific demonstrations of blindsight in normal observers (Meeres and Graves, 1990; Kolb and Braun, 1995) could simply represent special instances of this phenomenon. In this case, blindsight is simply a variant of what has traditionally been termed subliminal perception.

We would like to finish, however, with another line of speculation. Let us start with an empirical observation. Although cases where blindsight seems to extend across large areas of the visual field have proved to be few and far between, in our islands of residual vision, *blindsight seems to be the rule.* Altogether, we have now found seven islands of residual function distributed across five patients, and the criterion for blindsight — visual function without acknowledged awareness — has been met in every case. Saying that again slightly differently, we have seven cases of islands with blindsight, but no case of an island of vision with awareness. What is it about islands that makes blindsight happen?

We suggest that while awareness of the neural representation of a stimulus may depend in part upon signal to noise ratios, *it may also depend upon that representation being cohesive with the remainder of a person's visual world.* When attempting to elaborate this idea, it is useful to consider another phenomenon — hemispatial neglect. This is a syndrome where patients fail to acknowledge or respond to objects and events on one side of space. In acute cases, patients may copy only one side of a drawing, eat food from one side of their plate, read only half of a word, write on one side of a page. Neglect is a complex phenomenon; it may have motor as well as perceptual components, can operate within both spatiotopic and object-based reference frames, and can result from lesions to several different regions of the brain (For several reviews of neglect, see Jeannerod, 1987; for a review that specifically compares neglect and blindsight, see Driver and Mattingley, 1998.) The instances of neglect we are referring to are those that seem to entail a global unilateral loss of spatial awareness. In humans, this kind of neglect occurs primarily on the side of space contralateral to parietal lobe damage, and is more prevalent in cases of right parietal damage. In such cases, there are two broad classes of explanations that have been offered for the phenomenon. One is attentional — the argument is that patients are impaired at placing their attention on the neglected side (e.g. Posner et al., 1984; Heilman et al., 1987; Kinsbourne, 1987). The other approach, which has been less popular but which we find more interesting in the present context, is that neglect occurs because an internal representation of space has been disrupted (see Bisiach and Berti, 1987). In this case, unilateral neglect and hemianopia can be construed as complementary. Adopt for a moment the metaphor that our visual world is displayed on some kind of internal screen. In patients with cortical blindness due to an interruption of the geniculostriate pathway, part of the projection beam has been interrupted. In patients with hemispatial neglect, the image is being projected but part of the screen has been torn away. In both cases, the neural networks responsible for visual consciousness are confronted with a void.

Certainly, hemianopes do not ignore one side of space in the way neglect patients may — they know the world extends into the regions they cannot see, are sensitive to non-visual inputs from those regions, and develop strategies to deal with their restricted fields. Nevertheless, we suggest that blindsight, like neglect, can result from the constriction of a visual spatial framework. If one stands in total darkness, that darkness still extends to fill a visual space. In the absence of a geniculostriate input, more than a sensory overlay is lost. Hemianopes do not, so far as we can tell, perceive the region within their scotomas as a large empty areas. These regions are simply not visually represented, like the space behind one's head. Consider the case of JC, who for 35 years did not know she had a visual impairment.

The representation of space within the visual system is normally continuous. When there are small spatial gaps in the sensory input to this representation — as in the case of the natural blind spot or a focal scotoma — the visual system fills in this gap with extrapolated information, so that the representation appears unbroken. When a large region of the visual field is lost, the representation contracts. We propose that small islands of information which are outside the borders of the contracted representation, and therefore isolated from it, are excluded from visual awareness. In effect, islands of visual information that would normally map to the scotomous regions are not seen because there is no visual spatial substrate into which they can be incorporated. Because they are disconnected from the integrated representation of a patients visual world, they are also disconnected the conscious experience of that world.

We can speculate just a bit further about what physiology might be commensurate with this proposal. If an island of intact tissue is able to influence behavior, then output connections from that island must be present, presumably via axonal tracts. However, the continuity of the visual space may depend on lateral connections within visual cortex, which serve to link each topographically mapped location to adjacent locations. Gilbert and his associates have argued that such lateral connections mediate the disappearance of small visual scotomas (e.g. Gilbert, 1995; Darian-Smith and Gilbert, 1995). We argue that when an island of functioning tissue has output connections to other neural modules but does not have the lateral connections needed to bind it to the remainder of a persons visual field, blindsight may be the consequence.

This view is commensurate with the observation that patients generally are aware of degraded representations which lie at the borders of their seeing fields. Even weak and noisy visual signals from such regions may have an improved chance of entering consciousness because they are neurally bound to a subject's seeing field. In addition, if the output from a island is sufficiently strong, it might still impinge on consciousness but in a non-visual way. The patient might say something like, "I didn't see anything but I felt something." Weiskrantz's patient DB appears to have had experiences of this sort (Weiskrantz, 1986).

Our data and these speculations do not imply that *all* cases of blindsight are attributable to islands. We are only arguing that the neural conditions which result in islands of residual function may also make blindsight very likely. In patients like GY, other patterns of neural pathology may lead to visual function without awareness, although the completeness of the dissociation between function and awareness in this patient has recently been questioned (Benson et al., 1998; Zeki and Ffytche, 1998). Kentridge et al. (1997) have mapped out an ordered transition from preserved vision with awareness to apparent blindsight to total blindness in GY. This suggests that diffuse sparing in dysfunctional primary cortex could be the substrate of GY's blindsight, although Kentridge et al. do not favor this view. Our own observations suggest that when V1 is truly gone, most patients are profoundly blind. But this may be a rule with exceptions, especially when conditions have favored neural re-organization. If it does turn out that there are cases where blindsight is mediated by a secondary system, the general argument that blindsight occurs when stimulation maps onto cortical regions that are isolated from the phenomenal representation of visual space could still apply. In such instances, a loss of geniculostriate function would still account for the loss of the visual representation, while the secondary system would be the source of the stimulation. In any case, the contributions of secondary systems to residual vision and the conditions that result in blindsight are issues that can be dissociated. It is on the latter more general issue that the significance of blindsight for our understanding of the neural substrate of consciousness depends.

References

Azzopardi, P. and Cowey, A. (1998) Blindsight and visual awareness. *Conscious. Cogn.*, 7: 292–311.

Barbur, J.L., Ruddock, K.H. and Waterfield, V.A. (1980) Human visual responses in the absence of the geniculo-calcarine projection. *Brain*, 103: 905–928.

Barbur, J.L., Forsyth, P.M. and Findlay, J.M. (1988) Human saccadic eye movements in the absence of the geniculocalcarine projection. *Brain*, 111: 63–82.

Barbur, J.L., Watson, J.D.G., Frackowiak, R.S.J. and Zeki, S. (1993) Conscious visual perception without V1. *Brain*, 116: 1293–1302.

Benson, P.J., Guo, K. and Blakemore, C. (1998) Direction discrimination of moving gratings and plaids and coherence in dot displays with primary visual cortex (V1). *Eur. J. Neurosci.*, 10: 3767–3772.

Bermant, R.I. and Welch, R.B. (1976) The effect of degree of visual–auditory stimulus separation and eye position upon the spatial interaction of vision and audition. *Percept. Motor Skills*, 43: 487–493.

Bisiach, E. and Berti, A. (1987) Dyschiria. An attempt at its systematic explanation. In: M. Jeannerod (Ed.), *Advances in Psychology*. Vol. 45, *Neurophysiological and Neuropsychological Aspects of Spatial Neglect*. Elsevier, Amsterdam, pp. 183–201.

Bittar, R.G., Ptito, M., Faubert, J., Dumoulin, S.Q. and Ptito, A. (1999) Activation of the remaining hemisphere following stimulation of the blind hemifield in hemispherectomized subjects. *NeuroImage*, 10: 339–346.

Blyth, I.M., Bromley, J.M., Kennard, C. and Ruddock, K.H. (1986) Visual discrimination of target displacement remains after damage to the striate cortex in humans. *Nature*, 320: 619–621.

Blyth, I.M., Kennard, C. and Rudduck, K.H. (1987) Residual vision in patients with retrogeniculate lesions of the visual pathways. *Brain*, 110: 887–905.

Bridgeman, B. and Staggs, D. (1982) Plasticity in human blindsight. *Vision Res.*, 22: 1199–1203.

Campion, J., Latto, R. and Smith, Y.M. (1983) Is blindsight an effect of scattered light, spared cortex and near threshold vision? *Behav. Brain Sci.*, 6: 423–486.

Corbetta, M., Marzi, C.A., Tassinari, G. and Aglioti, S. (1990) Effectiveness of different task paradigms in revealing blindsight. *Brain*, 113: 603–616.

Cowey, A. and Stoerig, P. (1991) The neurobiology of blindsight. *Trends Neurosci.*, 14: 140–145.

Cowey, A. and Stoerig, P. (1995) Blindsight in monkeys. *Nature*, 373: 247–249.

Cowey, A. and Stoerig, P. (1997) Visual detection in monkeys with blindsight. *Neuropsychologia*, 35: 929–939.

Cowey, A., Stoerig, P. and Perry, V.H. (1989) Transneuronal retrograde degeneration of retinal ganglion cells after damage to striate cortex in Macaque monkeys: selective loss of Pβ cells. *Neuroscience*, 29: 65–80.

Darian-Smith, C. and Gilbert, C.D. (1995) Topographic reorganization in the striate cortex of the adult cat and monkey is cortically mediated. *J. Neurosci.*, 15: 1631–1647.

Driver, J. and Mattingley, J.B. (1998) Parietal neglect and visual awareness. *Nat. Neurosci.*, 1: 17–22.

Faubert, J., Diaconu, V., Ptito, M. and Ptito, A. (1999) Residual vision in the blind field of hemidecorticated humans predicted by a diffusion scatter model and selective spectral scatter of the human eye. *Vision Res.*, 39: 149–157.

Fendrich, R., Wessinger, C.M. and Gazzaniga, M.S. (1992) Residual vision in a scotoma: implications for blindsight. *Science*, 258: 1489.

Gilbert, C.D. (1995) Dynamic properties of adult visual cortex. In: M.S. Gazzaniga (Ed.), *The Cognitive Neurosciences*. MIT Press, Cambridge, MA, pp. 73–90.

Gross, C.G. (1991) Contribution of striate cortex and the superior colliculus to visual function in area MT, the superior temporal polysensory area and inferior temporal cortex. *Neuropsychologia*, 29: 497–515.

Guzeldere, G., Flanagan, O. and Hardcastle, V.G. (2000) The nature and function of consciousness: lessons from blindsight. In: M.S. Gazzaniga (Ed.), *The New Cognitive Neurosciences*. MIT Press, Cambridge, MA, pp. 1277–1284.

Heilman, K.M., Bowers, D., Valenstein, E. and Watson, R.T. (1987) Hemispace and hemispatial neglect. In: M. Jeannerod (Ed.), *Advances in Psychology*. Vol. 45, *Neurophysiological and Neuropsychological Aspects of Spatial Neglect*. Elsevier, Amsterdam, pp. 115–150.

Holliday, I.E., Anderson, S.J. and Harding, G.F. (1997) Magnetoencephalographic evidence or non-geniculostriate visual input to human cortical area V5. *Neuropsychologia*, 35: 1139–1146.

Holtzman, J.D. (1984) Interactions between cortical and subcortical visual areas: evidence from human commissurotmy patients. *Vision Res.*, 24: 801–813.

Humphrey, N.K. (1974) Vision in a monkey without striate cortex: a case study. *Perception*, 3: 241–255.

Jeannerod, M. (Ed.) (1987) *Advances in Psychology*. Vol. 45, *Neurophysiological and Neuropsychological Aspects of Spatial Neglect*. Elsevier, Amsterdam.

Kentridge, R.W., Heywood, C.A. and Weiskrantz, L. (1997) Residual vision in multiple retinal locations within a scotoma: implications for blindsight. *J. Cogn. Neurosci.*, 9: 191–202.

Kinsbourne, M. (1987) Mechanisms of unilateral neglect. In: M. Jeannerod (Ed.), *Advances in Psychology*. Vol. 45, *Neurophysiological and Neuropsychological Aspects of Spatial Neglect*. Elsevier, Amsterdam, pp. 69–86.

Kolb, C.F. and Braun, J. (1995) Blindsight in normal observers. *Nature*, 377: 336–338.

Marcel, A.J. (1983) Conscious and unconscious perception: an approach to the relations between phenomenal experience and perceptual processes. *Cogn. Psychol.*, 15: 197–237.

Marcel, A.J. (1998) Blindsight and shape perception: deficit of visual consciousness or of visual function? *Brain*, 121: 1565–1588.

Marzi, C.A. (1999) Why is blindsight blind? *J. Conscious. Studies*, 6: 12–18.

Marzi, C.A., Tassinari, G., Aglioti, S. and Lutzemberger, L. (1986) Spatial summation across the vertical meridian in hemianopics: a test of blindsight. *Neuropsychologia*, 24: 749–758.

Meeres, S.L. and Graves, R.E. (1990) Localization of unseen visual stimuli by humans with normal vision. *Neuropsychologia*, 28: 1231–1237.

Mohler, C.W. and Wurtz, R.H. (1977) Role of striate cortex and superior colliculus in visual guidance of saccadic eye movements in monkeys. *J. Neurophysiol.*, 40: 1977.

Moore, T., Rodman, H.R., Repp, A.B. and Gross, C.G. (1995) Localization of visual stimuli after striate cortex damage in monkeys: parallels with human blindsight. *Proc. Natl. Acad. Sci. USA*, 92: 8215–8218.

Morris, J.S., Ohman, A. and Dolan, R.J. (1999) A subcortical pathway to the right amygdala mediating 'unseen' fear. *Proc. Natl. Acad. Sci. USA*, 96: 1680–1685.

Pasik, P. and Pasik, T. (1982) Visual functions in monkeys after total removal of visual cortex. In: W.D. Neff (Ed.), *Contributions to Sensory Physiology*, Vol. 7. Academic Press, New York, pp. 147–200.

Pöppel, E., Held, R. and Frost, D. (1973) Residual function after

brain wounds involving the central visual pathways in man. *Nature*, 243: 295–296.
Posner, M.I., Walker, J.A., Friedrich, F.J. and Rafal, R.D. (1984) Effects of parietal injury on covert orienting of attention. *J. Neurosci.*, 4: 1863–1874.
Ptito, M., Herbin, M., Boire, D. and Ptito, A. (1996) Neural basis of residual vision in hemicorticectomized monkeys. *Prog. Brain Res.*, 112: 385–404.
Rafal, R., Smith, J., Krantz, J., Cohen, A. and Brennan, C. (1990) Extrageniculate vision in hemianopic humans: saccadic inhibition by signals in the blind field. *Science*, 250: 118–121.
Rodman, H.R., Gross, C.G. and Albright, T.D. (1990) Afferent basis of visual response properties in area MT of the macaque. II. Effects of superior colliculus removal. *J. Neurosci.*, 10: 1154–1164.
Schneider, G.E. (1969) Two Visual Systems. *Science*, 163: 895.
Schaerli, H., Harman, A.M. and Hogben, J.H. (1999) Blindsight in subjects with homonymous hemianopia. *J. Cogn. Neurosci.*, 11: 52–66.
Sparks, D.L. and Groh, J.M. (1995) The superior colliculus: a window for viewing issues in integrative neuroscience. In: M.S. Gazzaniga (Ed.), *The Cognitive Neurosciences*. MIT Press, Cambridge, MA, pp. 565–584.
Stein, B.E. and Meredith, M.A. (1993) *The Merging of the Senses*. MIT Press, Cambridge, MA.
Stoerig, P. and Cowey, A. (1989) Wavelength sensitivity in blindsight. *Nature*, 342: 916–918.
Stoerig, P. and Cowey, A. (1992) Wavelength discrimination in blindsight. *Brain*, 115: 425–444.
Stoerig, P., Kleinschmidt, A. and Frahm, J. (1998) No visual responses in denervated V1: high-resolution functional magnetic resonance imaging of a blindsight patient. *NeuroReport*, 9: 21–25.
Torjussen, T. (1978) Visual processing in cortically blind hemifields. *Neuropsychologia*, 16: 15–21.
Warren, D.H. (1979) Spatial localization under conflict conditions: is there a single explanation. *Perception*, 8: 323–337.
Weiskrantz, L. (1986) *Blindsight: A Case Study and Implications*. Oxford University Press, Oxford.
Weiskrantz, L. (1987) Residual vision in a scotoma: a followup study of ‘form’ discrimination. *Brain*, 110: 77–92.
Weiskrantz, L., Warrington, E.K., Sanders, M.D. and Marshall, J. (1974) Visual Capacity in the hemianopic field following a restricted occipital ablation. *Brain*, 97: 709–728.
Weiskrantz, L., Cowey, A. and Passingham, C. (1977) Spatial responses to brief stimuli by monkeys with striate cortex ablations. *Brain*, 100: 655–670.
Welch, R.B. and Warren, D.H. (1986) Intersensory Interactions. In: K. Boff, L. Kaufman and Thomas, J. (Eds.), *Handbook of Perception and Human Performance*, Vol. 1. John Wiley and Sons, New York, pp. 25:1–25:36.
Wessinger, C.M., Fendrich, R. and Gazzaniga, M.S. (1997) Islands of residual vision in hemianopic patients. *J. Cogn. Neurosci.*, 9: 203–221.
Wessinger, C.M., Loback, E.L., Fendrich, R. and Gazzaniga, M.S. (1999) Residual vision following damage to the primary visual pathway: additional subjects, additional islands. *Soc. Neurosci. Abstr.*, 25: 1938.
Zeki, S. and Ffytche, D.H. (1998) The Riddoch syndrome: insights in the neurobiology of conscious vision. *Brain*, 121: 24–45.
Zeki, S., Guy, C.N. and Ffytche, D.H. (1996) Motion specific responses from a blind hemifield. *Brain*, 119: 1971–1982.
Zihl, J. and von Cramon, D. (1980) Registration of light stimuli in the cortically blind hemifield and its effect on localization. *Behav. Brain Res.*, 1: 287–298.

C. Casanova and M. Ptito (Eds.)
Progress in Brain Research, Vol. 134

CHAPTER 23

'Seeing' in the blind hemifield following hemispherectomy

Alain Ptito [1,*], Audrey Fortin [1,2] and Maurice Ptito [1,2]

[1] *Montreal Neurological Institute and Hospital, McGill University, 3801 University St., Montreal, PQ, H3A 2B4, Canada*
[2] *School of Optometry, University of Montreal, 3744 Jean-Brillant St., Montreal, PQ, H3C 3J7 Canada*

Abstract: Destruction of the striate cortex has traditionally been thought to lead to permanent blindness in the contralateral visual field and to the dogma that this region is indispensable for vision in primates. For over 25 years now, evidence has been accumulating that hemianopic human subjects and monkeys possess wide-ranging residual visual capacities or 'blindsight' in the blind part of their visual field. For some researchers, isolated islands of the striate cortex have been associated with patches of degraded vision and made responsible for blindsight. Artefacts such as light scatter, criterion effects, macular sparing, eccentric fixation and minute eye movements have also been linked with the residual vision. For others, the fact that certain aspects of the visual information can be processed without the geniculostriate pathway suggests mediation by the visual subsystems such as extrastriate visual cortical areas which receive visual information via subcortical pathways, that escaped the cortical damage. Subjects who have had a whole cerebral hemisphere removed or disconnected (for the treatment of uncontrollable epilepsy) and who show residual vision in their blind field offer a remarkable opportunity to help clear the controversy regarding the neural substrate of blindsight. Because it is certain that no functional striate or extrastriate cortex remains on the ablated side, these subjects have contributed significantly to identifying the critical pathways involved in blindsight.

Introduction

Evidence has been accumulating that residual visual functions remain after retrogeniculate lesions of the visual pathways. The types of visual processing elicited by stimulation of the blind field have been conveniently classified and described (Stoerig and Cowey, 1997). They include neuroendocrine responses such as melatonin suppression following exposure to a bright light (Czeisler et al., 1995), reflexive responses as shown by pupillary reaction to changes in illumination, implicit processing whereby presentation of a stimulus in the blind field affects performance in the normal visual field (Marzi et al., 1986; Torjussen, 1976) and, direct responses where the subject answers, usually with a forced-choice method, to stimuli restricted to the blind field. It is with the latter method, where subjects carry out visual discriminations without acknowledged awareness, that the term 'blindsight' has been applied. The visual abilities reported are far-ranging, they include target detection and localization by saccadic eye movements (Pöppel et al., 1973) or manual pointing (Weiskrantz et al., 1974), movement detection and direction as well as relative velocity discrimination (Barbur et al., 1980), stimulus orientation (Weiskrantz, 1986), and even in some cases, wavelength discrimination (Stoerig, 1987).

In contrast to good discrimination without awareness, some subjects also verbally report sensations in response to stimulation in the blind field. This residual vision whereby the subject is 'aware' has been

* Corresponding author: A. Ptito, Montreal Neurological Institute and Hospital, McGill University, 3801 University St., Montreal, PQ, H3A 2B4 Canada. Tel.: +1-514-398-8906; Fax: +1-514-398-1338;
E-mail: ptito@bic.mni.mcgill.ca

observed (Weiskrantz et al., 1995) in the well-known patient G.Y. who could, for example, consciously detect a fast-moving stimulus and its direction. This same patient also showed genuine blindsight, depending on the parameters of the stimuli used (e.g. wavelength discrimination, briefly presented slow-moving stimuli). More recently, he showed he was able, with awareness, to discriminate and match color and motion but not brightness between the normal and blind hemifields, although he denied seeing the stimuli (Morland et al., 1999). These positive results contrast with those of patients with retrogeniculate damage who show neither blindsight nor residual vision. Individual differences have been attributed to extent and location of lesions, which are not uniform across patients. Also, age at which the lesion occurred is important, the earlier injured being the more likely to show blindsight. Several authors (Weiskrantz et al., 1995) have, in addition, underlined the importance of the stimulus parameters used when testing for blindsight as well as the collaboration of the subjects. It is a fact that subjects who are convinced they are blind in a part of their visual field remain sceptical when they are still required to respond to presentations within their blind region.

Reports of blindsight in subjects with V1 lesions are not without controversy. Recently, some authors (Zeki and Ffytche, 1998) who also tested G.Y., concluded that blindsight is but a manifestation of a single syndrome referred to as the Riddoch syndrome, characterized by three inter-related states that depend on the coupling of discrimination and awareness. Their results using functional magnetic resonance imaging (fMRI) show that V5 is always active when moving stimuli, slow or fast, are presented in G.Y.'s blind field and that the activity in V5 co-varies with less intense activity in other cortical areas. The authors conclude that there is a clear relationship between awareness and activity, both in individual cortical areas, and in the reticular activating system. More recently, evidence of blindsight was found in only one of six subjects with damage in visual cortex when a forced-choice procedure was used (Scharli et al., 1999). In contrast to previous studies in subjects with homonymous field defects, none of these subjects showed a spatial summation effect. The fact that blindsight occurred in one small isolated area in the upper visual field of that subject and in some but not all locations in his lower visual field suggests to the authors that spared optic radiation geniculate fibers were responsible for the residual visual sensitivities.

Several researchers (Campion et al., 1983; Fendrich et al., 1992) have challenged the evidence and suggested that residual visual functions within scotomas, whether conscious or unconscious, may have sources other than simply mediation by subcortical structures and/or cortical reorganization. Methodological inadequacies such as inadvertent eye movements, scattered light, eccentric fixation as well as intra- and extra-ocular light scatter have been identified as possibly responsible for the residual visual abilities. In addition, given the variability of the lesions responsible for field defects in humans, it may be difficult to be certain that all of striate cortex is inoperative. In fact, fragments or islands of intact striate cortex, rather than extrastriate pathways, have been associated with residual visual abilities (Fendrich et al., 1992).

In order to eliminate the possibility that residual vision is mediated by spared striate cortex, our team in Montreal has been conducting for several years now a series of studies with two groups of hemispherectomy subjects who had undergone complete removal or deafferentation of a whole cerebral hemisphere. In these subjects, striate cortex has been entirely ablated or deafferented, such that explanations based on spared striate cortex and lateral geniculate (LGB) or collicular projection to ipsilateral extrastriate cortex are inapplicable. From autopsy studies (Ueki, 1966), it has been established that following hemispherectomy, there is retrograde degeneration of the entire thalamus on the ablated side, including the lateral geniculate body and other thalamic relays, and only those retinal ganglion cells projecting to midbrain structures remain. Therefore, these groups offered a valuable opportunity to evaluate residual vision mediated by the ipsilesional subcortical structures and/or the remaining cerebral hemisphere.

Cerebral hemispherectomy

In 1928, Dandy (in Villemure and Mascott, 1995) was first to report the results of a cerebral hemispherectomy on a hemiplegic adult patient who suffered from a malignant glioma. According to his description, the approach consisted in occluding the anterior and middle cerebral arteries at the carotid bifurcation and removing the hemisphere in two large fragments, including the caudate nucleus, basal ganglia and insula. Variations in the technique or in the extent of removal have been proposed by many neurosurgeons. They follow two different principles: excision in fragments (Dandy, Krynaw, Penfield) or en bloc (Obrador, Rasmussen), or disconnection (see Villemure and Mascott, 1995 for a review). Anatomical hemispherectomy consists in excising the entire hemisphere sparing the basal ganglia. Hemidecortication aims at preserving the ventricle by removing only the gray matter. Functional hemispherectomy and hemispherotomy are techniques where the hemisphere is only partially removed but completely disconnected from the rest of the brain, thus achieving the same physiological result as an anatomical hemispherectomy.

Hemispherectomy is indicated for control of pharmacologically refractory seizures in patients suffering from a diffuse unilateral hemispheric pathology, congenital or acquired (e.g. Rasmussen's encephalitis, the Sturge–Weber syndrome, hemimegalencephaly, infantile spasms, and the Lennox–Gastaux syndrome). Clinically, candidates for hemispherectomy demonstrate a severe unilateral hemispheric syndrome manifested by hemiplegia and hemianopia. Some have a milder neurological deficit at time of evaluation but may suffer from a progressive condition, such as Rasmussen encephalitis. Success with regard to seizure control has been high. Seventy-five to 80% of patients who underwent a hemispherectomy will become seizure-free while another 20% will improve by 80% in their seizure frequency. In well-selected cases, hemispherectomy is dramatic in controlling the epilepsy and will lead to an improvement in motor performance, behavior, cognitive functions and social integration. For these reasons, the identification of the candidate and the operation at an early age are essential for maximum benefit (Fig. 1 and Table 1).

Candidates for hemispherectomy offer a valuable opportunity to investigate brain plasticity. For instance, Wilson (1970) has underlined that in cases where the hemiplegia was present before language acquisition, no major verbal deficit is observed, irrespective of the hemisphere removed. When the hemiplegia appears after language acquisition, removal of the left hemisphere results in deficient verbal functions with subsequent considerable recuperation in the majority of cases. Increases in intellectual functions have been reported and it is possible that in some cases, hemispherectomy arrests and reverses underlying pathological processes that might otherwise result in mental retardation.

TABLE 1
Characteristics of hemispherectomized subjects

Subjects	Etiology	Symptoms	Surgery			Age at test (years)	IQ at time of testing		
			Type	Age (years)	Side		VIQ	PIQ	FSIQ
DR	Rasmussen's chronic encephalitis	Seizures L-hemiparesis L-hemianopia	FH	17	R	20	87	83	83
SE	Neuronal migration disorder	Seizures L-hemiparesis L-hemianopia	FH	25	R	28	90	84	99
IG	Middle cerebral artery occlusion	Seizures L-hemiparesis L-hemianopia	AH	13	R	42	84	75	79
JB	Congenital porencephalic cyst	Seizures R-hemiparesis R-inferior Quadrantanopia	FH	20	L	29	90	88	88

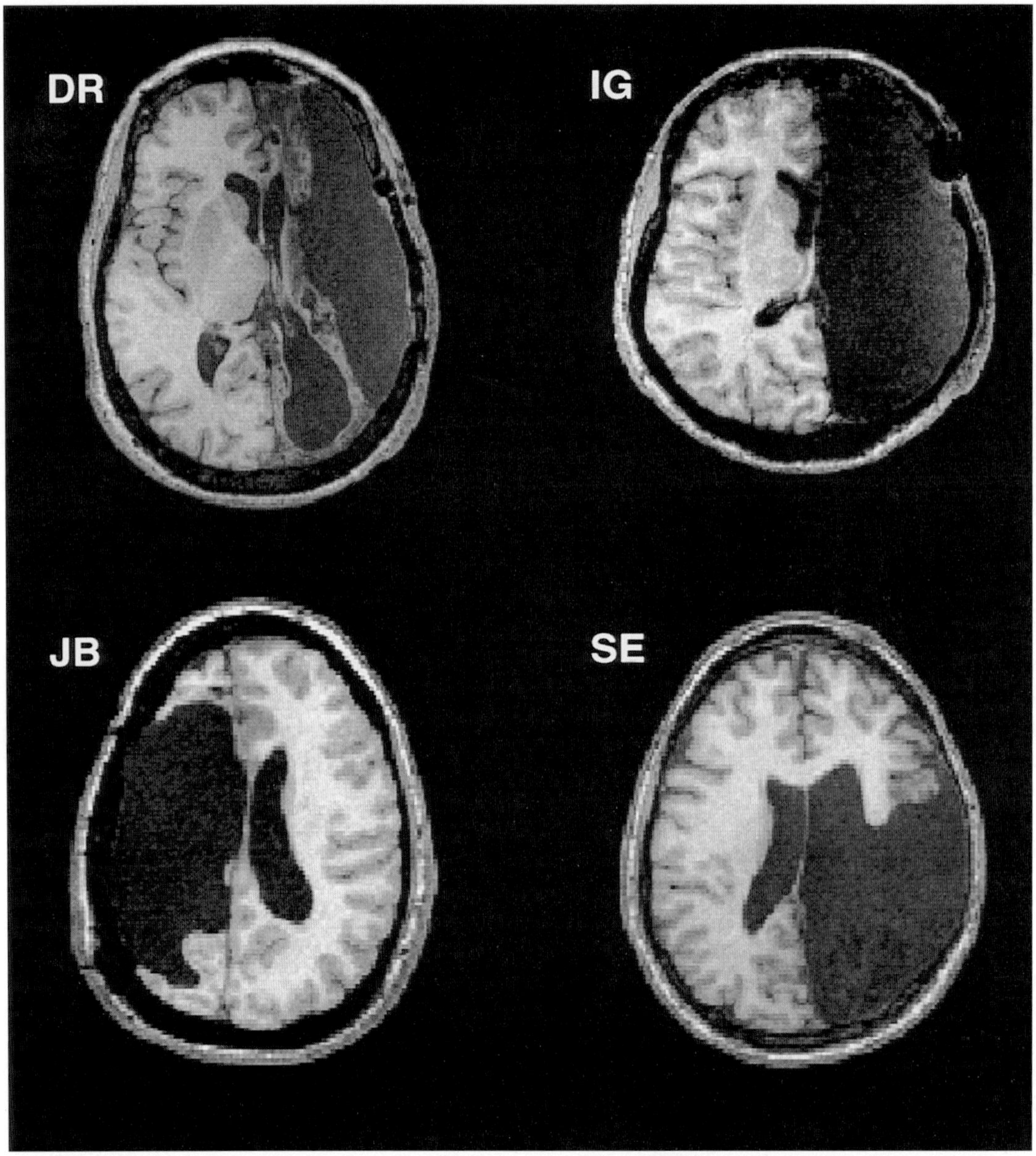

Fig. 1. Magnetic resonance axial images of our second group of subjects showing the surgical ablation.

Psychophysical studies

Detection and localization with awareness

The first group of subjects we tested had undergone complete anatomical hemispherectomy for the relief of uncontrollable seizures. All had suffered severe head injury shortly after birth except for one who developed seizures at the age of 2.5 years following an episode of encephalitis. Although all had IQ ratings below average, their general level of function was good overall. The experiments (Ptito et al., 1991) were carried out monocularly and eye movements were monitored with Beckman EOG electrodes. Any movement of the eye that exceeded 5° interrupted stimulus presentation and produced automatic rejec-

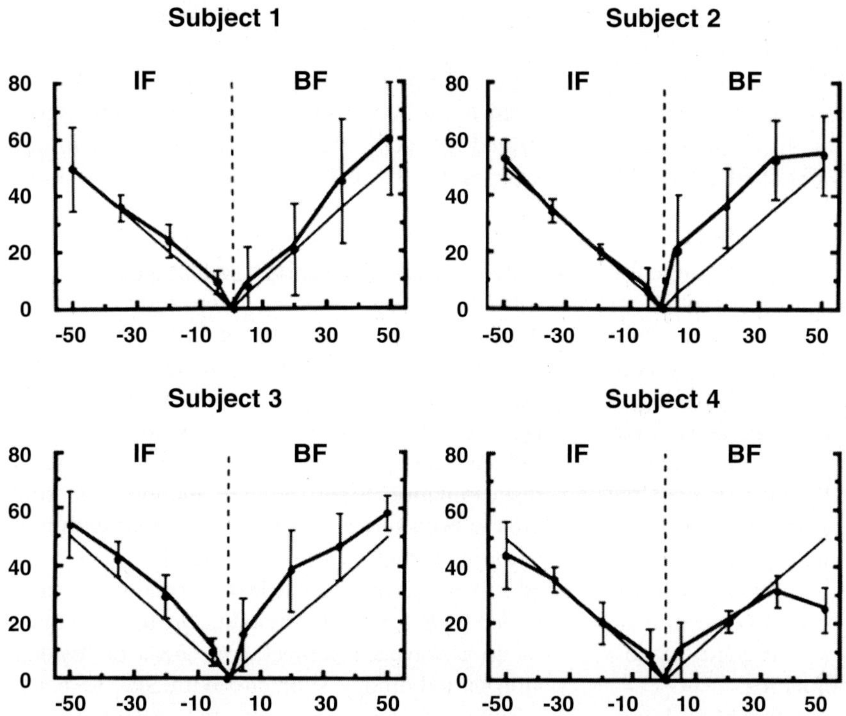

Fig. 2. Accuracy of localization of combined stationary, moving and flashing targets for four subject. Horizontal axis, target position; vertical axis, responses. IF, intact field; BF, blind field. (Adapted from Ptito et al., 1991.)

tion of the trial. In addition, fixation was ensured by requiring the subject to fixate a centrally presented row of eight randomly flickering light-emitting diodes (LEDs) superimposed at intervals of 2.5 cm and to tap on the table as soon as one of the LEDs remained on. The tapping response was picked up by a microphone and relayed to a microprocessor, which then triggered within 5 ms, the presentation of the stimulus. With this rigorous control of eye fixation, we showed, as others had, that the extent and quality of the residual vision vary among subjects and type of task investigated. In the first task, all could detect and localize with reasonable accuracy in their blind field a moving, flashing or stationary stimulus presented during 150 ms (Fig. 2). They rarely denied that a stimulus had been presented and all experienced little difficulty in distinguishing blank trials (absence of the visual stimulus). They were therefore aware of the presence of the stimulus without, however, specifying its nature. This contrasted with the forced-choice techniques used to circumvent the subjects' denial of the presence of a stimulus and we were probably measuring residual vision rather than blindsight as described at the time (Weiskrantz et al., 1974). In a second experiment, we asked the subjects to indicate the presence or absence of a grating and, in the affirmative, to report if it was moving or not. Again, all detected without error blank trials but individual differences with regard to performances in the blind field emerged. Whereas all were capable of detecting the presence of the grating, and two out of three could distinguish between a 'rapidly' moving grating (2.6 cycles/s) and a stationary one, none could detect a slow movement (0.3 cycles/s). In the second part of this experiment we assessed relative velocity discrimination and found a modest but still significant ability. One subject (case 2) was able to discriminate large and median differences in stimulus velocity, but remained at chance when the gratings moved at the same speed. In contrast, case 3 could only detect an absence of difference between velocities while case 1 remained at chance in all conditions involving his blind field. When the gratings were presented simultaneously in both hemifields, similar results were obtained. In a third experiment, we asked the subjects to report whether the direction of displacement of the stimuli presented in the intact field, in the blind field or in both fields simultaneously were the same or different. Results showed that while the subjects obtained over 90% correct responses in their intact field, none were able to discriminate, in the blind field or in both fields simultaneously, direction of movement, a function associated with area MT (putative V5), absent in our subjects (Table 2).

With a second group of hemispherectomy subjects, we showed in a collaborative study (King et al., 1996a) an insensitivity to visual displays simulating motion-in-depth, presented in the hemianopic field and an inability to verbally discriminate the direction of motion of the target patterns. This incapacity to respond to motion-in-depth information in the blind field we interpret as consistent with the inability of our first group of subjects to discriminate movement direction as well as with their modest ability to discriminate relative velocities.

The positive visual functions in the blind hemifield of hemispherectomized subjects has been put into doubt by some control experiments suggesting that there may have been stray light entering the intact hemifield (King et al., 1996b). Subsequently, we showed the importance of controlling intraocular light scatter since spectral sensitivity within the blind field can be reduced considerably and yet, high intensity stimuli can be detected probably by foveal receptors (Stoerig et al., 1996), and we presented a model that could explain the effects of scatter properties of the eye on the visual sensitivities obtained with hemispherectomy subjects (Faubert et al., 1999).

In a well-controlled study, we nevertheless confirmed the existence of residual vision, *with awareness*, in the blind field, that could not be linked to light scatter, eccentric fixation or eye movements (Fendrich et al., 1996; Wessinger et al., 1996). We tested two hemispherectomized subjects with a double Purkinje eye tracker, which allows the stimulus displays to be stabilized retinally with a mirror deflector system and eliminates artifacts due to eye motion. Using a forced-choice method and black stimuli (<1 cd/m^2) on a gray background (10 cd/m^2) to reduce light scatter, we tested stimulus detection and discrimination. Stabilized field mapping identified an area in both subjects' hemianopic field within which stimulus detection was possible. The area consisted of a band along the vertical meridian generally not wider than 3.5°, but extending up to 6° at one field location for each subject. The areas of residual vision varied among subjects. With SE, the band was within both visual quadrants, but only above the horizontal meridian for JB. The subjects were aware of their residual vision and mean confidence values in areas with sparing were significantly higher than in those areas without sparing. Within the areas of residual vision, both subjects readily discriminated simple stimuli such as square and diamond figures and, although they were poorer at discriminating complex stimuli, they still performed above chance. Both were also able to verbally identify squares and

TABLE 2

Percentage of correct responses to movement, velocity differences and movement direction

		Case 1			Case 2			Case 3		
		Intact field	Blind field	Both fields	Intact field	Blind field	Both fields	Intact field	Blind field	Both fields
Movement detection	Stationary	90	20 [a]		100	65		95	93	
	Slow	30 [a]	10 [a]		100	35 [a]		85	5 [a]	
	Rapid	90	10 [a]		100	65		100	95	
	Blank trials	100	100	100	100	100	100	100	100	100
Velocity differences	Same	83	20 [a]	56 [a]	89	30 [a]	29 [a]	100	94	94
	Medium	79	42 [a]	41 [a]	92	83	67 [a]	58 [a]	29 [a]	42 [a]
	Large	92	67 [a]	25 [a]	92	75	75	100	50 [a]	75
Direction of movement		90	50 [a]	54 [a]	100	52 [a]	50 [a]	100	58 [a]	46 [a]

[a] At or below chance level.

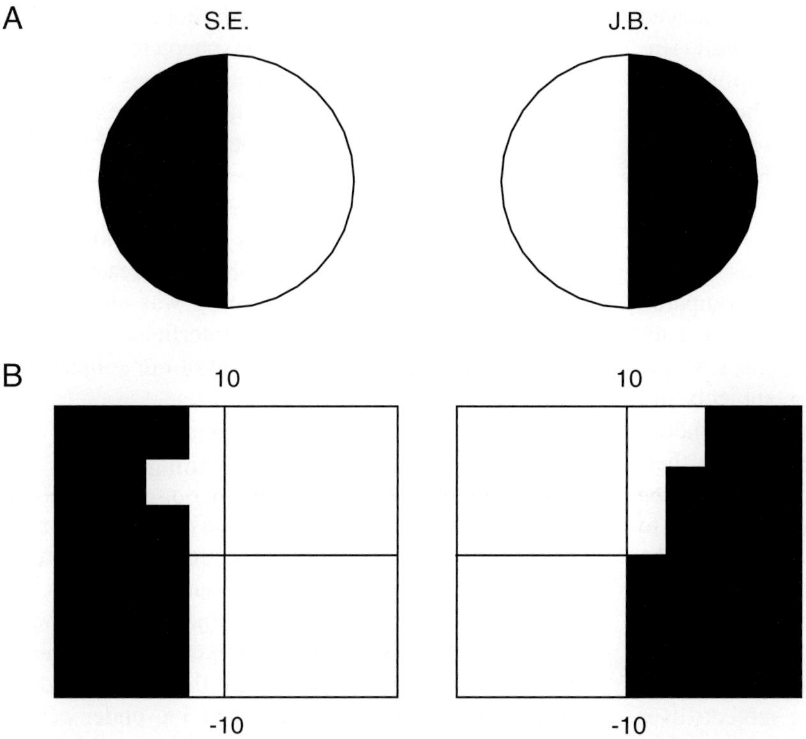

Fig. 3. Schematic representation of (A) perimetric test results of subjects SE and JB showing contralateral hemianopia without macular sparing; and (B) stabilized visual field detection results for SE and JB. (Adapted from Wessinger et al., 1996.)

diamonds presented within the zone of sparing, but neither could identify similarly presented complex figures. In both the discrimination and identification tasks, the subjects performed at chance when stimuli were outside the areas with spared detection while they were always identified correctly in each subject's seeing field (Fig. 3 and Table 3).

Vision without awareness: blindsight

Recently we used a paradigm by which blindsight could not be explained by the use of a lax decisional criterion. We tested four hemispherectomy subjects on a protocol based on the redundant-target effect, a summation phenomenon well-known in experimental psychology (Raab, 1962), whereby the simultaneous presentation of two or more stimuli results in a faster reaction time than that to a single stimulus. This indirect procedure allowed us to observe whether unseen stimuli in the blind field can influence the subject's response to stimuli in the intact field. This is so because the subject responds to stimuli in the normal hemifield only and is not asked to guess about the presence of a

TABLE 3

Percentage of correct responses on discrimination and identification of simple and complex stimuli within and outside areas of residual vision in the blind field

	Discrimination				Identification			
	Simple		Complex		Simple		Complex	
Subject:	SE	JB	SE	JB	SE	JB	SE	JB
Upfar	45	52	50	42	50	60	0	–
Upclose	93 [a]	97 [a]	46	77 [a]	90 [a]	100 [a]	0	0
Downfar	50	52	54	46	61	45	0	–
Downclose	88 [a]	60	63 [a]	35	92 [a]	55	0	0

Upfar, presentation in upper quadrant outside zone of sparing; Upclose, presentation in upper quadrant within zone of sparing; Downfar, presentation in lower quadrant outside zone of sparing; Downclose, presentation in lower quadrant within zone of sparing (SE only).

[a] At or above chance level.

stimulus in the hemianopic field. Results showed that none of the patients were aware of stimuli (single or double) presented in their blind hemifield. As a group, the summation effect across the vertical meridian was not a consistent finding, but single case analysis again revealed the presence of individual differences. First, all but one subject (JB) showed a summation effect in their seeing visual field. When reaction times elicited by the simultaneous display in the normal and blind hemifield were compared to single presentations in the intact field, two subjects (SE and DR) showed faster responses in the double stimulus condition. The other subjects did not show significantly faster reaction times when a second flash was simultaneously presented in their blind hemifield. Furthermore, we conducted a second experiment with normal control subjects in order to confirm that light scatter could not be a factor in the results obtained with the experimental subjects. To do so, we positioned a LED (40 cd/m2) to stimulate the blind spot of the right eye of each subject (~12.5° lateral to the fixation spot and on the same horizontal axis as the other LED's). None of the subjects ever responded to the flashes presented in their blind spot, indicating that light scatter was at most restricted to an area not larger than the blind spot (~5°). This conclusion was further supported by the absence of a difference between responses to a single stimulus versus the double stimulus condition where one was delivered into the blind spot (Fig. 4).

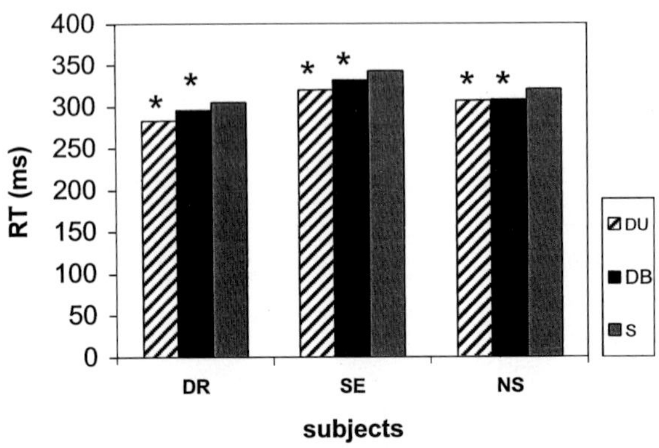

Fig. 4. Mean reaction times (RT) for two hemispherectomy subjects and a normal control subject who showed spatial summation. DU, double unilateral flash; DB, double bilateral flash; S, single flash; *, statistically significant difference with a single flash ($P = 0.05$). (Adapted from Tomaiuolo et al., 1997.)

These results are at odds with those of King et al. (1996b) who tested their hemispherectomy patients for interfield effects on reaction times to simple visual stimuli. They reported no evidence of spatial summation across the visual fields but their negative results may be explained by the fact that they used a very limited number of trials (40 for each condition of stimulus presentation versus at least 1800 for each condition in our study). Also, the mean reaction time of the patients in the latter study was slower than that of our subjects showing interfield summation and approximately similar to that of our subjects not showing such an effect.

Functional magnetic resonance imaging

The results we have been discussing so far reinforce the common observation that with regard to blindsight and residual vision with awareness, individual differences among subjects exist. While some demonstrate total blindness, the phenomenological experience reported in the blind field by others appears context-dependent i.e. under certain experimental conditions there could be a conscious experience qualified as 'residual vision' (Ptito et al., 1987 and Ptito et al., 1991; Wessinger et al., 1996) while in others there is an unconscious visual sensitivity (Herter et al., 1998; Tomaiuolo et al., 1997). The question remains as to which cerebral structures could mediate the residual vision in hemispherectomized subjects. Whereas ipsilesional extrastriate cortices have been proposed as responsible for blindsight in subjects with restricted posterior lesions, we have suggested subcortical structures (such as the superior colliculi and/or the pulvinar thalami) possibly in conjunction with the remaining hemisphere, as likely contenders in hemispherectomized subjects (Ptito et al., 1991).

To investigate more directly the neural pathways involved in blindsight and/or residual vision, we recently conducted an fMRI experiment (Bittar et al., 1999) with three hemispherectomized subjects (JB, IG and DR) who participated in the Tomaiuolo et al. study (Tomaiuolo et al., 1997). To the best of our knowledge, this was the first functional neuroimaging study with hemispherectomized subjects aiming to visualize the cerebral regions involved in blindsight.

The baseline condition comprised viewing computer-generated randomly moving dots (1 Hz; 128 luminance gray levels). The activation condition consisted of a black and white semicircular ring (inner radius 8°, outer radius 11°) with two embedded gratings (1.5°) moving vertically in opposite directions (8 Hz), presented unilaterally on the background of randomly moving dots. This stimulus was specifically designed to prevent Lambertian intraocular scatter in a model whereby intraocular light scatter can account for human sensitivity values obtained in the blind field of hemispherectomized subjects (Faubert et al., 1999).

Blood oxygen level-dependent (BOLD) fMRI was used to examine the pattern of activation in each occipital lobe upon stimulation of the contralateral visual hemifield. Multislice $T2^*$-weighted gradient echo (GE) echo-planar imaging (EPI) images (TR/TE = 4 s/45 ms, flip angle 90°) were acquired with a Siemens Magnetom Vision 1.5T MRI scanner in planes through the occipital cortex, parallel to the calcarine sulcus (10–12 contiguous 6-mm slices). In all subjects, a T1-weighted anatomical MRI scan (TR = 18 ms; TE = 10 ms; flip angle 30°) was acquired and the images were mapped into a common standard (stereotaxic) space. An activation minus baseline subtraction was performed, and the acquired t-statistic map transformed into the stereotaxic coordinate space of Talairach and Tournoux (1988).

As expected for normal subjects, activation patterns were symmetrical and consistent across subjects, with statistically significant ($P < 0.05$) activation in the contralateral areas V1/V2, V3/V3A, VP, and V5. After the results of right hemifield activation were averaged, significant activation foci ($P < 0.01$) were observed in V1/V2 (calcarine sulcus; Talairach coordinates −10, −86, 4.6), V3/V3A (occipital pole; −17, −93, 22), VP (lingual gyrus; −15, −77, −2.9), and V5 (parieto-temporo-occipital junction; −50, −72, 7.5). The statistically significant activation was produced in homologous regions of the right occipital lobe with left hemifield stimulation. In all studies, activation was confined to the cerebral hemisphere contralateral to the stimulated visual field.

Stimulation of the intact hemifield in hemispherectomized subjects resulted in several areas of statistically significant activation ($P < 0.01$) exclusively within the contralateral occipital lobe. Stimulation of the anopic hemifield in the two subjects who did not exhibit blindsight in the Tomaiuolo et al. study (Tomaiuolo et al., 1997), failed to yield statistically significant activation. Stimulation of the hemifield contralateral to the hemispherectomy resulted in statistically significant activation in the ipsilateral occipital lobe in one subject with blindsight. Four activation foci were obtained in this subject with right hemispherectomy (DR): (1) left temporo-occipital junction (putative V5); $t = 10.7$; −48, −75, −2; (2) left occipital pole (V3/V3A); $t = 7.9$; −24, −93, −2; (3) left cuneus (V3/V3A); $t = 7.7$; −12, −87, 16; and (4) left occipital pole (V3/V3A); $t = 6.4$; −24, −86, 24 (Fig. 5). The subject reported awareness of something moving on her left, but could not describe it. A directed search did not reveal significant activation within the superior colliculi or pulvinar of either the experimental or control subjects.

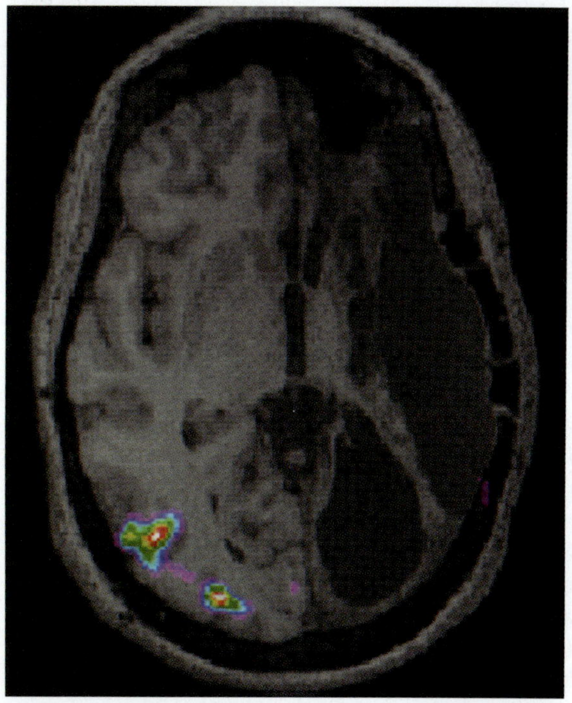

Fig. 5. Stimulation of the blind hemifield in DR (who had been shown previously to possess blindsight) resulted in statistically significant activation foci in V5, V3 and V3A.

Potential anatomical substrates of blindsight

The results so far are consistent with the possibility that the remaining hemisphere plays a role in the mediation of blindsight and/or residual visual abilities in the blind field. This would be achieved either by a process of cortical plasticity and/or by utilization of existing neural pathways such as subcortical nuclei.

Several observations have provided support for the superior colliculi as a likely mediator of residual visual function following removal or destruction of the striate and extrastriate cortices. Monkeys who have had their striate cortex removed are able to localize visual stimuli in the blind hemifield, perform wavelength discrimination, simple shape and pattern discrimination, as well as velocity discrimination (reviewed in Ptito et al., 1996). These abilities are abolished following the additional destruction of the ipsilateral superior colliculus (Rodman et al., 1990). In hemispherectomized infant monkeys that could detect stimuli in their blind hemifield, anatomical and histochemical studies revealed transneural retrograde degeneration of many retinal ganglion cells, a large reduction in volume of the ipsilateral dLGN, but only a very slight reduction in volume of the ipsilateral superior colliculus (Ptito et al., 1996). In monkeys, the superior colliculi receive direct input from both the retina and the striate cortex, and contain a complete representation of the visual field (Schiller, 1972). The two superior colliculi, at least in the cat, communicate with each other via tecto-tectal projections (Behan and Kime, 1996), and provide a potential channel to the extrastriate visual cortices, most notably area MT (or V5), via the pulvinar (Cowey et al., 1994). Cells in the superior colliculi respond most vigorously to moving objects (Moors and Vendrik, 1979). In primates, area MT contains a large contingency of direction-selective neurons, and these neurons remain direction-selective following ablation of the striate cortex (Rodman et al., 1989). Subsequent collicular ablation extinguishes this direction-selectivity (Rodman et al., 1990). Thus the ability to discriminate the direction of motion relies upon the integrity of not only the superior colliculus, but also the extrastriate cortex. This would explain why hemispherectomized patients (with an absence of striate and extrastriate cortex, but a presumably intact superior colliculus) demonstrate an inability to discriminate the direction of motion in their blind field (horizontal motion or motion-in-depth; Perenin, 1991; Ptito et al., 1991; King et al., 1996a).

Evidence that the superior colliculi are involved in the spatial summation effect across the vertical meridian has been demonstrated (Zihl and Von Cramon, 1979; Reuter-Lorenz et al., 1995). Preservation of the superior colliculi following hemispherectomy, in the face of degeneration of structures involved in the geniculocalcarine pathway, adds weight to their putative role in the mediation of residual visual functions in monkeys (Ptito et al., 1996) and humans (Ueki, 1966).

Another possible explanation of residual visual abilities in hemispherectomized subjects is cortical plasticity. For example, topographical remapping of sensory space can occur after primary inputs are removed even in undamaged brains after learning (Buonomano and Merzenich, 1998). Visual function may improve substantially with time following striate cortex destruction (Weiskrantz et al., 1974; Zihl, 1981; Weiskrantz, 1986; Ptito et al., 1999a,b) and receptive fields in primary visual cortex appear to vary in response to changes in recent stimulus history (Gilbert, 1998). Serial PET-studies in children following hemispherectomy have shown that glucose metabolism in the caudate nucleus ipsilateral to the resection initially decreased, but partially or completely returned to their preoperative levels over the next couple of years (Chugani and Jacobs, 1994). This recovery of metabolic activity was taken as evidence of anatomical reorganization. A case of hemispherectomy in a 20-year-old woman which was not followed by hemianopia has been reported (Damasio et al., 1975). This patient had sustained a severe closed head injury at 5 years, and had bilateral optic nerve atrophy and concentric retraction of both visual fields prior to surgery. Following the resection, the patient actually demonstrated an increased visual field in one eye. Although this was a single case report, it furnishes some evidence that the human visual system is capable of adaptation or reorganization following major structural misadventure.

Whilst the anatomical and physiological basis of blindsight in hemidecorticated subjects may be a combination of both the retinotectal system as well as plasticity of the unaffected cerebral cortex, the potential role of the intact occipital cortex should be considered. A vital issue is the route by which information from one visual hemifield reaches the ipsilateral cortex. Aside from transcallosal pathways, there are no known direct pathways for the transmission of visual information to the ipsilateral occipital lobe. It is conceptually possible for such information to occur via tecto-tectal pathways, with eventual arrival at the ipsilateral extrastriate cortices after passing through the pulvinar. V5 is said to possess up to 15° of representation in the ipsilateral visual field (Maunsell and Van Essen, 1983), although the mechanism of this is unclear. Activation of V5 and V3/V3A in our hemispherectomized subjects with blindsight supports the role of the ipsilateral extrastriate cortex in the mediation of residual vision.

Conclusion

Hemispherectomy patients present a unique opportunity to evaluate the anatomical substrates of residual vision observed in their blind field. We show that residual vision with and without awareness is subject to experimental conditions and to intra- and inter-patients variability. We propose that the remaining hemisphere contributes to these visual residual functions in the blind hemifield in conjunction with ipsilesional subcortical structures.

Acknowledgements

This work was supported by grants from le Fond Formation de Chercheurs et Aide à la Recherche (FCAR) and the National Science and Engineering Research Council of Canada (NSERC).

References

Barbur, J.L., Ruddock, K.H. and Waterfield, V.A. (1980) Human visual responses in the absence of the geniculo-calcarine projection. *Brain*, 103: 905–928.

Behan, M. and Kime, N.M. (1996) Spatial distribution of tectotectal connections in the cat. *Prog. Brain Res.*, 112: 131–142.

Bittar, R.G., Ptito, M., Faubert, J. and Ptito, A. (1999) Activation of the remaining hemisphere following stimulation of the blind hemifield in hemispherectomized subjects. *NeuroImage*, 10: 339–346.

Buonomano, D.V. and Merzenich, M.M. (1998) Net interaction between different forms of short-term synaptic plasticity and slow-IPSPs in the hippocampus and auditory cortex. *J. Neurophysiol.*, 80: 1765–1774.

Campion, J., Latto, R. and Smith, Y.M. (1983) Is blindsight an effect of scattered light, spared cortex and near-threshold vision? *Behav. Brain Sci.*, 6: 423–486.

Chugani, H.T. and Jacobs, B. (1994) Metabolic recovery in caudate nucleus of children following cerebral hemispherectomy. *Ann. Neurol.*, 36: 794–797.

Cowey, A., Stoerig, P. and Bannister, M. (1994) Retinal ganglion cells labelled from the pulvinar nucleus in macaque monkeys. *Neuroscience*, 61: 691–705.

Czeisler, C.A., Shanahan, T.L., Klerman, E.B., Brotman, D.J., Emens, J.S., Klein, T. and Rizzo, J.F. (1995) Suppression of melatonin secretion in some blind patients by exposure to bright light. *New Engl. J. Med.*, 332: 6–11.

Damasio, A.R., Lima, A. and Damasio, H. (1975) Nervous function after right hemispherectomy. *Neurology*, 25: 89–93.

Faubert, J., Diaconu, V., Ptito, M. and Ptito, A. (1999) Residual vision in the blind field of hemidecorticated humans predicted by diffusion scatter model and selective spectral absorption of the human eye. *Vision Res.*, 39: 149–157.

Fendrich, R., Wessinger, C.M. and Gazzaniga, M.S. (1992) Residual vision in scotoma: implication for blindsight. *Science*, 258: 1489–1491.

Fendrich, R., Wessinger, C.M. and Gazzaniga, M.S. (1996) Nasotemporal overlap at the retinal vertical meridian: investigations with a callosotomy patient. *Neuropsychologia*, 34: 637.

Gilbert, C.D. (1998) Adult cortical dynamics. *Physiol. Rev.*, 78: 467–485.

Herter, T., Ptito, A. and Guitton, G. (1998) Visuo-oculomotor capabilities of hemidecorticate patients. *Soc. Neurosci. Abst.*, 24: 1144.

King, S.M., Frey, S., Villemure, J.G., Ptito, A. and Azzopardi, P. (1996a) Perception of motion-in-depth in patients with partial or complete cerebral hemispherectomy. *Behav. Brain Res.*, 76: 169–180.

King, S.M., Azzopardi, P., Cowey, A., Oxbury, J. and Oxbury, S. (1996b) The role of light scatter in the residual visual sensitivity of patients with complete cerebral hemispherectomy. *Vis. Neurosci.*, 13: 1–13.

Marzi, C.A., Tassinari, G., Aglioti, S. and Lutzemberger, L. (1986) Spatial summation across the vertical meridian in hemianopics: a test of blindsight. *Neuropsychologia*, 24: 749–758.

Maunsell, J.H. and Van Essen, D.C. (1983) The connections of the middle temporal visual area (MT) and their relationship to a cortical hierarchy in the macaque monkey. *J. Neurosci.*, 3: 2563–2586.

Moors, J. and Vendrik, A.J. (1979) Responses of single units in the monkey superior colliculus to moving stimuli. *Exp. Brain Res.*, 35: 349–369.

Morland, A.B., Jones, S.R., Finlay, A.L., Deyzac, E., Le, S. and Kemp, S. (1999) Visual perception of motion, luminance and colour in a human hemianope. *Brain*, 122: 1183–1198.

Perenin, M.T. (1991) Discrimination of motion direction in perimetrically blind fields. *NeuroReport*, 2: 397–400.

Pöppel, E., Held, R. and Frost, D. (1973) Residual visual function after brain wounds involving the central visual pathways in man. *Nature*, 243: 295–296.

Ptito, A., Lassonde, M., Ptito, M. and Lepore, F. (1987) Visual discrimination in hemispherectomized patients. *Neuropsychologia*, 25: 869–879.

Ptito, A., Lepore, F., Ptito, M. and Lassonde, M. (1991) Target detection and movement discrimination in the blind field of hemispherectomized patients. *Brain*, 114: 497–512.

Ptito, M., Herbin, M., Boire, D. and Ptito, A. (1996) Neural bases of residual vision in hemicorticectomized monkeys. *Prog. Brain Res.*, 112: 385–404.

Ptito, M., Dalby, M. and Gjedde, A. (1999a) Visual field recovery in a patient with bilateral occipital lobe damage. *Acta Neurol. Scand.*, 99: 252–254.

Ptito, M., Johannsen, P., Faubert, J. and Gjedde, A. (1999b) Activation of human extrageniculostriate pathways after damage to area V1. *NeuroImage*, 9: 97–107.

Raab, D. (1962) Statistical facilitation of simple reaction time. *Trans. New York Acad. Sci.*, 43: 574–590.

Reuter-Lorenz, P.A., Nozawa, G., Gazzaniga, M.S. and Hughes, H.C. (1995) Fate of neglected targets: a chronometric analysis of redundant target effects in the bisected brain. *J. Exp. Psychol. Hum. Percept. Perform.*, 21: 211–230.

Rodman, H.R., Gross, C.G. and Albright, T.D. (1989) Afferent basis of visual response properties in area MT of the macaque I Effects of striate cortex removal. *J. Neurosci.*, 9: 2033–2050.

Rodman, H.R., Gross, C.G. and Albright, T.D. (1990) Afferent basis of visual response properties in area MT of the macaque II Effect of the superior colliculus removal. *J. Neurosci.*, 10: 1154–1164.

Scharli, H., Harman, A.M. and Hogben, J.H. (1999) Blindsight in subjects with homonymous visual field defects. *J. Cogn. Neurosci.*, 11: 52–66.

Schiller, P.H. (1972) The role of the monkey superior colliculus in eye movement and vision. *Invest. Ophthalmol.*, 11: 451–460.

Stoerig, P. (1987) Chromaticity and achromaticity evidence for a functional differentiation in visual field defects. *Brain*, 110: 869–886.

Stoerig, P. and Cowey, A. (1997) Blindsight in man and monkey. *Brain*, 120: 535–559.

Stoerig, P., Faubert, J., Ptito, M., Diaconu, V. and Ptito, A. (1996) No blindsight following hemidecortication in human subjects? *NeuroReport*, 12: 1990–1994.

Talairach, J. and Tournoux, P. (1988). *Co-Planar Stereotaxis Atlas of the Human Brain*, Thieme, New York.

Tomaiuolo, F., Ptito, M., Marzi, C.A., Paus, T. and Ptito, A. (1997) Blindsight in hemispherectomized patients as revealed by spatial summation across the vertical meridian. *Brain*, 120: 795–803.

Torjussen, T. (1976) Residual function in cortically blind hemifields. *Scand. J. Psychol.*, 17: 320–323.

Ueki, K. (1966) Hemispherectomy in the human with special reference to the preservation of function. *Prog. Brain Res.*, 21: 285–338.

Villemure, J.G. and Mascott, C.R. (1995) Peri-insular hemispherotomy: surgical principles and anatomy. *Neurosurgery*, 37: 975–981.

Weiskrantz, L. (1986) *Blindsight: a Case Study and Implications*, Clarendon Press, Oxford.

Weiskrantz, L., Warrington, E.K., Sanders, M.D. and Marshall, J. (1974) Visual capacity in the hemianopic field following a restricted occipital ablation. *Brain*, 97: 709–728.

Weiskrantz, L., Barbur, J.L. and Saraie, A. (1995) Parameters affecting conscious versus unconscious visual discrimination with damage to the visual cortex (V1). *Proc. Natl. Acad. Sci. USA*, 92: 6122–6126.

Wessinger, C.M., Fendrich, R., Ptito, A., Villemure, J.G. and Gazzaniga, M.S. (1996) Residual vision with awareness in the field contralateral to a partial or complete functional hemispherectomy. *Neuropsychologia*, 34: 1129–1137.

Wilson, P.J. (1970) Cerebral hemispherectomy for infantile hemiplegia. A report of 50 cases. *Brain*, 93: 47–80.

Zeki, S. and Ffytche, D.H. (1998) The Riddoch syndrome: insight into the neurobiology of conscious vision. *Brain*, 121: 25–45.

Zihl, J. (1981) Recovery of visual functions in patients with cerebral blindness. Effect of specific practice with saccadic localization. *Exp. Brain Res.*, 44: 159–169.

Zihl, J. and Von Cramon, D. (1979) Restitution of visual function in patients with cerebral blindness. *J. Neurol. Neurosurg. Psychiatry*, 42: 312–322.

C. Casanova and M. Ptito (Eds.)
Progress in Brain Research, Vol. 134

CHAPTER 24

Visual pathways following cerebral hemispherectomy

Denis Boire [1], Hugo Théoret [3] and Maurice Ptito [1,2,*]

[1] *École d'Optométrie, Université de Montréal, CP, 6128, succursale Centre-ville, Montréal, PQ, H3C 3J7 Canada*
[2] *Centre de Recherche en Sciences Neurologiques, Université de Montréal, CP, 6128, succursale Centre-ville, Montréal, PQ, H3C 3J7 Canada*
[3] *Groupe de Recherche en Neuropsychologie Expérimentale, Université de Montréal, CP, 6128, succursale Centre-ville, Montréal, PQ, H3C 3J7 Canada*

Abstract: The anatomical consequences of unilateral cerebral hemispherectomy in some animal models are reviewed. We have shown that the retinogenigulate pathway undergoes severe degenerative changes in hemispherectomized monkeys, greater than those shown in cats and we proposed that remaining retinal terminals to the dorsal lateral geniculate nucleus have little potential for conveying visual information any further. All subdivisions of the pulvinar undergo severe degeneration following hemispherectomy showing that the ascending tectofugal pathway is also shut off. On the other hand, the retina subserving the blind field is not depleted of ganglion cells which still send normal appearing terminals to the midbrain pretectum and superior colliculus. Visual information from the blind hemifield can thus gain access to the brain and could potentially reach the contralateral cerebral cortex through the midbrain commissure and possibly through thalamic commissural cells.

Introduction

The purpose of this contribution is to shortly review the anatomical consequences of unilateral cerebral hemispherectomy. Although cerebral hemispherectomy has been used primarily in an experimental context, it is now performed in humans as a surgical treatment of intractable epilepsy and other early congenital malformations of one cerebral hemisphere. Its success in controlling seizures and the quality of life gained by patients has sparked renewed interest in the behavioral and anatomical consequences of this procedure. One particularly persisting question concerns the visual capabilities of hemispherectomy patients (see A. Ptito et al., 2001, this volume). We will not review the literature on blindsight in patients with lesions to the primary visual cortex (see Fendrich et al., 2001, this volume) or in hemispherectomy patients (see A. Ptito et al., 2001, this volume), but rather concentrate on the anatomy of the visual system following hemispherectomy and discuss the differences between the outcomes observed in animal models of this procedure. This will point out similarities and differences in the organization of the visual system which will help in understanding the fundamentals of visual processing by subcortical visual components and possible pathways for residual visual capabilities.

Being interested in the consequences of hemispherectomy in humans, we consider non-human primates as the best model. The most striking feature of the primate forebrain is undoubtedly the great development in size and areal diversification of the isocortex. We might therefore gain information on the effects of removing the large and highly differentiated isocortex in primate and man compared to ablating isocortical equivalents in cats. It is clear

[3] Present address: Laboratory for Magnetic Brain Stimulation, Behavioral Neurology Unit, Beth Israel Deaconess Medical Center, Harvard Medical School, 330 Brookline Ave KS-454, Boston, MA 02215, USA.
* Corresponding author: M. Ptito, École d'Optométrie, Université de Montréal, CP, 6128, succursale Centre-ville, Montréal, PQ, H3C 3J7 Canada. Tel.: +1-514-343-6052; Fax: +1-514-343-2382; E-mail: ptito@psy.umontreal.ca

that, when one removes the isocortex of a man, monkey, carnivore or rodent, the ablated tissue shares common 'themes' and many intricate differences. It is increasingly believed that the basic circuitry of sensory systems in the forebrain is similar in amniotes (see Karten, 1997 and Medina and Reiner, 2000 for an overview), the differences resting mainly in the laminar organization of cells and areal differentiation of cortical fields involved in higher processing. For example, it is generally agreed that all extant amniotes possess an isocortical equivalent of the primary visual cortex (see Medina and Reiner, 2000), but there is much debate on the homologies beyond V1 (see Rosa and Krubitzer, 1999 and Kaas and Lyon, 2001, this volume). In ablating the whole isocortex on one side of the brain, one is removing not only the equivalent of V1, but up to 20 or 30 different visual cortical areas in a primate compared to a handful of differentiated visual fields in rodents and a few more in carnivores.

Removing visual cortices

Behavioral effects

Processing of visual information or any other sensory information is increasingly being seen as the result of simultaneous activity of distributed brain regions rather than in terms of sequential processing. Although much attention is focused on the interactions between cortical fields, the studies of Schneider (1969) defining a cortical 'what' and a midbrain 'where', have addressed the question on the behavioral abilities to perform visual discrimination and orienting responses in animals with cortical and midbrain lesions. These and subsequent lesion studies indicate that the midbrain and forebrain visual systems may play complementary roles in visual behavior (Schneider, 1967, 1969) and that the function of the midbrain system is significantly influenced by the forebrain (Sprague, 1966; Sherman, 1977; Wallace et al., 1989, 1990).

There is ample literature on visual cortex lesions in rodents and reviewing even some of it would be quite lengthy (see Dean, 1990 and Goodale and Carey, 1990). Hamsters (Schneider, 1969) and rats (Spear and Barbas, 1975; Dean, 1978, 1981 see also Dean, 1990) with large bilateral lesions of visual cortices (including extrastriate areas) lose pattern discrimination capabilities, but are still able to orient to visual stimuli. Hamsters (Schneider, 1969; Carman and Schneider, 1992) and rats (Dyer et al., 1976; Milner et al., 1979) with bilateral ablations of the superior colliculi lose visual orienting capabilities, but retain pattern discrimination abilities (see also Goodale et al., 1978). Bilaterally decorticate rats have been shown to be able to learn to locate a visible platform in a water maze and display head movements typical of searching behavior (Whishaw and Kolb, 1984). To make things simple, rodents with posterior cortical lesions retain some visual orientation capabilities.

Numerous studies have detailed the residual visual behaviors of cats with lesions of areas 17/18. Despite a performance below that of normal cats, many visual functions are preserved in these animals. In their review on the subject, Payne et al. (1996) mention the following: visual acuity (Berkeley and Sprague, 1979; Lehmkhule et al., 1982; Hughes and Sprague, 1986), line orientation discrimination (Berkeley and Sprague, 1979; Orban et al., 1988, 1990), form and motion discrimination (Pasternak and Maunsell, 1992; Pasternak et al., 1995), depth perception (Cornwell et al., 1976, 1980a); Shupert et al., 1993), stereopsis (Kaye et al., 1981; Ptito et al., 1992), detection of patterns in the presence of noise or texture (Hughes and Sprague, 1986; Kruger et al., 1986, 1988; De Weerd et al., 1994), learning of complex pattern discrimination (Doty, 1971; Cornwell et al., 1980a,b, 1989), orientation to new stimuli introduced in the peripheral visual field (Shupert et al., 1993) and optokinetic nystagmus (Shupert et al., 1993). When a lesion of areas 17/18 is accompanied by the ablation of parts of extrastriate cortex, visual deficits are more severe than those seen in destriate animals (Ptito et al., 1988 and review by Payne et al., 1996).

In the monkey, it has been known for many decades that some visual behaviors are spared following lesions of area V1 (Kluver, 1936, 1942, 1949). These behaviors include manual (Keating, 1975; Feinberg et al., 1978) and saccadic (Mohler and Wurtz, 1977; Seagraves et al., 1987) localization, target detection (Pasik and Pasik, 1973) and orientation (Keating, 1975) and luminosity (Schilder et al., 1971) discriminations. Many studies have also demonstrated the presence of simple form discrimination in those animals (Pasik and Pasik, 1982; Dineen and Keating, 1981; Humphrey, 1974). However, the number of trials required to reach criteria is high and performance drops dramatically when certain stimulus parameters are modified. Similarly to the cat, behavioral impairments are more severe following additional ablation of extrastriate areas (Pasik and Pasik, 1971; Keating, 1975). Anatomical and electrophysiological evidence also suggest an important role for extrastriate cortex in residual vision. There are numerous parallel pathways to the geniculo-striate projection which bypass area V1. There is, among others, the direct geniculo-extrastriate projection, the direct retino-pulvino-extrastriate pathway and the indirect pathways involving mesencephalic structures such as the superior colliculus (SC) and the pulvinar (Stoerig and Cowey, 1997). Electrophysiological studies have also shown that extrastriate areas remain functional following removal or inactivation of area V1 (Girard and Bullier, 1989; Rodman et al., 1989, 1990; Girard et al., 1991, 1992; Gross, 1991).

Anatomical considerations

Early lesions of area 17/18 in the cat result in important modifications of the visual pathways. The retino-geniculate pathway is particularly affected by visual cortex lesions. There is massive retrograde degeneration of layer A and A1 cells within the dorsal lateral geniculate nucleus (dLGN) whereas many layer C neurons are spared (Payne et al., 1988; Lomber et al., 1993). It is assumed that the C layer cells survive because of their projections to extrastriate cortex. The geniculate cell loss is accompanied by the death of a majority of Pβ retinal ganglion cells (Pearson et al., 1981; Kalil, 1984; Payne et al., 1984) which project exclusively to the degenerate A and A1 layers of the dLGN. Pα and Pγ RGC are mostly spared due to their projections to the C layers of the LGN and to the SC (Bowling and Michael, 1984; Leventhal et al., 1985). In addition to neuronal loss, ablations of areas 17/18 are accompanied by the amplification of certain pathways: expansion of the thalamo-extrastriate, cortico-cortical and descending extrastriate pathways (Kalil et al., 1991; Sun et al., 1994; Lomber et al., 1995; MacNeil et al., 1996). It is believed that this reorganization results in increased visual information reaching extrastriate cortex neurons which maintain similar receptive field properties to those of normal cats (Guido et al., 1990, 1992; Payne and Cornwell, 1994).

The anatomical consequences of ablation of area V1 in the monkey are similar to those observed in the cat. Namely, it is assumed that residual visual functions in these animals are mediated by visual pathways which escape neuronal degeneration (Stoerig and Cowey, 1997). Almost 80% of Pβ RGC die following destriation while Pα and Pγ cells are spared (Cowey, 1974; Cowey et al., 1989; Niida et al., 1990). In the dLGN, only about 1% of the projection neurons survive the ablation (Mihailovic et al., 1971) and are believed to be maintained by their projection to extrastriate cortex (Yukie and Iwai, 1981; Cowey and Stoerig, 1989). Retinal projections to the SC, on the other hand, do not seem to be modified following the lesion (Dineen et al., 1982; Cowey et al., 1994).

To summarize, anatomical and behavioral data in cats, monkeys and humans (see Fendrich et al., 2001, this volume) show that some visually guided behaviors are maintained following the removal of primary visual cortex. Area 17/18 lesions are accompanied by the important degeneration of the retino-geniculo-striate pathway and the relative sparing of secondary pathways projecting to extrastriate areas, which have been shown to remain active following the ablation. This converging evidence shows that residual vision is subserved by extra geniculo-striate pathways, which include the direct geniculo-striate projection and the retino-collicular projection reaching extrastriate cortex through the pulvinar. This in turn suggests that extrastriate cortices play a fundamental role in residual vision. If this were to be true, a lesion which encompasses, in addition to primary visual cortex, all extrastriate cortical areas should abolish all residual visual functions. One model which provides such a possibility is hemispherectomy, a surgical procedure in which the entire cortical mantle on one side of the brain is removed.

Hemispherectomy as an experimental paradigm

Originally, hemispherectomies have been performed in a variety of mammals in order to shed light onto thalamocortical connections based on retrograde and anterograde degenerations. In early experiments, hemidecortication was instrumental in the classification of thalamic nuclei based on the presence and magnitude of cell degeneration (Walker, 1935, 1938; Papez, 1938; Lashley, 1941; Bodian, 1942; Rose and Woolsey, 1943; Mettler, 1943; Combs, 1949; Powell, 1952; Peacock and Combs, 1965). Following cortical removal, some thalamic nuclei undergo severe degeneration, whereas others are either partially or totally spared. In general, anterior, lateral and posterior thalamic cell masses suffer severe cell loss compared to midline, medial and intralaminar nuclei (see Macchi, 1967). Among the structures involved in visual thalamo-cortical relationships, the LGNd and the pulvinar generally exhibit important cell loss, whereas the ventral lateral geniculate is relatively spared by cortical ablations. These degeneration techniques have been used in attempts to decipher thalamo-cortical connections. It is clear, however, that some nuclei that do project to the cerebral cortex do not exhibit such massive retrograde degeneration, e.g. intralaminar nuclei (see Jones, 1999 p. 59). The severity of cell loss varies, however, between species. For example, a near total depletion of LGN neurons has been reported in the rat, rabbit, monkey and man (Polyak, 1932; Walker, 1935; Lashley, 1941; Powell, 1952; Chow and Dewson, 1966; Ralston and Chow, 1973) and 15% survival cell survival has been shown in the LGN in cats with total chronic cortical disconnection (Madarasz et al., 1983). Hemidecortication is clearly not the most powerful tool to decipher thalamo-cortical connections, the advent of numerous sensitive substances for detailed tract tracing greatly surpass in power degeneration techniques. However, unilateral cerebral hemispherectomy could shed light on the capabilities of the subcortical visual relays in processing visual information in absence of all visual cortical fields.

Behavioral and anatomical consequences of hemispherectomy

There seems to be little doubt that hemispherectomy does not abolish all visually guided behaviors in cats. Although adult hemispherectomy results in complete contralateral hemianopia, neonatally lesioned animals (less than 2 weeks of age) can orient to stimuli presented up to 45° in the affected hemifield (Hovda and Villablanca, 1990). Similar results were obtained in the monkey, where some animals hemispherectomized as infants might also detect and orient to stimuli presented up to 45° in the blind hemifield (Ptito et al., 1996). It is important to note, however, that Tusa et al. (1986) reported that monkeys with large occipital lesions could not produce visually guided saccades to the contralesional visual field. These contradictory results in monkeys are reminiscent of those obtained in human hemispherectomy patients (see A. Ptito et al., 2001, this volume) where presence of residual vision has not always been reported.

As in primary visual cortex lesioned animals and humans, residual orienting and discriminative capabilities will depend upon the state of the surviving pathways. In early lesioned cats, functional sparing of orienting behaviors is accompanied by a smaller decrease of the SC oxidative metabolism compared to adult lesioned animals in which no visual functions persist (Villablanca and Hovda, 1989; Hovda et al., 1992, 1996). Furthermore, neuronal densities in the ipsilesional SC of neonatally hemispherectomized cats are not significantly different from those of normal animals (Villablanca and Hovda, 1989). Retinal ganglion cells which project to retinorecipient nuclei of the midbrain in cats also seem to be spared following hemispherectomy (Théoret et al., 1997). This suggests that the retino-collicular pathway is relatively well preserved in those animals and could contribute to orienting behaviors in cats which sustained massive occipital ablations. Hemispherectomy in adult cats is also accompanied by severe retrograde degeneration of dLGN neurons, where volume and mean number of neurons are reduced by 33 and 80%, respectively (Shook and Villablanca, 1991). On the other hand, neonatal lesions result in a statistically insignificant volume reduction (23%) and a decrease in mean number of neurons of 43% (Shook and Villablanca, 1991).

In primates, data on the anatomical consequences of hemispherectomy are scarce. Some older studies have reported the complete degeneration of the dLGN, with the exception of magnocellular layers in monkeys (Walker, 1935, 1938; Mettler, 1943; Peacock and Combs, 1965) and humans (Powell, 1952). However, detailed quantitative anatomical analysis of the residual subcortical visual system of hemispherectomized monkeys were not carried out.

We will overview in the following sections quantitative studies of the retina of hemispherectomized cats and monkeys. Moreover, we describe the organization of some subcortical retinorecipient nuclei in the hemispherectomized monkey.

The retina and central projections following hemispherectomy

The cat retina

Early visual cortex lesions induce transneuronal retrograde degeneration of a substantial number of β, or X-type retinal ganglion cells (Pearson et al., 1981; Tong et al., 1982; Callahan et al., 1984; Kalil, 1984; Payne et al., 1984;). However, cell death is less important following lesions incurred later than 1 month of age compared to that in animals lesioned within days of birth (Callahan et al., 1984). Cortical ablations involving all or most of extrastriate regions as well as primary areas 17 and 18 result in greater degeneration of dLGN (especially the C-complex), a reduction in retinal projections to the dLGN and a greater ganglion cell loss in the retina (Lomber et al., 1993). The magnitude of RGC degeneration induced by a unilateral cerebral hemispherectomy earlier or later in life cannot be readily predicted by the repercussions of lesions restricted to primary visual areas. For example, a greater number of layer A and A1 dLGN neurons survive in hemispherectomized than in visual cortex lesioned kittens (Shook and Villablanca, 1991). The question arose whether the pattern of ganglion cell degeneration reflects the altered pattern of connections that develops following limited lesions restricted to the visual cortex, or would the pattern of neuron degeneration reflect more closely the different pattern of degeneration reported in the dLGN of cats which sustained hemispherectomy?

Following hemispherectomy on postnatal day 16 (P16), there is a significant loss of ganglion cells in the peripheral retina (Fig. 1B) and no significant cell loss in the central retina. In the P25 animal (Fig. 1C), the ganglion cell density maps appear unaltered compared to a normal cat (Fig. 1A). This shows that the critical period where ganglion cells are vulnerable to the cortical ablation has all but ended at P25, much like the visual cortex lesioned cat.

We have shown (Théoret et al., 1997) that the magnitude of cell loss in a P16 hemispherectomized kitten is very similar to that reported by Payne et al. (1984) in P1, 2, 3 or 5 striate cortex lesioned cats. This suggests that a hemispherectomy results in more retrograde degeneration of RGCs than a lesion of areas 17–18 performed at the same age. Given that the total population of RGCs in the normal cats' retina comprises 45–55% of X-type cells (Stone et al., 1980; Illing and Wassle, 1981), one would expect this to be the maximum percentage of cell loss if all X-cells degenerate and if the W- and Y-type cell populations remain intact. The 41% cell loss throughout the whole nasal hemiretina of the P16 cat could then be explained by the loss of 90–100% of retinal X-cells. This is unlikely since the majority of these cells are concentrated in the area centralis (Stone et al., 1980) and that no cell degeneration was observed therein. Alternatively, one can hypothesize that in addition to X-cells, a number of Y- or W-cells also degenerate following hemispherectomy. Although most studies argue that transneuronal degeneration of RGCs following visual cortex lesions is restricted to X-cells, Rowe (1990) suggested that W-cells are also lost following lesions of areas 17–18. The possible disappearance of W-cells in the present study could be supported by the greater degeneration of target cells within the dLGN, particularly the C-complex. As was shown by Lomber et al. (1993), a lesion which involves extrastriate areas as well as areas 17–18 results in greater degeneration of the C-complex of the dLGN than a lesion restricted to areas 17–18. It is also known that the C-complex receives a majority of inputs from retinal W-cells. It is then reasonable to assume that the hemispherectomy results in an important degeneration of the C-complex, which could in turn have resulted in the death of a number of retinal W-cells.

The monkey retina

Lesions of the optic radiations or striate cortex in monkeys induce a near total retrograde degeneration of the corresponding dLGN (Mihailovic et al., 1971) and extensive transneuronal degeneration of

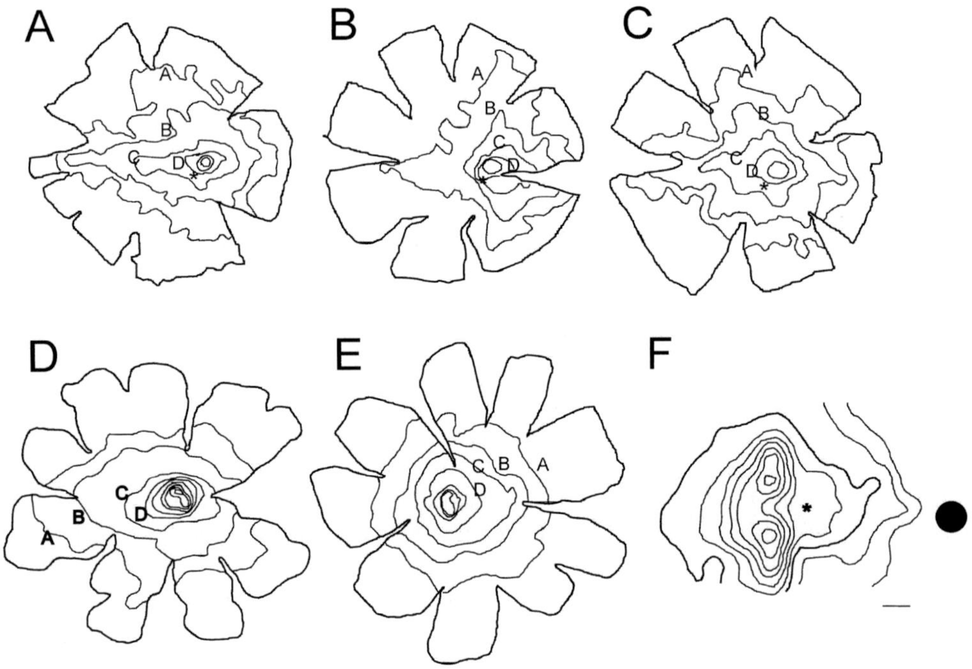

Fig. 1. Retinal ganglion cell isodensity maps in cats and monkeys. Right eye of A, normal cat B, of a P16 and C, of a P25 left hemispherectomized cats. Isodensity contours are labeled from the periphery: A = 125 RGCs/mm^2; B = 250 RGCs/mm^2; C = 500 RGCs/mm^2; D = 1000 RGCs/mm^2. Subsequent central contours represent 2000, RGCs/mm^2 or more (in 1000 RGCs/mm^2 steps). Central contours have been omitted for clarity, but cell density in the area centralis is in the order of 5000 RGCs/mm^2. The asterisk represents the optic disk. Nasal is to the left, temporal to the right. There is only mild cell loss in the temporal retinal of the left eye in the P16 hemispherectomized cat (not shown here). Ganglion cell isodensity map of the whole retina of D, a normal monkey and E, the whole retina and F, foveal region of the right eye of a monkey with a left unilateral cerebral hemispherectomy performed at 4 months. In D, A = 500 RGC/mm^2, B = 1000 RGCs/mm^2, C = 2000 RGCs/mm^2, D = 5000 RGCs/mm^2 subsequent contours increase by 5000 RGCs/mm^2. In F, the bold line represents isodensity curves at 10,000 RGCs/mm^2 and subsequent lines represent a 5000-RGCs/mm^2 increase in density. The filled circle represents the location of optic disk. The asterisk represents the location of the foveola. In F, the scale bar represents 1 mm. Note the clear unilateral loss of cells in the fovea and immediate surroundings with no apparent cell loss in the rest of the retina.

retinal ganglion cells (RGCs) in the corresponding hemiretina of each eye (Stoerig and Cowey, 1997). It is well documented that the speed of this degenerative process is dependent upon the age of the animal at the time of the ablation and the length of the postoperative survival period (Cowey, 1974; Cowey et al., 1989; Weller and Kaas, 1989; Niida et al., 1990). These studies were carried out in monkeys with lesions circumscribed to the striate cortex and little was known concerning the effects of removing all the visual cortical areas of one hemisphere on the retina.

We have shown that in hemispherectomized monkeys, RGC loss is circumscribed to the foveal and parafoveal regions (Herbin et al., 1999). The periphery was not affected in any of our lesioned cases (Fig. 1D–F). The RGC loss in the affected hemiretinae within 7° eccentricity is 70% at 4 months, 63% at 6 months, 28% at 8 months. and 11% at 9 months. These results clearly show that transneuronal retrograde degeneration in the retina of hemispherectomized monkeys is directly correlated with age at the time of the lesion. This degeneration is maximal when the lesion is induced in the first 4–6 months of life, and despite a long postoperative survival period, the RGC loss remains at about 70% (Fig. 2).

These results on hemispherectomized monkeys are similar to those observed in monkeys with striate cortex lesions (Weller and Kaas, 1989). Our results show that following hemispherectomy the most significant cell loss occurs when lesions are suffered prior to 8 months of age. Dineen and Hendrickson

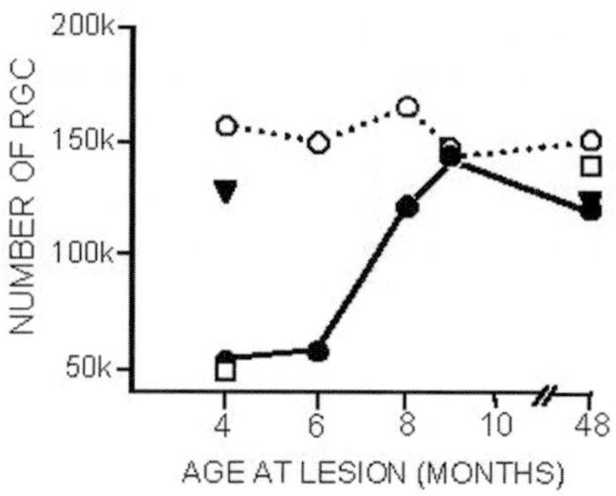

Fig. 2. Number of RGC at 7.5° eccentricity as a function of the age at which hemispherectomy is performed in monkeys. Open circles, intact nasal retina of the left eye; filled circles, deafferented temporal retina of the left eye; open squares, deafferented nasal retina of the right eye; filled triangles, intact temporal retina of the right eye. Note the inverse relationship between cell loss and age at lesion.

(1981) found in striate cortex ablated *M. nemestrina* 80 and 65% cell loss at 12 and 15 months, respectively. This led to the hypothesis (Weller and Kaas, 1989) that RGCs survival following cortical lesions changes from days to months to years over the first 1.5 postnatal years. We confirmed this hypothesis in showing that susceptibility to degeneration changes rapidly between 8 and 9 months in *C. aethiops*.

We also demonstrated that the consequences of hemispherectomy on transneuronal loss of RGCs are similar to those reported on destriate monkeys. Recently, Cowey et al. (1999) re-evaluated the effects of the size of the striate cortex lesion and involvement of extrastriate cortex in transneuronal degeneration of retinal ganglion cells in monkeys. Their results indicate that variance in RGC degeneration after visual cortex lesions which cannot be explained by either the age at which cortical lesions were performed or the postsurgical survival time, is correlated with lesion size. In particular, monkeys with lesions involving ventral occipito-temporal regions are those exhibiting degeneration of RGCs of the same magnitude as hemispherectomized monkeys. Because postsurgical survival is equally long in these groups of cases, this suggest that lesions involving ventral extrastriate cortices could result in greater RGC loss than lesions restricted to striate cortex, and that larger lesions do not result in a detectable additional cell loss. We insist on the fact that further cell loss cannot be ruled out even though it has not been detected. Most studies are based on relatively small samples comprising just a few cases with comparable lesions sizes and survival periods, and the methodologies of quantification employed differ between laboratories. Therefore, this conclusion is not supported by sufficient statistical power. Nevertheless, one cannot exclude that extrastriate lesions in combination with a near total ablation of striate cortex could lead to some supplemental loss of RGCs.

Summarizing, these results show that retinal ganglions cells in cats and monkeys do not follow similar patterns of degeneration following either restricted visual cortex lesions or unilateral cerebral hemispherectomy. Although it is generally accepted that β-type cells are affected by lesions of the visual cortex, we presented some evidence that other cell types might also degenerate following cerebral hemispherectomy in cats. In monkeys, lesions of all the visual cortices appear to induce some cell loss that would not be expected following a complete removal of primary visual cortex and we find no evidence for involvement of other than β-type cells. The most significant difference between the two species is in the distribution of cell loss, whereas in cat the central retina appears unaffected by a cortical ablation, in monkeys RGC degeneration is circumscribed to the fovea and its immediate surround.

Although all these studies generally focus on the fact that cells are lost, we insist on the fact that the retina of the blind hemifield in hemispherectomized cats and monkeys are far from being depleted of RGCs. There is some evidence, however, that the surviving population of RGCs might exhibit altered functional properties. The degenerated retinal sectors show increased GABA immunoreactivity in the ganglion and amacrine cell layers as well as in the inner plexiform layer (Kisvàrday et al., 1991; see also Rowe, 1988). Cell densities in the peripheral retina of hemispherectomized monkeys are not different than those of normal monkeys and the central visual field is still sampled by at least 30% of the normal numbers of RGC. There is no evidence for any loss of photoreceptors in the 'blind' hemifovea. From the inspection of the retina only, one might expect that visual capabilities could be altered, but by no means completely abolished.

In order to further understand the potential for residual functions in the visual system of hemispherectomized subjects, we engaged in studies of retinal projections and quantitative studies of cell numbers in some subcortical visual structures, namely the dLGN nucleus and the SC.

The lateral geniculate nucleus

The fact that Pβ cells are mainly affected by the lesion, whereas other RGC types escape retrograde degeneration (Weller et al., 1979; Dineen and Hendrickson, 1981) has been explained by the sustaining collateral theory which states that Pβ cells are more susceptible to transneuronal degeneration because they project exclusively to the parvocellular layers of the LGNd, whereas the other retinal ganglion cell types rely on projections to the SC or other targets for their survival (Weller et al., 1979; Weller and Kaas, 1984, 1989). Lesions made in infant macaques result in a nearly complete depletion of retinal terminals in parvocellular layers, whereas the density and distribution of labeled terminals found in magnocellular and interlaminar layers following long postsurgical survival are much less affected (Weller and Kaas, 1989). The normal density of retinal afferents to magnocellular layers has been explained by a superior resistance of Pα cells to transneuronal degeneration imparted by the sustaining collaterals they send to targets other than the dLGN. Nevertheless, some retinal projections are found in parvocellular layers of striate cortex lesioned monkeys indicating that they might find therein some available and appropriate postsynaptic sites. The few remaining neurons in the LGNd of striate cortex ablated monkeys could be local interneurons (Pasik et al., 1973) and/or parvocellular neurons projecting to extrastriate cortices (Benevento and Yoshida, 1981; Yukie and Iwai, 1981; Cowey and Stoerig, 1989). If retinal projections to LGNd in destriate monkeys are maintained by geniculo-extrastriate pathways, the question then arises whether retinal projections to LGNd could be maintained in the absence of extrastriate cortices.

The degenerate LGNd in hemispherectomized monkeys continues to receive laminar eye-specific retinal input (Boire et al., 2000) (see Fig. 3). In visual cortex lesioned monkeys, retinal projections which are maintained could be attributed to geniculo-extrastriate projections. In hemispherectomized monkeys, all striate as well as extrastriate cortices have been removed. In the normal monkey, LGNd retinal terminals are presynaptic to both relay cells and interneurons and participate in the formation of triades (Colonnier and Guillery, 1964; Szentágothai, 1973; Hámori et al., 1974; Wilson, 1989). In striate cortex ablated monkeys, the remaining relay cells can be retrogradely labeled from extrastriate visual cortices (Hendrickson and Dineen, 1982; Cowey and Stoerig, 1989). In addition, there are no direct synaptic contacts between retinal afferents and these extrastriate projecting cells. Retinal input to these remaining cells could be provided indirectly through the SC projection to the LGNd and through interneurons (Kisvàrday et al., 1991). Assuming that all relay cells degenerate following hemispherectomy and that some interneurons remain, they could be postsynaptic targets to retinal terminals that would be maintained even though they would constitute a functional dead-end.

Maintained retinal projections in the LGNd of hemispherectomized monkeys allow for two possible explanations. Firstly, if the degenerate LGNd ipsilateral to the cortical ablation comprises a population of relay cells that convey information to targets other than ipsilateral extrastriate cortex, the retinal projections could have been sustained by a residual population of neurons comprising both projection and internuncial cells. Some relay cells appear to survive in the LGNd of cats with a total cortical disconnection (Madarasz et al., 1983). Some relay cells appear to develop presynaptic sites on their dendrites. Dendritic axonization has been proposed as a factor explaining the survival of relay cells following axotomy (Hámori and Silakov, 1980, 1981; Madarasz et al., 1983). There is no evidence for such survival of relay cells in monkeys (Walker, 1935; Kisvàrday et al., 1991). There is evidence, however, that LGNd relay cell axons emit intrinsic collaterals to interneurons in cats (Friedlander et al., 1981), but not in monkeys. Relay cells do, however, emit collaterals to the thalamic reticular nucleus (see Garey et al., 1991); however, it is not known whether a relay cell can survive with its sole retrograde support coming from this collateral. Secondly, the LGNd could be a residual structure devoid of relay cells and comprising only residual interneurons, from which no outside projections emerge. The residual retinal projections arrive here in a dead end situation. Their failure to degenerate completely could be attributed either to the availability of postsynaptic sites on the few remaining neurons or to the fact that the retinal terminals become at one point independent of their target in order to survive as demonstrated in striate cortex ablated cats (Lomber et al., 1993).

The superior colliculus

The SC ipsilateral to the cortical ablation suffers moderate cell loss in hemispherectomized monkeys (Théoret et al., 2001). These results are commensurate with those reported in hemispherectomized cats (Hovda et al., 1992; see also Huffman et al., 1999 on the opossum). The cross-sectional area of the ipsilesional SC is reduced by 45.1% in adult-lesioned cats and by 28.7% in neonatal-lesioned cats (Villablanca and Hovda, 1989). This is close to the 28.2% volume reduction we observed in the young hemispherectomized monkeys. Furthermore, neuronal densities in the ipsilesional SC of neonatally hemispherectomized cats are not significantly different from those of normal animals (Villablanca and Hovda, 1989). Again, this corresponds well to the data obtained in hemispherectomized monkeys where no differences in neuronal density were observed between the right and left SC of lesioned

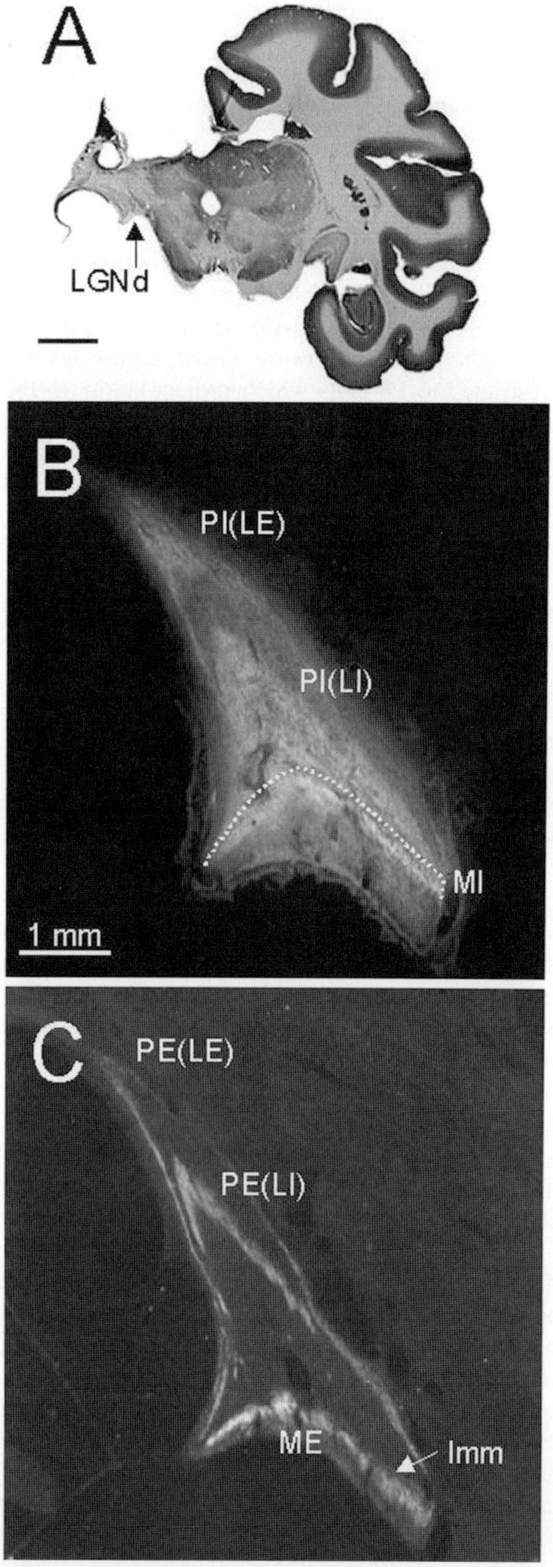

Fig. 3. (A) Coronal section through the thalamus in a monkey hemispherectomized at the age of 8 months. Note the shrunken aspect of the entire diencephalon ipsilateral to the cortical ablation and the small but conspicuous remnant of the LGNd. Scale bar: 5 mm. (B) Darkfield digital photomicrographs of autoradiograph and (C) HRP-labeled retinal projections from the same monkey shown in A, in the LGNd ipsilateral to the cortical ablation (left side). Uncrossed retinal projections in the left LGNd are shown by the location of transported protein following an intraocular injection of [^{3}H]proline in the left eye. Crossed retinal projections in the left LGNd are TMB histochemistry revealing anterogradely transported WGA–HRP injected in the right eye. Dotted line indicates the border between MI and PI(LI). MI, internal magnocellular layers; PI, internal parvocellular layers; LI, internal leaflet; LE, external leaflet; Imm, magnocellular interlaminar zone.

monkeys. Finally, metabolic imbalance between the SC of hemispherectomized cats as measured with cytochrome oxidase was reported to be mild (Hovda and Villablanca, 1990), which is commensurate with our own results.

Retinal input is maintained to both SC following hemispherectomy (Fig. 4). Retinal projections to the SC appear to maintain a normal distribution pattern in monkeys with lesions limited to striate cortex (Dineen et al., 1982; see also Kahn et al., 2000). Given that retrograde degeneration of retinal ganglion cells following visual cortex lesions is restricted to Pβ cells which project solely to the dLGN (Cowey et al., 1989), it is not surprising that Pα and Pγ cells, which escape degeneration, maintain their normal projections to midbrain nuclei and diencephalon (Leventhal et al., 1981; Perry et al., 1984).

The small reduction in volume and cell number, unaltered distribution pattern of oxidative metabolism and presence of retinal terminals in the SC ipsilateral to the cortical ablation suggest that this structure maintains visual processing capabilities. This is in agreement with studies attributing an important role to the SC in residual vision following hemispherectomy (Perenin and Jeannerod, 1978; Ptito et al., 1991, 1996; Braddick et al., 1992; Tomaiuolo et al., 1997).

These results are also in agreement with the hypothesis that the SC mediates the auditory gap effect reported in hemispherectomy human subjects (Reuter-Lorenz et al., 1999) which is believed to be mediated by the SC (Dorris and Munoz, 1995). The question remains as to why residual vision is not ubiquitous in patients with a unilateral cerebral hemispherectomy.

Alternate routes for vision without one cerebral hemisphere

Our results on hemispherectomized monkeys have shown retinal projections to the dLGN in normal complementary eye specific layers as well as in the SC and pretectal targets (not shown). The question remains, however, on how visual information from the blind hemifield might reach the contralateral hemisphere for higher processing. There is evidence for cortical activation by visual stimuli presented in the anopic visual hemifield as shown by using fMRI (Bittar et al., 1999). Significant activation was observed in MT and areas V3/V3A in hemispherectomized patients (op. cit.). Even though the dLGN receives retinal projections, we have no evidence for geniculate output in absence of its normal cortical target. One could speculate on axon sprouting outside the geniculate, but this seems unlikely. The most likely route for conveying visual information to the contralateral forebrain is through the intertectal commissure.

Commissural fibers between the mesencephalic tectum are present throughout vertebrate phyla, from fish to mammals (see Ariens-Kappers et al., 1936; Vanegas, 1984; Nieuwenhuys et al., 1998), but have received relatively little attention. The description of the Sprague effect (see below), has sparked more acute interest in the midbrain tectum commissure, whose function remains nevertheless unknown. The most striking feature of the commissure of the superior colliculus (CSC) is the great variation between species in the rostro-caudal distribution of commissural cells. Tectal commissural cells are deemed absent in rabbits (Nagata et al., 1980), confined to the rostral tectum in hamsters (Rhoades et al., 1981, 1986; Fish et al., 1982), rats (Yamasaki et al., 1984) and cats (Edwards, 1977; Magalhäes-Castro et al., 1978; Behan and Kime, 1996; Olivier et al., 1998) and distributed throughout the rostro-caudal extent of the SC in monkey (Olivier et al., 1998) and fish (Herrero et al., 1999). It has been suggested that this pathway is involved in motor functions (Behan and Kime, 1996; Olivier et al., 1998) and that the distribution of commissural cells is related to the oculomotor range (Olivier et al., 1998). Others have suggested that species differences are related to variance in visual and somatosensory tectal maps (Edwards, 1977; Magalhäes-Castro et al., 1978; Nagata et al., 1980; Fish et al., 1982). Neither the sensory or motor hypothesis yet explain species differences in tectotectal cell distribution (see Olivier et al., 1998 and Herrero et al., 1999). Also there is clear evidence that commissural cells of the tectum consist in a heterogeneous population of units some of which respond to visual or cutaneous stimuli in hamsters (Rhoades et al., 1986) and cat (McIlwain, 1991). Given that the functions of the CSC are not well understood in normal intact animals we do not know how its structure and development might be affected by an early unilateral

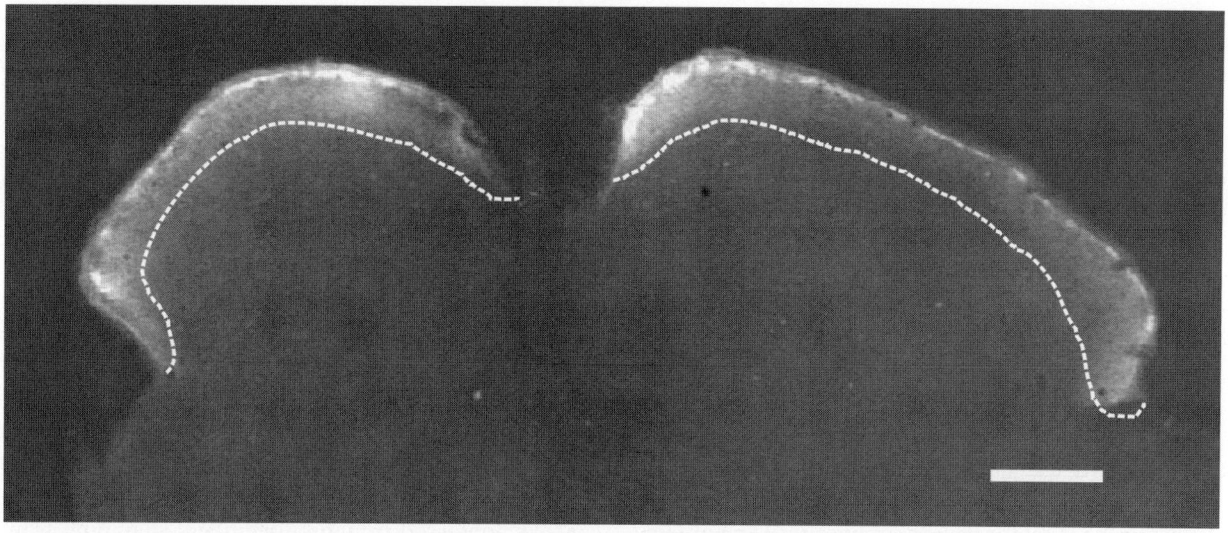

Fig. 4. Photomicrograph showing retinal projections to the superior colliculus of a monkey hemispherectomized at 8 months, [^{3}H]proline was injected in the left eye. The left superior colliculus (to the left) is ipsilateral to the cortical ablation. Scale bar: 1 mm.

ablation of the cortex. Furthermore, there is evidence that visually responsive commissural cells receive direct retinal input in cats (Moschovakis and Karabelas, 1985) possibly from Y-type retinal ganglion cells (McIlwain, 1991). Evidence in monkeys as in cats indicates that tectotectal cells consist in a heterogeneous population comprising both excitatory and inhibitory projections (see Olivier et al., 1998). The main axon of 80% of tectotectal cells courses through the predorsal bundle and provides an excitatory input to the brainstem saccade generator of the contralateral reticular formation (Moschovakis et al., 1988a,b). In cats, some tectotectal cells exhibit GABA immunoreactivity (Appell and Behan, 1990; Olivier et al., 1997) and terminals with morphologies suggestive of inhibitory input (Behan, 1985). These observations suggest that tectal commissural connections are involved in some complex manner, not restricted to inhibitory influences, in the modulation of the output from both colliculi mediated by vision as well as somatosensory and possibly other sensory modalities. Because in monkeys commissural cells are distributed throughout the collicular surface they could transfer visual input from the whole contralateral visual field to the other side of the brain. However, although commissural cells in monkeys are found in all layers of the SC only a few cells are located in the superficial gray layers which receive direct retinal input. (Olivier et al., 1998). In addition most commissural terminals appear to be confined to intermediate and deep collicular layers as well as to the contralateral periaqueductal gray, although some have been seen in superficial layers (Behan and Kime, 1996). The question here is whether visual information from the SC ipsilateral to the cortical ablation can gain access to the contralateral cortex.

Electrophysiological (Berson and McIllwain, 1982) and anatomical studies have suggested the presence of retinal input into intermediate layers in the cat, rat and monkey (Beckstead and Frankfurter, 1983) and also ground squirrel (Agarwala et al., 1989). However, other studies do not support this possibility (Graybiel, 1975; Harting and Guillery, 1976). We have recently seen clear evidence for a direct retinal projection to intermediate layers of the SC in cat using anterograde transport of the cholera toxin B fragment (unpublished observation) and whether this retinal projection is also present in monkeys and man remains to be confirmed. Visual information can also be available to intermediate layer cells which can subsequently be transferred to the SC contralateral to the cortical ablation. Dendrites of deep SC neurons have been shown to extend to superficial layers and axons of superficial layer neurons have been traced to intermediate and deep layers in hamsters, cat, squirrel monkeys and tree shrew (Mooney et al., 1984, 1988; Moschovakis and Karabelas, 1985; Rhoades et al., 1985; Highstein et al., 1986; Karabelas et al., 1986; Moschovakis et al., 1988a; Behan and Appell, 1992; Hall and Lee, 1993). From the deep and intermediate layers, ascending pathways exist to a host of diencephalic and mesencephalic targets (see Sparks and Hartwich-Young, 1989 for review). Thalamic nuclei which receive ascending collicular projection (suprageniculate, medial geniculate, medial dorsal, ventral anterior, lateral posterior and intralaminar) do not in turn project to V1, but to a wide range of cortical fields. It is thus quite possible that in certain circumstances hemispherectomized subjects submitted to visual detection tasks under a forced choice paradigm, respond correctly above chance levels without really having a conscious visual percept of the stimuli.

In addition to the above described trans-collicular pathway, other paths to the contralateral cortex could be activated in hemispherectomy subjects, although their activation by visual input is quite speculative. Visual information can reach non-specific nuclei of the thalamus (central lateral and paracentral nuclei) through the SC and also the pretectal nuclei to the ventral lateral geniculate nucleus (see Garey et al., 1991) which still receive visual input from the retina in hemispherectomized monkeys. Several studies have shown that midline and intralaminar nuclei are relatively spared in hemispherectomized monkeys and humans. From the midline thalamic nuclei ipsilateral to the cortical ablation visual impulses could be transferred to the contralateral cortex by crossed thalamocortical projections. Crossed thalamocortical connections have been shown to originate from mediodorsal, anteromedial and midline nuclei and macaques (Preuss and Goldman-Rakic, 1987). Whether such crossed thalamocortical pathways are involved in visual processing in normal or in hemispherectomized subjects is unknown.

The Sprague effect hypothesis

Negative results as to the presence of residual vision in the affected hemifield of hemispherectomy subjects suggest that extrastriate cortex is necessary for residual visual functions. However, it might also be argued that removal of cortical areas per se do not abolish all visual functions but that the cortical ablation produces imbalances in the residual subcortical system of lesioned animals which inhibit visual responses. The introduction of a salient stimulus in the visual field of normal animals will induce an orienting response. In cats, this response can be abolished by the ablation of all visual cortical areas contralaterally to the stimulus presentation. In a seminal paper, Sprague (1966) demonstrated that the orienting response could be restored in visual cortex lesioned cats by the subsequent destruction of the contralesional SC or by transection of the CSC. This phenomenon was later named the Sprague effect. Sprague originally hypothesized that following the cortical ablation, activity within the ipsilesional SC is depressed by inhibitory fibers stemming from the contralateral SC and coursing through the CSC. Recovery of orienting behaviors following SC ablation or CSC destruction was thus believed to occur through disinhibition of the ipsilesional SC. It was later shown that disinhibition of the SC was probably causing the recovery, but that the critical inhibitory fibers did not originate from the contralateral SC. Wallace et al. (1989) reported that transection of tectotectal fibers within the CSC (which are located rostrally) did not produce an orienting response recovery. Destruction of caudal fibers, however, did produce the recovery. Furthermore, ibotenic acid lesions of the contralesional SC, which destroy cell bodies but spare coursing fibers, also did not produce a recovery. This suggested that the inhibitory influences were originating from another subcortical nucleus which was sending axons through the SC and the CSC en route to the ipsilesional colliculus. In a subsequent study, Wallace et al. (1990) showed that lesions of the contralesional substantia nigra pars reticulata, which sends projections to the contralateral SC, did result in the restoration of orienting behaviors. Finally, the SC disinhibition theory was given additional support when it was shown that disinhibiting the ipsilesional SC through injections of a GABA agonist, bicuculline methiodine, also restored orienting responses in hemianopic cats (Ciaramitaro et al., 1997).

These data thus suggest that the SC plays an active role in residual visual capabilities of the cat following massive ablations of occipital cortex. Could a similar phenomenon modulate residual visual behaviors in primates? The role of the monkey SC in residual vision is well documented. Visually guided saccades can be generated in the absence of primary visual cortex, but are abolished following subsequent destruction of the ipsilesional SC (Mohler and Wurtz, 1977). In adolescent monkeys (2.5–3.5 years old), Tusa et al. (1986) reported that following unilateral decortication encompassing all visual cortical areas, monkeys can no longer make reflexive and visually guided saccades in the defective visual field. The removal of extrastriate cortical areas thus seems to create complete contralateral hemianopia. In one animal, the same authors sectioned the intertectal commissure but, contrary to what is seen in cats, there was no recovery of orienting behaviors.

Our own data show anatomical sparing within the SC of hemispherectomized monkeys (Ptito et al., 1996; Théoret et al., 2001). Furthermore, the SC continues to receive near-normal retinal input and metabolic activity is similar in normal and hemispherectomized animals. Evidently, the SC retains some potential functional capabilities following hemispherectomy in primates. The SC can thus process, or at least receive, visual information in the absence of ipsilateral cortical structures. This implies that a mechanism similar to that observed in cats (Sprague, 1966; Ciaramitaro et al., 1997) might be present in the hemispherectomized monkey. According to this hypothesis, a still functional SC can process visual information without ipsilateral cortical support and relay motor signals to subcortical structures of the brainstem to generate saccadic eye movements to the affected hemifield. In addition, the substantia nigra, which is believed to mediate the Sprague effect, is also spared following hemispherectomy in monkeys (Théoret et al., 1999). It is thus possible that Sprague effect-like mechanisms might explain the absence of residual function in the affected hemifield of primates, including humans. At least in the monkey, one can hypothesize that the contralateral SN is inhibiting some critical parts of the ipsilesional SC, thus preventing orienting responses. It would be of great interest to thoroughly evaluate the effects of CSC transection or SN ablation in the primate model of hemispherectomy.

Conclusion

Although substrate pathways to the contralateral cortex are present, the visual information they convey might not be in a format or of sufficient strength to activate visual cortices and result in a conscious visual percept. They might contribute in producing a non-conscious "different kind of nothing" (see Stoerig and Cowey, 1997) as demonstrated by forced choice paradigms.

In closing, we would like to make two points on the significance and limitations of animal models of cerebral hemispherectomy. As we have shown in this brief review, anatomical and behavioral consequences of hemispherectomy differ quite significantly between animals. Each animal model has revealed fundamental knowledge on the functions of subcortical and cortical fields in the production of conscious vision and visual orienting behaviors. Nevertheless, the anatomical consequences of a cerebral hemispherectomy in primates are clearly different than those in cats. Consequently primates are the best model for the understanding of cerebral hemispherectomy in humans.

All animal studies of hemispherectomy rely on cortical ablations performed at various developmental stages. One has to keep in mind that human candidates for hemispherectomy undergo surgery long after the onset of their pathology, often in utero. In view of the fact that earlier lesions lead to better outcomes in animal models as well as in humans, neuroanatomical data on primates with early and prenatal brain lesion would provide baseline information on how the brain react to very early insults and any evaluation of therapeutics for repair. Presently, all studies on cerebral hemispherectomies in primates are based on lesions performed at times which are not representative of the onset of pathologies which require early surgical treatment.

There is no doubt that, however dramatic a hemispherectomy may sound to the general public and to families, patients greatly benefit from this intervention. Several hundred hemispherectomies are performed yearly and these are increasingly done at an early age. In the years to come, we hope that careful postmortem preparation of hemispherectomized patients' brains will be available for study in order to provide even better outcomes and years of quality time for the future patients as well as further understanding of the fundamentals of visual consciousness.

Acknowledgements

Supported by grants from the National Science and Engineering Research Council of Canada (NSERC).

References

Agarwala, S., Petry, H.M. and May, J.G. (1989) Retinal projections in the ground squirrel (*Citellus tridecemlineatus*). *Vis. Neurosci.*, 3: 537–549.

Appell, P.P. and Behan, M. (1990) Sources of subcortical GABAergic projections to the superior colliculus in the cat. *J. Comp. Neurol.*, 302: 143–158.

Ariens-Kappers, C.U., Huber, G.C. and Crosby, E.C. (1936) *The Comparative Anatomy of the Vertebrate Nervous System of Vertebrates, Including Man.* Hafner, New York.

Beckstead, R.M. and Frankfurter, A. (1983) A direct projection from the retina to the intermediate gray layer of the superior colliculus demonstrated by anterograde transport of horseradish peroxidase in monkey, cat, and rat. *Exp. Brain Res.*, 52: 261–268.

Behan, M. (1985) An EM-autoradiographic and EM-HRP study of the commissural projection of the superior colliculus in the cat. *J. Comp. Neurol.*, 234: 105–116.

Behan, M. and Appell, P.P. (1992) Intrinsic circuitry in the cat superior colliculus: projections from the superficial layers. *J. Comp. Neurol.*, 315: 230–243.

Behan, M. and Kime, N.M. (1996) Spatial distribution of tectotectal connections in the cat. *Prog. Brain Res.*, 112: 131–142.

Benevento, L.A. and Yoshida, K. (1981) The afferent and efferent organization of the lateral geniculo-prestriate pathways in the macaque monkey. *J. Comp. Neurol.*, 203: 455–474.

Berkeley, M.A. and Sprague, J.M. (1979) Striate cortex and visual acuity functions. *J. Comp. Neurol.*, 187: 679–702.

Berson, D.M. and McIllwain, J.T. (1982) Retinal Y-cell activation of deep layer cells in the superior colliculus of the cat. *J. Neurophysiol.*, 47: 700–714.

Bittar, R.G., Ptito, M., Faubert, G. and Ptito, A. (1999) Activation of the remaining hemisphere following stimulation of the blind hemifield in hemispherectomized subjects. *Neuroimage*, 10: 339–346.

Bodian, D. (1942) Studies on the diencephalon of the Virginia opossum: Part III: Thalamo-cortical projections. *J. Comp. Neurol.*, 77: 525–571.

Boire, D., Théoret, H., Herbin, M., Casanova, C. and Ptito, M. (2000) Retinogeniculate projections following early cerebral hemispherectomy in the vervet monkey. *Exp. Brain Res.*, 135: 373–381.

Bowling, D.B. and Michael, C.R. (1984) Termination patterns of single physiologically characterized optic fibers in the cat's lateral geniculate nucleus. *J. Neurosci.*, 4: 198–216.

Braddick, O., Atkinson, J., Hood, B., Harkness, W., Jackson, G. and Vargha-Khadem, F. (1992) Possible blindsight in infants lacking one hemisphere. *Nature*, 360: 461–463.

Callahan, E.C., Tong, L. and Spear, P.D. (1984) Critical period for the loss of retinal X-cells following visual cortex damage in cats. *Brain Res.*, 323: 302–306.

Carman, L.S. and Schneider, G.E. (1992) Orienting behavior in hamsters with lesions of superior colliculus, pretectum and visual cortex. *Exp. Brain Res.*, 90: 79–91.

Chow, K. and Dewson, J.H. (1966) Numerical estimates of neurons and glia in lateral geniculate body during retrograde degeneration. *J. Comp. Neurol.*, 128: 63–74.

Ciaramitaro, V.M., Todd, W.E. and Rosenquist, A.C. (1997) Disinhibition of the superior colliculus restores orienting to visual stimuli in the hemianopic field of the cat. *J. Comp. Neurol.*, 387: 568–587.

Colonnier, M. and Guillery, R.W. (1964) Synaptic organization in the lateral geniculate nucleus of the monkey. *Z. Zellforsch.*, 62: 333–355.

Combs, C.M. (1949) Fibers and cell degeneration in the albino rat after hemidecortication. *J. Comp. Neurol.*, 90: 373–394.

Cornwell, P., Overman, W.H., Levitsky, C., Shipley, J. and Lezynski, B. (1976) Performance on the visual cliff by cats with marginal gyrus lesions. *J. Comp. Physiol. Psychol.*, 90: 996–1010.

Cornwell, P., Overman, W.H. and Campbell, A. (1980a) Subtotal lesions of visual cortex impair discrimination of hidden figures by cats. *J. Comp. Physiol. Psychol.*, 94: 289–304.

Cornwell, P., Overman, W.H. and Ross, C. (1980b) Lesions of visual cortex impair discrimination of hidden figures by cats. *Physiol. Behav.*, 24: 533–540.

Cornwell, P., Herbein, S., Corso, C., Eskew, R., Warren, J.M. and Payne, B.R. (1989) Selective sparing after lesions of visual cortex in newborn cats. *Behav. Neurosci.*, 103: 1176–1190.

Cowey, A. (1974) Atrophy of retinal ganglion cells after removal of striate cortex in a rhesus monkey. *Perception*, 3: 257–260.

Cowey, A. and Stoerig, P. (1989) Projection patterns of surviving neurons in the dorsal lateral geniculate nucleus following discrete lesions of striate cortex: implications for residual vision. *Exp. Brain Res.*, 75: 631–638.

Cowey, A., Stoerig, P. and Perry, V.H. (1989) Transneuronal retrograde degeneration of retinal ganglion cells after damage to striate cortex in macaque monkeys: selective loss of P beta cells. *Neuroscience*, 29: 65–80.

Cowey, A., Stoerig, P. and Bannister, M. (1994) Retinal ganglion cells labeled from the pulvinar nucleus in macaque monkeys. *Neuroscience*, 61: 691–705.

Cowey, A., Stoerig, P. and Williams, C. (1999) Variance in transneuronal retrograde ganglion cell degeneration in monkeys after removal of striate cortex: effects of the size of the cortical lesion. *Vision Res.*, 39: 3642–3652.

Dean, P. (1978) Visual acuity in hooded rats: effects of superior colliculus and posterior neocortical lesions. *Brain Res.*, 156: 17–31.

Dean, P. (1981) Visual pathways and acuity in hooded rats. *Behav. Brain Res.*, 3: 239–271.

Dean, P. (1990) Sensory cortex: visual perceptual functions. In: B. Kolb and R.C. Tees (Eds.), *The Cerebral Cortex of the Rat.* MIT Press, Cambridge.

De Weerd, P., Sprague, J.M., Vandenbussche, E. and Orban, G.A. (1994) Two stages in visual texture segregation: a lesion study in the cat. *J. Neurosci.*, 14: 929–948.

Dineen, J.T. and Hendrickson, A.E. (1981) Age correlated differences in the amount of retinal degeneration after striate cortex lesions in monkeys. *Invest. Ophthalmol. Vis. Sci.*, 21: 749–752.

Dineen, J.T. and Keating, E.G. (1981) The primate visual system after bilateral removal of striate cortex. Survival of complex pattern vision. *Exp. Brain Res.*, 41: 338–345.

Dineen, J.T., Hendrickson, A. and Keating, E.G. (1982) Alterations of retinal inputs following striate cortex removal in adult monkey. *Exp. Brain Res.*, 41: 338–345.

Dorris, M.C. and Munoz, D.P. (1995) A neural correlate for the gap effect on saccadic reaction times in monkey. *J. Neurophysiol.*, 73: 2558–2562.

Doty, R.W. (1971) Survival of pattern vision after removal of striate cortex in the adult cat. *J. Comp. Neurol.*, 143: 341–369.

Dyer, R.S., Marino, M.F., Johnson, C. and Kruggel, T. (1976) Superior colliculus lesions does not impair orientation to patterns. *Brain Res.*, 112: 176–179.

Edwards, S.B. (1977) The commissural projection of the superior colliculus in the cat. *J. Comp. Neurol.*, 173: 23–40.

Feinberg, T.E., Pasik, T. and Pasik, P. (1978) Extrageniculostriate vision in the monkey. VI. Visually guided accurate reaching behaviors. *Brain Res.*, 152: 422–428.

Fendrich, R., Wessinger, C.M. and Gazzaniga, S. (2001) Speculations on the neural basis of islands of blindsight. In: C. Casanova and M. Ptito (Eds.), *Vision: From Neurons to Cognition. Progress in Brain Research*, Vol. 134. Elsevier, Amsterdam, pp. 353–366.

Fish, S.E., Doodman, D.K., Kuo, D.C., Polcer, J.D. and Rhoades, R.W. (1982) The intercollicular pathway in the golden hamster: an anatomical study. *J. Comp. Neurol.*, 204: 6–20.

Friedlander, M.J., Lin, C.S., Stanford, L.R. and Sherman, S.M. (1981) Morphology of functionally identified neurons in the lateral geniculate nucleus of the cat. *J. Neurophysiol.*, 46: 80–129.

Garey, L.J., Dreher, B. and Robinson, S.R. (1991) The organization of the visual thalamus. In: B. Dreher and S.R. Robinson (Eds.), *Neuroanatomy of the Visual Pathways and their Development. Vision and Visual Dysfunction*, Vol. 3, CRC Press, Boston, pp. 176–234.

Girard, P. and Bullier, J. (1989) Visual activity in area V2 during reversible inactivation of area 17 in the macaque monkey. *J. Neurophysiol.*, 62: 1287–1302.

Girard, P., Salin, P.A. and Bullier, J. (1991) Visual activity in areas V3a and V3 during reversible inactivation of area V1 in the macaque monkey. *J. Neurophysiol.*, 66: 1493–1503.

Girard, P., Salin, P.A. and Bullier, J. (1992) Response selectivity of neurons in area MT of the macaque monkey during reversible inactivation of area V1. *J. Neurophysiol.*, 67: 1437–1446.

Goodale, M.A. and Carey, D.P. (1990) The role of cerebral cortex in visuomotor control. In: B. Kolb and R.C. Tees (Eds.), *The Cerebral Cortex of the Rat.* MIT Press, Cambridge, MA, pp. 309–340.

Goodale, M.A., Foreman, N.P. and Milner, A.D. (1978) Visual orientation in the rat: a dissociation of deficits following cortical and collicular lesions. *Exp. Brain Res.*, 31: 445–457.

Graybiel, A.M. (1975) Anatomical organization of retinotectal afferents in the cat: an autoradiographic study. *Brain Res.*, 96: 1–23.

Gross, C.G. (1991) Contribution of striate cortex and the superior colliculus to visual function of area MT, the superior temporal polysensory area and inferior temporal cortex. *Neuropsychologia*, 29: 497–515.

Guido, W., Spear, P.D. and Tong, L. (1990) Functional compensation in the lateral suprasylvian visual area following bilateral visual cortex damage in kittens. *Exp. Brain Res.*, 83: 219–224.

Guido, W., Spear, P.D. and Tong, L. (1992) How complete is physiological compensation in extrastriate cortex after visual cortex damage in kittens? *Exp. Brain Res.*, 91: 455–466.

Hall, W.C. and Lee, P. (1993) Interlaminar connections of the superior colliculus in the tree shrew. I. The superficial gray layer. *J. Comp. Neurol.*, 332: 213–223.

Hámori, J. and Silakov, V.L. (1980) Plasticity of relay neurons in dorsal lateral geniculate nucleus of the adult cat: morphological evidence. *Neuroscience*, 5: 2073–2077.

Hámori, J. and Silakov, V.L. (1981) Myelinated perikarya and dendrites in lateral geniculate nucleus of the cat following chronic cortical deafferentation. *J. Neurocytol.*, 10: 879–888.

Hámori, J., Pasik, T., Pasik, P. and Szentágothai, J. (1974) Triadic synaptic arrangements and their possible significance in the lateral geniculate nucleus of the monkey. *Brain Res.*, 80: 379–393.

Harting, J.K. and Guillery, R.W. (1976) Organization of retinocollicular pathways in the cat. *J. Comp. Neurol.*, 166: 133–144.

Hendrickson, A.E. and Dineen, J.T. (1982) Hypertrophy of neurons in the dorsal lateral geniculate nucleus following striate cortex lesions in infant monkeys. *Neurosci. Lett.*, 30: 217–222.

Herbin, M., Boire, D., Théoret, H. and Ptito, M. (1999) Transneuronal degeneration of retinal ganglion cells in early hemispherectomized monkeys. *NeuroReport*, 10: 1447–1452.

Herrero, L., Pérez, P., Núnez Abadez, P., Hardy, O. and Torrez, B. (1999) Tectotectal connectivity in goldfish. *J. Comp. Neurol.*, 411: 455–471.

Highstein, S.M., Moschovakis, A.K. and Warren, J.D. (1986) Morphophysiology of vertical medium lead burst neurons in the alert squirrel monkey. *Soc. Neurosci. Abstr.*, 12: 1186.

Hovda, D.A. and Villablanca, J.R. (1990) Sparing of visual field perception in neonatal but not adult cerebral hemispherectomized cats. Relation with oxidative metabolism of the superior colliculus. *Behav. Brain Res.*, 37: 119–132.

Hovda, D.A., Villablanca, J.R. and Adelson, P.D. (1992) Anatomical and metabolic corticotectal neuroplasticity after neonatal cerebral hemispherectomy: correlations with visual field sparing. *Brain Dysfunct.*, 5: 3–26.

Hovda, D.A., Villablanca, J.R., Chugani, H.T. and Phelps, M.E. (1996) Cerebral metabolism following neonatal or adult hemineodecortication in cats: I. Effects on glucose metabolism using [^{14}C]2-deoxy-D-glucose autoradiography. *J. Cereb. Blood. Flow Metab.*, 16: 134–146.

Huffman, K.J., Molnár, Z., Van Dellen, A., Kahn, D.M., Blakemore, C. and Krubitzer, L. (1999) Formation of cortical fields on a reduced cortical sheet. *J. Neurosci.*, 19: 9939–9952.

Hughes, H.C. and Sprague, S.M. (1986) Cortical mechanisms for local and global analysis of visual space. *Exp. Brain Res.*, 61: 332–354.

Humphrey, N.K. (1974) Vision in a monkey without striate cortex: a case study. *Perception*, 3: 241–255.

Illing, R.B. and Wassle, H. (1981) The retinal projection to the thalamus in the cat: a quantitative investigation and a comparison with the retinotectal pathway. *J. Comp. Neurol.*, 202: 265–285.

Jones, E.G. (1999) Making brain connections: neuroanatomy and the work of TPS Powell, 1923–1996. *Annu. Rev. Neurosci.*, 22: 49–103.

Kaas, J.H. and Lyon, D.C. (2001) Visual cortex organization in primates: theories of V3 and adjoining visual areas. In: C. Casanova and M. Ptito (Eds.), *Vision: From Neurons to Cognition. Progress in Brain Research*, Vol. 134. Elsevier, Amsterdam, pp. 285–295.

Kahn, D.M., Hunt, D.L., Greene, M.J., Molnár, Z., Huffman, K.J., Usrey, W.M. and Krubitzer, L. (2000) Retinal projections in adult *Monodelphis domestica* following cortical lesions in early postnatal development. *Soc. Neurosci. Abstr.*, 26: 1699.

Kalil, R.E. (1984) Removal of visual cortex in the cat: effects on the retino-geniculo-cortical pathway. In: J. Stone, B. Dreher and D.E. Rappaport (Eds.), *Development of Visual Pathways in Mammals.* Alan R. Liss, New York, pp. 257–274.

Kalil, R.E., Tong, L.L. and Spear, P.D. (1991) Thalamic projections to the lateral suprasylvian visual area in cats with neonatal or adult visual cortex damage. *J. Comp. Neurol.*, 314: 512–525.

Karabelas, A.B., Moschovakis, A.K. and Highstein, S.M. (1986) Morphological classification of intracellularly HRP injected efferent neurons of the deeper layers of the primate superior colliculus. *Soc. Neurosci. Abstr.*, 12: 1185.

Karten, H.J. (1997) Evolutionary developmental biology meets the brain: the origins of mammalian cortex. *Proc. Natl. Acad. Sci. USA*, 94: 2800–2804.

Kaye, M., Mitchell, D.E. and Cynader, M. (1981) Selective loss of binocular depth perception after ablation of cat visual cortex. *Nature*, 293: 60–62.

Keating, E.G. (1975) Effects of prestriate and striate lesions on the monkey's ability to locate and discriminate visual forms. *Exp. Neurol.*, 47: 16–25.

Kisvàrday, Z.F., Cowey, A., Stoerig, P. and Somogyi, P. (1991) Direct and indirect retinal input into degenerated dorsal lateral geniculate nucleus after striate cortical removal in monkey: implications for residual vision. *Exp. Brain Res.*, 86: 271–292.

Kluver, H. (1936) An analysis of the effects of the removal of the occipital lobes in monkeys. *J. Psychol.*, 2: 46–61.

Kluver, H. (1942) Functional significance of the geniculo-striate system. *Biol. Symp.*, 3: 253–299.

Kluver, H. (1949) Visual functions after removal of the occipital lobes. *J. Psychol.*, 11: 23–45.

Kruger, K., Heitlander-Fansa, H., Dinse, H. and Berlucchi, G. (1986) Detection performance of normal cats and those lacking areas 17 and 18: a behavioral approach to analyse pattern recognition deficits. *Exp. Brain Res.*, 63: 233–247.

Kruger, K., Donicht, M., Muller-Kusdian, G., Kiefer, W. and Berlucchi, G. (1988) Effects on the cat's performance in a binary detection task. *Exp. Brain Res.*, 72: 510–516.

Lashley, K.S. (1941) Thalamo-cortical connections of the rat's brain. *J. Comp. Neurol.*, 75: 67–121.

Lehmkhule, S., Kratz, K.E. and Sherman, S.M. (1982) Spatial and temporal sensitivity of normal and amblyopic cats. *J. Neurophysiol.*, 48: 372–387.

Leventhal, A.G., Rodieck, R.W. and Dreher B. (1981) Retinal ganglion cell classes in the Old World monkey: morphology and central projections. *Science*, 213:1139–1142.

Leventhal, A.G., Rodieck, R.W. and Dreher, B. (1985) Central projections of cat retinal ganglion cells. *J. Comp. Neurol.*, 237: 216–226.

Lomber, S.G., Payne, B.R., Cornwell, P. and Pearson, H.E. (1993) Capacity of the retinogeniculate pathway to reorganize following ablation of visual cortical areas in developing and mature cats. *J. Comp. Neurol.*, 388: 432–457.

Lomber, S.G., MacNeil, M.A. and Payne, B.R. (1995) Amplification of thalamic projections to middle suprasylvian cortex following ablation of immature primary visual cortex in cat. *Cereb. Cortex*, 5: 166–191.

Macchi, G. (1967) Les relations thalamo-corticales dans la phylogénèse: rapport sur les projections thalamo-corticales chez les mammifères. In: R. Hassler and H. Stephan (Eds.), *Evolution of the Forebrain; Phylogenesis and Ontogenesis of the Forebrain.* Plenum Press, New York, pp. 356–376.

MacNeil, M.A., Lomber, S.G. and Payne, B.R. (1996) Rewiring of transcortical projections to middle suprasylvian cortex following early removal of cat areas 17 and 18. *Cereb. Cortex*, 6: 362–376.

Madarasz, M., Somogyi, J., Silakov, V.L. and Hámori, J. (1983) Residual neurons in the lateral geniculate nucleus of adult cats following chronic disconnection from the cortex. *Exp. Brain Res.*, 52: 363–374.

Magalhäes-Castro, H.H., de Lima, A.D., Saraiva, P.E.S. and Magalhäes-Castro, B. (1978) Horseradish peroxidase labeling of cat tectotectal cells. *Brain Res.*, 148: 1–13.

McIlwain, J.T. (1991) Visual input to commissural neurons of the cat superior colliculus. *Vis. Neurosci.*, 7: 389–393.

Medina, L. and Reiner, A. (2000) Do birds possess homologues of the mammalian primary visual, somatosensory and motor cortices? *Trends Neurosci.*, 23: 1–12.

Mettler, F.A. (1943) Extensive unilateral cortical removals in the primate: physiologic effects and resultant degeneration. *J. Comp. Neurol.*, 115: 185–245.

Mihailovic, L.T., Drakoslava, C. and Dekleva, N. (1971) Changes in the numbers of neurons and glial cells in the lateral geniculate nucleus of the monkey during retrograde cell degeneration. *J. Comp. Neurol.*, 142: 223–229.

Milner, A.D., Goodale, M.A. and Morton, M.C. (1979) Visual sampling after lesions of the superior colliculus in rats. *J. Comp. Physiol. Psychol.*, 93: 1015–1023.

Mohler, C.W. and Wurtz, R.W. (1977) Role of striate cortex and superior colliculus in visual guidance of saccadic eye movements in monkeys. *J. Neurophysiol.*, 40: 74–94.

Mooney, R.D., Klein, B.G., Jacquin, M.F. and Rhoades, R.W. (1984) Dendrites of deep layer, somatosensory superior collicular neurons extend into the superficial laminae. *Brain Res.*, 324: 361–365.

Mooney, R.D., Nikoletseas, M.M., Hess, P.R., Allen, Z., Lewin, A.C. and Rhoades, R.W. (1988) The projection from the superficial to deep layers of the superior colliculus: an intracellular horseradish peroxidase injection study in the hamster. *J. Neurosci.*, 8: 1384–1399.

Moschovakis, A.K. and Karabelas, A.B. (1985) Observations on the somatodendritic morphology and axonal trajectory of intracellularly HRP-labeled efferent neurons located in the deeper layer of the superior colliculus of the cat. *J. Comp. Neurol.*, 239: 276–308.

Moschovakis, A.K., Karabelas, A.B. and Highstein, S.M. (1988a) Structure–function relationships in the primate superior colliculus. I. Morphological classification of efferent neurons. *J. Neurophysiol.*, 60: 232–262.

Moschovakis, A.K., Karabelas, A.B. and Highstein, S.M. (1988b) Structure–function relationships in the primate superior colliculus. I. Morphological identity of presaccadic neurons. *J. Neurophysiol.*, 60: 263–302.

Nagata, T., Magalhäes-Castro, H.H., Saraiva, P.E.S. and Magalhäes-Castro, B. (1980) Absence of tectotectal pathway in the rabbit: an anatomical and electrophysiological study. *Neurosci. Lett.*, 17: 125–130.

Nieuwenhuys, R., ten Donkelaar, H.J. and Nicholson, C. (1998) *The Central Nervous System of Vertebrates*. Springer-Verlag, Berlin.

Niida, T., Mukuno, K., Ishikawa, S. and Iwai, E. (1990) Transneuronal retrograde degeneration in adult monkey retina following ablation of striate cortex. In: E. Iwai and M. Mishkin (Eds.), *Vision, Memory and the Temporal Lobe*. Elsevier, New York, pp. 369–375.

Olivier, E., Pauluis, Q., Hardy, H., Missal, M. and Corvisier, J. (1997) Evidence for excitatory tectotectal neurons in the cat superior colliculus. An immunohistochemical study. *Soc. Neurosci. Abstr.*, 23: 510.

Olivier, E., Porter, J. and May, P.J. (1998) Comparison of the distribution and somatodendritic morphology of tectotectal neurons in the cat and the monkey. *Vis. Neurosci.*, 15: 903–922.

Orban, G.A., Vandenbussche, E., Sprague, J.M. and DeWeerd, P. (1988) Stimulus contrast and visual cortical lesions. *Exp. Brain Res.*, 72: 191–194.

Orban, G.A., Vandenbussche, E., Sprague, J.M. and DeWeerd, P. (1990) Orientation discrimination in the cat: a distributed function. *Proc. Natl. Acad. Sci. USA*, 87: 1134–1138.

Papez, J.W. (1938) Thalamic connections in a hemidecorticate dog. *J. Comp. Neurol.*, 69: 103–120.

Pasik, T. and Pasik, P. (1971) The visual worlds of monkeys deprived of striate cortex: effective stimulus parameters and the importance of the accessory optic system. *Vision Res. (Suppl.)*, 3: 419–435.

Pasik, T. and Pasik, P. (1973) Extrageniculostriate vision in the monkey. IV. Critical structures for light vs. no-light discrimination. *Brain Res.*, 56: 165–182.

Pasik, P. and Pasik, T. (1982) Visual functions in monkeys after total removal of visual cerebral cortex. *Contrib. Sens. Physiol.*, 7: 147–200.

Pasik, P., Pasik, T., Hámori, J. and Szentágothai, J. (1973) Golgi type II interneurons in the neuronal circuit of the monkey lateral geniculate nucleus. *Exp. Brain Res.*, 17: 18–34.

Pasternak, T. and Maunsell, J.H.R. (1992) Spatio-temporal sensitivity following lesions of area 18 in the cat. *J. Neurosci.*, 12: 4521–4529.

Pasternak, T., Tomkins, J. and Olson, C.R. (1995) The role of striate cortex in visual functions of the cat. *J. Neurosci.*, 15: 1940–1950.

Payne, B.R. and Cornwell, P. (1994) System-wide repercussions of damage to the immature visual cortex. *Trends Neurosci.*, 3: 126–130.

Payne, B.R., Pearson, H.E. and Cornwell, P. (1984) Transneuronal retrograde degeneration of beta retinal ganglion cells in the cat. *Proc. R. Soc. Lond. B*, 222: 15–32.

Payne, B.R., Pearson, H.E. and Cornwell, P. (1988) Development of connections in cat visual and auditory cortex. In: A. Peters and E.G. Jones (Eds.), *Cerebral Cortex, Vol. 7, Development and Maturation of Cerebral Cortex*. Plenum Press, New York, pp. 309–389.

Payne, B.R., Lomber, S.G., MacNeil, M.A. and Cornwell, P. (1996) Evidence for greater sight in blindsight following damage of primary visual cortex early in life. *Neuropsychologia*, 34: 741–774.

Peacock, J.H. and Combs, C.M. (1965) Retrograde cell degeneration in diencephalic and other structures after hemidecortication of rhesus monkeys. *Exp. Neurol.*, 11: 367–399.

Pearson, H.E., Labar, D.R., Payne, B.R., Cornwell, P. and Aggarwal, N. (1981) Transneuronal retrograde degeneration in the cat following neonatal ablation of visual cortex. *Brain Res.*, 212: 470–475.

Perenin, M.T. and Jeannerod, M. (1978) Visual function within the hemianopic field following early cerebral hemidecortication in man. I. Spatial localization. *Neuropsychologia*, 16: 1–13.

Perry, V.H., Oelher, R. and Cowey, A. (1984) Retinal ganglion cells that project to the dorsal lateral geniculate nucleus in the macaque monkey. *Neuroscience*, 12: 1101–1123.

Polyak, S. (1932) *The Main Afferent Fiber Systems of the Cerebral Cortex*. Univ. California Press, Berkeley, CA.

Powell, T.P.S. (1952) Residual neurons in the human thalamus following hemidecortication. *Brain*, 75: 571–584.

Preuss, T.M. and Goldman-Rakic, P.S. (1987) Crossed corticothalamic and thalamocortical connections of macaque prefrontal cortex. *J. Comp. Neurol.*, 257: 269–281.

Ptito, A., Lepore, F., Ptito, M. and Lassonde, M. (1991) Target detection and movement discrimination in the blind field of hemispherectomized patients. *Brain*, 114: 497–512.

Ptito, A., Fortin, A. and Ptito, M. (2001) 'Seeing' in the blind hemifield following hemispherectomy. In: C. Casanova and M. Ptito (Eds.), *Vision: From Neurons to Cognition. Progress in Brain Research*, Vol. 134. Elsevier, Amsterdam, pp. 367–378.

Ptito, M., Lepore, F., Tremblay, F. and Guillemot, J.P. (1988) Initial acquisition of visual discriminations following selective cortical lesions in cats. *J. Hirnforsch.*, 29: 279–287.

Ptito, M., Lepore, F. and Guillemot, J.P. (1992) Loss of stereopsis following lesions of cortical areas 17–18 in the cat. *Exp. Brain Res.*, 89: 521–530.

Ptito, M., Herbin, M., Boire, D. and Ptito, A. (1996) Neural bases of residual vision in hemicorticectomized monkeys. *Prog. Brain Res.*, 112: 385–404.

Ralston, H.D. and Chow, K.L. (1973) Synaptic reorganization in the degenerating lateral geniculate nucleus of the rabbit. *J. Comp. Neurol.*, 147: 321–350.

Reuter-Lorenz, T., Herter, M., Ptito, A., Ptito, M. and Guitton, D. (1999) The effect of hemispherectomy on pro- and anti-saccades to auditory targets in the gap paradigm. *Soc. Neurosci. Abstr.*, 25: 657.

Rhoades, R.W., Fish, S.E. and Voneida, T.J. (1981) Anatomical and functional characteristics of commissural neurons in the superior colliculus of the hamster. *Neurosci. Lett.*, 21: 255–260.

Rhoades, R.W., Klein, B.G. and Mooney, R.D. (1985) Correlations between structure and function for single visual cells in the superficial layers of the hamster's superior colliculus. *Soc. Neurosci. Abstr.*, 11: 1006.

Rhoades, R.W., Mooney, R.D., Szczepanik, A.M. and Klein, B.G. (1986) Structural and functional characteristics of commissural neurons in the superior colliculus of the hamster. *J. Comp. Neurol.*, 253: 197–215.

Rodman, H.R., Gross, C.G. and Albright, T.D. (1989) Afferent basis of visual response properties in area MT of the macaque. I. Effects of striate cortex removal. *J. Neurosci.*, 9: 2033–2050.

Rodman, H.T., Gross, C.G. and Albright, T.D. (1990) Afferent basis of visual response properties in area MT of the macaque. II. Effects of superior colliculus removal. *J. Neurosci.*, 10: 1154–1164.

Rosa, M.G.P. and Krubitzer, L.A. (1999) The evolution of visual cortex: where is V2? *Trends Neurosci.*, 22: 242–248.

Rose, J.E. and Woolsey, C.N. (1943) A study of thalamo-cortical relations in rabbits. *Bull. Johns Hopkins Hosp.*, 2: 65.

Rowe, M.H. (1988) Changes in inner plexiform layer thickness following neonatal visual cortical ablation in cats. *Brain Res.*, 439: 345–349.

Rowe, M.H. (1990) Evidence for degeneration of W cells following early visual cortical removal in cats. *Brain Behav. Evol.*, 35: 253–267.

Schilder, P., Pasik, T. and Pasik, P. (1971) Extrageniculostriate vision in the monkey. II. Demonstration of brightness discrimination. *Brain Res.*, 32: 383–398.

Schneider, G.E. (1967) Contrasting visuomotor functions of tectum and cortex in the golden hamster. *Psych. Forsch.*, 31: 52–62.

Schneider, G.E. (1969) Two visual systems. *Science*, 163: 895–902.

Seagraves, M.A., Goldberg, M.E., Deng, S.Y., Bruce, C.J., Ungerleider, L. and Mishkin, M. (1987) The role of striate cortex in guidance of eye movements in the monkey. *J. Neurosci.*, 7: 3040–3058.

Sherman, S.M. (1977) The effect of superior colliculus lesions upon the visual fields of cats with cortical ablations. *J. Comp. Neurol.*, 172: 211–230.

Shook, B.L. and Villablanca, J.R. (1991) Quantitative cytoarchitectural analysis of cellular degeneration in the dorsal lateral geniculate nuclei of cats and kittens with cerebral hemispherectomy. *Exp. Neurol.*, 111: 80–94.

Shupert, C., Cornwell, P. and Payne, B.R. (1993) Differential sparing of depth perception, orienting and optokinetic nystagmus after neonatal versus adult lesions of cortical areas 17, 18, 19 in the cat. *Behav. Neurosci.*, 107: 633–650.

Sparks, D.L. and Hartwich-Young, R. (1989) The deep layers of the superior colliculus. In: Wurtz and Goldberg (Eds.), *The Neurobiology of Saccadic Eye Movements*. Elsevier, Amsterdam, pp. 213–255.

Spear, P.D. and Barbas, H. (1975) Recovery of pattern discrimination ability in rats receiving serial or one-stage visual cortex lesions. *Brain Res.*, 94: 337–346.

Sprague, J.M. (1966) Interaction of cortex and superior colliculus in mediation of visually guided behavior in the cat. *Science*, 53: 1544–1547.

Stoerig, P. and Cowey, A. (1997) Blindsight in man and monkey. *Brain*, 120: 535–559.

Stone, J., Leventhal, A., Watson, C.R., Keens, J. and Clarke, R. (1980) Gradients between nasal and temporal areas of the cat retina in the properties of retinal ganglion cells. *J. Comp. Neurol.*, 192: 219–233.

Sun, J.S., Lomber, S.G. and Payne, B.R. (1994) Expansion of suprasylvian cortex projections in the superficial layers of the superior colliculus following damage of areas 17 and 18 in developing cats. *Vis. Neurosci.*, 11: 13–22.

Szentágothai, J. (1973) Neuronal and synaptic architecture of the lateral geniculate body. In: R. Jung (Ed.), *Handbook of Sensory Physiology*, Springer, Berlin, pp. 141–176.

Théoret, H., Herbin, M., Boire, D. and Ptito, M. (1997) Transneuronal retrograde degeneration of retinal ganglion cells following cerebral hemispherectomy in cats. *Brain Res.*, 775: 203–208.

Théoret, H., Boire, D., Herbin, M. and Ptito, M. (1999) Stereological evaluation of substantia nigra cell number in normal and hemispherectomized monkeys. *Brain Res.*, 835: 354–359.

Théoret, H., Boire, D., Herbin, M. and Ptito, M. (2001) Anatomical sparing in the superior colliculus of hemispherectomized monkeys. *Brain Res.*, Brain Res. 894:274–280.

Tomaiuolo, F., Ptito, M., Marzi, C.A., Paus, T. and Ptito, A. (1997) Blindsight in hemispherectomized patients as revealed by spatial summation across the vertical meridian. *Brain*, 120: 795–803.

Tong, L., Spear, P.D., Kalil, R.E. and Callahan, E.C. (1982) Loss of retinal X-cells in cats with neonatal or adult visual cortex damage. *Science*, 217: 72–75.

Tusa, R.J., Zee, D.S. and Herdman, S.J. (1986) Effect of unilateral cerebral cortical lesions on ocular motor behavior in monkeys: saccades and quick phases. *J. Neurophysiol.*, 56: 1590–1625.

Vanegas, H. (1984) *The Comparative Neurobiology of the Optic Tectum*. Plenum Press, New York.

Villablanca, J.R. and Hovda, D.A. (1989) Quantitative study of neural degeneration following neonatal or adult cerebral hemispherectomy in cats. II. Transsynaptic effects in the superior colliculus and mammillary nuclei. *Brain Dysfunct.*, 2: 237–254.

Walker, A.E. (1935) The retrograde cell degeneration in the thalamus of *Macacus rhesus* following hemidecortication. *J. Comp. Neurol.*, 62: 407–419.

Walker, A.E. (1938) The thalamus of the chimpanzee. II. Its nuclear structures, normal and following hemidecortication. *J. Comp. Neurol.*, 69: 467–507.

Wallace, S.F., Rosenquist, A.C. and Sprague, J.M. (1989) Recovery from cortical blindness mediated by destruction of nontectotectal fibers in the commissure of the superior colliculus of the cat. *J. Comp. Neurol.*, 284: 429–450.

Wallace, S.F., Rosenquist, A.C. and Sprague, J.M. (1990) Ibotenic acid lesions of the lateral substantia nigra restore visual orientation behavior in the hemianopic cat. *J. Comp. Neurol.*, 269: 222–252.

Weller, R.E. and Kaas, J.H. (1984) Developmental changes in susceptibility to retinal ganglion cell loss after lesions of visual cortex in primates and other mammals. In: J. Stone, B. Dreher and D.H. Rapaport (Eds.), *Development of Visual Pathways in Mammals*. Alan R. Liss, New York, pp. 289–302.

Weller, R.E. and Kaas, J.H. (1989) Parameters affecting the loss of ganglion cells of the retina following ablations of striate cortex in primates. *Vis. Neurosci.*, 3: 327–349.

Weller, R.E., Kaas, J.H. and Wetzel, A.B. (1979) Evidence for the loss of X-cells of the retina after long-term ablation of visual cortex. *Brain Res.*, 160: 134–138.

Whishaw, I.Q. and Kolb, B. (1984) Decortication abolishes place but not cue learning in rats. *Behav. Brain Res.*, 11: 123–134.

Wilson, J.R. (1989) Synaptic organization of individual neurons in the macaque lateral geniculate nucleus. *J. Neurosci.*, 9: 2931–2953.

Yamasaki, D.S., Krauthamer, G. and Rhoades, R.W. (1984) Organization of the intercollicular pathway in rat. *Brain Res.*, 300: 368–371.

Yukie, M. and Iwai, E. (1981) Direct projection from the dorsal lateral geniculate nucleus to prestriate cortex in macaque monkeys. *J. Comp. Neurol.*, 201: 81–97.

C. Casanova and M. Ptito (Eds.)
Progress in Brain Research, Vol. 134

CHAPTER 25

From visual consciousness to spectral absorption in the human retina

Jocelyn Faubert * and Vasile Diaconu

École d'optométrie, Université de Montréal, 3744 rue Jean-Brillant, Montréal, PQ H3T 1P1, Canada

Abstract: In this paper, we present work that started as an interest in visual consciousness with the study of the blindsight phenomena and color processing. This led us to develop an intraocular reflection and absorption model of the human eye that is sufficient to account for luminance and color detection in blindsight subjects. Luminance and color thresholds were obtained in the good and blind field of hemidecorticated patients under controlled conditions. To determine the role of internal scatter and absorption properties of the human eye we tested the model predictions in three ways. By psychophysical means, by measuring absorption and scatter properties of the human eye, and by building an electromechanical sensor apparatus mimicking Lambertian reflection in the eye. The results of the simulations and measurements support the notion that the sensitivity functions obtained with the hemidecorticated patients can be explained by reflection and absorption properties of the human eye that have not been fully accounted for in the blindsight literature. In the light of such findings, future blindsight experiments must necessarily account for intraocular absorption and reflective properties of the human eye of the type described.

Introduction

A main concern for humanity is to determine what makes them different from other organisms, in particular, other animal species. It has been proposed by philosophers and scientists alike that one of the distinctions between humans and other animal species may reside in a unique structure of human intelligence that gives rise to consciousness. For this reason the study of consciousness has been a major focus by a number of researchers in an attempt to elucidate its biological determinants. This interest is epitomized in the study of the 'blindsight' phenomenon. For the past two decades, there has been substantial evidence that patients whose primary visual cortex has been destroyed or disconnected can demonstrate a variety of residual visual functions in the corresponding cortically blind visual field (see Weiskrantz, 1986; Stoerig and Cowey, 1995 for reviews). The interest in blindsight is natural given the simplicity of its logic. That is, if the destruction of a cortical area removes the conscious awareness of a visual event without eliminating the capacity of processing the information, then visual consciousness must be the consequence of processing within that cortical structure.

The support for blindsight has been challenged by evidence that the hemianopic field determined by standard perimetry may in fact still have functional islands of vision not detected by standard perimetry (Fendrich et al., 1992). Blindsight was also challenged by Campion et al. (1983) where they suggested that blindsight could be the result of either scattered light, near-threshold vision, or spared cortex. However, the suggestion related to spared neural tissue cannot explain the residual vision observed in the blind field of patients in whom the whole cerebral hemisphere has been removed or deaffer-

* Corresponding author: J. Faubert, École d'Optométrie, Université de Montréal, 3744 rue Jean-Brillant, Montréal, PQ, H3T 1P1 Canada.
E-mail: jocelyn.faubert@umontreal.ca;
http://mapageweb.umontreal.ca/faubert/jocelyn_labo/

ented (Perenin and Jeannerod, 1978; Ptito et al., 1987; Perenin, 1991; Ptito et al., 1991). In recent papers, we have proposed that intraocular diffusion and scatter are the probable sources of residual visual functions (Faubert et al., 1995; Stoerig et al., 1996; Faubert et al., 1999). We extrapolated further that, under photopic conditions, the most common site of light detection as a result of scatter must be the central visual field area (CVFA) for a target positioned in the blind field, and we also suggested that spectral absorption in the eye must be considered (Faubert et al., 1995; Faubert et al., 1999). Controlling for extraocular scatter properties in studies with hemicorticectomized patients (as discussed by King et al., 1996) is insufficient because scatter within the eye is more significant than scatter outside of it. We assessed the validity of our model in the following three ways: an electromechanical system that simulates Lambertian light scatter properties; psychophysical experiments that address the notion of where the light signal is detected relative to the stimulated area; and spectroreflectometry measurements of the retinal area to characterize absorption properties.

Model components and assumptions

To understand the model, we must first elaborate the assumptions made about the reflective and absorption properties of the human eye and how light energy would be distributed in the case of hemidecorticated patients.

Lambertian scatter

In the human eye there is an important source of Lambertian (diffuse) scatter and not just specular reflection (LeGrand, 1958). Specular reflection implies that light rays are reflected with 'mirror-like' properties. The geometry of the incident light determines the direction of specular reflection in a similar way to the blinding effect you get when pointing a flashlight perpendicular to a mirror because the light rays bounce right back towards the original light source. Lambertian scatter, on the other hand, implies that the light energy is distributed at all angles simultaneously because of irregularities of the reflective surface. The mere fact that we can observe structures of the eye with an ophthalmoscope implies that there is a strong source of diffuse scatter, otherwise we would only perceive specularly reflected light.

Central visual field detectors

It is well known that sensitivity to light changes with eccentricity. In photopic conditions, the best sensitivity is in the central area of the visual field and decreases with eccentricity (Hood and Finkelstein, 1986). This is often referred to as the 'island of vision' because the sensitivity profile of the visual field appears like an island with a peak in the central visual field and a decrement with eccentricity. If we assume that light was distributed evenly at all angles from its original point of reflection (diffuse scatter) then the most likely place within the visual field where the slightest energy changes should be detected under photopic conditions, would be the central portion containing the fovea. As it will be demonstrated later, this assumption only holds true for reflected lights that are beyond 10° from the vertical midline. Stimulation at 10° or less will generate lateral scatter easily detected by detectors from the opposite visual field as evidenced by both simulated and patient data results presented below. The central detector assumption above relates to luminance detection under controlled conditions because any portion of the functional retina can potentially respond to the scatter emanating from stimuli presented at suprathreshold luminance levels.

Selective spectral absorption of retinal tissues

The model we propose assumes that when a light source is presented in the blind field, it is redirected to a portion of the visual field that has not been affected by cortical damage (most probably the central detectors as mentioned above). The spectral composition of the light that is redirected must change as a function of the absorption and reflective properties of the retinal layer in the blind field (Faubert et al., 1995, 1999). We must therefore, characterize these properties of the eye in our model. The classic way of measuring the absorption properties of the eye is by using spectroreflectometry procedures (Rushton, 1962). Spectroreflectometry is a method for measuring the properties of the reflected light in relation to the properties of the original light source. The difference between the reflected light and the original incident light, gives an estimate of what has been absorbed by the reflecting surface. In simplified terms, what is missing is what was absorbed by the reflecting object. In the eye, there are many layers of absorption as the light travels through the eye and back out when reflected. Below we will elaborate how we have measured the absorption characteristics of the retina.

Testing the model

We have tested the model in several ways. (1) We built an electromechanical system that simulates Lambertian light scatter properties to determine whether this simple apparatus could mimic results obtained with hemidecorticated patients. (2) We then conducted psychophysical experiments that address the notion of where the light signal is detected relative to the stimulated area. This is to test the assumption that the light source is redistributed prior to being detected by the good field. (3) We obtained spectroreflectometry measurements of the retinal area that was stimulated in patients to assess whether we could explain the relative differences obtained between the blind and good field performances by the absorption properties of the retina.

The electromechanical simulation

Fig. 1 illustrates the setup in which a Ganzfeld field was used to simulate the internal human eye. This is an obvious oversimplification of the scatter properties of the eye as a whole given that we did not take into consideration the scatter generated from the optics of the eye. Nevertheless, the model does allow us to simulate and isolate the role of diffusion scatter properties.

We cut a hole in the center of the Ganzfeld and placed an integrative cosine detector to act as our central receptors. In this way, we could project a stimulus at different locations in the Ganzfeld and directly measure the energy level at the detector site. The amount of energy measured by the radiometer (Optronic Spectroradiometer model 736) receiving its input from the cosine detector is the sensitivity measure for the system. The measures obtained with the present model were compared with our patient data previously reported (Stoerig et al., 1996; Faubert et al., 1999). Essentially, these data were obtained under conditions where the entire visual field

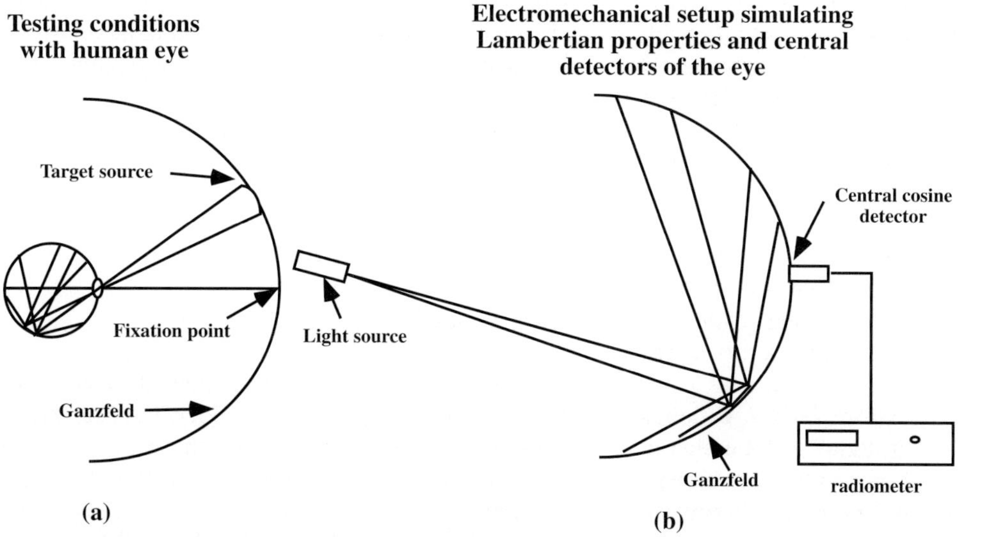

Fig. 1. Simplified schematic representation of the eye facing a Ganzfeld in the testing conditions (a) and the mechanical scatter diffusion setup (b). A cosine detector was placed in the center of the model retina (Ganzfeld) and was interfaced with a radiometer. Stimuli were projected in different areas of the Ganzfeld as a function of different target sizes. The amount of energy measured by the radiometer was taken as the sensitivity value for the simulation setup.

was adapted with a 45 cd/m^2 white background, and the light source was generated from behind the adaptive surface while the size of the target was controlled by an aperture. This was done to avoid producing scatter within the adaptive field itself.

Electromechanical model results

Typical responses obtained when testing the blind visual field of our hemidecorticated patients is represented in Fig. 2a plotted on an energy scale as opposed to a luminance scale for comparison with the setup data (Fig. 2b).

The right portion of Fig. 2a shows a sharp drop-off of sensitivity from the fovea to about 10° of retinal eccentricity where it then stabilizes for a given target size (subject fixation corresponds to the zero point on the x-axis). On the other hand, the data obtained from the good field of the patients, shown in the left portion of Fig. 2a, shows a continual drop of sensitivity as a function of increasing eccentricity as expected for a normal observer. The simulation data shown in Fig. 2b are very similar to the blind hemifield data of our patients. Up to 10° eccentricity, there is a sharp drop-off of sensitivity followed by a leveling off for further eccentricities.

The patient blind field (Fig. 2a, right) and electromechanical setup (Fig. 2b) data show what appears as spatial summation (better sensitivity with increasing target size). Under similar experimental conditions used to test our patients (400 ms and 1° target sizes or greater), we should expect no spatial summation in a normal visual system since these conditions are beyond Ricco's area (Hood and Finkelstein, 1986). We argue that the spatial summation effect in the blind field is observed because the data are represented as relative density measures (e.g. cd/m^2) and that in the light of the scatter hypothesis, the data must be analyzed in terms of the total energy entering the eye.

To make our point, we can replot the patient's data represented in Fig. 2a in terms of total energy entering the eye from actual physical measurements made at the level of the pupil (Fig. 2c). When we represent the data in this fashion, we now have two overlapping functions for the different target sizes in the blind hemifield, whereas the good field shows spatial summation (Fig. 2c). Fig. 2d shows that when we replot the simulation data factoring in the target size to represent the total energy generated by the various target sizes for a given threshold, we obtain overlapping functions just like the blind field data of the patient shown in Fig. 2c.

Electromechanical simulation discussion

What we have demonstrated from this simulation is that the luminance and target size threshold response profiles obtained in the blind field of hemidecorticated patients can be mimicked by a Lambertian scatter electromechanical model with central detectors. What this implies, therefore, is that the detection thresholds obtained in the blind field of our patients must derive from a response in the good field and not from the original point of stimulation. It is possible to test this model assumption psychophysically and the next section will precisely test this prediction.

Psychophysical evaluation of the model predictions

The first prediction we can test is that of spatial summation in the good and blind field obtained in hemidecorticated patients. As predicted from the model, we should always obtain spatial summation in the blind field as a function of different target sizes while data in the good field data should demonstrate a constant sensitivity profile for relatively large stimuli. This is expected because the model predicts that the blind field sensitivity should be the result of the total energy of the stimulus, which is a consequence of the target size, while the patients should respond to the relative density of the stimulus energy in the good field (Ricco's area).

Psychophysical results

Fig. 3 demonstrates that the patient data are consistent with these predictions. What is observed in this figure is that as we increase the target size, the patient thresholds in the good field show no changes as demonstrated by the flat function. Conversely, the data obtained from the blind field of the patients show a constant increase as a function of target size increase as predicted from the total energy assumption of the model.

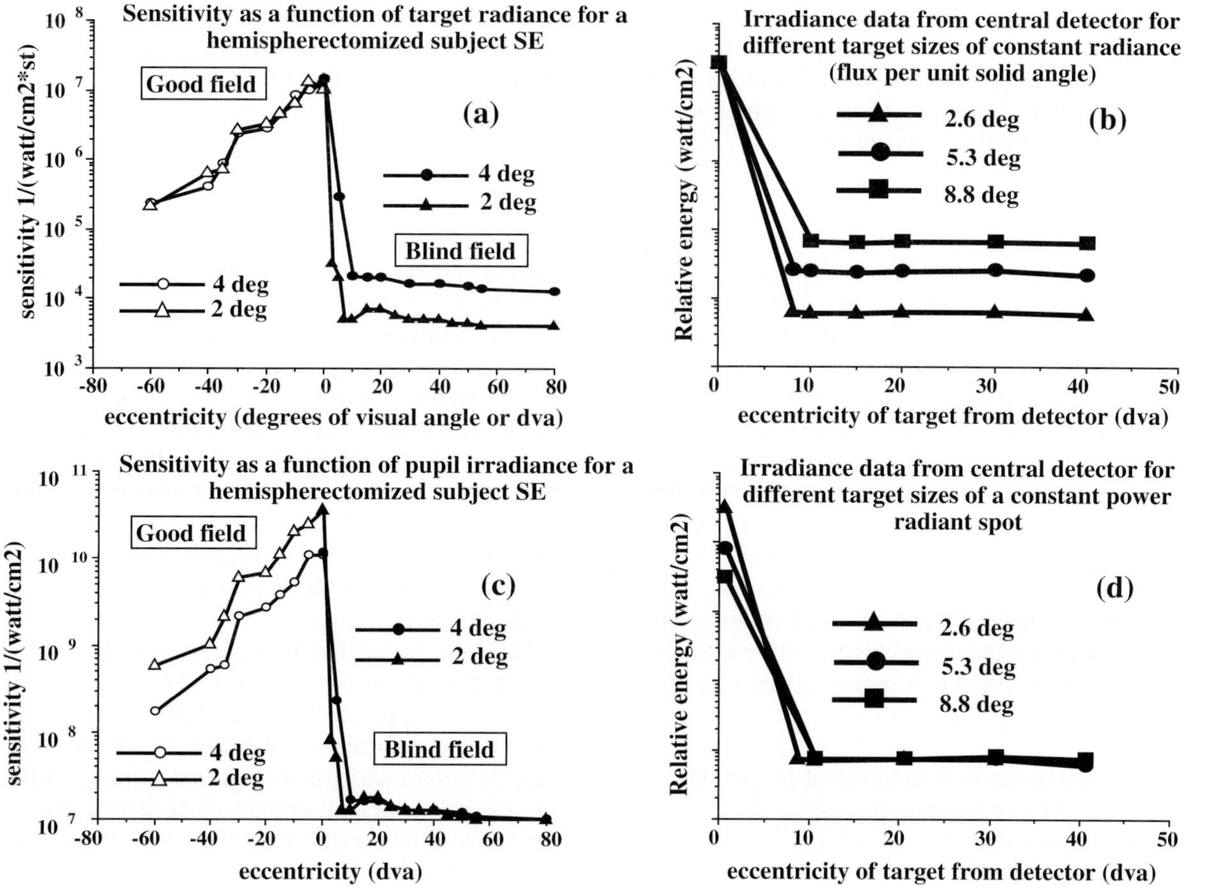

Fig. 2. Sensitivity as a function of eccentricity in the good and blind field of partially hemidecorticated patient SE (a, adapted from Faubert et al., 1999) and for the electromechanical setup (b). Two target sizes were evaluated for SE and three target sizes for the electromechanical setup. The data in a represent sensitivity values computed from target radiance. b illustrates the data obtained from the central detector for different targets of constant radiance (same flux per unit solid angle). The same data are represented for the patient in c where the sensitivity values are computed from pupil irradiance. This corresponds to the relative total energy required to obtain a threshold for a given testing condition. The total energy representation for the model (when the size of the target is factored in) is presented in d. This corresponds to the electromechanical setup data obtained for different target sizes generated from a constant power radiant spot. Note that the setup data corresponds with the data obtained in the blind field of SE.

The next model assumption that we can test is whether the sensitivity values obtained in the scotoma actually derives from detection in some other location of the visual field. The model predicts that the sensitivity data obtained from stimulation in the blind field is actually generated from detection in some other part of the visual field that receives Lambertian scatter. If this is the case, the point of stimulation in the blind field should show no or little response to its state of local adaptation. On the other hand, if detection is truly coming from a local response in the blind field, then the background adaptation state (luminance level) should influence the thresholds as it would be expected for any visual detector. Fig. 4a illustrates how the sensitivity varies as a function of local background adaptation for the good and blind field of a hemidecorticated subject. In this case, we have changed the intensity level of a 4° local background and tested thresholds for a 2° target superimposed on the background. The data clearly show that the sensitivity profile obtained in the good field is directly proportional to the intensity level of the background. As the intensity level of the background increases, the sensitivity for the target stimulus decreases as expected. The blind field data show no correspondence with the local background intensity, which is inconsistent with the notion that the detection of the target is generated at the retinal site where the stimulus is directly projected. Rather, it is perfectly consistent with the model prediction that detection is scatter based and only corresponds to the absolute change of the total energy of the target stimulus.

If the detection thresholds obtained when stimulating the blind field in fact come from a different area of the visual field as predicted from the model, then we can further test this notion by adapting the entire visual field and determine how this influences the sensitivity profile. If, in this case, the sensitivity values obtained in the blind field change as a consequence of the entire field adaptation, this would be further evidence that detection is not local and that the sensitivity in fact is the consequence of visual detectors positioned somewhere in the good field where light is redistributed by Lambertian scatter. Fig. 4b shows that the results confirm the model prediction in that the total background adaptation has a

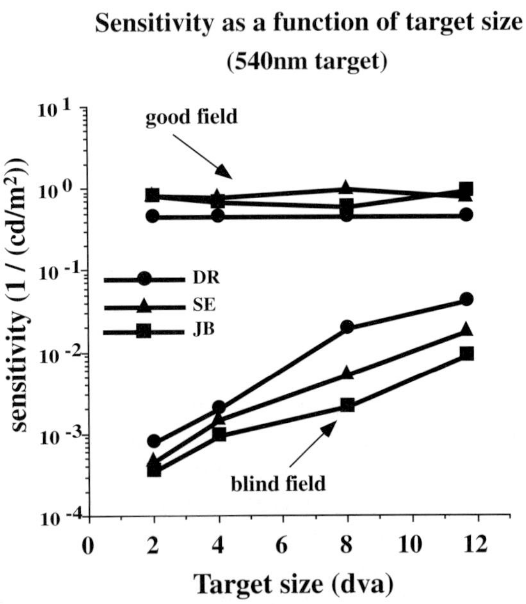

Fig. 3. Spatial summation data obtained at 20° eccentricity in the blind and good fields of three hemidecorticated (DR, SE, and JB) patients. The good field data show flat functions as expected when target sizes are beyond Ricco's area of spatial summation. Data from the blind field show what wrongly appears to be spatial summation in the blind field. See text for details.

direct influence on sensitivity in the blind field as it does for the local and global background adaptation conditions in the good field.

Psychophysical evaluation discussion

The results of the psychophysical tests using global (full field) and local background adaptation procedures are perfectly consistent with the model predictions. When the blind field of a patient is stimulated, the light is diffusely redistributed and detected somewhere else in the visual field where visual detectors are functional. Furthermore, the properties of the sensitivity profiles follow the notion that detection when stimulating the blind field is based on the total energy of the stimulus (scatter model prediction) while the sensitivity profile of the good field, under the same conditions, exhibits properties consistent with a local density system as expected from normal visual processes.

The final prediction from the model pertains to the selective absorption of retinal layers. If the target light that is projected in the blind field is redistributed and detected somewhere else in the visual field, then that redistributed light must have a different spectral composition than when it first reaches the retina. The model would predict that the redistributed light must be lacking spectral energy components that correspond with the selective absorption of the reflected surface. When we tested our hemidecorticated subjects for spectral sensitivity functions under photopic conditions, we obtained a relative decrease in sensitivity for the middle wavelength region of the visible spectrum in their blind field as compared to their good field as shown in Fig. 5 (Stoerig et al., 1996; Faubert et al., 1999). The next section will discuss this in detail and show whether the spectroreflectometry and the spectral sensitivity measurements made in these subjects are consistent with the model.

Selective retinal absorption model prediction

As mentioned above, if light projected on the blind field is reflected to other areas of the visual field and subsequently detected, the detection thresholds for lights of different wavelength components should reflect the absorption characteristics of the reflecting

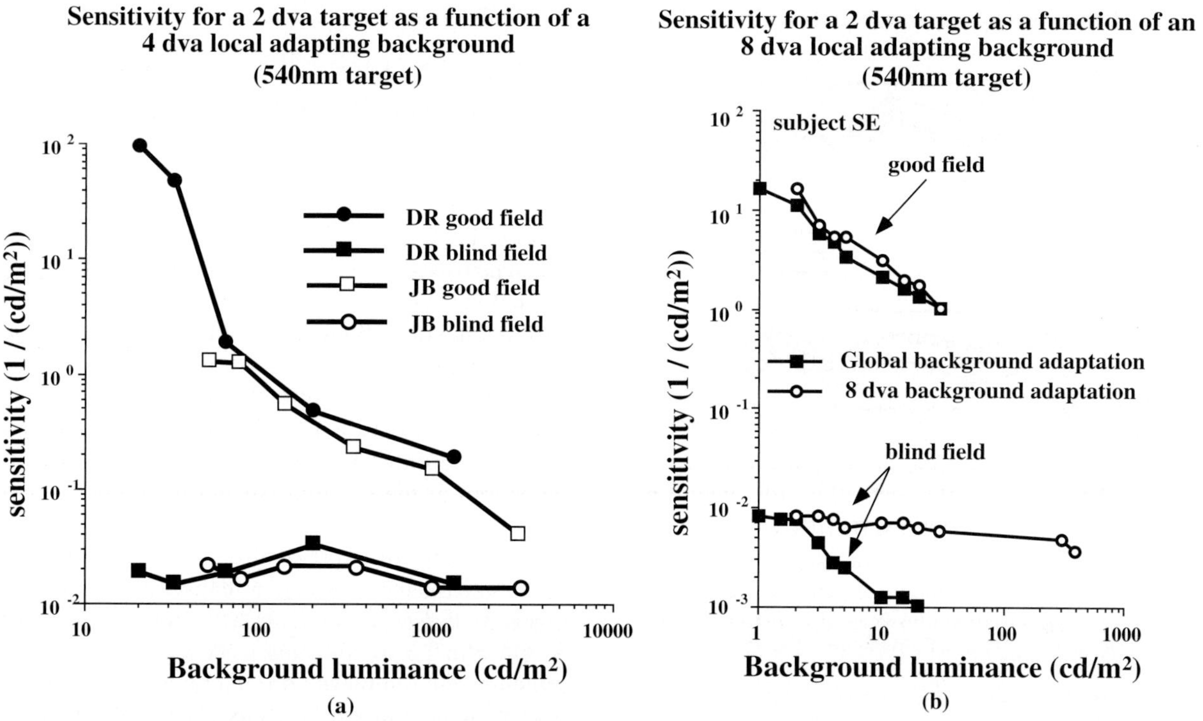

Fig. 4. Sensitivity values obtained in the good and blind fields of two patients (DR and JB) for a 2° target superimposed on a 4° local adapted background of different intensities (a). Note that the good field data show the expected decreased sensitivity with increasing background intensity while the blind field data show flat functions implying that the detection of the target was in fact occurring somewhere else in the visual field. (b) Shows sensitivity values obtained in the good and blind fields of patient SE for local (2° target superimposed on an 8° local adapted background) and global (2° target superimposed on the Ganzfeld) background adaptation conditions. Note that when the entire background changes in intensity, the sensitivity slope of the blind field is the same as that of the good field while this is not the case for the local background condition. This is evidence that the detection of the stimulus in the blind field takes place somewhere else then where the target is projected. See text for details.

surface, namely, the retina. To understand the absorption and reflective properties of the human eye we must first elaborate on these properties.

Model representation of scattered light in the human eye

Fig. 6 shows the different retinal layers and the path of scattered light in the human eye.

The model can be quantitatively represented by the following formula described in Faubert et al. (1999):

$$I_1(\lambda) = I_o(\lambda) \times 10^{-(2\alpha_1 d_1 + 2\alpha_p d_p)} \times \left[r_1 + r_2(1 - r_1)^2 \times 10^{-(2\alpha_3 d_3 + 2\alpha_4 d_4)}\right] \times C(\Omega) \quad (1)$$

where $I_1(\lambda)$ represents the spectral luminance flux reflected by the pigment epithelium and the sclera at the level of the pupil exit, $I_o(\lambda)$ represents the initial spectral luminance flux, and $C(\Omega)$ is a constant which depends on the measurement geometry. For most of the reflection measurements obtained at the pupil exit we can assume that $C(\Omega)$ equals 10^{-3}. We can simplify Eq. (1) by regrouping the coefficients corresponding to the retinal components and rewrite Eq. (1) as the following formula:

$$I_1(\lambda) = I_o(\lambda) \times 10^{-(2\alpha_1 d_1)} \times 10^{-(2\alpha_p d_p)} \times \left[r_1 + r_2(1 - r_1)^2 \times 10^{-(2\alpha_3 d_3 + 2\alpha_4 d_4)}\right] \times C(\Omega) \quad (1')$$

which can be simplified further into the following

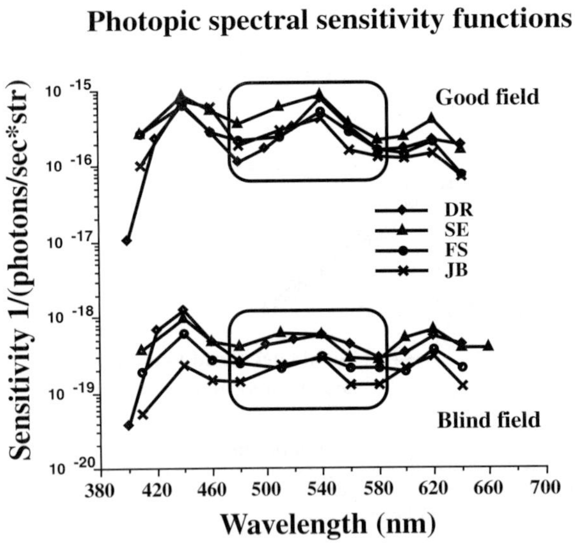

Fig. 5. Spectral sensitivity functions obtained in the blind and good fields of four hemidecorticated patients. Notice that there is a relative depression of sensitivity in the blind field relative to the good field in the middle portion of the spectrum. The model predicts that this difference is a consequence of the selective spectral absorption of the human retina before light is redistributed to the good field where it is subsequently detected.

formula:

$$I_1(\lambda) = I_o(\lambda) \times 10^{-(2\alpha_1 d_1)} \times r(\lambda) \qquad (1'')$$

where

$$r(\lambda) = 10^{-(2\alpha_p d_p)} \times \left[r_1 + r_2(1 - r_1)^2 \times 10^{-(2\alpha_3 d_3 + 2\alpha_4 d_4)}\right] \times C(\Omega).$$

Simplified in this way, $r(\lambda)$ corresponds to a coefficient that is characteristic of the retinal reflection and absorption and $10^{-(2\alpha_1 d_1)}$ corresponds to the absorption within the ocular media.

If we apply these formulations to the specifics of our scatter-based model for residual vision in the blind field we can say that we use two different procedures to measure the resulting reflection at the CVFA derived from scatter of a stimulus presented at 15° of eccentricity. One method is to compare the luminance flux $I_o(\lambda)$ (which is our reference light) with $I_1(\lambda)$ (which is the light reflected by the back of the eye) as measured by a spectroradiometer. $I_o(\lambda)$ and $I_1(\lambda)$ are measured at the pupil entrance and at the pupil exit respectively. Therefore the absorption is calculated as:

$$A_1(\lambda) = I_1(\lambda)/I_o(\lambda) = 10^{-(2\alpha_1 d_1)} \times r(\lambda).$$

The second method is to measure the luminance flux $I'_o(\lambda)$ (the reference light) and $I'_1(\lambda)$ (the light reflected by the back of the eye) by using the CVFA detectors of the patient (as represented by our model in Fig. 1). In this case, $I'_o(\lambda)$ represents the spectral sensitivity function obtained in the good field of the patient while $I'_1(\lambda)$ represents the spectral sensitivity function obtained in the bad field. As we have suggested previously, the model assumes that the detection of the stimulus presented in the bad field is in fact detected by the good field. It follows that the absorption in this case is represented as $A_2(\lambda) = I'_1(\lambda)/I'_o(\lambda)$ which should have the shape of $r(\lambda)$.

To be able to express $A_2(\lambda)$ and to compare it with $A_1(\lambda)$ it is necessary to first express $I'_o(\lambda)$ as a function of $I_o(\lambda)$, and $I'_1(\lambda)$ as a function of $I_1(\lambda)$. At the retinal level, the luminance flux $I'_o(\lambda)$ is represented as the luminance flux $I_o(\lambda)$ attenuated by the ocular media and measured as a spectral sensitivity function $F(\lambda)$ of the photoreceptors. Therefore:

$$I'_o(\lambda) = F(\lambda) \times I_o(\lambda) \times 10^{-\alpha_1 d_1}.$$

Similarly, $I'_1(\lambda)$ is represented as the luminance flux $I_1(\lambda)$ attenuated by the ocular media and measured as a spectral sensitivity function $F(\lambda)$ of the photoreceptors (Kitahara et al., 1987).

It follows that:

$$I'_1(\lambda) = F(\lambda) \times I_1(\lambda) \times 10^{+\alpha_1 d_1} = F(\lambda) \times I_o(\lambda) \times 10^{-\alpha_1 d_1} \times r(\lambda).$$

Therefore:

$$A_2(\lambda) = I'_1(\lambda)/I'_o(\lambda) = r(\lambda).$$

In this way, it is possible to derive that the difference between $A_1(\lambda)$ and $A_2(\lambda)$ is the factor $10^{-(2\alpha_1 d_1)}$ which represents the ocular media.

We can summarize and simplify the mathematical formulations by stating that we propose two ways of measuring the selective absorption of the retinal tissues which ultimately are represented as data in Fig. 7a and b. One method is by using the detection thresholds of the good and bad fields of our patients (Fig. 7a) and the other is by spectroreflectometry (Fig. 7b).

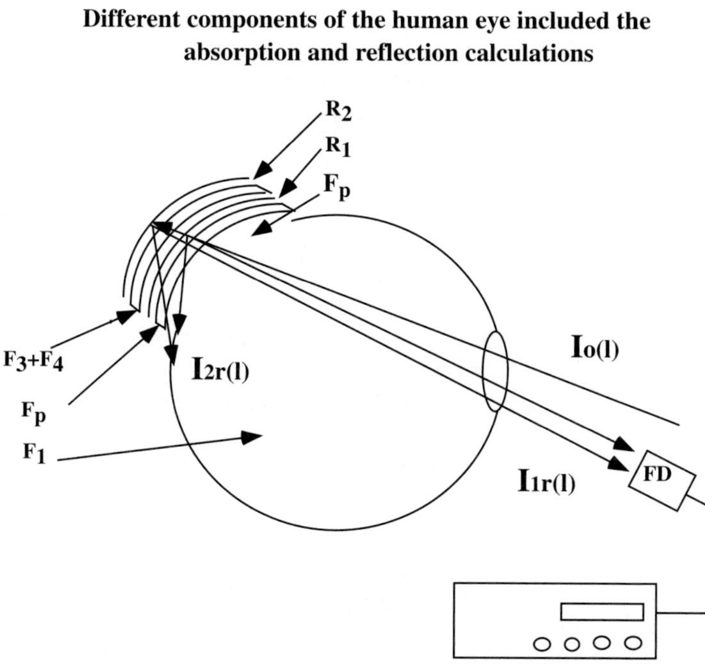

Fig. 6. Illustration of the eye and its different components which influence absorption and reflection of light in our model for residual vision. F_1 represents the ocular medium; α_1 represents linear absorption coefficient of F_1; d_1 represents the thickness of F_1; F_p represents the photopigment layer; α_p represents linear absorption coefficient of F_p; d_p represents the thickness of F_p; F_3 represents the melanin pigment; α_3 represents linear absorption coefficient of F_3; d_3 represents the thickness of F_3; F_4 represents the hemoglobin; α_4 represents linear absorption coefficient of F_4; d_4 represents the thickness of F_4. R_1 represents the epithelium and r_1 corresponds to the reflection coefficient for R_1 $(0 < r_1 < 1)$; R_2 represents the sclera and r_2 corresponds to the reflection coefficient for R_2 $(0 < r_2 < 1)$. See text for equation details.

To compare the methods directly we must trace the light rays for the two types of 'reflectometry' measurements proposed above. In the first method, we compare the detection thresholds in the good field with those of the bad field. In both the good field and bad field data we can argue that the light travels through the ocular media for the entire length of the eye only once before it reaches the detectors. In this case the ocular media factor can be simplified out of the good field/bad field (gf/bf) ratio and there is no need to correct for ocular media when comparing the results between the two fields. Essentially, it is argued that the light reaches the retina of the bad field, there is absorption by the retina, and then the light is redirected to the good field less some energy at specific wavelengths corresponding to the specific light components absorbed within the retinal layers. These data are represented in Fig. 7a and show that the relative absorption as measured by the ratio between the good and blind spectral sensitivity functions is within the middle wavelength region of the visible spectrum (green portion).

In the second method, we compare the light measured at the pupil entry with the light which exits the pupil (see method and apparatus in Faubert et al., 1999). In this case, the light rays reach the retina, some component is absorbed just like the gf/bf method mentioned above, and then the light is reflected back out of the eye. The difference in this case is that we must take into consideration the absorption of the ocular media twice for the reflected light because it travels the entire length of the eye going in and once again when it is reflected back out of the eye while the reference light (at pupil entry) never enters the eye and therefore is not affected by ocular media. We tested this assumption by making spectroreflectometry measurements in the eyes of the same patients, represented in Fig. 7a, in order to determine if selective wavelength absorption of the eye could account for the relative decrease of sensitivity

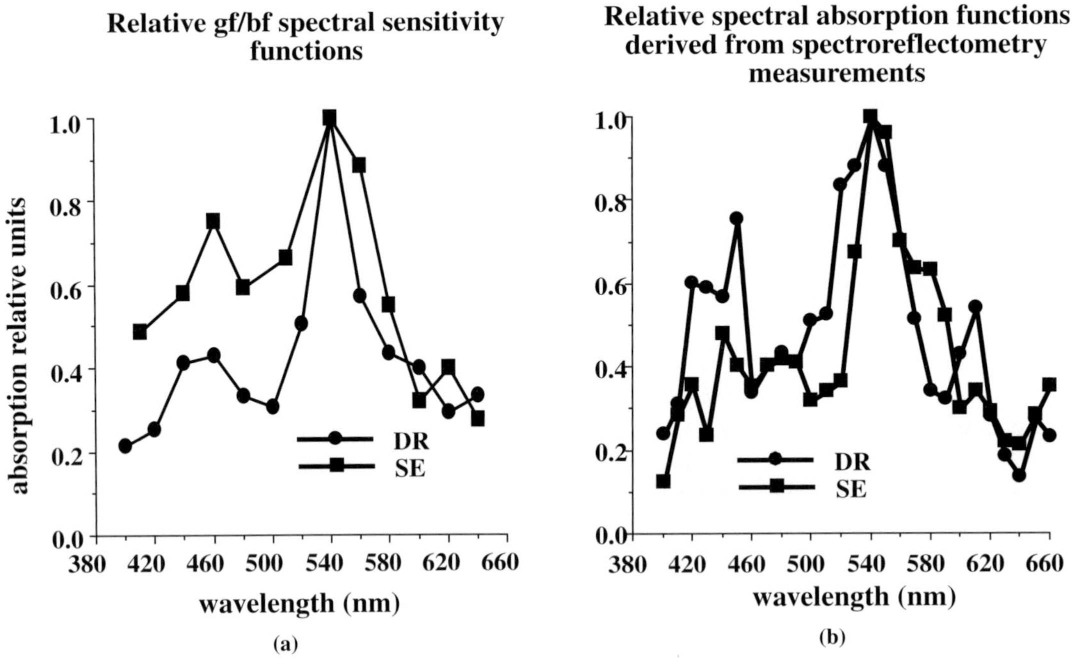

Fig. 7. Good/blind field sensitivity ratios for patients DR and SE (a). These ratios show that there is a relative loss of sensitivity in the middle wavelengths of the visible spectrum in the blind field as compared to the good field. In vivo spectroreflectometry measurements made in the eyes of the same two patients are shown in b. These measurements are obtained by establishing the relative difference between the energy entering the eye and the energy coming out of the eye while taking into account the energy absorbed by the optics of the eyes.

in the middle wavelength region of the spectrum and the results are shown in Fig. 7b (Faubert et al., 1995, 1999).

Selective spectral absorption discussion

When comparing the methods obtained from the two methods shown in Fig. 7a and b it is clear that the relative decrease observed in the spectral sensitivity measures of the blind field is attributable to selective spectral absorption at the retinal level before light is redistributed to the good field. We must conclude, therefore, that the predictions made by the Lambertian scatter model of blindsight in hemidecorticated patients are all supported by our data.

General discussion

The present data suggest that the sensitivity profiles obtained in the blind field of hemidecorticated patients may be accounted for by Lambertian diffusion scatter properties and selective spectral absorption of the eye. The model presented above is in itself sufficient to explain the results obtained with our hemidecorticated patients. It is important to note that, even under well controlled conditions which eliminate extraocular scatter, it is possible to obtain sensitivity values in the blind field of hemidecorticated patients solely on the basis of diffusion scatter within the eye. Whether one obtains a sensitivity value or not depends on the size of the stimulus. For instance, if the stimulus target size used is 5° in diameter, it may require a luminance difference of 3 log units between the good and blind field to obtain thresholds, but if a target size of 10° is used then it may require half that amount in relative difference. This occurs because changing the size of a given target also modifies the total energy entering the eye and as a consequence less energy is required to produce the same stimulation for a given unit of area.

In essence, it appears that the sensitivity measures obtained in the good and blind fields function on two different mechanisms. The good visual field functions according to the amount of energy for a given area; the residual vision in the blind field depends upon the total amount of energy entering the eye because the central receptors detect the energy which has been scattered from its original site of projection. The present model is consistent with the fact that we could not change the sensitivity in the blind field of patients when we modify only a local adapting background, whereas the sensitivity values change in a normal fashion when the entire visual field is adapted.

In conclusion, we present a model to explain the potential effects of scatter properties of the eye on visual sensitivities obtained with hemidecorticated patients. The model clearly demonstrates that the sensitivity profiles obtained in the blind field of these patients may be derived from receptors in the good field (most probably central visual field). The model successfully demonstrates that intraocular Lambertian scatter off the back surface of the eye is probably the main source for the sensitivity obtained in the blind field of these patients when extraocular light scatter is controlled. Furthermore, the model predicts that it is theoretically possible to obtain very similar sensitivities from the normal and blind fields if large enough targets and/or eccentricities are used. We also demonstrate that the relative difference observed in the middle wavelength sensitivities between the good and blind hemifields of hemidecorticated patients is a result of selectively greater absorption of the eye for these wavelengths. Finally, we recommend, for future blindsight studies, that an experiment similar to the local and global background adaptation experiment mentioned above should be conducted in such a population to eliminate all doubts as to where detection is actually taking place.

Acknowledgements

This project was supported by FCAR (Québec), NSERC (Canada), and MRC (Canada).

References

Campion, J., Latto, R. and Smith, Y.M. (1983) Is blindsight the effect of scattered light, spared cortex, and near-threshold vision? *Behav. Brain Sci.*, 6: 423–448.

Faubert, J., Diaconu, V., Ptito, M. and Ptito, A. (1995) Modeling visual scatter in the human eye: implications for residual vision. *Invest. Ophthalmol. Vis. Sci.*, 36: s633.

Faubert, J., Diaconu, V., Ptito, M. and Ptito, A. (1999) Residual vision in the blind field of hemidecorticated humans predicted by a diffusion scatter model and selective spectral absorption of the human eye. *Vision Res.*, 39: 149–157.

Fendrich, R., Wessinger, C.M. and Gazzaniga, M.S. (1992) Residual vision in a scotoma: implications for blindsight. *Science*, 258: 1489–1491.

Hood, D.C. and Finkelstein, M.A. (1986) Sensitivity to light. In: K.N. Boff, L. Kaufman and J.P. Thomas (Eds.), *Handbook of Perception and Human Performance*. Vol. I, *Sensory Processes and Perception*, Wiley, New York, Chapt. 5.

King, S.M., Azzopardi, P., Cowey, A., Oxbury, J. and Oxbury, S. (1996) The role of light scatter in the residual visual sensitivity of patients with complete cerebral hemispherectomy. *Vis. Neurosci.*, 13: 1–13.

Kitahara, K., Kandatsu, A., Tamaki, R. and Matsuzaki, H. (1987) Spectral sensitivities on a white background as a function of retinal eccentricity. *Doc. Ophthalmol. Proc. Ser.*, 49: 651–655.

LeGrand, Y. (1958) *Light, Colour and Vision*. Chapman and Hall, London.

Perenin, M.T. (1991) Discrimination of motion direction in perimetrically blind fields. *NeuroReport*, 2: 397–400.

Perenin, M.T. and Jeannerod, M. (1978) Visual function within the hemianopic field following early cerebral hemidecortication in Man. I. Spatial localization. *Neuropsychologia*, 16: 1–13.

Ptito, A., Lassonde, M., Leporé, F. and Ptito, M. (1987) Visual discrimination in hemispherectomized patients. *Neuropsychologia*, 25: 869–879.

Ptito, A., Lepore, F., Ptito, M. and Lassonde, M. (1991) Target detection and movement discrimination in the blind field of hemispherectomized patients. *Brain*, 114: 497–512.

Rushton, W.A.H. (1962) Visual pigments in man. *Sci. Am.*, 207: 120–132.

Stoerig, P. and Cowey, A. (1995) Visual perception and phenomenal consciousness. *Behav. Brain Res.*, 71: 147–156.

Stoerig, P., Faubert, J., Ptito, M., Diaconu, V. and Ptito, A. (1996) No blindsight following hemidecortication in human subjects? *NeuroReport*, 12: 1990–1994.

Van Nooren, D. and Tiemeijer, L.F. (1986) Spectral reflectance of the human eye. *Vision Res.*, 26: 313–320.

Weiskrantz, L. (1986). Blindsight: *A Case Study and Implications*. Oxford University Press, Oxford.

Wyszecki, G. and Stiles, W.S. (1982) *Color Science*. Wiley, New York.

C. Casanova and M. Ptito (Eds.)
Progress in Brain Research, Vol. 134

CHAPTER 26

Tickling the brain: studying visual sensation, perception and cognition by transcranial magnetic stimulation

Alan Cowey * and Vincent Walsh

University of Oxford, Department of Experimental Psychology, South Parks Road, Oxford OX1 3UD, UK

Abstract: Transcranial magnetic stimulation (TMS) is a means of stimulating the brain from outside the skull with little, and occasionally no discomfort for the subject. A single TMS pulse, lasting less than 1 ms, can briefly disrupt the normal activity of a targeted region of the brain for tens of milliseconds, allowing the effects of disruption on specific perceptual and cognitive tasks to be measured behaviorally. Rapid, repeated pulses can disrupt activity for correspondingly longer periods. The reversibility of the effects make it possible to create 'virtual patients' who can be tested in the same way as actual patients with real brain damage in order to explore regional functional specialization. Although several aspects of TMS continue to be evaluated, such as its safety, the extent and localization of the effective region of induced electrical current, the importance of the waveform of the pulse, the configuration and positioning of the coil, its productivity has been firmly established in little more than 10 years of systematic use. Examples of the latter are given from investigations of the nature of visual phosphenes produced by TMS applied to different regions of the visual cortex in normal subjects and subjects with occipital or ocular damage in an attempt to reveal the role of visual cortex in visual awareness.

Backdrop

When discussing transcranial magnetic stimulation (TMS) with colleagues and students the same questions occur repeatedly, for example: "is it safe?"; "can it be localized?"; "is it repeatable?"; "how does it work?"; "does it show anything we did not know already?". Sometimes the questions are framed more like assertions, such as: "surely it can't be very useful because the effects can't be localized!" or "all it does is disrupt activity in the brain and that can't be helpful!". Before describing some of the discoveries that have been made with respect to visual perception by using TMS, we will therefore address the problems that seem to us to trouble both the would-be user and the sceptic. We emphasize that what follows is a thumb-nail sketch of TMS and not a detailed technical account. There are several of the latter, mostly in technical journals, but surprisingly few of the former, despite the fact that most interested scientists want the former, at least initially.

What is TMS?

TMS is pulsed magnetic stimulation applied to the brain through the skull, muscle and skin that cover it. It is no different in kind from magnetic stimulation applied to any other part of the body, for example to peripheral nerves. TMS was first used on the human motor cortex by Barker et al. (1985), which means that it is still a relatively modern technique. But its antecedents are ancient by comparison. Like so many applications of electrochemistry, magnetic nerve stimulation stems from the discoveries of Michael Faraday, who demonstrated in 1831 that when an *electric* current was turned on or off in a (primary) coil of wire, another current was induced

* Corresponding author: A. Cowey, University of Oxford, Department of Experimental Psychology, South Parks Road, Oxford OX1 3UD, UK. Tel.: +44-1865-271353; Fax: +44-1865-310447;
E-mail: alan.cowey@psy.ox.ac.uk

in a neighboring (secondary) coil by the fluctuating *magnetic* field around the primary coil. An important aspect of this famous demonstration is that it is the sudden change in current, and thence magnetic field, that is responsible for induction. Despite jumping ahead slightly, this immediately answers one common question, namely "why don't we all experience TMS when we lie in a powerful magnetic field like that of a modern magnetic brain scanner?". The powerful magnetic field is not changing, therefore there is no stimulation; it is the pulsed radiofrequency waves that change in a scanner.

"But why does a fluctuating magnetic field affect the brain at all?", is another frequently asked question. The answer is that a current is induced in the brain, which is therefore acting like Faraday's secondary coil. Although the current is weak, the flow of ions can depolarize or hyperpolarize nerve cell membranes where the direction of the current is across the membrane. If the depolarization exceeds some level, the nerve cell will discharge. The effectiveness of the stimulation depends on the strength of the magnetic field produced by the stimulating coil (typically 1–2 Tesla), the shape of the pulse (notably monophasic or biphasic but also its rate of change) and the frequency of the pulses (still single pulse in most applications but increasingly repetitive- or rapid-pulse and typically around 10–15 Hz). Interestingly, but frequently misunderstood, it is not the fluctuating magnetic field itself that stimulates the tissue, but the current it induces. Right from its birth, the term TMS was therefore a misnomer. The term is so evocative that the solecism seems slight, but it has led to a confusion between electrical and magnetic stimulation. TMS works by a brief magnetic field which induces an electric field which in turn causes ionic current flow, whereas electrical stimulation directly produces a flow of ions between the stimulating electrodes. Not surprisingly, electrical stimulation can be more precisely localized because there is no doubt about the position of the electrodes whereas pinpointing the effective locus of action of TMS is far more difficult, as discussed below. However, TMS has major advantages in that indwelling electrodes are avoided and, with minor exceptions, the discomfort or pain produced by electrical stimulation from electrodes on the scalp is absent.

A brief history

It was 65 years after Faraday's discovery that d'Arsonval (1896) persuaded a subject to place his head inside a coil pulsed at 42 Hz. The subject experienced flashing lights (now called magnetophosphenes) but mercifully little else apart from dizziness. This finding was confirmed several times, notably by Thompson (1910), shown in Fig. 1, who attributed the phosphenes to direct stimulation of the visual centers of the brain. Given the size and disposition of the stimulating coil and what we now know to be the great sensitivity of the retina to induced current, it is almost certain that the early investigators were stimulating the eyes and not the visual cortex at the opposite end of the head, which must be on a par with confusing the North and South poles. The anecdote is amusing but it does highlight the possibility of mislocalization.

It was nearly a half century later that investigators began to use magnetic stimulation to investigate the properties of nerves — whole nerves not individual axons — in both animals and human subjects. They showed that peripheral nerves in the arm could be stimulated and that by placing the coil on the skin over different, and even quite deep nerves, different muscles in the hand could be made to twitch. The early stimulators could not produce strong magnetic fields and brief sharp pulses and it was only in the last 30 years that technical developments led to the introduction of stimulating coils that were compact yet could produce a magnetic field of up to 2-Tesla and a pulse with a rise time of about 100 μs and a total duration about 400 μs. Such coils are in common use today. With such a coil, Barker (1976), one of the pioneers of modern magnetic stimulation, activated nerves in the wrist and elicited both muscle twitches in the hand and tingling sensations in the same parts of the hand. Clearly, nerve impulses were being propagated proximally and distally from the area of stimulation and were leading to the appropriate movements and feelings. The brief pulses also allowed them to record evoked potentials at distant points and measure conduction velocity (Polson et al., 1982).

Could the same kind of thing be done with the brain? The first account of TMS applied to motor cortex swiftly followed (Barker et al., 1985). Using

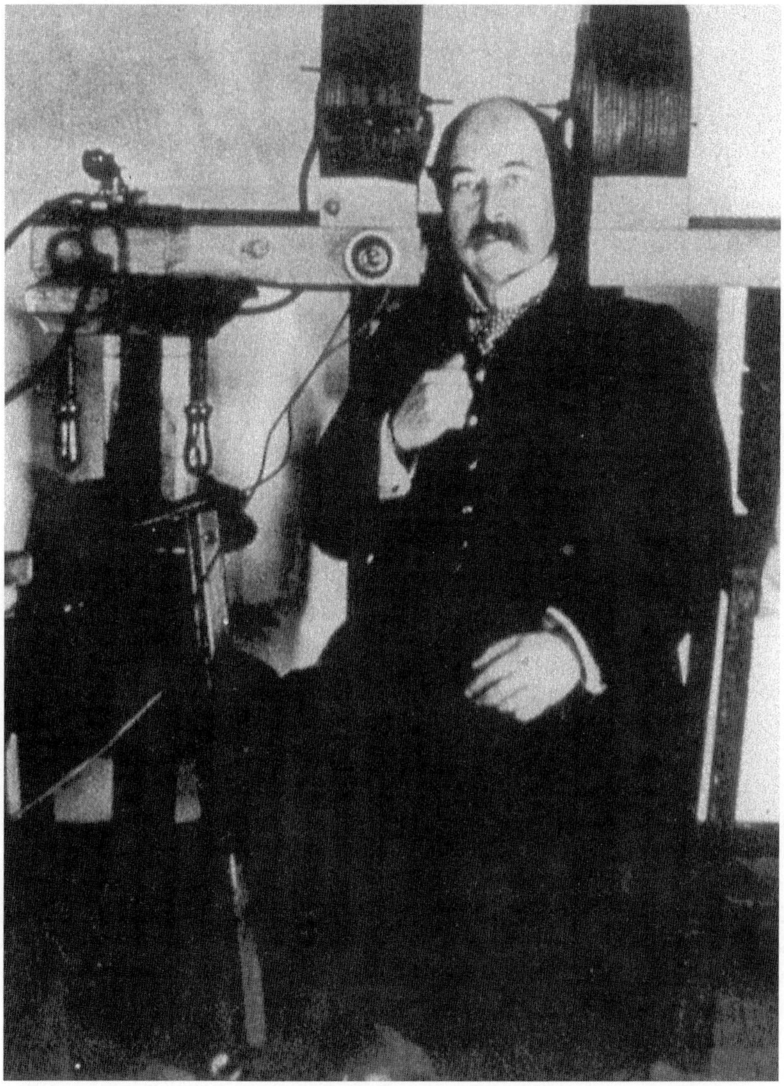

Fig. 1. Sylvanus P. Thompson in his laboratory with his head between the two large coils he used to stimulate his own brain in 1910.

a circular coil centered on the vertex (which produces maximal stimulation beneath the rim of the coil, not the vertex, as explained later) they elicited hand movements and recorded the associated muscle potentials from the fingers. The trickle of papers quickly became a stream as investigators discovered that they could stimulate visual, somatosensory and auditory cortex and produce illusory sensory perceptions. Just as importantly, by using TMS parameters that did not yield illusory percepts and stimulation aimed at other than classical sensory or motor cortex, they were able to influence the performance of subjects on a wide range of perceptual and cognitive abilities such as visual search, visual neglect, motion perception and memory (for reviews see Amassian et al., 1993; Walsh and Cowey, 1998; Pascual-Leone et al., 1999).

Why coil design and position of the coil matter

It is now possible to buy magnetic stimulators and coils off the shelf. Spending a few minutes to think about their properties is well worth the effort. They all work by charging one or more capacitors up to a high voltage, which takes a few seconds, then discharging the capacitor into the coil as one single pulse or as several pulses when the experimenter presses a switch. The early models discharged the capacitor in a single pulse, delivering all the power in a single monophasic pulse, peaking at about 100 μs and decaying within 1.0 ms. The induced electric field is almost monophasic and is effectively over in about 0.5 ms. In summary, all the delivery is over within 1.0 ms. The problem with single-pulse stimulators is that although the effects on nerve cells can last much longer than 1.0 ms, several seconds are needed before the next pulse can be delivered. It is therefore difficult to disrupt brain activity that might last longer than this or influence performance on tasks that might take up to a second to present, for example several frames of a display of visual motion or a static display in which the observer is searching for a particular feature.

Rapid rate stimulation (rTMS) produces a series of biphasic magnetic pulses (but the series can be a single pulse if necessary). Its main advantage is that a biphasic (oscillatory) waveform can activate nerve cells at lower magnetic field strengths than that of monophasic pulses, with the result that less energy needs to be discharged and the stimulator can therefore produce pulses more frequently, sufficiently often to stimulate the brain over the period of seconds required for many perceptual tasks. Many experiments are only possible with rTMS.

The simplest TMS coil is an insulated circular winding, with a handle, as shown schematically in Fig. 2. The arrow shows the overall direction in which the current flows in the coil during each pulse. This current creates a magnetic field around the coil, which in turn induces an electric field in the tissue beneath the coil. This electric field is indicated schematically in Fig. 2, right, by the curved arrows, whose length crudely represents the field strength. The first thing to note is that the induced current flow is opposite to that in the coil. The second thing to note is that the electric field is weakest in the center of the coil and at progressively eccentric points from the rim. But there is no single 'point' where the field is stronger than anywhere else. It is therefore an exaggeration to refer to TMS with a simple coil as focal; it can not be brought to a focus. But TMS can properly be described as local in that the induced field is not everywhere strong enough to depolarize nerve cells and appropriate placement of the coil on the scalp can lead to selective effects beneath it. For example shifts in position of as little as 1 cm over visual cortex can lead to a perceived change in position and intensity and quality of a visual phosphene (Cowey and Walsh, 2000).

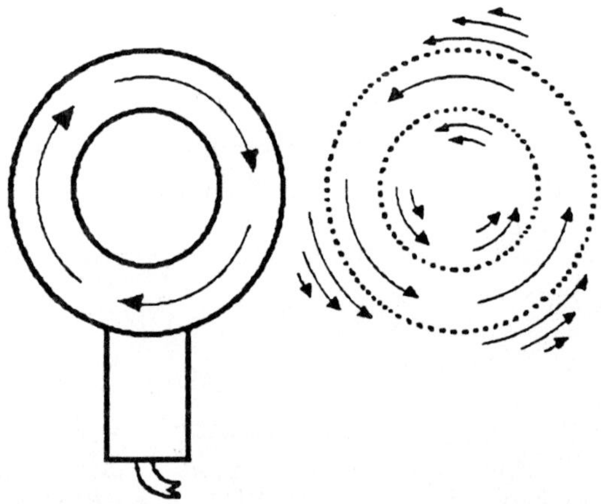

Fig. 2. Left: outline of a simple circular stimulating coil. The arrows indicate the direction of current flow in the coil. Right: a highly schematic representation of the induced electric field in the tissue beneath the coil, which has been moved sideways for clarity. The arrows show the direction of current flow, which is opposite to that in the stimulating coil. The length of the arrows crudely indicates the magnitude of the induced current, which declines towards the center of the coil and away from the perimeter of the coil. The depiction assumes a homogenous medium beneath the coil which will never be true when the coil is placed against the skull.

The orientation of the coil is also important. For example, Fig. 3 (modified from Barker, 1999) schematically shows a circular coil placed above a nerve, N1. The arrows indicate the flow of current in the tissue beneath the coil, not in the coil itself. Nerve cells can only be depolarized with TMS by a *change* in electric field which will correspondingly change the current flowing across cell membranes. The higher the rate of change the better, which is why the temporal properties of the pulse are so crucial. In Fig. 3, nerve N1 will be maximally exposed to a change in current in the vicinity of points A and B. At A, the membrane change will be in the direction of depolarization, i.e. tending to cause the nerve to discharge, and at B it will be hyperpolarization. Note that if the coil is turned over, depolarization

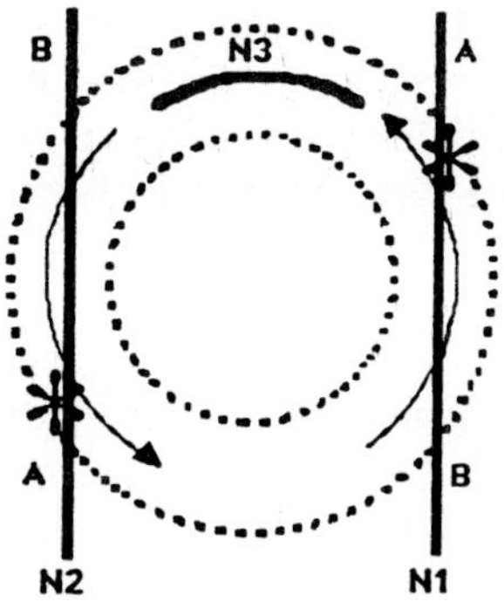

Fig. 3. Schematic representation of the effects of magnetic stimulation through a circular coil on a nerve tracts beneath the coil. The arrows on the coil indicate the current flow in the tissue beneath it, i.e. they are really like Fig. 2, right. Beneath the coil are three nerves. Nerve N1 will be maximally depolarized at the 'virtual cathode', marked with an asterisk, near position A and hyperpolarized near B. Beneath the other side of the coil a similar nerve will be maximally excited in a different position, where the 'virtual cathode' is again marked with an asterisk. Nerve N3 is shown as following a curved path in which the radius of curvature happens to be the same as that of the coil. This hypothetical nerve will be barely if at all excited because the current flow does not cross the axons. (Based on a figure from Barker, 1999.)

will now occur at B, which can be a considerable distance away. Nerve N2 beneath the opposite side of the coil will depolarize at a point closer to the bottom edge of the coil. Nerve N3 has a different configuration in that it is curved and follows the contour of the coil so precisely that there is little or no change in electric field across the nerve. Nerve N3 will not discharge and will not even experience any change in potential difference across the cell membranes of its axons.

By analogy with direct extracellular electrical stimulation, where it is the cathode that excites the cell, A and B for nerves N1 and N2 at the coil configuration shown in Fig. 3 are sometimes called the virtual cathode and virtual anode, respectively. Fig. 3 depicts the field around three hypothetical peripheral nerves, two straight, one curved. But brain tissue is not like this and in this instance it works to our advantage. First, the cortex contains rounded or fusiform or pyramidal cell bodies, often with dendrites oriented in many directions. This means that no matter what the orientation of the coil, several parts of the cell membrane will experience a sharp change in flow of current. Second, there are axons oriented in all directions in a particular piece of cortex, although not equally in all directions. Third, it would be difficult even in the white matter to find anything like the discrete peripheral nerve depicted in Fig. 3. However, there are some long and relatively unconvoluted white matter tracts, for example the visual radiations from the dorsal lateral geniculate nucleus to the striate cortex and the shorter but compact projections from striate cortex (V1) to several surrounding extrastriate areas. Here the problem of coil orientation is non-trivial.

It is sometimes thought that the problem of identifying the effective part of the circular coil in a given investigation could be overcome by positioning the coil at right angles to the skull, so that only a small part of its outer rim rests on the skull and only a small part of its magnetic field can influence the brain directly beneath it. If only this were a practical possibility! When the coil is positioned in this way, the total magnetic field, and, therefore, induced electric field, in the brain is reduced to such an extent that much higher stimulating energies would be required, far above those provided by conventional machines.

Fortunately, the problems just discussed can be reduced by using different types of coil, notably the figure-of-eight coil introduced in 1988 by Ueno et al. (1998). The idea is simple. Two round coils are placed next to each other and wired so that the current travels in opposite directions in the two coils. The highest electric field in the tissue beneath is induced at the center, where the coils abut, and is roughly twice as strong as beneath the most effective part of a single coil. One can be fairly confident with the figure-of-eight coil that the TMS is having its effect beneath the center, as long as each of the component coils is not large. Why the proviso? If each of the component coils is large, it is likely that one of them will be distant from the skull at some part of its circumference and its magnetic field will be too far from the brain to induce a sufficiently high electric field in the tissue, rather like the effect of applying a single coil at right angles to the skull. The outcome is that the effective stimulation is now being provided solely by one of the two coils and the effective region might no longer be beneath its junction with the other coil. Angling the two coils towards each other so that they approximate the contours of the skull can help, but in practice a given angle is not optimal for all positions on the skull because the head is not spherical. Smaller component coils could in theory solve the problem and one like a four-leaf clover has been used to concentrate the peak field even further. But smaller coils have weaker fields and therefore poorer penetration compared to a conventional single coil of about the same total diameter.

As usual, life is a compromise. A simple coil will serve well enough for most purposes, especially if there is some independent indication of localization, such as which part of the body is made to move or where in the visual field a phosphene appears. Simple coils might even be better when one wishes to stimulate a large body of cortex, e.g. area 46 of the frontal lobe. A figure-of-eight coil of about 8 cm across gives concentrated stimulation that is effective down to about 2 cm below its center and this is good enough for most purposes (Barker, 1999).

How deeply into the brain can one stimulate?

A rough and ready answer to this question is: "A few centimeters". The answer is rough because the brain tissue beneath any coil is not uniform in density or biophysical properties and it also depends on the size of the coil or component coils. For a simple commercial coil about 8 cm across and with a maximum field strength of 2T, the induced field where the current would stimulate a given and acceptable proportion of nerve cells is more or less hemispherical and the pole is about 2.5 cm from the surface of the skull. Given the thickness of the skull, this means that most brain tissue is not sensitive to TMS. We are unlikely to encounter any studies of the amygdala, using present TMS technology. The field beneath a figure-of-eight coil is more complex in shape but the region of most concentrated stimulation penetrates a little further as well as ending more abruptly. However, it should never be overlooked that the areas of secondary stimulation beneath each of the component coils can be as intense at shallower depths, say 1 cm. In studying some particular effect of TMS it would be easy to conclude that the effective locus of stimulation was the cortex beneath the center of the dual coil that was involved, whereas it could be cortex several cm lateral and in an unknown direction. But at least one could be confident that it was not a deep site. For an excellent detailed discussion of these issues see Barker (1999) and Ruohonen and Ilmoniemi (1999).

How safe is it?

Any artificial stimulation of the brain is potentially dangerous and there is a duty to assess the danger and minimize it to the point where it is negligible. Unfortunately, safety is not an exact science. We know of no evidence that single-pulse TMS delivered by the stimulators presently available leads to undesirable short-term or long-term effects (Wassermann, 1998; Lorberbaum and Wasserman, 2000). It has been used on thousands of subjects and some, like ourselves, have served as subjects in experiments for several years and received thousands of single, i.e. widely separated, pulses. Possible short-term effects could be epilepsy, long-term could involve memory. So far, single-pulse TMS has a clean bill of health. Rapid, or repetitive, TMS poses more problems for it has occasionally led to seizures in a few subjects, although without any evident long-term effects. However, in these subjects, the rTMS was delivered at an intensity close to the threshold for eliciting movements of the limbs. The best practice is never to use subjects with a personal or family history of epilepsy and always to use a stimulating intensity close to the threshold for eliciting movement in that subject (see Wassermann et al., 1996; Chen et al., 1997, for details of internationally accepted guidelines). In following these guidelines, we have used rTMS on ourselves at frequencies of up to 10 Hz, again for thousands of pulses, without undesirable effects.

Safety addresses discomfort as well as physical harm. TMS can stimulate superficial nerves on the scalp and produce uncomfortable tingling or even pain. The problem is much greater with stimulation at the base of the skull, level with the ears and especially close to the nape of the neck. It is best to avoid these regions or to choose a coil orientation that minimizes the discomfort, or only to use oneself as a subject. The noise — a sharp crack — from the coil with each pulse can also be unpleasant and ear plugs should be worn. Even if it does not sound particularly loud, the plugs should be used because for a brief moment the sound pressure level can reach well over 100 dB and subjective loudness of such brief pulses is not a good guide to their potentially dangerous effects on the inner ear. The answer to the general question about safety is that, in the right hands, it as safe as many other investigative techniques.

Using TMS to study visual processing

The time course of action of a single pulse

Since TMS is most commonly used in visual studies to interfere with cortical visual processing it is important to establish the timing and duration of its effectiveness. Amassian et al. (1989) were the first to demonstrate the disruptive effects of TMS in relation to the identification of brief visually presented letters that subjects had to identify. They found that a single pulse of TMS delivered over the occipital pole, where the fovea is represented in striate cortex (V1) and also in V2, maximally impaired letter recognition when it was delivered between 80 and 100 ms after the stimulus had been presented. Several other investigators have reported essentially similar results (Beckers and Homberg, 1991, 1992; Masur et al., 1993; Beckers and Zeki, 1995; Epstein and Zangaladze, 1996; Miller et al., 1996; Kastner et al., 1998). Although the pulse lasts for less than 1.0 ms, its detectable effects on performance can be at least 20 times longer. In order to explore the latter and in addition to see whether effects could occur at even earlier and later times with respect to stimulus presentation, we used single-pulse TMS in 10-ms steps at times from −100 ms (i.e. before the stimulus was presented) to +200 ms after it had been presented (Corthout et al., 1999a). The task was to identify a letter, from a set of ten roughly equally identifiable letters, presented with negative contrast (dark on bright) for 10 ms. Each letter subtended only 0.35° and was viewed foveally 250 ms after the disappearance of a fixation cross. Immediately after the presentation of the letter, there was a black square of similar negative contrast in order to make the task more difficult. Each subject had 600 trials in which letters and delays were randomized. The outer perimeter of the coil next to the handle was held against the head at a point 2 cm above the inion. TMS intensity was between 80 and 90% of the maximum of 2 Tesla, depending on the results of pilot experiments on each subject.

The mean results of three subjects are shown in Fig. 4, top. The most noteworthy finding is that there are two broad periods during which TMS is effective in impairing performance, with maximum reduction in percentage correct approaching or even reaching chance levels (10%) at delays of around −30 and +90 ms. Such a result does not 'explain' the reason for the effect of TMS of course. One uninformative possibility is that the TMS exerts a non-specific effect on visual identification almost wherever it is delivered over visual cortex. A second experiment, using the same subjects and a sub-set of delays and four different coil positions, showed that the effect was certainly sensitive to the latter. Fig. 4, bottom, shows that the effect of TMS delivered 60 or 50 ms before the presentation of the visual stimulus was the same at coil positions 1, 3, 5 and 7 cm above the inion but that at −10, +10 and +100 ms it severely impaired performance only at the 1- and 3-cm positions. In other words, the location of the coil was important in relation to the second broad dip, but not to the first one.

One unexpected feature of the experiment just described is that the dips in the performance curves were so broad. A further investigation with new subjects was therefore made in which more trials were given at and around the peaks and troughs and the stimulus display was altered by using positive contrast (bright letters on a dark surround) and the post-stimulus masking was removed. One reason for doing the latter is that TMS might influence the potency of the masking and therefore the ability to identify the letter. The number of targets was also reduced to 5 (chance = 20% correct). TMS intensity as a percentage of maximum varied from 55 to 70%. Some subjects showed two dips in performance and some showed three (Corthout et al., 1999b). Fig. 5 shows typical results from subjects in the latter category. There are dips centered at −70, +20 and +110. The initial dip almost certainly reflects the effects of blinking (Corthout et al., 2000a,b); the later dips — referred to as visual dips by the authors — seem, respectively, to relate to the first stage of processing in V1 (and perhaps V2/V3 as well) and to a later stage that could involve some or all of the feedback projections to V1 from extrastriate visual cortex.

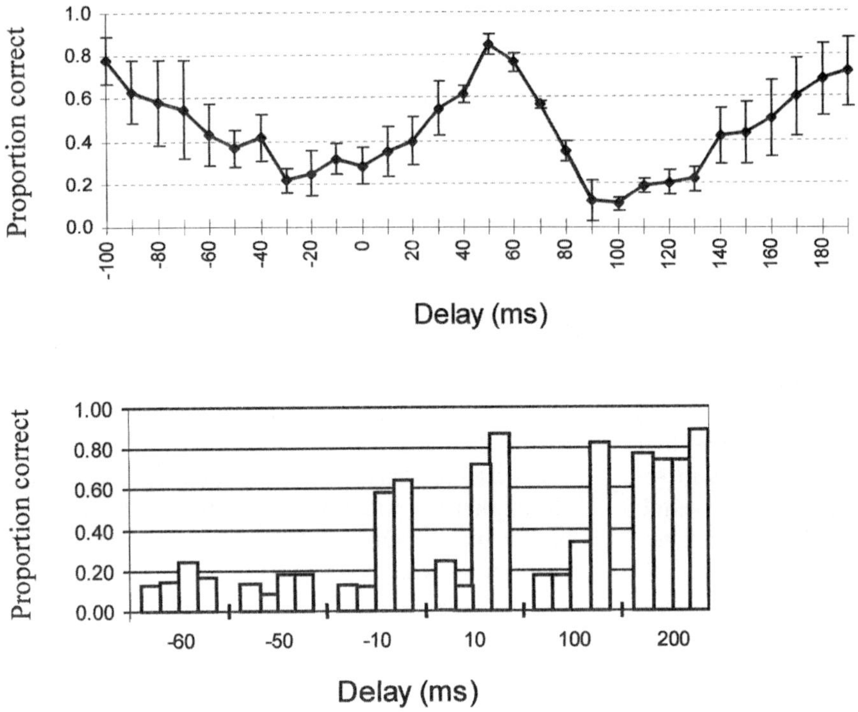

Fig. 4. Top: the mean proportion of letters correctly identified as a function of the delay, averaged across three subjects. The delay refers to the time of onset of a single magnetic pulse minus the time of onset of the visual stimulus. Negative values thus indicate that the magnetic stimulus preceded the visual stimulus. The error bars denote ±1 standard error of the mean. Bottom: the mean proportion of letters correctly identified as a function of selected delays for different coil locations, averaged across the same three subjects. At each delay is a set of four bars, which correspond respectively to a distance of 1, 3, 5, and 7 cm between the lower end of the coil and the inion. (Redrawn from Corthout et al., 1999a.)

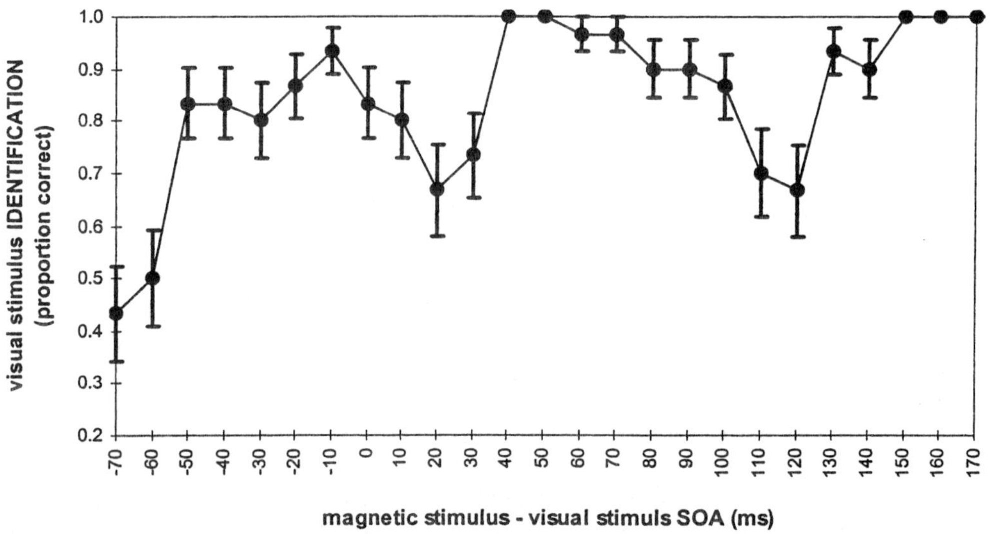

Fig. 5. Proportion of letters correctly identified as a function of the delay for a subject showing three dips. Each point is the mean of 30 trials and error bars denote ±1 SEM. (Redrawn from Corthout et al., 1999b.)

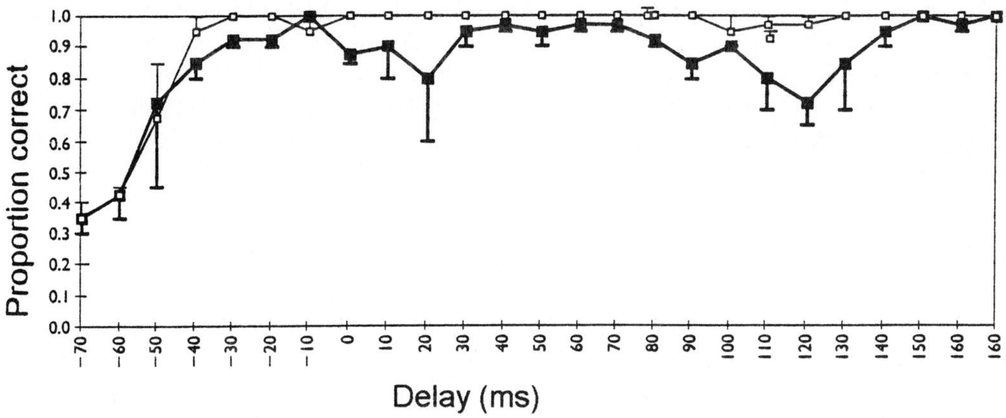

Fig. 6. The proportion of letters correctly identified as a function of the delay, averaged for two subjects. The performance curve shown by the solid squares was obtained 1 week before the curve shown by the unfilled squares. Chance level is 20%, indicated by the dashed line. Error bars indicate ± 1 SEM. Note that there was no improvement in performance with practice at a delay of −70 ms, which corresponds to the dip associated with blinking. (Redrawn from Corthout et al., 2000a.)

A further characteristic of TMS is that its effectiveness can diminish with extensive practice in the same subject performing the same task. Can this tell us anything interesting? In a further experiment, Corthout et al. (2000a) repeated the procedure of the experiment described in the previous paragraph but gave repeated testing over a period of several weeks (Fig. 6). The performance of the subjects improved, despite the TMS, but only at the delays coinciding with the second and third dips. There was no improvement around the initial (blinking) dip. Since the impairment at the later dips could be reinstated by reducing the contrast of the stimulus letters, the most likely explanation for the change in effectiveness of TMS with repeated testing is that the improved sensory coding believed to underlie perceptual learning must involve early visual cortex (V1, V2, V3). This is discussed in detail by Corthout et al. (2000a).

Phosphenes

"To see or not to see; that is the question". The misquotation alludes to phosphenes, the illusory visual percepts produced by stimulating the visual cortex directly, whether by a blow on the back of the head (seeing stars) or by electrical means. But whether TMS can induce phosphenes from different occipital sites provides a means of studying the contributions of different visual areas to the conscious perception of visual events. For example, and bearing in mind the results of electrophysiological recordings in different visual areas in monkeys, would phosphenes induced by stimulating V1 and V2 be predominantly colored and static but those induced by stimulating area MT/V5 be chiefly achromatic and moving? Would phosphenes induced by stimulation beyond V1 survive removal of V1? The answer to the last question should be "yes" according to some theories of the role of area MT/V5 in visual awareness of motion (see Ffytche and Zeki, 1995, for review) but "no" according to other views of the role of V1 in phenomenal visual awareness (for review see Stoerig and Cowey, 1997). In an attempt to address these questions we studied phosphenes in several normal subjects and in two subjects with damage to the eyes or to the visual cortex.

The first systematic studies of phosphenes were carried out by direct electrical stimulation of the brains of neurological patients who were being assessed for surgery to alleviate intractable epilepsy (Penfield and Rasmussen, 1957). Although most of the stimulating sites were in the temporal lobes and the phosphenes were often complex and meaningful images or sequences of images, Penfield and Rasmussen systematically stimulated parts of the occipital lobe in a few subjects. For example, in three patients (Penfield and Rasmussen, 1957, pp. 136–147) stimulation produced phosphenes whose position, color and shape varied according to the position of the electrode. Some of them even moved. Many years later Brindley and Lewin (1968) implanted an array of electrodes sub-durally over the medial surface of one occipital lobe in a patient peripherally blinded by acute glaucoma. When electrically stimulated in turn through the electrodes the patient experienced simple phosphenes whose size and eccentricity with respect to the blind fovea depended on the position of the electrode over what was almost certainly parts of V1 and V2 representing the lower quadrant of the contralateral visual hemifield. Knowing the distance between the electrodes and the angular separation of the phosphenes, it was possible to calculate the human magnification factor for the first time (Cowey and Rolls, 1974). The phosphenes were bright flashes and, with rare exceptions, had no structure or clear orientation. Is it possible to induce localizable phosphenes by TMS and would the characteristics of the phosphenes depend on which extrastriate regions are stimulated?

In the experiments concerned with the effects of TMS on letter recognition the intensity of the magnetic field was deliberately kept low and only single pulses from a simple round coil were used. If higher fields and/or repeated pulses are used subjects experience phosphenes, although the proportion of subjects in which they can be elicited from caudomedial occipital sites varies from small (e.g. Amassian et al., 1989) to almost 100% (e.g. Kammer, 1999). In our own experiments, we have encountered very few subjects who do not experience clear and repeatable phosphenes with TMS delivered in pulse trains of from 1 to 5 Hz over the occipital cortex via a figure-of-eight coil (Stewart et al., 1999).

We therefore attempted to induce phosphenes by TMS to assess the integrity of visual cortex in a subject who became totally retinally blind following a traffic accident and to compare the results with those obtained by stimulating the same regions in normally sighted individuals and in a well-documented hemianopic subject who shows blindsight in his impaired field. The purpose of this was to test the hypothesis that in the absence of area V1, the retinal projection to visual area MT/V5, via the mid-brain and the pulvinar nucleus, is sufficiently effective to give rise to conscious visual impressions, especially of moving stimuli (Barbur et al., 1993; Benson et al., 1998; Zeki and Ffytche, 1998).

The peripherally blind subject PS had a road accident that transected one optic nerve and crushed the other and has been totally blind for over 8 years. He does not know when the lights in a room are turned on or off and shows no pupillary response to any change in illumination, even when measured with a pupillometer that can detect changes of as little 1% in diameter. He volunteered to take part in TMS experiments to see whether his visual cortex remained excitable. Patient GY is a well-known hemianope who suffered almost complete destruction of left striate cortex (V1), with some additional damage to dorsal parts of extrastriate areas V2 and V3 in a traffic accident at the age of eight. Now in his forties, he has been a subject in many experiments on blindsight, reviewed by Stoerig and Cowey (1997). In order to discover whether these two patients and several undamaged subjects could localize any phosphenes induced by TMS they were asked to fixate the center of a tilted drawing board placed 57 cm in front of them, and to describe and draw, with respect to the fixation point, any visual sensations produced by the TMS.

All six fully sighted subjects experienced phosphenes and drew them in different locations that depended on the site of the figure-of-eight stimulating coil. As the stimulating coil was moved forwards from the inion and just to one side of the mid-line the phosphenes became progressively more eccentric in the contralateral lower visual quadrant. As the coil was moved left/right on the scalp with respect to the mid-line the phosphenes were in roughly mirror image correspondence in the right/left visual field, respectively. An example is shown in Fig. 7a. In all six normal subjects, the phosphenes produced by TMS near the mid-line were sometimes colored, although invariably unsaturated, and were rarely described as moving.

The peripherally blind subject also reported phosphenes (initially to his astonishment) from TMS applied over and around the occipital pole but in all three testing sessions, several months apart, the phosphenes were unusual (Fig. 7b) in that they were clustered around the center of 'fixation', which was his finger tip placed in the center of his 'visual field' on the drawing board. But like normal subjects, he frequently described them as colored, most often using the descriptions "red, green, blue, silver, gold,

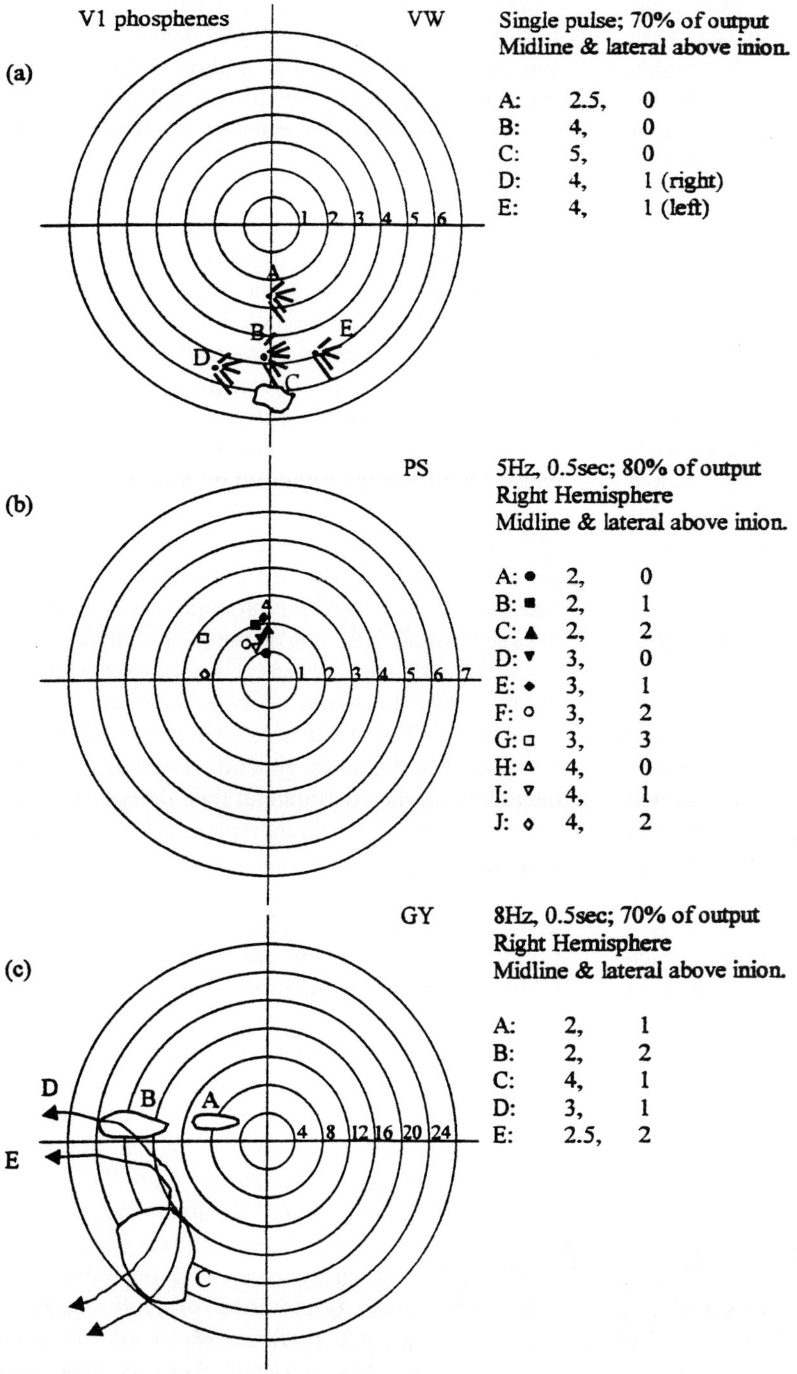

Fig. 7. Examples of phosphenes produced by TMS at and near the occipital pole in a normal subject (a), in a retinally blind subject (b) and in a hemianopic subject with blindsight (c). In the case of the blindsighted subject (c), the stimulation was delivered over his intact right hemisphere and all the phosphenes are in the intact left visual hemifield. It was not possible to produce phosphenes in his blind hemifield. The retinally blind subject (b) drew all his phosphenes in and around the center of the display board in front of him, which he could not see, but onto which he could imagine his phosphenes, close to his fingertip which he 'looked at' with his blind eyes. Note the different scales for eccentricity for a and b and for c. For each phosphene, the first number refers to the distance above the inion and the second number to the distance from that point laterally along the scalp. (From Cowey and Walsh, 2000, with permission.)

orange, or brown". Despite exploring all sites at intervals of 1 cm up to 6 cm forward of the inion and up to 3 cm lateral to the midline on each side the retinally blind subject never reported phosphenes beyond a few degrees of his finger on the center of the board in front of him. In striking contrast, the hemianope showed normal spatial organization in the hemifield contralateral to his normal occipital lobe (Fig. 7c) but when TMS was applied over his damaged left occipital region within 1–2 cm of the mid-line, it was not possible to elicit phosphenes, even with repetitive pulse TMS (rTMS) of up to 10 Hz, 0.5 s and maximal stimulator output.

We next explored functional specialization in TMS induced phosphenes. We have shown elsewhere (Stewart et al., 1999) that rTMS applied over visual area MT/V5 can produce moving phosphenes. Our six sighted subjects consistently perceived movement in the visual field contralateral to the hemisphere of stimulation when TMS was applied at and around a point 3 cm in front of inion and 5–6 cm laterally. (e.g. Fig. 8a). However, the reports of movement were variable, even in the same subject. In some subjects, the phosphene was a single elongated blob which jumped in one direction but in another subject it was like the visual noise on a de-tuned TV screen. Sometimes the phosphene consisted of sparkling elements that jumped in one direction then in another. They were usually described as "silvery, cloudy, sparkling, grayish, like pepper and salt, a snowstorm" and only rarely had any color, which was always faint. In this sense they were different from the often colored phosphenes elicited from sites closer to the occipital pole. In all subjects other than the retinally blind subject, the movement tended to have an overall centrifugal or centripetal direction. The retinally blind subject also reported movement (Fig. 8b), but whereas sighted subjects often reported discrete and unidirectional perceptions of movement, his phosphenes often swirled or shimmered, and changed direction and position from trial to trial at the same scalp location. Whereas the phosphenes produced by stimulation near the mid-line were close to the fovea, those produced by stimulating over area MT/V5 were more eccentric, like those of normal subjects.

Blindsighted subject GY also perceived moving phosphenes when TMS was applied over MT/V5 of his intact right hemisphere (Fig. 8c), but not from TMS over his damaged left hemisphere. To be certain that we had actually applied TMS to V5 on that side, we used published structural and functional images of his brain (Barbur et al., 1993; Baseler et al., 1999; Zeki and Ffytche, 1998) to establish the position of MT/V5 in relation to the skull. We then applied TMS at and around this region at 100% of stimulator output for 1 s at 10 Hz. Such dense sampling and intense stimulation around this area makes it unlikely that we failed to stimulate MT/V5. On only three trials (out of more than 100) in which rTMS was applied to left hemisphere V5, he reported faint phosphenes but they were in the in the *ipsilateral* normal visual field. Presumably the TMS had weakly activated neurons in the normal hemisphere via callosal connections — an interpretation consistent with the neuroimaging study of Baseler et al. (1999). These faint ipsilateral phosphenes were stationary, and could not be reproduced on a subsequent testing session. It is not disputed that area MT/V5 is essential for normal perception of visual motion, but it is clear that shorn of its major input from V1, activity in V5 alone, at least when it is induced by TMS, is insufficient to generate a visual percept of movement in the contralateral field defect.

Conclusion

TMS is in theory straightforward but in practice tricky, like many other common techniques used to investigate brain function, e.g. event-related potentials, functional magnetic resonance imaging, positron emission tomography, electrical stimulation through indwelling electrodes. Many apparently trivial considerations, such as the angle at which the coil is held against the head or which side of the coil is closer to the skull, can substantially influence the outcome of stimulation. By controlling and standardizing these factors TMS has been successfully used to investigate the role of, especially, dorsolateral cortical areas in visual perception, sensory awareness and neglect, the generation of movement, and plasticity following brain damage. Other cognitive abilities such as language, memory, emotions and planning have been less intensively investigated, but there is no reason why they should not be unless the underlying functional networks are either too ex-

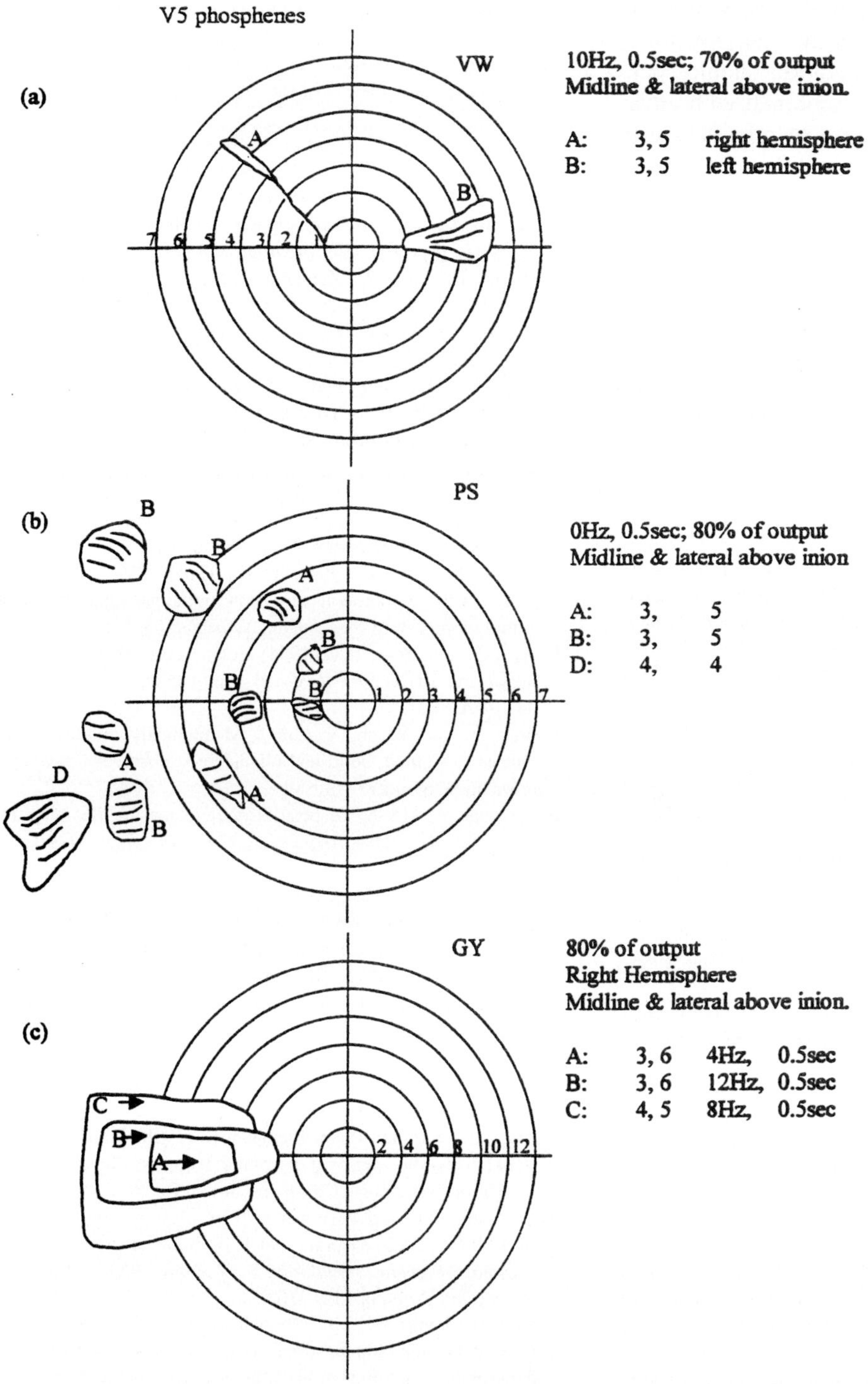

Fig. 8. Examples of moving phosphenes produced by stimulating above and around area MT/V5 in the same three subjects as depicted in Fig. 7. Moving phosphenes were easily produced in the retinally blind subject (Fig. 7b) but could only be produced in the blindsighted subject (Fig. 7c) by stimulating his intact hemisphere. In all three subjects, many more positions were stimulated than could be shown on the figure. The positions shown are those where phosphenes were subjectively most prominent. (From Cowey and Walsh, 2000, with permission.)

tensive or too inaccessibly deep in the brain, or both. Given the impressive advance in the successful use of TMS in the last decade, the answer should soon be known. TMS has also been combined with other techniques — fMRI and EEG — in relatively few studies. This is likely to change rapidly in the near future.

Acknowledgements

This work was supported by the UK Medical Research Council and by a Royal Society Research Fellowship to V.W. We thank Erik Corthout, Amanda Ellison and Carolyne LeMare for their help in preparing the figures.

References

Amassian, V.E., Cracco, R.Q., Maccabee, P.J., Cracco, J.B., Rudell, A.P. and Eberle, L. (1989) Suppression of visual perception by magnetic coil stimulation of human occipital cortex. *Electroencephalogr. Clin. Neurophysiol.*, 74: 458–462.

Amassian, V.E., Cracco, R.Q., Maccabee, P.J., Cracco, J.B., Rudell, A.P. and Eberle, L. (1993) Unmasking human visual perception with the magnetic coil and its relationship to hemispheric asymmetry. *Brain Res.*, 605: 312–316.

Barbur, J.L., Watson, J.D., Frackowiak, R.S. and Seki, S. (1993) Conscious visual perception without V1. *Brain*, 116: 1293–1302.

Barker, A.T. (1976) Determination of the Distribution of Conduction Velocities in Human Nerve Trunks. Ph.D. Thesis, University of Sheffield.

Barker, A.T. (1999) The history and basic principles of magnetic nerve stimulation. *Electroencephalogr. Clin. Neurophysiol.*, Suppl. 51: 3–21.

Barker, A.T., Jalinous, R. and Freeston, I.L. (1985) Non-invasive magnetic stimulation of the human motor cortex. *Lancet*, 1: 1106–1107.

Baseler, H., Morland, A.B. and Wandell, B. (1999) Topographic organization of human visual areas in the absence of input from primary visual cortex. *J. Neurosci.*, 19: 2619–2627.

Beckers, G. and Homberg, V. (1991) Impairment of visual perception and short term memory scanning by transcranial magnetic stimulation of occipital cortex. *Exp. Brain Res.*, 87: 421–432.

Beckers, G. and Homberg, V. (1992) Cerebral visual motion blindness: transitory akinetopsia induced by transcranial magnetic stimulation of human area V5. *Proc. R. Soc. Lond. B.*, 249: 173–178.

Beckers, G. and Zeki, S. (1995) The consequences of inactivating areas V1 and V5 on visual motion perception. *Brain*, 118: 49–60.

Benson, P.J., Guo, K. and Blakemore, C. (1998) Direction discrimination of moving gratings and plaids and coherence in dot displays without primary visual cortex (V1). *Eur. J. Neurosci.*, 10: 3767–3772.

Brindley, G.S. and Lewin, W.S. (1968) The sensations produced by electrical stimulation of the visual cortex. *J. Physiol.*, 196: 479–493.

Chen, R., Gerloff, C., Classen, J., Wassermann, E.M., Hallett, M. and Cohen, L.G. (1997) Safety of different inter-train intervals for repetitive transcranial magnetic stimulation and recommendations for safe ranges of stimulation parameters. *Electroencephalogr. Clin. Neurophysiol.*, 105: 417–421.

Corthout, E., Uttl, B., Ziemann, U., Cowey, A. and Hallett, M. (1999a) Two periods of processing in the (circum)striate visual cortex as revealed by transcranial magnetic stimulation. *Neuropsychologia*, 37: 137–145.

Corthout, E., Uttl, B., Walsh, V., Hallett, M. and Cowey, A. (1999b) Timing of activity in early visual cortex as revealed by transcranial magnetic stimulation. *NeuroReport*, 10: 2631–2634.

Corthout, E., Uttl, B., Walsh, V., Hallet, M. and Cowey, A. (2000a) Plasticity revealed by transcranial magnetic stimulation of early visual cortex. *NeuroReport*, 11: 1–5.

Corthout, E., Uttl, B., Juan, C.-H., Hallett, M. and Cowey, A. (2000b) Suppression of vision by transcranial magnetic stimulation: a third mechanism. *NeuroReport*, 11: 2345–2349.

Cowey, A. and Rolls, E.T. (1974) Human cortical magnification factor and its relation to visual acuity. *Exp. Brain Res.*, 21: 447–454.

Cowey, A. and Walsh, V. (2000) Magnetically induced phosphenes in sighted, blind and blindsighted observers. *NeuroReport*, 11: 3269–3273.

d'Arsonval, A. (1896) Dispositifs pour la mesure des courants alternatifs de toutes frequences. *C.R. Soc. Biol. (Paris)*, 3: 450–457.

Epstein, C.M. and Zangaladze, A. (1996) Magnetic coil suppression of extrafoveal visual perception using disappearance targets. *J. Clin. Neurophysiol.*, 13(3): 242–246.

Ffytche, D.H. and Zeki, S. (1995) The parallel visual motion inputs into areas V1 and V5 of human cerebral cortex. *Brain*, 118: 1375–1394.

Kammer, T. (1999) Phosphenes and transient scotomas induced by magnetic stimulation of the occipital lobe: their topographic relationship. *Neuropsychologia*, 37: 191–199.

Kastner, S., Demmer, I. and Ziemann, U. (1998) Transient visual field defects induced by transcranial magnetic stimulation over human occipital pole. *Exp. Brain Res.*, 118: 19–26.

Lorberbaum, J.P. and Wasserman, E.M. (2000) Safety concerns of TMS. In: M.S. George, and R.H. Bellmaker (Eds.), *Transcranial Magnetic Stimulation in Neuropsychiatry*. American Psychiatric Press, pp. 141–162.

Masur, H., Papke, K. and Oberwittler, C. (1993) Suppression of visual perception by transcranial magnetic stimulation — experimental findings in healthy subjects and patients with optic neuritis. *Electroencephalogr. Clin. Neurophysiol.*, 86: 259–267.

Miller, M.B., Fendrich, R., Eliassen, J.C., Demirel, S. and Gazzaniga, M.S. (1996) Transcranial magnetic stimulation: delays in visual suppression due to luminance changes. *NeuroReport*, 7: 1740–1744.

Pascual-Leone, A., Bartres, Faz, D., and Keenan, J.P. (1999) Transcranial magnetic stimulation: studying the brain–behaviour relationship by induction of 'virtual lesions'. *Phil. Trans. R. Soc. Lond.*, 354: 1229–1238.

Penfield, W. and Rasmussen, T. (1957) *The Cerebral Cortex of Man*. Macmillan, New York, pp. 1–248.

Polson, M.J.R., Barker, A.T. and Freeston, I.L. (1982) Stimulation of nerve trunks with time-varying magnetic fields. *Med. Biol. Eng. Comput.*, 20: 243–244.

Ruohonen, J. and Ilmoniemi, R.J. (1999) Modelling of the stimulating field generation in TMS. *Electroencephalogr. Clin. Neurophysiol.*, Suppl. 51: 30–40.

Stewart, L., Battelli, L., Walsh, V. and Cowey, A. (1999), Motion perception and perceptual learning studied by magnetic stimulation. *Electroencephalogr. Clin. Neurophysiol.*, Suppl. 51: 334–350.

Stoerig, P. and Cowey, A. (1997) Blindsight in man and monkey. *Brain*, 120: 535–559.

Thompson, S.P. (1910) A physiological effect of an alternating magnetic field. *Proc. R. Soc. Lond. B.*, 82: 396–398.

Ueno, S., Tashiro, T. and Harada, K. (1998) Localised stimulation of neural tissue in the brain by means of a paired configuration of time-varying magnetic fields. *J. Appl. Phys.*, 64: 5862–5864.

Walsh, V. and Cowey, A. (1998) Magnetic stimulation studies of visual cognition. *Trends Cogn. Sci.*, 2: 103–110.

Walsh, V., Ellison, A., Battelli, L. and Cowey, A. (1998) Task-specific impairments and improvements following magnetic stimulation of human visual area V5. *Proc. R. Soc. Lond. B.*, 265: 537–543.

Wassermann, E.M. (1998) Risk and safety of repetitive transcranial magnetic stimulation. Report and recommendations from the International Workshop on the Safety of Repetitive Transcranial Magnetic Stimulation, June 5–7, 1966. *Electroenceph. Clin. Neurophysiol.*, 108: 1–16.

Wassermann, E.M., Cohen, L.G., Flitman, S.S., Chen, R. and Hallett, M. (1996) Seizures in healthy people with repeated 'safe' trains of transcranial magnetic stimuli. *Lancet*, 347: 825–826.

Zeki, S. and Ffytche, D.H. (1998) The Riddoch syndrome: insights into the neurobiology of consciousness. *Brain*, 121: 25–45.

C. Casanova and M. Ptito (Eds.)
Progress in Brain Research, Vol. 134

CHAPTER 27

The metamodal organization of the brain

Alvaro Pascual-Leone * and Roy Hamilton

Behavioral Neurology Unit, Department of Neurology, Beth Israel Deaconess Medical Center, Harvard Medical School, 330 Brookline Avenue, Boston, MA 02215, USA

Introduction

Confronted with the question of how we perceive the world, we are often taught that we have a series of distributed systems structured according to the sensory modalities that they process. We talk about a visual system, a somatosensory or tactile system, an auditory system, and so forth. Certainly, the existence of specialized detectors or receptors for different sensory modalities grants us the opportunity to process different forms of energy and hence capture different 'views' of the world in parallel. Some experiences are uniquely unimodal. Hue can only be experienced by sight, tickle can only be felt by touch, and pitch can only be differentiated by audition. Nevertheless, our perceptual experience of the world is richly multimodal as eloquently elaborated by Barry Stein and Alex Meredith (Stein and Meredith, 1993). We are able to extract information derived from one sensory modality and use it in another; we can, for example, know a shape by touch and identify it correctly by sight. This is reminds us of Molyneaux's question, and raises the broad issue of internal versus experiential influences in the organization of the brain. Furthermore, we are able to integrate into a richer percept the impressions generated by different sensory modalities. Such intersensory perceptual phenomena (Stein and Meredith, 1993) are many and there is no question that the experience in one sensory modality influences the experience in another. Think, for example, of listening to music over the radio or while watching an orchestra perform. The melody played by the violins seems to 'sound' much clearer when we see the instrumentalists and watch their fingering and bowing than when we do not. The 'ventriloquism effect' broadly refers to this phenomenon on which much of our knowledge of the world and an entire entertainment industry is based (Howard and Templeton, 1966; Stein and Meredith, 1993). Multimodal association areas that contain multisensory neurons are thought to provide a neural substrate for integrating ('merging') sensory experiences, modulating the saliency of stimuli, assigning experiential and affective relevance, and providing the substrate for the true perceptual experience of our rich world (Stein and Meredith, 1993).

However, studies on early blind subjects and visually deprived sighted subjects raise questions about the organization of the brain in parallel unimodal sensory systems that are eventually integrated in multimodal association cortical regions. One may argue that early blindness represents a pathological state resulting in substantial cross-modal brain plasticity (Rauschecker, 1995; Hamilton and Pascual-Leone, 1998; Kujala et al., 2000), but the findings in visually deprived sighted subjects are difficult to account for with such an argument. After providing a historical backdrop for the topic and reviewing the experimental data, we will hypothesize that the brain might actually represent a metamodal structure

* Corresponding author: A. Pascual-Leone, Behavioral Neurology Unit, Department of Neurology, Beth Israel Deaconess Medical Center, 330 Brookline Avenue, Boston, MA 02215, USA. Tel.: +1-617-667-0203; Fax: +1-617-975-5322;
E-mail: apleone@caregroup.harvard.edu

organized as operators that execute a given function or computation regardless of sensory input modality. Such operators might have a predilection for a given sensory input based on its relative suitability for the assigned computation. Such predilection might lead to operator-specific selective reinforcement of certain sensory inputs, eventually generating the impression of a brain structured in parallel, segregated systems processing different sensory signals. In this view, the 'visual cortex' is only 'visual' because we have sight and because the assigned computation of the striate cortex is best accomplished using retinal, visual information. Similarly, the 'auditory cortex' is only auditory in hearing individuals and only because the computation performed by the temporal, perisylvian cortex is best implemented on cochlear, auditory signals. However, in the face of visual deprivation, the 'striate cortex operator' will unmask its tactile and auditory inputs to implement its assigned computation using the available sensory information.

Molyneaux's question

In 1688, the Irish philosopher William Molyneux posed a question in a letter to John Locke that would capture the attention of cognitive psychologists and philosophers of mind for more than three centuries (Degenaar, 1996). Probably motivated to some degree by the fact that his own wife was blind, Molyneaux posed the following question to his English contemporary:

> Suppose a man born blind, and now adult, and then taught by his touch to distinguish between a cube and a sphere of the same metal, and the same bigness, so as to tell, when he felt one and the other, which is the cube, which is the sphere. Suppose then, the cube and the sphere placed on a table, and the blind man to be made to see. Query, whether by sight, before he touched them, he could distinguish, and tell, which is the globe, which is the cube?

Molyneux's question has served as the touchstone for over three centuries of debate over the role of experience in the development of perception and the existence of innate or acquired cross-modal relationships between the senses. Molyneux himself came to the conclusion that the blind subject of his thought experiment would not be able to equate his tactile experience to visual percepts. Locke considered Molyneux's query in his 1690 Essay Concerning Human Understanding, and stated that "the blind man, at first, would not be able with certainty to say which was the globe, which the cube . . . "

Molyneux was certainly not the first to ponder the relationship between vision and touch in the mind. In a famous passage in his Dioptrics (1637), Rene Descartes considers how a blind man might build up a perceptual world by tapping objects around him with a stick. He first considers a sighted person using a stick in darkness, and says:

> . . . without long practice this kind of sensation is rather confused and dim; but if you take men born blind, who have made use of such sensations all their life, you will find they feel things with perfect exactness that one might almost say that they see with their hands . . .

Descartes goes on to argue that normal vision resembles a blind man exploring and building up his sense by successive probes with his stick. In 1709, Bishop George Berkeley agreed that there was no necessary connection between a tactile world and a sight world, that a connection between them could only be established through experience. Over a century and a half later, William James argued similarly that perceptions of space across different modalities have intrinsically different properties that make it impossible for cross-modal information to be relayed between sight and touch without experience (James, 1890).

Not all great thinkers agreed that Molyneux's question can be answered in the negative. The respected and versatile scholar Gottfried Wilhelm Liebniz wrote a critical commentary on Locke's empirical approach to visual and tactile perception. Leibniz argued that while visual and tactile sensations of forms are different, the accompanying concepts underlying their perceptions are the same or share something critical in common. Leibniz makes an explicit distinction between images and ideas, and argues that a person blind from birth would be capable of distinguishing a sphere from a cube using his understanding and the knowledge acquired through the sense of touch with the aid of exact ideas of the forms of both objects. Francis Hutcheson, another Irish philosopher, gave a similar answer to Molyneux's question. According to Hutcheson, we can, by virtue of our ideas about form, judge by touch what the visual extension of a touched object will be when we open our eyes, although we cannot tell by touch which color we will see.

Surgical answers to a philosophical debate

Molyneux's question was approached experimentally in 1728, when William Cheselden, an English surgeon, removed the cataracts from the eyes of a 13-year-old boy born blind. Cheselden's celebrated case was, by no means the first successful operation of its kind: the earliest reported dates from A.D. 1020, of a 30-year-old man operated upon in Arabia, and several other cases were reported between that first operation and the one performed by Cheselden. Chelselden's commentary on the case, however, stands out for its consideration of the changes in percept experienced post-surgically by the patient.

> When he first saw, he was so far from making any Judgement about Distances, that he thought all Objects whatever touched his Eyes, (as he expressed it) as what he felt, did his Skin; and thought no Objects so agreeable as those which were smooth and regular, though he could form no Judgment of their Shape, or guess what it was in any Object that was pleasing to him:

Despite his high intelligence and youth, the boy encountered profound difficulties with the simplest visual perceptions. He had no idea of space or size, and found it remarkably difficult to recognize and remember the visual form of objects, and had to constantly relate them to his previously acquired tactile impressions.

> He knew not the Shape of any Thing, nor any one thing from another, however different in Shape, or Magnitude; but upon being told what Things were, whose Form he before knew from feeling, he would carefully observe, that he might know them again; but having too many Objects to learn at once, he forgot many of them; and (as he said) at first he learned to know, and again forgot a thousand Things a Day. One particular only (though it might appear trifling) I will relate; Having forgot which was the Cat, and which was the Dog, he was ashamed to ask; but catching the Cat (which he knew by feeling) he was observed to look at her steadfastly, and then setting her down, said, So Puss! I shall know you another Time.

It has been similar with other patients in the 250 years since Cheselden's operation: nearly all had experienced the most profound, Lockean confusion and bewilderment. The best known and most influential account of these patients is provided by Von Senden (1932). Reporting on 60 cases, Von Senden attempted to investigate whether the tactile impressions of blind people provide them with any spatial awareness and he also sought to discover how spatial awareness develops in blind people who have been surgically treated.

Von Senden came to the conclusion that immediately after the operation the patients were able to distinguish objects one from the other and could localize them at a distance, but they could not identify any objects. When it appeared that they could identify objects, he attributed it to the fact that they were using other senses or had prior knowledge of the situation. Psychologists Richard Gregory and Jean Wallace dispute Von Senden's conclusions on the grounds of their own study of a blind person who had been operated on (Gregory and Wallace, 1963) and could recognized day-to-day objects, such as tables and chairs, immediately after the operation. Experimental approaches to Molyneux's problem have included visual deprivation in animals and the use of 'sensory substitution systems' which represent visual scenes and objects tactually (Morgan, 1977). However, we still lack unequivocal evidence with which to answer Molyneux's 300-year-old conundrum.

It seems clear from the experimental evidence as well as from a careful philosophical dissection of the question itself, that there are indeed two different problems posed: " ... whether by sight, before he touched them, he could **distinguish**, and **tell**, which is the globe, which is the cube". In order to 'distinguish' Molyneaux's hypothetical subject would merely need to differentiate the two stimuli on the basis of sight. In order to 'tell' the subject would have to learn by matching the newly experienced visual sensation to the old concept formed by touch alone. It is likely the subject would only be able to 'distinguish', just as Chelsenden's patient could differentiate between his cat and his dog by looking at them but needed to touch them to know (to 'tell') which one was actually the cat and which the dog. Hence, we may conclude that senses are merged perhaps at different levels. Knowledge ('telling') requires the high-order integration of what is perceived with what is recalled. Therefore, the patients of Von Senden and others actually experienced a visual agnosia, the inability of using information in one sensory modality (vision) to access metamodal knowledge. Obviously, not knowing how to use specific sensory information for knowledge does not imply that merging of the senses does not occur.

How merged are the senses?

The notion of information from different sensory modalities being merged and even being processed together in the same brain areas is far from new[1 1]. The medieval model of the mind contained within it the concept of a 'sensus communis', a place in the brain where information from all modalities was summed into an integrated whole that could be utilized by the higher cognitive faculties of reason and memory. Since medieval 'neuroscientists' could not believe something as grand as consciousness could emerge from the mere physical tissues of the brain, this so-called 'common sense' was thought to be located in the lateral ventricles, which early anatomists collapsed into a single ventricle. The sensations merged in the sensus communis yielded images, and thus, fantasy and imagination were often located here as well. The second or middle ventricular space was the site of cognitive process: reasoning, judgment, and thought; the third was the site of memory (Gross, 1998). With the exception of some minor alterations, the multimodal view of sensory processing remained popular among intellectuals throughout the Middle Ages and Renaissance. For example, in his Treatise on Man (1662), Renee Descartes, proposed that sensory information from different modalities meets in the pineal gland, and that information from one sensory modality interacts with information processing from another modality (Descartes, 1976).

Unimodal models of sensory processing did not emerge until it had become clear that different brain regions were responsible for mediating different functions. Localization of cognitive processes to particular regions of the brain began in early 19th century with Francis Gall and J.C. Spurzheim, who postulated that there were "about thirty-five affective and intellectual faculties" in the brain (Gall and Spurzheim, 1835). In one of the best known misapplications of an essentially good idea, Gall and Spurzheim subsequently founded the study of phrenology. The central ideas of their phrenological system were that the brain was an elaborately wired machine for producing behavior, thought, and emotion, and that the cerebral cortex was a set of organs with different functions. They postulated that the faculties of the brain were localized in specific organs of the cerebral cortex and that the development or prominence of these faculties was a function of their activity, such that the amount of activity would be reflected in the size of the cortical organ. They thus reasoned that the size of each cortical organ, and hence the prominence of mental faculties would be reflected by the prominence of cranial bumps on the overlying skull (Gall and Spurzheim, 1835).

Phrenology had wide appeal, especially in England and the United States, and among many leading intellectuals, but met considerable opposition from the religious, political, and scientific establishments of the day. The most important and influential scientific critique of Gall came from Pierre Fluorens, later professor of natural history at the Sorbonne in Paris. Starting in the 1820s and continuing for over 20 years, he carried out a series of experiments on the behavioral effects of brain lesions, particularly in pigeons. Fluorens reported that lesions of the cerebral hemisphere had devastating effects on willing, judging, remembering, and perceiving but that the site of lesions seemed irrelevant: all regions of the hemispheres contributed to these functions. The only exception was vision, in that unilateral, focal lesions produced only contralateral blindness (Clarke and Jacyna, 1987; Gross, 1998). Despite the fact that these holistic results tended to eclipse Gall's ideas of discreet localization, the overall impact of Fluo-

[1] Much of the information discussed in the following section is derived from Charles Gross' superb book on the history of the Neurosciences. The readers are encouraged to read this source (Gross, 1998).

rens' work was to support Gall's broader notion that cognitive function could be localized to the cerebral cortex. By the third quarter of the 19th century, Gall's general ideas had been confirmed by Broca's demonstration of an association between damage of the frontal lobes and aphasia, and again by Fritsch and Hitzig's experiments on stimulation of the motor cortex (Gross, 1998). Thus while the practice of phrenology is no longer held in high esteem as an index of mental faculties, the notion of cognitive function being subdivided and routed to different regions of the brain has remained a central idea in neural science and a fundamental principle in the clinical practice of neurology.

The last quarter of the 19th Century saw an intense search for localization of the sensory centers in the cortex. Interestingly, a notable shift occurred from the concept of function-specific centers to modality-specific brain regions. A major spur in the search for modality-specific cortical regions was Johannes Müller's doctrine of specific nerve energies. This doctrine had three elements. The first and most important was the revolutionary notion that persons are aware of the states of their sensory nerves, not of the state of the outside world itself. Secondly, when a given nerve type or nerve energy was excited, the same type of experience is produced no matter what the stimulus. The third element of this doctrine was that the same physical stimulus applied to different sense organs gives rise to different sensations. Hence, a similar blow to the eye and to the ear produce visual and auditory sensations, respectively (Müller, 1965). Subsequently Hermann von Helmholtz, the renowned physician, physicist, and psychologist, and a student of Müller, argued that the specificity of nerve energies could be attributed to the specific brain regions upon which they terminate. He compared nerves to wires through which impulses between modalities are essentially identical, but take on different meaning based on the portion of the brain to which they are routed. Emil Du Bois-Reymond, another of Müller's students, and the discoverer of the action potential, went one step further and claimed that if it were possible to cross-connect the auditory and optic nerves, we would see with our ears and hear with our eyes (Gross, 1998). Müller's doctrine of specific nerve energies thus became directed toward the cortex as the locus of specific nerve energies. Under the influence of this doctrine, in the later part of the 19th century, neural pathways were traced from the sense organs into the brain to find the specific regions in which they ended. The cortex was divided up into separate centers or organs on the basis of the pattern of its structure, thereby yielding the techniques of cytoarchitectonics and myeloarchitectonics. Cortical lesions were made in animals to find the sensory centers, and in close parallel, attempts were made to correlate sensory losses in humans with sites of cortical damage. Nowadays, for each of the sensory modalities, we assume that there exists a hierarchically organized system that begins with specialized receptors that 'feed' unimodal, primary cortical. A series of secondary areas unimodally integrate different aspects of the processed information. Eventually, multimodal association areas integrate the processed signals with information derived from other sensory modalities. Certainly, top-down influence from multimodal association areas can change the function of 'hierarchically lower' unimodal cortical regions. Furthermore, in a modern-age experimental testing and refinement of von Helmholtz's and Du Bois-Reymond's hypotheses, Sur and colleagues have shown the enormous dependence of cortical development on external influences (Sur et al., 1990; Merzenich, 2000). Sur and colleagues rewired the brain of young ferrets so that the retinal nerves were directed to grow into the auditory thalamus, which was deprived of its normal auditory inputs. This intervention results in the emergence of a functional primary visual cortex in the brain area destined to develop into the primary auditory cortex (Sur et al., 1990; Roe et al., 1990; Sharma et al., 2000). The 'new' visual cortex is topographically organized and its neurons are selective for differently oriented visual stimuli and are arranged in visual orientation columns, much like it would be expected in the 'normal' primary visual cortex. Furthermore, this 'new visual cortex' shows behavioral functionality (Melchner et al., 2000). Using a variant of this original paradigm, Melcher and colleagues rewired cortical circuits on only one side of ferrets' brains, using inputs to the unaffected hemisphere as a control. They then trained ferrets on a task in which different responses elicited different rewards depending on whether the stimulus was visual or auditory. They found that when light stimuli were presented in the portion of the visual field that is mediated only by rewired projection, the ferrets responded as though they perceived the stimuli to be visual rather than auditory. Literally, the rewired ferrets 'see' with the brain area that was meant to be the primary auditory cortex. Importantly, these animals do not become confused nor display behavior that might suggest synaesthetic merging of the senses. Rather, they appear to have developed a fully functional visual cortex with its appropriate, source-specific perceptual qualities.

This functional 'redefinition' of the 'auditory' cortex into a new 'visual' cortex requires rewiring of the retinal, visual inputs and depriving the medial geniculate nucleus in the thalamus of its cochlear, auditory inputs. Furthermore, the experiments by Sur and colleagues are successful in very young ferrets that are born very early in their neural development Sur et al., 1990). Could it be, that in fact, in normal development, multimodal sensory inputs feed into all cortical regions and that external influences and predefined functional superiority of given cortical areas shape the brain? Could it be the case that the brain is actually metamodal, and that the impression of hierarchically structured unimodal systems is only the consequence of selection of functions by groups of neural networks that compete with each other in order to acquire specific processes? One might envision a cortical region with a functional role in spatial discrimination, that might therefore be predisposed to perform the kinds of processes that vision requires. In this setting, from early development onward, sight would be progressively selected as the input signal for such an 'operator'. Eventually such an operator might appear to be 'visual cortex' by virtue of its dominant input, when in fact, under certain conditions, the presence of metamodal inputs could be unmasked. In the present article we advance such a hypothesis, based on a series of experiments in early blind subjects and visually deprived sighted volunteers.

Functional brain organization in the early and congenitally blind

Loss of vision due to injury to the eyes results in deafferentation of very large areas of the human cortex and poses striking demands on other sensory systems to adjust to blindness in a society that relies heavily on vision. Blind subjects need to extract crucial spatial information from touch and hearing. Perhaps the most instructive approach to the experience of blindness is reading the several excellent accounts of the experiences of adults who became blind and had to adapt to their disability. One of the most compelling and lucid accounts of blindness, is John Hull's autobiography 'Touching the Rock'. Several passages should be underscored. For example, Mr. Hull relates how he 'knows' his youngest son, born after Hull became blind due to diabetes differently than he 'knows' his other children whom he saw being born and growing up. Another remarkable passage is the description of how he enjoys stepping outside in the rain. It is the sound that the rain makes on the different objects and planes that allows him to create a mental image of the space that surrounds him. Indeed, blind people often do not describe space, but rather describe specific objects and routes that can guide a listener around the room or from one place to another: "As you enter my house you will be able to feel the light switches on the left, by the door frame. If you then turn to the left and take a couple of short steps there will be a coat rack and next to it, on the right, you will feel the door opening to the kitchen ... ". There is a lack of more global space perception, and substitution with a percept that inches along, guided by touch.

Braille reading provides blind subjects with the opportunity to read and write communication, thus greatly expanding their integration into society and their opportunities for employment. Braille reading requires the processing of tactile information into meaningful shapes. Subjects have to discriminate small patterns of raised dots with the pad of their index finger and extract spatial information through touch rather than vision. In order to accomplish this task, subjects move their index finger from side to side at a controlled speed so that the sensory skin receptors are maximally activated by the raised dots and as much information as possible is obtained. Therefore, learning to read Braille poses a great demand on sensory and motor representations from a rather small part of the body, the distant pad of the index finger, and stresses the spatial coding capabilities of tactile exploration. Blind, Braille readers do not have a lower peripheral sensory threshold in the pad of the reading index finger than blind, non-Braille reading controls or sighted volunteers (Pascual-Leone and Torres, 1993). However, the sensory and motor representations of the reading index finger in the brain are significantly larger for Braille readers than for blind or sighted non-Braille readers (Pascual-Leone and Torres, 1993; Pascual-Leone et al., 1993). This enlarged sensorimotor representation in blind Braille readers develops slowly, over the course of months (Pascual-Leone et al., 1993, 1996) and is modulated by the preceding activity (Pascual-Leone et al., 1995). Therefore, changes in representation of the reading finger in the brain cortex seem to play a critical role in the acquisition of the Braille reading skill (Hamilton and Pascual-Leone, 1998).

Peripherally blind subjects also have very large areas of their brain cortex deafferented from input and hence parts of the former visual cortex are available to be recruited for the processing of tactile and auditory information. Indeed, proficient Braille reading by blind subjects activates the dorsal and ventral portion of the occipital cortex (Fig. 1A) (Sadato et al., 1996; Sadato et al., 1998). Furthermore, there is suppression of parietal operculum and activation of the ventral portion of the occipital cortex in blind subjects during tactile discrimination tasks, opposite to the pattern of activation observed in sighted subjects (Sadato et al., 1996, 1998). Studies using event-related potentials, cerebral blood flow, and magnetoencephalography also suggest occipital cortex activation by tactile stimuli activation in early blind humans (Hamilton and Pascual-Leone, 1998; Kujala et al., 2000). Participation of the striate 'visual' cortex in a tactile task seems related to the difficulty of the tactile discrimination regardless of whether there is a lexical component to it or not (Sadato et al., 1996). These findings suggest that the pathway for tactile discrimination changes with blindness. Indeed, in the congenitally blind, interference with the function of the occipital cortex during Braille reading using repetitive transcranial magnetic stimulation (rTMS) results in disruption of the Braille reading skill (Fig. 1B) (Cohen et al., 1997). Subjects were aware that they had felt Braille characters, but during rTMS to their occipital cortex were unable to discriminate them. In fact, some of the subjects reported phantom tactile sensations, feeling Braille dots that were not there or distortions of the Braille symbols evoked by TMS. In sighted subjects, rTMS to the visual cortex does not interfere with the ability to detect or discriminate embossed roman letters by touch. Therefore, it would appear that Braille reading in the blind is an example of true 'cross-modal sensory plasticity' by which the deafferented, formally visual cortex, is recruited for demanding tactile tasks, thus enhancing the sensory discrimination abilities of the blind subjects and making the acquisition of tactile Braille reading skill possible.

Further support for the role of striate cortex in the perception of complex tactile stimuli comes from the findings in a most unfortunate patient (Hamilton et al., 2000). She had been blind since birth due to retinopathy of prematurity. She was a highly proficient Braille reader who used Braille at her work. She was a proof reader for the newsletter for the Spanish Organization for the Blind, and thus read Braille for 4–6 hours per day. At age 62, she had an acute neurological event that resulted in coma from which she recovered but was left unable to read Braille. She had no difficulties discriminating textures or identifying everyday objects by touch, but she was greatly impaired in tactile discriminations that required complex spatial decoding. She made frequent errors trying to identify even single Braille letters and she was completely unable to read Braille words. She described being able to 'feel' the Braille dots, but she could not 'make sense' of what she was touching. She complained that it felt "as if I had never learned Braille at all." Her neurological examination was otherwise unremarkable, and her MRI showed a bilateral occipital stroke (Fig. 2). Therefore, the findings in this case, emphasize the role that the occipital cortex plays in Braille reading in early blind subjects.

Cohen et al. argue for a critical period for this plasticity (Cohen et al., 1997), such that beyond age 14, the striate cortex is no longer recruited for the processing of tactile information. They base this argument on the study of late-blind subjects who became blind after age 15, in whom tactile stimulation failed to reveal activation of the striate cortex on PET, and in whom rTMS to the striate cortex did not interfere with reading of embossed Roman characters. Nevertheless there are a number of other potential confounders. For example, late blind individuals are often less skillful Braille readers, and

A

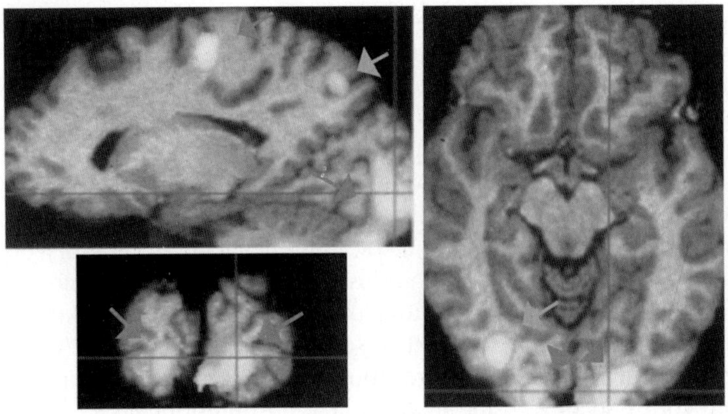

B

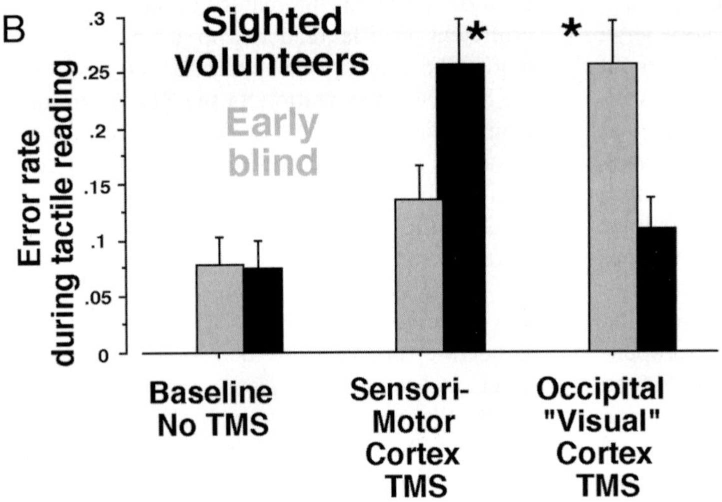

Fig. 1. (A) Modified from Sadato et al. (1996, 1998). Activation of the occipital cortex in congenitally and early blind subjects during tactile Braille reading as demonstrated by positron emission tomography (PET). (B) Modified from Cohen et al. (1997). Effects of repetitive transcranial magnetic stimulation (TMS) to the occipital or somatosensory cortex on tactile Braille reading ability in early blind subjects and on tactile perception of embossed Roman letter in sighted controls.

among the five subject studied, four had residual vision that could well affect the plastic changes that can take place in the brain.

A relationship between tactile discrimination ability and the amount of activation of the striate cortex in the blind is suggested by recent results in early and congenitally blind subjects. Behaviorally, early blind subjects show significant superiority to age-matched sighted controls in a gratings-orientation discrimination task (Fig. 3) (Van Boven et al., 2000). A gratings-orientation threshold was determined for the tip of several fingers using the Johnson, Van Boven, Phillips (JVP) Domes. Blind subjects had a lower mean threshold of 1.04 mm (SD = 0.19) compared to 1.46 mm (SD = 0.46) for the sighted group ($F = 10.78$, df = 1,28, $P = 0.003$). Interestingly, there was a significant Group × Finger interaction ($F = 3.03$; df = 3,84; $P = 0.034$) indicating that the extent of the difference in thresholds between the two groups was not the same across fingertips. Post hoc comparisons revealed that among the blind subjects, there were significant differences in threshold for the different fingers, such that their preferred Braille reading finger has the lowest threshold (Fig. 3). Sighted controls showed no threshold differences across fingers.

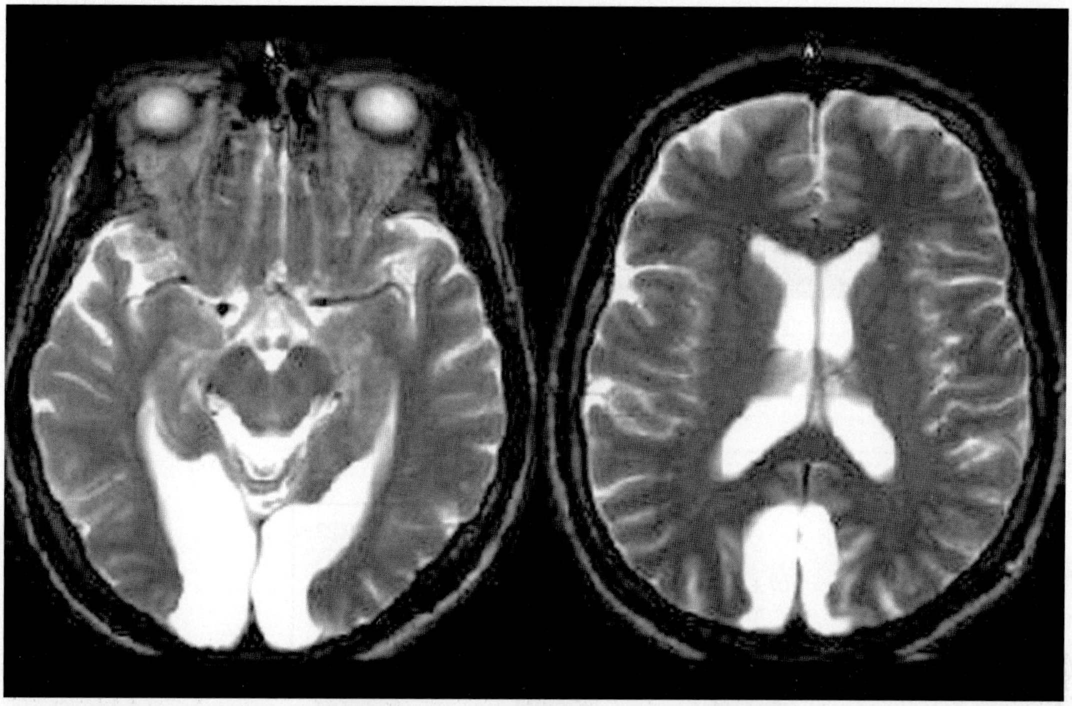

Fig. 2. Modified from Hamilton et al. (2000). T2-weighted brain magnetic resonance imaging (MRI) of early blind woman with sudden onset of alexia for Braille. Note the large, bilateral occipital stroke in distribution of bilateral posterior cerebral arteries.

In these same 15 early blind subjects, we found a significant correlation between the amount of activation in striate and peri-striate cortex to tactile stimulation of the finger pads as measured by functional magnetic resonance imaging (fMRI) and the gratings-orientation thresholds for their different fingers (Kiriakopoulos et al., 1999). The blood-oxygen level dependent (BOLD) activation in occipital cortex was significantly greater during stimulation of the preferred reading finger than during stimulation of adjacent fingers in the same hand or of the homologous finger in the other hand (Fig. 3).

There are certainly alternative explanations as to how, in the blind, primary cortical areas that normally mediate vision can become responsive during tactile tasks. One possibility is that occipital activation in these tasks reflects mental imagery. Kosslyn and colleagues have repeatedly shown that visual imagery in normal subjects activates primary occipital cortical regions (Kosslyn, 1994). An argument could therefore be made that subjects who activate occipital networks during tactile tasks may, to some extent, be building visual representations of stimuli encountered by touch. There are, however, a few pieces of evidence that suggest that visual imagery is not the phenomenon underlying activity across sensory modalities. In the absence of further evidence, it seems unlikely that early blind subjects, who in many cases have never had any vision whatsoever, are receiving top-down projections of visual percepts that then allow them to construct visual impressions of tactile stimuli. Furthermore, studies with late blind subjects, who often do remember the visual appearance of objects, suggest that these individuals may not activate occipital cortical networks during tasks, although this finding is still a topic of debate (Büchel et al., 1998).

More interestingly, it may be the case that occipital activation in the blind for tactile tasks does not represent visual imagery, but instead represents what can be thought of as 'tactile imagery'. According to this hypothesis, top-down processes rather than afferent inputs may be driving occipital cortical response. Although such a model postulates a different 'direction of flow' of information from the bottom-up architecture being hypothesized, this view

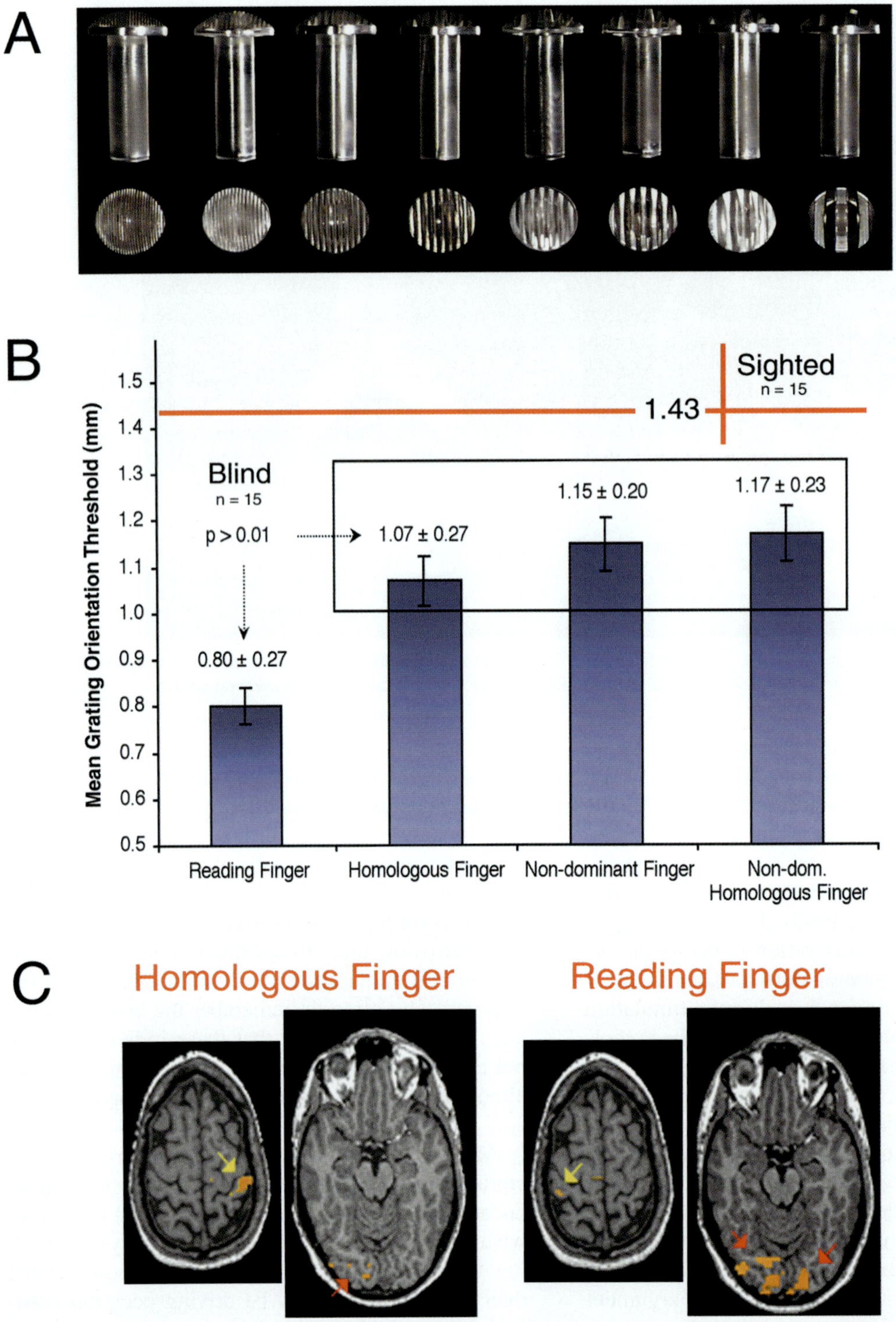

Fig. 3. (A) JVP Domes used for grating orientation discrimination testing. (B) Histogram displaying the thresholds for gratings orientation discrimination in early blind and sighted control subjects. Note the marked superiority (lower thresholds) of the blind subjects in general and in particular of their dominant Braille reading finger. Modified from Van Boven et al. (2000). (C) Modified from Kiriakopoulos et al. (1999). Representative example in one early blind subject of the differential activation of somatosensory and occipital cortex during tactile stimulation of the Braille reading finger and of the homologous finger in the other hand. Note the relative hypoactivity of the somatosensory cortex and the activation of the occipital cortex during stimulation of the reading finger.

is, nonetheless, entirely consistent with a metamodal model of the brain. The localization of tactile imagery to the occipital region would imply that complex reconstruction of aspects of a stimulus gained via touch are being represented in the occipital cortex, possibly because expert networks of neurons in that region of cortex have acquired, through competition, the ability to perform that operation.

Therefore, it seems that the occipital cortex in early blind and congenitally blind subjects is engaged in spatial tactile processing: it is both required for it and its activation is correlated with performance on behavioral measures. Is this the case in only the blind? Is seems tempting to consider the possibility that such a role of the occipital cortex is present in all of us, sighted or blind, but that visual input masks detectable evidence of processing of information from other sensory modalities. If so, visual deprivation by blindfolding might unmask the metamodal role of the 'visual cortex'.

The subjective experience of instructors for the blind in Spain

For a number of years, aspiring instructors for the blind in Spain were required to undergo a period of complete blindfolding "to get a first hand experience of what being blind really is like." These future instructors of the blind lived at a boarding school and spent 1 week blindfolded. The blindfold was put on before getting up from bed in the morning and was worn all day until retiring for the night. The students were required to leave the blindfold on until they were in bed and the lights had been switched off. Most likely all of them cheated some, tampered with the blindfold and sneaked a peak into the light occasionally. However, this was likely held to a minimum since bright light bothered their eyes, which had adapted to darkness.

Most of these trainees report noticing improved abilities to orient to sounds and judge distance by sound by the end of the blindfolded week. For example, several describe becoming able to identify people quickly and accurately as they started talking or even as they simply walked by due to the cadence of their steps. Several learned to differentiate cars by the sounds of their motors, and one described the "joy of telling motorcycles apart by their sound." A few felt that they had become able to detect objects or furniture in their paths by the "echos of sounds". Similarly, most of them noted an improved ability to differentiate surfaces and identify objects by touch during the 7 blindfolded days.

Interestingly, at the end of the week, removal of the blindfold required a period of several hours for readjustment to a visual world, during which time these persons experienced difficulties in visual spatial information decoding. Frequently subjects experienced the greatest difficulties when attempting to cross the street after the blindfold had been removed: "it was difficult to judge the height of the curb and it was very anxiety provoking not to be confident about the time it would take for an approaching car to close in. I would question whether I had the time to cross the street safely because I could not judge the speed of the cars or how long it would take them to get to me".

The blindfold experiment

In order to follow-up on these anecdotal reports by instructors for the blind in Spain in a systematic and controlled fashion, we are conducting a study in which normal sighted volunteers are visually deprived for 5 days (Maguire et al., 1999; Schlaug et al., 1999; Kauffman et al., 2000; Schlaug et al., 2001). During this time they are kept at the General Clinical Research Center (GCRC) at Beth Israel Deaconess Medical Center and are intensively trained in tactile and auditory spatial discrimination tasks. In addition to behavioral testing, subjects undergo serial fMRI studies to tactile and acoustic stimuli. Subjects are fitted with a specially designed blindfold that completely prevents all light perception. Potential tampering with the blindfold by the subjects is controlled with the use of a piece of photographic paper attached to the inside of the blindfold and analyzed for possible exposure to light at the end of the experiment. Non-blindfolded control subjects are blindfolded temporarily for all serial MRI and behavioral experiments.

MR Imaging is performed using a whole body 1.5 T Siemens Vision EPI system. A 3-D T1-weighted MR sequence ($1.0 \times 1.0 \times 1.0$ mm) is acquired for co-localization with functional images. A set of 18 functional MR images ($2.5 \times 2.5 \times 4$ mm) parallel to the ACPC plane is acquired every 5 s for a total of 40 s/epoch. For the auditory fMRI studies, volunteers perform a tone matching task and a motor control task in counterbalanced order. Each task is repeated 8 times. The matching task consisted of a series of tones and subjects have to compare each tone with the previous one, stating whether it is the same or different using a button press. In the motor control task, subjects are instructed to alternate button presses between the two responses. For the tactile stimulation task, pairs of Braille symbols are presented to the pad of the right index finger and the subject has to report whether they are the same or different. A motor control task of alternating button presses is again used as control. Image analysis is done using the AFNI software package (2.2) using '3dvolreg' for motion correction. All images are spatially standardized into the Talairach space. A two-factorial 3D ANOVA analysis is performed on each of the two groups, i.e. blind-folded and control group, with the first factor being 'condition' (tone, rest) and the second factor being 'scan' (before, during, after blindfolding). The F-tests and planned contrasts are corrected for multiple comparisons.

Behaviorally, subjects have been tolerating the blindfolded period well, though all of them have developed visual hallucinations that generally met criteria for Charles–Bonnet syndrome (Maguire et al., 1999). All subjects lacked a history of psychopathology, sensory disorders, or ocular pathology, and all were readily cognizant of their complex, often colorful, hallucinations. Visual hallucinations began shortly after individuals were blindfolded. Subjects were instructed to keep a daily journal of their thoughts, dreams, and perceptions throughout the blindfolded period. Hallucinations were reported as incidences of intrusive visual hallucinations that varied in onset, duration, and content. Additionally, images also varied in complexity, ranging from Lilliputian figures to landscapes and cartoon figures. Hallucinations most often occurred during the subject's ambulatory movements, such as when walking to and from the rest room, and also between testing sites within the research unit. No obvious memory sources were associated with the hallucinations, nor did they have a tendency to repeat themselves.

One subject, a 24-year-old male, experienced a broader range of images, which commenced a few hours after blindfolding and persisted for several hours after the blindfold was removed at the end of the study week. Hallucinations at first included flashing lights, mirrors, lamps, trees, and full landscapes. By the conclusion of the second day of blindfolding, the images grew in such complexity that the subject experienced difficulty walking due to the 'obstacles' he saw. While taking a walk outside, he reported seeing "a ground of dirt rows, mounds of pebbles, or little small stones that were running from upper left to lower right field of view and between them was running a small stream of water." Furthermore, the images became a constant presence to the subject, and by the end of the study week developed into ornate buildings of whitish green marble and cartoon-like figures. All of the hallucinations were recognized as such, and could consciously be cleared by the subject, if desired.

Another subject, a 20-year-old female, experienced an array of hallucinations that first appeared approximately 12 h after blindfolding and lasted throughout the course of the study week until moments before the blindfold was removed. The hallucinations seemed to appear suddenly and transform into a series of different images much like in a dream "a butterfly becomes a sunset, that becomes an otter, that becomes a flower, that becomes several different types of animals, and it all is kind of this big stream." Hallucinations varied in type from landscapes, such as cities, skies and sunsets, to objects that, as in the example transcribed above, frequently morphed into one another. The subject often described the visions as if looking at a kaleidoscope, with bright colors and shapes that moved in a continual rhythm: "if there is a sunset or a sunrise I couldn't look at the sun — because it was too bright ... It would seem like all of this light would just collect where the sun was and I just couldn't look there ... would get like a spot and it would turn into something else." The subject also stressed that the hallucinations were beautiful ("it is like art, sometimes they are much prettier I think than anything I've ever seen .... I really wish I could paint.") and that motion was always involved.

However, the most exciting aspect of these results is that the serial fMRI studies of these subjects showed activation of the visual cortex during tactile and auditory stimulation of the fingers. These data suggest that the appearance of visual hallucinations in these subjects may be the result of modifications made by the visual cortex in processing both tactile and other non-visual sensory information. As illustrated in Fig. 4 over the course of the blindfolded period, the striate and peri-striate cortex becomes increasingly activated during the tactile stimulation. On the first day of the blindfolding period there is activation in the contralateral somatosensory cortex, but none in the occipital cortex. On the second and particularly on the fifth day of blindfolding the activation in the somatosensory cortex is less, but there is increasing BOLD activation in occipital, 'visual', regions. Similarly, activation of striate cortex during auditory stimulation is seen at the end of the blindfold period and was absent prior to the blindfolding or in the control subjects (Schlaug et al., 1999, 2001).

Strikingly, the occipital activation with tactile or auditory stimulation disappears 12–24 h following removal of the blindfold (Fig. 4), even though for the purpose of the fMRI the subjects wear the blindfold again. In other words, removing the blindfold and being exposed to the seeing world for 12–24 h is sufficient to revert all changes induced by the 5 days of blindfolding.

A TMS experiment (Kauffman et al., 2000) serves to explore the behavioral significance of the findings (Fig. 5). At the last day of blindfolding, rTMS to the occipital cortex of the volunteers significantly disrupts their newly acquired tactile Braille symbol discrimination ability. The findings are similar to those found in early blind subjects. The sighted, non-blindfolded control subjects do not show such results. Interestingly, and in accordance with the fMRI results, 1 day after removal of the blindfold, disruption of the occipital cortex by rTMS no longer impairs tactile Braille reading ability.

These results suggest that the occipital cortex had become recruited for processing tactile and auditory information when it was deafferented of visual input. However, as soon as visual input became available, even transiently, the induced changes rapidly reversed to baseline. The speed of these changes is such that establishment of new connections is not possible. Therefore, it must be assumed that tactile and auditory input into 'visual cortex' is present in all of us and can be unmasked if behaviorally desirable.

Anatomical support

Such a hypothesis requires some anatomical support. One might expect that multimodal sensory responses of neurons in primary 'visual' cortex ought to be demonstrable and that tracing studies would have already revealed pathways relating information from the medial lemniscus, somatosensory thalamus, medial geniculate, or other structures to the striate cortex. In fact, the evidence is rather scarce.

A number of possible explanations can be discussed to account for the paucity of supporting evidence from animal models, including, for example, choice of the animal models and anesthetic agent. Most importantly, however, the competitive selection among expert systems that may determine the functional specificity of cortical modules would be expected to powerfully suppress less suitable inputs. Hence, experiments in selectively sensory deprived animals might be needed.

There is some evidence available that has indicated that neurons in striate cortex have auditory and tactile in addition to visual inputs. However, these results have been debated and gone largely without reliable reproduction by other investigators. Frank Morell (Morell, 1972) studied visual and acoustic responses of neurons in parastriate (18 and 19) areas in adult cats using microelectrode recording techniques. Seventy of 169 neurons recorded (41.4%) were responsive to visual and acoustic stimulation. Interestingly, none of these neurons demonstrated a frequency tuning curve analogous to those of the 'primary auditory cortex' to acoustic stimuli of 5–50 kHz. However, the responsiveness of 'visual cells' to acoustic stimuli depended on the location of the sound source in space. Fishman and Michael (Fishman and Michael, 1973) studied striate cortex (area 17) also using microelectrode recordings in unanesthetized cats, and similarly found that 38% of the recorded cells responded to both auditory and visual stimuli. As in the study by Morell (1972), bimodal cells had coincident acoustic and visual receptive fields and were distributed in functionally segregated, anatomically distinct clusters. Several previous studies had yielded similar findings (Lomo and Mollica, 1962; Jung et al., 1963; Murata et al., 1965; Spinelli et al., 1968). Therefore, these findings argue that neurons in striate and peristriate cortex might be engaged in the spatial

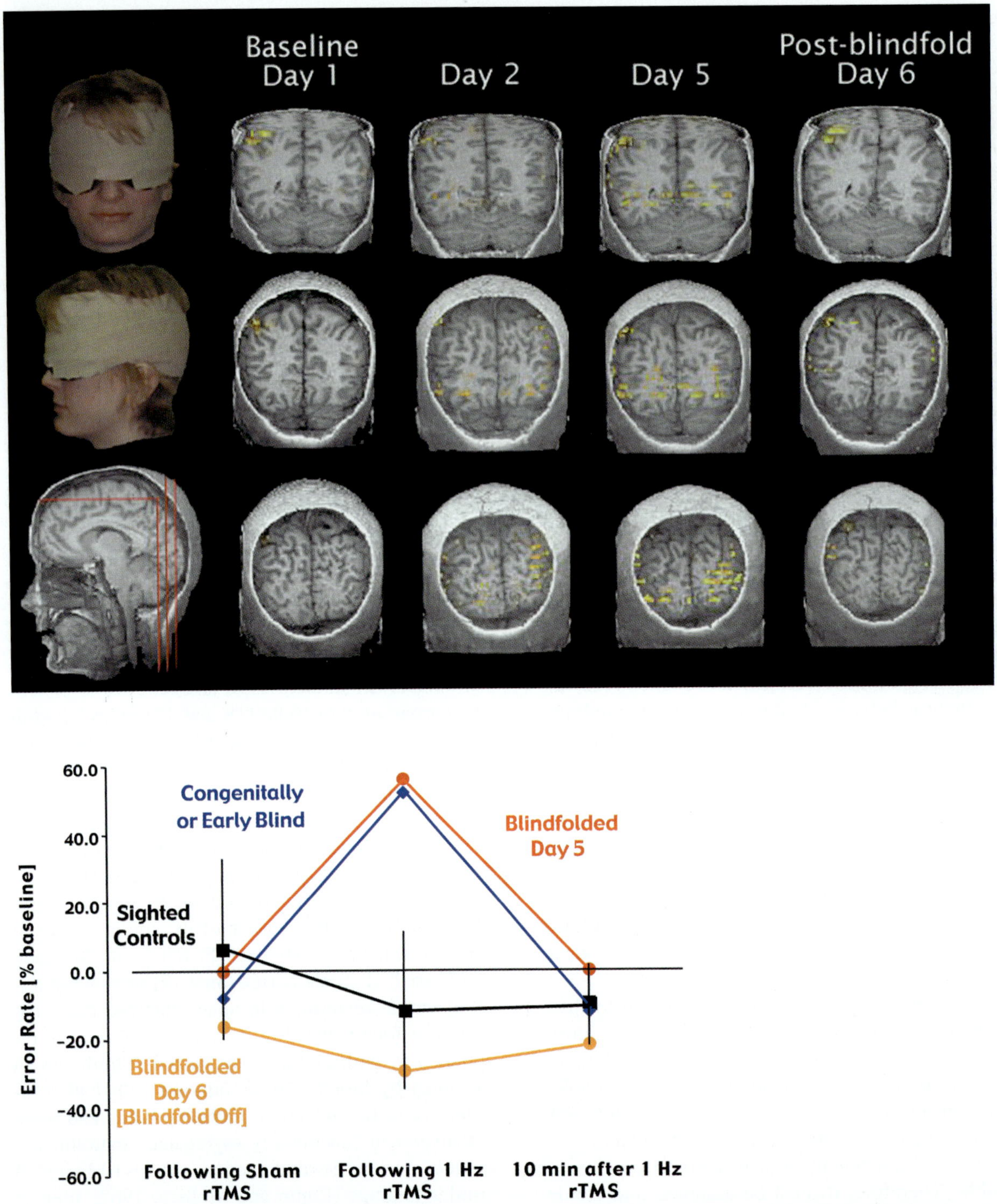

Fig. 5. Modified from Kauffman et al. (2000). Representative example of the effects of repetitive TMS to the occipital cortex onto the tactile Braille symbol discrimination ability in a subject after 5 days of complete visual deafferentation through blindfolding. Note the comparison with a subject undergoing the same experimental procedures but never blindfolded and with a congenitally blind control.

Fig. 4. Representative example of the changes in BOLD activation on functional brain MRI over the course of 5 days of complete visual deafferentation through blindfolding. Note the increasing activation of occipital cortex, including striate cortex by the fifth day of blindfolding and the dramatic return to baseline following removal of the blindfold for a single day (despite testing with the blindfold on).

localization of stimuli regardless of sensory modality and might indeed be tuned to specific topography along orientation columns. The anatomical pathways by which acoustic or tactile information reaches striate cortex are unclear. Thalamo-cortical or cortico-cortical pathways can be hypothesized but neither has been demonstrated to date.

Metamodal brain

Based on the data presented, the visual cortex seems to be a metamodal structure that receives not only visual, but also auditory and tactile stimuli. These inputs can be unmasked and functionally demonstrated as they gain functional relevance during visual deafferentation. Throughout these changes the 'visual cortex' appears to subserve spatial discrimination tasks regardless of the sensory input processed. Based on this example of the visual cortex, we propose that the brain, in a revised version of the views of the early 19th Century, is made up of metamodal operators. These operators are local neural networks defined by a given computation that is applied regardless of the sensory input received. This does not mean that there are not preferred sensory modalities for specific computations (and hence operators). Indeed, this is the case and the reason that the cortex gives the illusion of being built around sensory modalities rather than operators. We shall propose a model by which such a cortical architecture built around operators, rather than sensory modalities might be generated. This proposal is based on Robert Jacobs' 'mixture of experts' (ME) architecture (Jacobs, 1999).

Mixtures of experts architecture

The ME architecture implicitly contains two important notions. The first is that there are structure–function correspondences in the brain. Because the structural properties of different brain regions differ (e.g. different patterns of neural connectivity), different brain regions are best at performing particular types of functions. The second notion is that brain regions compete for the ability to perform a set of tasks. This competition leads to functional specialization of brain regions but also in the progressive segregation of the best suited inputs. This competition is not an altogether fair fight. It is biased by the structure–function correspondences; each region tends to win the competition for those functions for which its structure makes it particularly well-suited.

ME architecture incorporates the two ideas of competition and structure–function correspondences in a model that consists of two types of networks: expert networks and a gating network. The system is designed to try to learn training patterns, which consist of an input along with a desired output. The expert networks compete with each other to learn training patterns, while the gating network mediates this competition. The output of the entire architecture, denoted y, is the linear combination of the experts' outputs:

$$y_{i-1}^{n} = \sum g_i y_I$$

where y_I denotes the output of the i-th expert network and g_i is the gating network output corresponding to the i-th expert. The connection strengths of the expert and gating networks are adjusted simultaneously during training. Each expert network's output is compared with the target output at each time step. The expert whose output most closely matches the target is called the winner; the others are losers. The winning expert wins information and thus learns a lot about the current training pattern; the losers receive little or no information, and thus learn little about the current training pattern. The gating network receives information about the relative performances of the experts on the current pattern. It adjusts the connection strengths so that when the current input (or similar input) recurs in the future the activation of its output unit corresponding to the winning expert will be larger and the activation of its remaining output units will be smaller. This learning process has a positive feedback effect that ensures that an expert system that won the competition for a particular learning pattern will be most likely to win the same pattern in the future. This positive feedback loop also forces different expert networks to learn different tasks, since no expert network aside from the one that won before will ever be more likely to win in the future. Conversely, as an expert network receives and incorporates the information it receives from the gating network in order to become specialized for a particular task, it will become less likely to compete well on patterns from unrelated tasks.

Does ME architecture actually work, and can networks configured with ME architecture learn to make the kinds of distinctions that functionally distinct brain modules seem to be able to make? Naturally, the only way to find out would be to attempt to train these networks on tasks that mimic the kinds of processes we believe occur in brains. Jacobs and Kosslyn (1994) speculated that different subsystems in the brain are responsible for making categorical and coordinate visual judgements. In other words, they hypothesized that different neural agencies (or 'operators' in our terminology) using different kinds of information are responsible for classifying a stimulus (e.g. object A is a building) versus identifying a stimulus as a particular exemplar (e.g. object A is the Leaning Tower of Pisa). They hypothesized that systems that make categorical judgements would be more efficient if they monitored visual neurons with small non-overlapping receptive fields (and thus with low-resolution representation of visual objects), whereas systems that make coordinate visual judgements should be more efficient if they monitor neurons with large, overlapping receptive fields (high-resolution representation). Jacobs and Kosslyn used computer simulations to support this theoretical structure–function relationship, demonstrating that neural networks with small receptive learn category tasks more quickly, while networks with large receptive fields learn coordinate tasks more quickly. They then trained competing networks using small or large receptive field sizes and ME architecture and found that networks with small receptive fields tended to win the competition for category tasks while networks with large receptive fields won the competition for coordinate tasks. This set of simulations demonstrates that structure–function relationships and competition between networks can lead to functional specialization of processing, and suggests that ME architecture is a plausible and computationally efficient model for achieving this specialization.

For the purposes of applying ME architecture to biological systems, it is important to note that there is no need to determine which neural structure corresponds to the gating network. This is because the ME architecture is computationally and thus functionally equivalent to another architecture that does not contain gating networks, but instead contains inhibitory connections between expert networks that suppress each other's output. The strengths of the inhibitory connections depend on the value of the current input pattern, such that, depending on the task at hand, different expert networks would be more or less capable of winning the competition for that task. At the end of training, the expert that won the competition in the context of the current input, or closely related inputs, strongly suppresses the outputs of other experts. Experts that are the losers in the competition for a particular task suppress the outputs of other experts weakly or not at all.

Given what is currently known about how ME architecture works, it is not difficult to theorize how particular regions of the cortex might have acquired functional specificity using a network that approximates this architecture. One must first assume that there exist initial differences between competing neural modules. The occipital cortex, for example, might obtain the domain of visual processing because it is best suited for computations that may benefit from the information best supplied by vision. The data transformations at which the occipital cortex may initially excel might not be vision, per se. Instead, the occipital cortex may initially be a region of the brain with structural and functional qualities that enable it to excel at tasks which require high-acuity processing of spatial information. If this were the case, one would anticipate that the occipital cortical regions would constitute the expert network that would win the competition for vision, a sensory modality that provides tremendous amounts of distance and spatial information (as compared, for example, with sound or touch). As the occipital cortex continues to win the competition between expert networks for the input of vision, it is able to perform its task (spatial decoding) more and more accurately and hence adapts to become better and better at it, reinforcing visual input while increasingly suppressing inputs from other sensory modalities. Eventually, the occipital cortex may become so specialized for vision that it seems as though it is a 'visual' cortex, designed for the specific task of further subdividing and processing visual information. As evidenced in the studies of Sur and colleagues discussed earlier (Sur et al., 1990; Merzenich, 2000), the input to a brain region is a powerful bias that helps to determine the nature of the processing that the module ultimately performs. If ME architecture bears any resemblance to the development of functional brain modules, it may not be the visual cortex that determines what the act of seeing will be like. Rather, it is the task of seeing that instructs the functional modules of the developing brain regarding what vision will be like, and how it must be processed.

If the development of functional specificity of cortical modules is the result of competition between expert networks that have distinct structural and functional properties, it becomes possible to suggest a mechanism by which apparent 'crossmodal neuroplasticity' might occur. In the case of early blind subjects, for example, the brain loses a major source of sensory input, which normally constitutes a complex task, or set of tasks, that is normally 'won' by occipital networks. Without training from visual input, occipital cortical areas may not become specific for the particular functions involved in seeing. Furthermore, since occipital cortical networks may be initially structurally and functionally predisposed to excel at tasks that require high-acuity and high-fidelity processing of spatial information, they may begin to win the competition for other tasks that make these kinds of processing demands. Tactile discrimination or auditory localization may represent just such kinds of tasks. As a result, the occipital cortex may begin to subserve the functions of touch and hearing, which it would not have been able to do nearly as well if the demanding and specific needs of visual processing still had to met.

In light of the aforementioned model of modular specificity and the hypothesis of plasticity across sensory modalities that emerges from it, it seems that referring to the kinds of cortical changes seen in blind Braille readers and other subjects as cross-modal plasticity is something of a misnomer. Function-specific brain modules do not appear to have preordained roles that simply get 'switched' when the kinds of input received are radically altered. Rather, if cortical modules compete with each other to perform particular processing tasks, they should be thought of as being 'metamodal' brain centers that perform particular computational operations without specific reference to type of sensory input. It is these processes, and hence the cortical modules performing them, that are subsequently exploited and shaped by the demands of the sensory modalities that require them. Thus the many studies that demonstrate processing of sensory information outside of the classically recognized cortical boundaries for that modality may not be examples of the brain being redundant or 'getting its wires crossed,' but instead may represent the workings of an efficient metamodal brain, which uses inputs to those cortical regions (operators) that seem best suited to execute their computations successfully.

Acknowledgements

We wish to thank Alfonso Carammazza, Eduardo Fernandez, Jordan Grafman, Stephen Kosslyn, Margaret O'Connor, Daniel Press, and Robert Stickold for insightful comments. Our research was supported in part by the National Eye Institute (RO1EY12091), the National Institute for Mental Health (RO1MH57980, RO1MH60734), and the Harvard-Thorndike General Clinical Research Center (NCRR MO1 RR01032).

References

Büchel, C., Price, C., Frackowiak, R.S.J. and Friston, K. (1998) Different activation patterns in visual cortex of late and congenitally blind subjects. *Brain*, 121: 409–419.

Clarke, E. and Jacyna, L.S. (1987) *Nineteenth-Century Origins of Neuroscientific Concepts.* University of California Press, Berkeley, CA.

Cohen, L.G., Celnik, P., Pascual-Leone, A., Corwell, B., Falz, L., Dambrosia, J., Honda, M., Sadato, N., Gerloff, C., Catala, M.D. and Hallett, M. (1997) Functional relevance of cross-modal plasticity in blind humans. *Nature*, 389: 180–183.

Cohen, L.G., Weeks, R.A., Sadato, N., Celnik, P., Ishii, K. and Hallett, M. (1999) Period of susceptibility for cross-modal plasticity in the blind. *Ann. Neurol.*, 45: 451–460.

Degenaar, M. (1996) *Molyneux's Problem: Three Centuries of Discussion on the Perception of Forms.* Kluwer Academic, Dordrecht.

Descartes, R. (1976/1662) *Treatise on Man.* Harvard University Press, Cambridge.

Fishman, M.C. and Michael, C.R. (1973) Integration of auditory information in the cat's visual cortex. *Vision Res.*, 13: 1415–1419.

Gall, F.J. and Spurzheim, J.C. (1835) *On the Function of the Brain and Each of its Parts: with Observations on the Possibility of Determining the Instincts, Propensities and Talents, or the Moral and Intellectual Dispositions of Men and Animals, by the Configuration of the Brain and Head.* Marsh, Capen, and Lyon, Boston.

Gregory, R.L. and Wallace, J. (1963) *Recovery From Early Blindness: A Case Study*, Heffer and Sons.

Gross, C.G. (1998) In: C.G. Gross (Ed.), *Brain, Vision, Memory: Tales in the History of Neuroscience.* MIT Press, Cambridge, MA.

Hamilton, R.H. and Pascual-Leone, A. (1998) Cortical plasticity associated with Braille learning. *Trends Cogn. Sci.*, 2: 168–174.

Hamilton, R., Keenan, J.P., Catala, M.D. and Pascual-Leone, A. (2000) Alexia for Braille following bilateral occipital stroke in an early blind woman. *NeuroReport*, 11: 237–240.

Howard, I.P. and Templeton, W.B. (1966) *Human Spatial Orientation*, Wiley, London.

Jacobs, R.A. and Kosslyn, S.M. (1994) Encoding shape and spatial relations: the role of receptive field size in coordinating complementary representations. *Cogn. Sci.*, 18: 361–386.

Jacobs, R. (1999) Computational studies of the development of functionally specialized neural modules. *Trends Cogn. Sci.*, 3: 31–38.

James, W. (1890) *The Principles of Psychology.* Henry Holt, New York.

Jung, R., Kornhuber, H.H. and Da Fonseca, J.S. (1963) Multisensory convergence on cortical neurons: neuronal effects of visual, acoustic and vestibular stimuli in the superior convolutions of the cat's cortex. In: G. Moruzzi, A. Fessard and H.H. Jasper (Eds.), *Progress in Brain Research.* Elsevier, Amsterdam, pp. 207–240.

Kauffman, T., Hamilton, R., Warde, A., Keenan, J.P. and Pascual-Leone, A. (2000) The role of visual cortex in tactile Braille reading: the early blind, the sighted, and the blindfolded. *Ann. Neurol.*, in press.

Kiriakopoulos, E., Baker, J., Hamilton, R. and Pascual-Leone, A. (1999) Relationship between tactile spatial acuity and brain activation on brain functional magnetic resonance imaging. *Neurology*, 52(Suppl. 2): A307.

Kosslyn, S.M. (1994) *Image and the Brain: The Resolution of the Imagery Debate.* MIT Press, Cambridge.

Kujala, T., Alho, K. and Näätänen, R. (2000) Cross-modal reorganization of human cortical functions. *Trends Neurosci.*, 23: 115–120.

Lomo, T. and Mollica, A. (1962) Activity of single units in the primary optic cortex in the unanesthetized rabbit during visual, acoustic, olfactory and painful stimulation. *Arch. Ital. Biol.*, 100: 86–120.

Maguire, D.P., Stickgold, R., Warde, A., Kiriakopoulos, E. and Pascual-Leone, A. (1999) Appearance of Charles Bonnet syndrome (CBS) following prolonged blindfolding and Braille training. *Soc. Neurosci. Abstr.*, 25: 1315.

Melchner, L.v., Pallas, S.L. and Sur, M. (2000) Visual behaviour medicated by retinal projections directed to the auditory pathway. *Nature*, 404: 871–876.

Merzenich, M. (2000) Seeing in the sound zone. *Nature*, 404: 820–821.

Morell, F. (1972) Visual system's view of acoustic space. *Nature*, 238: 44–46.

Morgan, M.J. (1977) *Molyneux's Question: Vision, Touch and the Philosophy of Perception.* Cambridge University Press, Cambridge.

Müller, J.M. (1965/1838) On the specific energies of nerves. In: R. Herrnstein and E. Boring (Eds.), *Sourcebook of the History of Psychology.* Harvard University Press, Cambridge, MA.

Murata, K., Cramer, H. and Bach-y-Rita, P. (1965) Neuronal convergence of noxious, acoustic and visual stimuli in the visual cortex of the cat. *J. Neurophysiol.*, 28: 1223–1240.

Pascual-Leone, A. and Torres, F. (1993) Plasticity of the sensorimotor cortex representation of the reading finger in Braille readers. *Brain*, 116: 39–52.

Pascual-Leone, A., Cammarota, A., Wassermann, E.M., Brasil-Neto, J.P., Cohen, L.G. and Hallett, M. (1993) Modulation of motor cortical outputs to the reading hand of Braille readers. *Ann. Neurol.*, 34: 33–37.

Pascual-Leone, A., Wassermann, E.M., Sadato, N. and Hallett, M. (1995) The role of reading activity on the modulation of motor cortical outputs to the reading hand in Braille readers. *Ann. Neurol.*, 38: 910–915.

Pascual-Leone, A., Tarazona, F. and Catala, M.D. (1996) Modulation of motor cortical output maps associated with the acquisition of the Braille reading skill. *Neuroimage*, 3: S554.

Rauschecker, J.P. (1995) Compensatory plasticity and sensory substitution in the cerebral cortex. *Tends Neurosci.*, 18: 36–43.

Roe, A.W., Pallas, S.L., Hahm, J.-O. and Sur, M. (1990) A map of visual world induced in primary auditory cortex. *Science*, 250: 818–820.

Sadato, N., Pascual-Leone, A., Grafman, J., Ibañez, V., Deiber, M.-P., Dold, G. and Hallett, M. (1996) Activation of the primary visual cortex by Braille reading in blind subjects. *Nature*, 380: 526–528.

Sadato, N., Pascual-Leone, A., Grafman, J., Deiber, M.-P., Ibanez, V. and Hallett, M. (1998) Neural networks for Braille reading by the blind. *Brain*, 121: 1213–1229.

Schlaug, G., Halpern, A.R., Press, D.Z., Baker, J., Edelman, R.R. and Pascual-Leone, A. (1999) Changes in cortical auditory processing after blindfolding. *Soc. Neurosci. Abstr.*, 25: 1628.

Schlaug, G., Chen, C., Press, D.Z., Warde, A., Chen, Q. and Pascual-Leone, A. (2001) Hearing with the mind's eye. *Hum. Brain Mapping*, in press.

Sharma, J., Angelucci, A. and Sur, M. (2000) Induction of visual orientation modules in auditory cortex. *Nature*, 404: 841–847.

Spinelli, D.W., Starr, A. and Barrett, T.W. (1968) Auditory specificity in unit recordings from cat's visual cortex. *Exp. Neurol.*, 22: 75–84.

Stein, B.E. and Meredith, M.A. (1993) *The Merging of the Senses.* MIT Press, Cambridge, MA.

Sur, M., Pallas, S.L. and Roe, A.W. (1990) Cross-modal plastic-

ity in cortical development: differentiation and specification of sensory neocortex. *Trends Neurosci.*, 13: 227–233.
Van Boven, R., Hamilton, R., Kaufman, T., Keenan, J.P. and Pascual-Leone, A. (2000) Tactile spatial resolution in blind Braille readers. *Neurology*, in press.
Von Senden, M. (1932) *Space and Sight: The Perception of Space and Shape in the Congenitally Blind Before and After Operation*. J.A. Barth.

C. Casanova and M. Ptito (Eds.)
Progress in Brain Research, Vol. 134

CHAPTER 28

When the auditory cortex turns visual

M. Ptito [1,*], J.-F. Giguère [2], D. Boire [1], D.O. Frost [3] and C. Casanova [1]

[1] *School of Optometry and CRIR, University of Montreal, CP 6128, Montreal, PQ, H3C 3JT Canada*
[2] *Department of Psychology, University of Montreal, CP 6128, Montreal, PQ, H3C 3JT Canada*
[3] *Department of Pharmacology and Experimental Therapeutics, Department of Anesthesiology, University of Maryland Medical School, Baltimore, MD 21201, USA*

Abstract: We studied visually guided behavior and the visual response properties of single auditory cortex (A1) neurons in neonatally operated hamsters with surgically induced, permanent, ectopic retinal projections to auditory thalamic nuclei and to visual thalamic nuclei which normally receive little direct retinal input. The surgically induced retino-thalamo-cortical pathways can mediate visual guided behaviors whose normal substrate, the pathway from the retina to the primary visual cortex via the primary thalamic visual nucleus, is missing. The visually evoked response properties of A1 neurons resemble in many respects those of neurons in V1 of normal hamsters: many A1 neurons have well-defined visual receptive fields and preferences for orientation or direction of movement. In addition, some visually responsive cells in A1 are bimodal — they also respond to auditory stimuli. The visually responsive neurons in A1 probably account for the capacity of the auditory cortex to mediate visual behavior in 'rewired hamsters'.

Introduction

Brain lesions that occur during development can produce abnormal neural connectivity patterns. Growing retinal axons form permanent, ectopic projections to auditory (medial geniculate, MG; (Schneider, 1973; Frost, 1981; Sur et al., 1988) or somatosensory (ventrobasal, VB; Frost, 1981) thalamic nuclei following combined lesions of retinal targets and ascending auditory or somatosensory pathways to the thalamus, respectively, in neonatal hamsters. Such lesions also induce robust retinal projections in the lateral posterior thalamic nucleus, that normally receives little direct retinal input but is the principal thalamic target of the superior colliculus (SC) (Schneider, 1973; Crain and Hall, 1980a,b; Frost, 1981; Sur et al., 1988). The surgically induced retinal projections are retinotopically organized (Frost, 1981) and make functional synapses (Kalil and Schneider, 1975; Campbell and Frost, 1987, 1988; Frost and Métin, 1985; Métin and Frost, 1989). This occurs due to the combined effects of 'pruning' retinal axons within their normal targets and of the increased availability of target tissue in MG or VB (Schneider, 1973). Neurons in the somatosensory cortex of animals with ectopic retinal projections have visual response properties that resemble those of neurons in the primary visual cortex (V1) of normal animals (Frost and Métin, 1985; Métin and Frost, 1989). Ferrets that have retino-MG projections but no visual cortex appear to perceive light stimuli as visual (Von Melchner et al., 2000). However, the contribution of the surgically induced pathways to visual pattern discrimination in neonatally operated ('rewired') animals has not been assessed. In hamsters, as in other mammals, multiple, parallel pathways mediate different aspects of visual processing (Schneider, 1973, 1975). In rodents, the ability to distinguish horizontal from vertical square wave gratings or horizontal from vertical rows of squares depends on the integrity of the retino-dorsal lateral geniculate

* Corresponding author: M. Ptito, École d'Optométrie, Université de Montréal, CP 6128, Montréal, PQ, H3C 3J7 Canada. Tel.: +1-514-343-6052; Fax: +1-514-343-2382; E-mail: ptito@psy.umontreal.ca

(LGd)-V1 pathway (Schneider, 1969; Rothblat and Schwartz, 1978). By contrast, discrimination of light from dark stimuli normally depends upon the pretectal nuclei (Blochert et al., 1976). Therefore, in order to study the functional efficacy of the surgically induced pathways, we asked whether animals that lack the normal retino-LGd-V1 circuit but that have ectopic retino-thalamo-cortical circuits can perform visual discrimination tasks (Frost et al., 2000). We also investigated electrophysiologically the visual response properties of single neurons in the auditory cortex of 'rewired' hamsters and compared them to those of neurons in the primary visual cortex of normal animals.

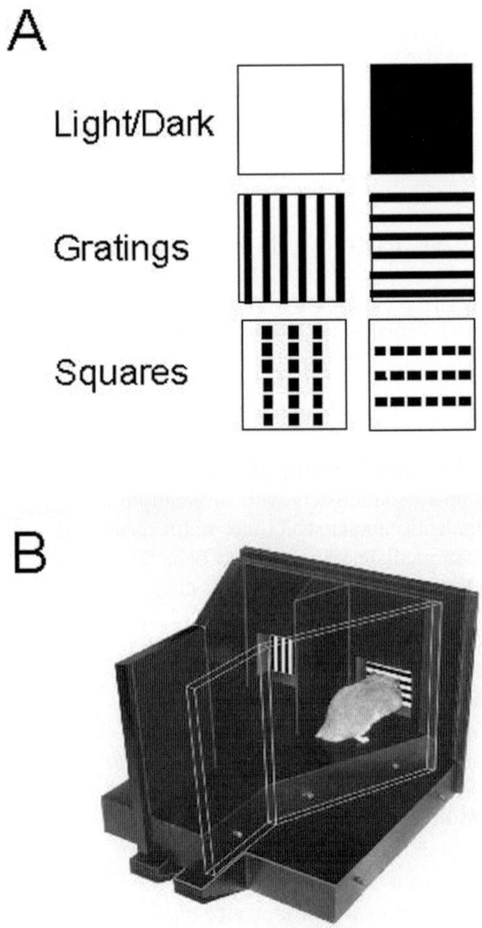

Fig. 1. Experimental set-up. (A) Test stimuli: the width of the stripes in the black and white gratings was 7 mm, which corresponds to a spatial frequency of 0.11 or 0.27 cycles/deg at distances of 9 or 22 cm, respectively, the distances over which the hamsters might have discriminated the stimuli. The size of the squares in each row was 10×10 mm ($= 6.34 \times 6.34°$ or $2.6 \times 2.6°$ at distances of 9 or 22 cm, respectively); there were six squares in each of the three rows, separated by a distance of 3 mm and each row was separated by 20 mm. Vertical and horizontal stimuli were identical except for their orientations. Each of the stimuli that constituted a pair to be discriminated was the rewarded stimulus for half of the hamsters in each group. (B) Testing apparatus.

Behavioral studies

Neonatal surgery

Newborn hamsters, anesthetized by hypothermia, received bilateral ablations of the SC made by applying a hot pin to the surface of the overlying skull. We transected the ascending auditory pathway to the thalamus and the brachium of the inferior colliculus (BIC) by inserting a razor knife into them through a small slit in the overlying skull. These procedures can induce the formation of permanent, ectopic retinal projections to the MG and robust retinal projections to the lateral posterior nucleus (LP) (Schneider, 1973; Frost, 1981; Sur et al., 1988; Crain and Hall, 1980a,b). At age 3–4 months, under Nembutal anesthesia, the animals received large, bilateral aspiration lesions of the occipital cortex. The lesions, were intended to ablate all of visual cortical (VC) areas V1, V2 and the medial visual area (Vm) (Tiao and Blakemore, 1976). After recovery ($\geq$2 weeks), these 'rewired' animals were tested on a light/dark discrimination and sequentially on the grating and rows of squares discriminations (Fig. 1A) in an open Y-maze illuminated by an overhead light bulb (40 or 25 W = 10.97 or 4.93 footcandles, respectively) (Fig. 1B). Ten trials were presented daily until a criterion of 85% correct (90% correct on one- and 80% correct on the other of two consecutive days) was attained or 500 trials were completed unsuccessfully. Testing was continued beyond 500 trials (with or without a change in ambient illumination) if and only if, a hamster's performance improved significantly over the first 500 trials, as determined by linear regression analysis ($P < 0.05$). As controls, we tested 22 normal adult hamsters on the same tasks. After testing, 'rewired' animals that had learned the grating discrimination received bilateral ablations (by aspiration) of the auditory cortex (AC; areas 41 and 22; Caviness, 1975; Caviness and Frost, 1980) and some normal animals were subjected to ablation of VC or AC. Following recovery, the animals were retested sequentially on the three discriminations. At the end of behavior testing, 'rewired' animals received bilateral intraocular injections of horseradish peroxidase (HRP) or cholera toxin B (CTB). After an appropriate survival time (24 h for HRP and 4 days for CTB), the hamsters were killed by an overdose of Nembutal, perfused and the brains sectioned frozen in the coronal plane. The outlines of cortical areas and thalamic nuclei were traced on the basis of standard cytoarchitectonic criteria (Caviness, 1975; Caviness and Frost, 1980) using a computer-assisted microscopy system.

Visual behavior in 'non-rewired' hamsters

After initially learning all three tasks, five animals received visual cortex lesions. After a minimum recovery period of 2 weeks, all of them relearned the light/dark discrimination, although their prior experience with this task did not result in 'post-operative savings'. Notably (and consistent with data of others; Schneider, 1969), neither of the two cases with small V1 remnants relearned the pattern discrimination tasks. Performance of the light/dark discrimination by hamsters with large VC lesions excludes a non-specific deficit in the relearning of all visual discriminations. In 'non-rewired' hamsters, lesions of the AC similar in size to those made in the visual cortex, do not prevent relearning of any of the three tasks. 'Non-rewired' hamsters subjected to AC lesions showed significant post-operative savings in relearning the light/dark discrimination and no significant pre-/post-operative difference in the rate at which they learned the grating- and rows of squares discriminations (see Fig. 2). Thus, in 'non-rewired' hamsters, the effects of cortical lesions on visual pattern discrimination performance are dependent upon the locus of the lesion.

Visual behavior in 'rewired' hamsters

Complete behavioral data and histological analysis confirming the total ablation of V1 were obtained from nine 'rewired' hamsters. All 'rewired' hamsters were able to learn all three discriminations (Fig. 3)

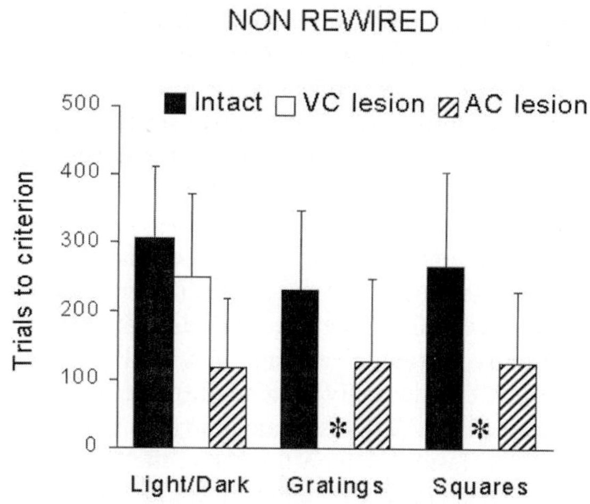

Fig. 2. Histograms showing trials to criterion on each task for normal hamsters. Following lesions of the primary visual cortex (VC), none of the animals reached learning criterion in the gratings and squares discriminations (*). Error bars indicate standard deviations.

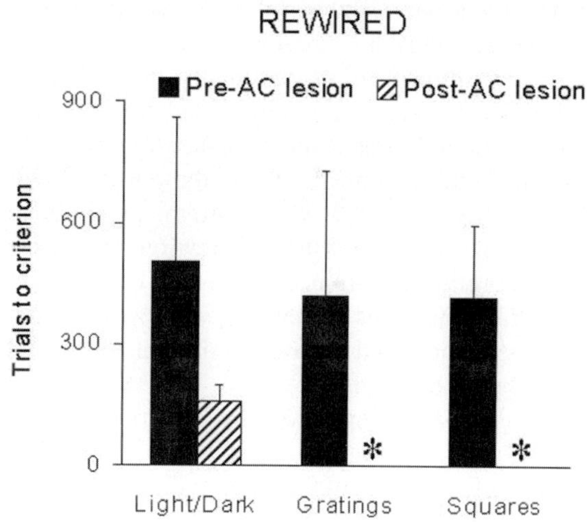

Fig. 3. Histograms showing trials to criterion on each task for 'rewired' hamsters. Asterisks indicate that rewired hamsters were not able to learn the grating or squares discriminations when the auditory cortex (AC) was ablated.

following VC lesions. Importantly, for all three tasks, there was no significant difference between 'rewired' hamsters and intact control hamsters with respect to the number of trials it took them to learn each task. Following behavior testing, 7/9 'rewired' hamsters received bilateral lesions of the AC. The two remaining 'rewired' animals were not subjected to further lesions or behavior testing so that the extent of the original cortical lesions could be assessed without enlargement by a second lesion. Following recovery from the AC lesion, all seven hamsters relearned the light/dark discrimination and their prior experience with this task significantly reduced the number of trials they required to reach criterion — i.e., there was 'post-operative savings'. Most of them could not relearn the gratings and squares discriminations (Fig. 3) except for those who had a small, cytoarchitecturally disrupted remnant of visual area V2, unilaterally or bilaterally. Retention of the ability to perform the light/dark discrimination after combined AC and VC lesions demonstrates that the lesions do not cause a non-specific deficit in the relearning of *all* visual discriminations.

Neural pathways mediating visual behavior in 'rewired' hamsters

The preceding data establish that surgically created retino-thalamo-cortical circuits can mediate visual pattern discriminations that normally depend upon the integrity of the missing retino-LGd-V1 pathway. To what extent is the residual behavioral capacity mediated by the retino-MG-AC or the retino-LP-V2 pathways, respectively? Post-mortem histological analysis (Fig. 4) showed that all 'rewired' hamsters had robust retino-LP projections and all but one had retino-MG projections of variable size. Correlation of the histological and behavioral data of individual cases suggests that *both* the retino-MG-AC pathway and the retino-LP-V2 pathway can contribute to visual pattern discrimination in 'rewired' hamsters (for details, see Frost et al., 2000).

Electrophysiological studies

Neonatal surgery

On the day of birth, all 17 animals used for single cell recordings were subjected bilaterally to ablations of the SC and lesions of the brachium of the inferior colliculus. This induced the formation of permanent, ectopic retinal projections to the MG and robust retinal projections to the lateral posterior nucleus (LP). Nine of the hamsters received an additional bilateral lesion of the occipital cortex 3–4 months later.

Animal preparation

Hamsters were premedicated with atropine (0.1 mg, s.c.) and dexamethasone (0.8 mg, i.m.) to prevent swelling of the brain and deeply anesthetized with urethane (210 mg/kg, i.p.; booster injections, 10% of the loading dose as required). The animals were tracheotomized and placed in a specially constructed stereotaxic frame that does not obscure the visual fields. All incisions were infiltrated with lidocaine hydrochloride (2%). The animals were then paralyzed with gallamine triethiodide (continuously infused through an i.p. catheter) and artificially ventilated (N_2O/O_2 = 70%/30%, supplemented with 0.5% halothane). The ECG was continuously monitored and rectal temperature was maintained at around 37°C using a feedback controlled heating pad. Atropine (1%) drops were topically applied to the eyes to dilate the pupils and the cornea was regularly hydrated by application of artificial tears (Alcon, Optifree). A skull flap was removed over the recording area, leaving the dura intact (visual cortex coordinates: A-P, 1 to −1; M-L, 0 to 4.5; auditory cortex coordinates: A-P, 3 to 0 mm; M-L, 5.5 to 7.5 mm). The craniotomy space was filled with warm agar to minimize brain pulsations and maintain hydration. Neuronal activity was recorded extracellularly using tungsten microelectrodes (impedance, 4–5 MΩ). Using a hand-held projector, the borders of single unit visual receptive fields (RFs) were plotted on a tangent screen located 28.5 cm from the animals' eyes. The units' response properties were first studied qualitatively and then quantitatively using computer-generated stimuli displayed on a CRT monitor at the same distance from the animals' eyes. For each neuron, flashing and moving bars as well as drifting gratings were used to assess orientation selectivity, motion sensitivity and direction selectivity. Cells were regarded as visually responsive if firing in response to an optimal stimulus was at least twice the spontaneous discharge rate. Cells were regarded as having a preference for orientation (or for direction), if, between the orientations (or directions) of maximum and minimum response, there was at least one orientation tested that produced a response of intermediate magnitude. The cells' responsiveness to natural auditory stimuli were qualitatively evaluated.

Upon completion of the recording session, the

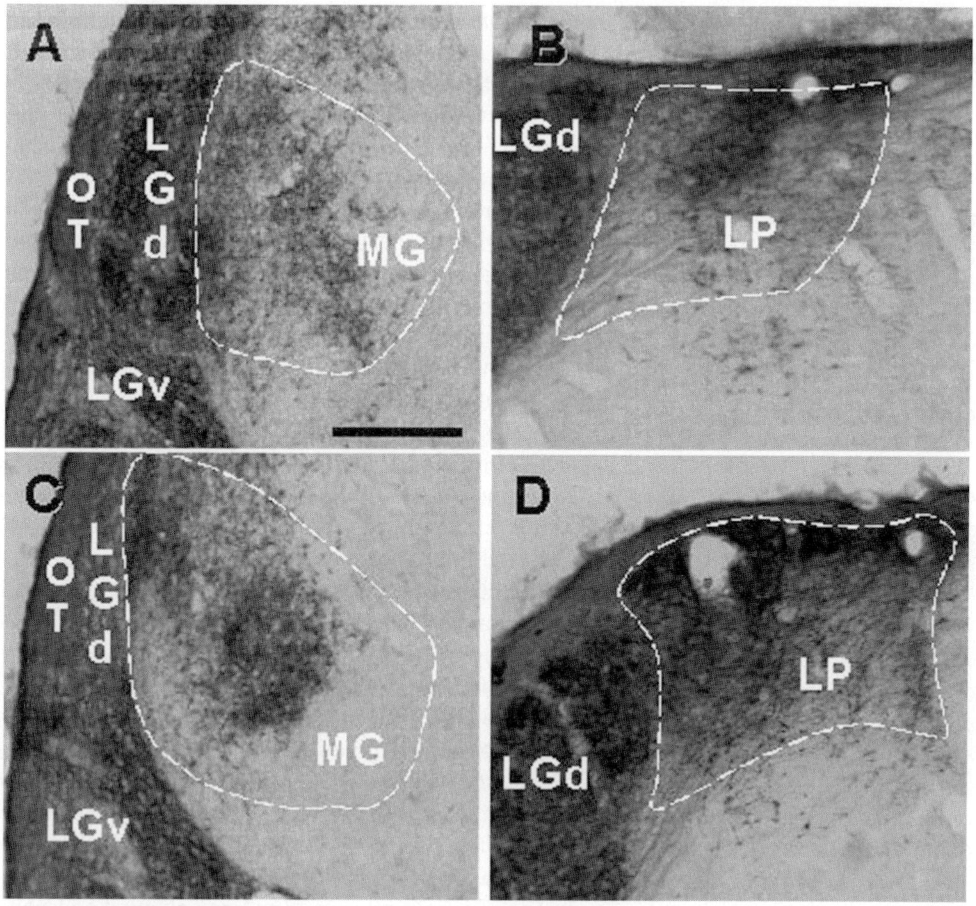

Fig. 4. Retinothalamic projections in 'rewired' adult hamsters. Video micrographs showing retino-MG projections (A and C) and retino-LP projections (B and D) for two animals. LGv, ventral lateral geniculate nucleus; LGd, dorsal lateral geniculate nucleus; OT, optic tract; MG, medial geniculate nucleus; LP, lateral posterior.

anesthetized animals were transcardially perfused with 10% formalin. Their brains were cryoprotected, sectioned frozen at 50 μm and stained with Cresyl violet. Some recording sites were marked by electrolytic lesions and the position of other sites in the same or other electrode penetrations were determined by interpolation.

We studied the receptive field properties of 112 visually responsive cells in the primary visual cortex (V1) of 31 normal hamsters. In two additional normal hamsters, we made multiple electrode penetrations in A1 while continuously sweeping the visual field with variously oriented bars of light. We did not obtain any single- or multi-unit visually evoked responses in these experiments. We also studied the receptive field properties of 38 visually responsive cells in A1 of 8 'rewired' hamsters. Of these cells, 9 (24%) were activated by auditory and visual stimuli (bimodal cells) (Fig. 5A).

Receptive field size

In V1 of normal hamsters, 85% of the neurons had distinct, well-defined RFs in the contralateral visual field. The mean RF size was 267 ± 22.3 deg^2. These data are consistent with those obtained from V1 of normal hamsters by Tiao and Blakemore (1976). By contrast, in A1 of operated hamsters, only 48% of the units had well defined RFs and these were significantly larger than those in V1 of normal hamsters (636 ± 120 deg^2; Mann–Whitney *U*-test, $P < 0.001$). Of the remaining units, 11% had RFs

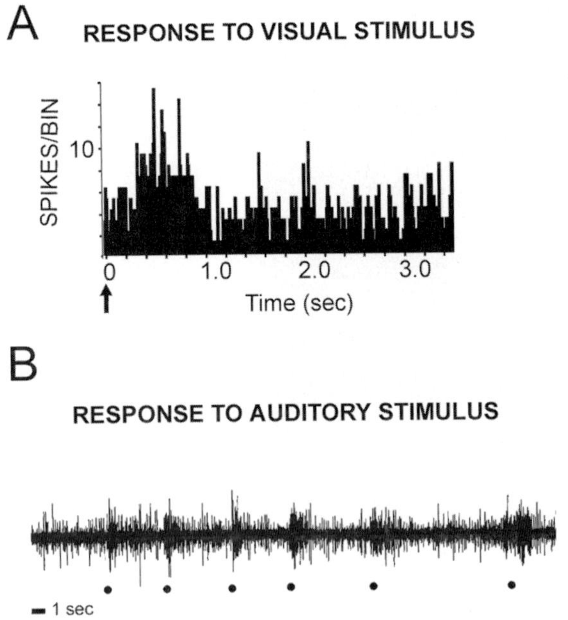

Fig. 5. (A) Response to visual (flash) and (B) auditory (e.g. hissing, jangling of keys, kissing sounds) stimulation of a bimodal unit recorded in AC of a 'rewired' hamster. The arrow indicates visual stimulus onset; dots represent the onset of the auditory stimulus. PSTH bin width is 10 ms.

with poorly defined borders and for 41% the limits of the RFs could not be determined with confidence.

Orientation selectivity

Orientation selectivity was determined using stationary, flashed bars of light. In V1 of normal hamsters, 20 (65%) of the 31 quantitatively studied neurons were orientation selective. Fig. 6A illustrates the distribution of preferred orientations for cells in area V1 of normal hamsters and shows a preference bias towards vertically oriented stimuli. An example of an orientation selective and a non-selective neurons in a normal animal is presented in Fig. 6B and C, respectively. In area A1 of operated hamsters 15 (54%) of the 28 quantitatively studied neurons were orientation selective and their distribution is shown in Fig. 6D. All orientations are still represented in rewired animals with no preference bias, although the proportions of non-orientation selective units seem to be higher. Examples of an orientation selective (90°) and a non-oriented cell are shown in Fig. 6E and F, respectively.

Direction selectivity

Cells' selectivity for the direction of stimulus movement was studied using bars of light and gratings moving in 12 directions. Non-selective (NS) units are those whose response magnitudes do not vary significantly as a function of the direction of stimulus movement. Direction selective units are those that respond preferentially to stimulus movement along a particular axis of the visual field. There are two types of direction selective units: unidirectional and bidirectional cells, that respond optimally to stimulus movement in, respectively, one or both directions along the preferred axis. Unidirectional and bidirectional units were distinguished using a direction index; DI = 1 − (response in the non-preferred direction/response in the preferred direction). Cells with DIs greater than 0.5 were regarded as unidirectional. Bidirectional cells were characterized by DI values lower than 0.5. In V1 of normal hamsters (Fig. 7A), 59 (80%) of the 74 quantitatively studied neurons were direction selective, (26 unidirectional and 33 bidirectional), whereas 15 (20%) had no preferred direction of movement (NS). In A1 of rewired hamsters (Fig. 7A), similar proportions were obtained: Of the 30 neurons recorded, 19 were direction selective (7 unidirectional and 12 bidirectional) and 11 (37%) were not direction selective. In Fig. 7B, examples of direction-selective and non-direction-selective neurons for normal and rewired are shown.

Spatial and temporal frequency tuning

100% contrast sine wave gratings drifting at optimal orientation and direction were used to assess the visual acuity of single neurons in areas V1 and A1 of normal and 'rewired' hamsters, respectively. For all 39 neurons recorded in V1 of normal hamsters, responses varied as a function of spatial frequency. Fig. 8A illustrates the distribution of preferred spatial frequencies in normal animals (mean = 0.12 ± 0.01 cycles/deg). All neurons showed a strong attenuation of their discharge at higher spatial frequencies and were considered 'low-pass' units (examples are shown in C, D and E). In A1 of 'rewired' hamsters, none of the 11 cells tested could be driven by drifting gratings.

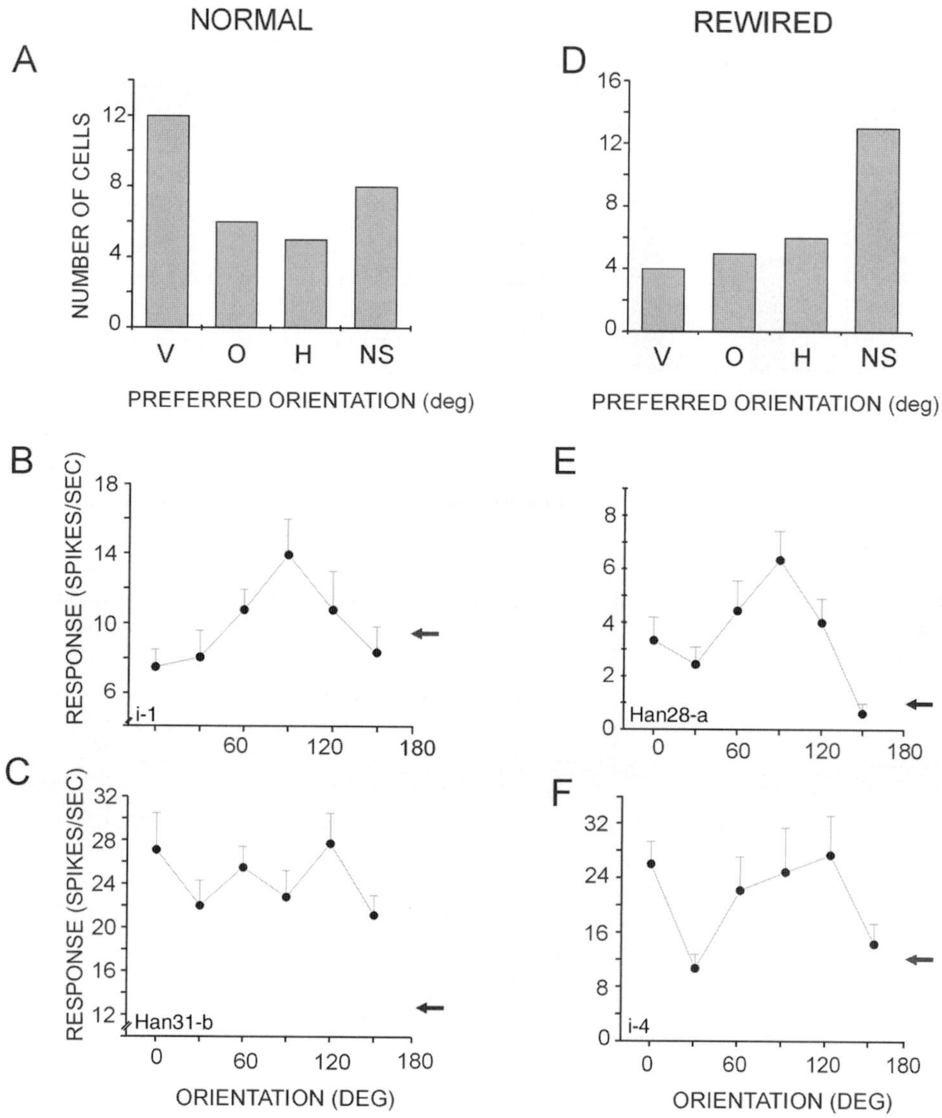

Fig. 6. Orientation selectivity of cells recorded in V1 of normal hamsters and A1 of operated ones. Distribution of preferred orientations in normal (A) and 'rewired' (D) hamsters. Note the bias towards the vertical orientation for normal hamsters and the increased number of non-selective cells (NS) in 'rewired' hamsters. V, vertical; H, horizontal; O, oblique stimulus orientations. (B and E) Examples of orientation tuning profiles from orientation-selective cells in normal and rewired hamsters. (C and F) Response profile of two non-orientation selective cells in normal and 'rewired' hamsters, respectively. The arrows indicate spontaneous activity levels; error bars represent SEM.

Fig. 7. Direction selectivity of cells recorded in V1 of normal and in AC of 'rewired' hamsters. (A) Histograms illustrating the percentage of unidirectional, bidirectional, and non-selective cells for both groups of animals (numbers in bars indicate the actual number of cells). (B) Examples of tuning profiles for normal and 'rewired' hamsters. The arrow indicates the level of spontaneous activity and error bars the SEM. BID, bidirectional cells; UNI, unidirectional cells; NS, non-selective.

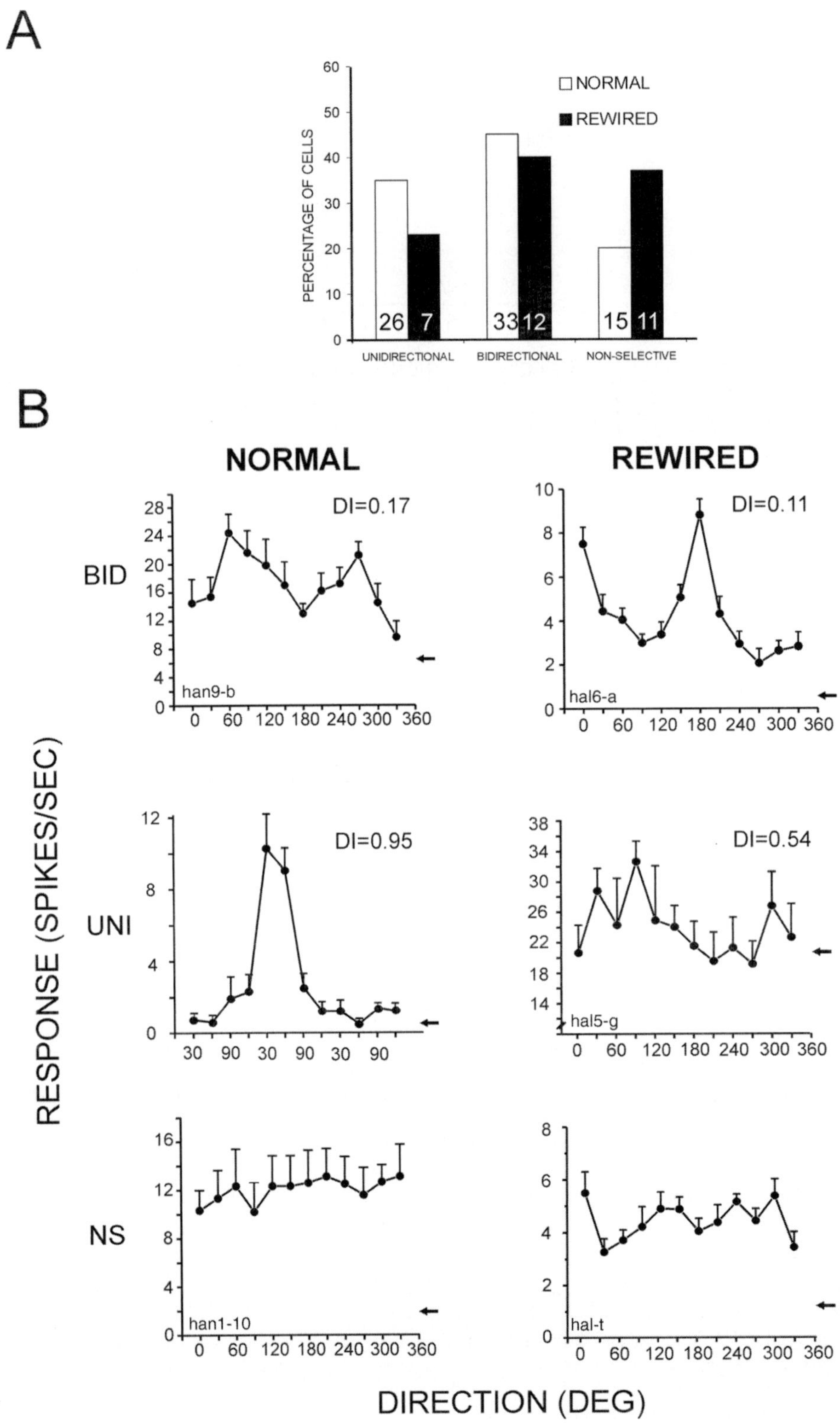
A
NORMAL
REWIRED
PERCENTAGE OF CELLS
26
7
33
12
15
11
UNIDIRECTIONAL
BIDIRECTIONAL
NON-SELECTIVE
B
NORMAL
REWIRED
BID
UNI
NS
DI=0.17
DI=0.11
DI=0.95
DI=0.54
han9-b
hal6-a
hal5-g
han1-10
hal-t
RESPONSE (SPIKES/SEC)
DIRECTION (DEG)

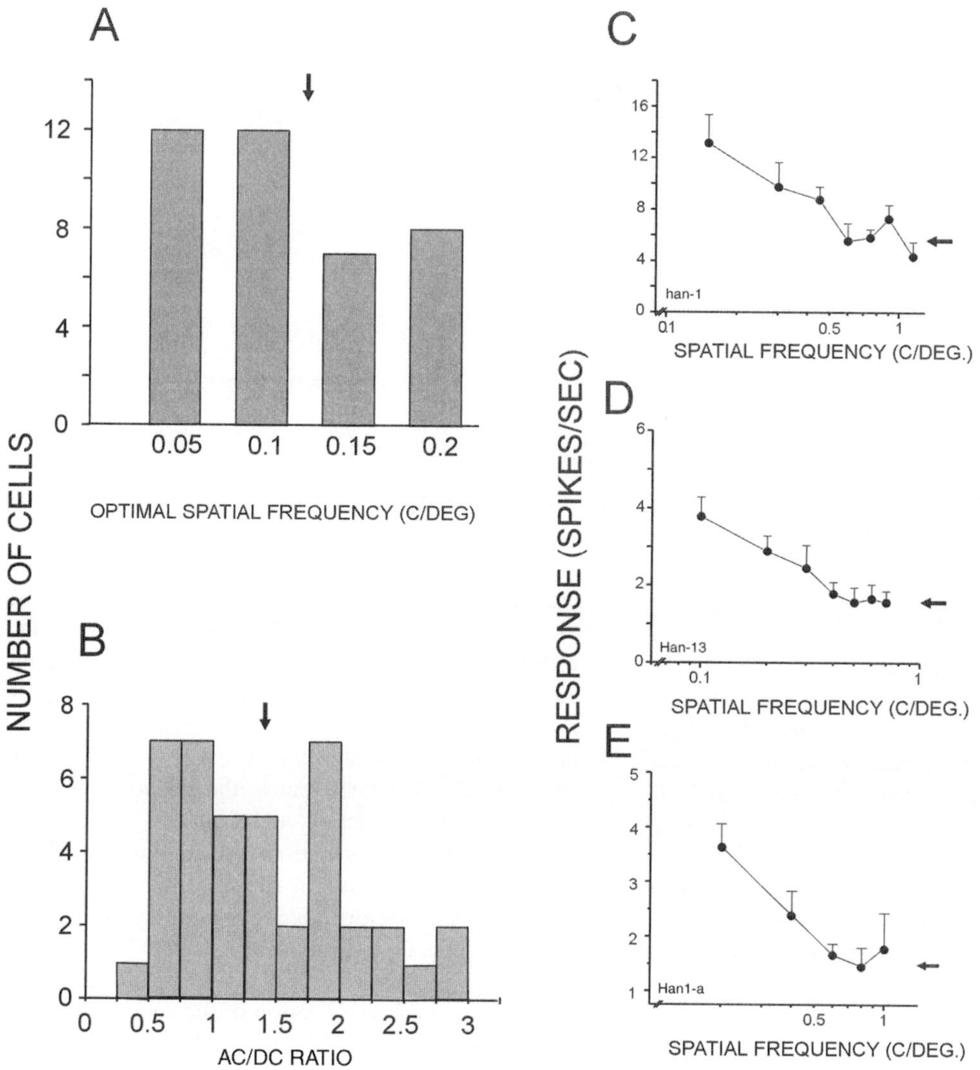

Fig. 8. Spatial frequency tuning of cells recorded in V1 of normal hamsters. (A) Distribution of optimal spatial frequencies. (B) Distribution of AC/DC ratios showing that most the cells have a ratio >1 indicating that they are simple. (C, D, and E) Examples of spatial frequency tuning curves. Horizontal arrows indicate spontaneous activity levels and errors bars represent SEM. Vertical arrows represent mean values.

A modulation index (MI) was also computed from the cells' responses evoked at the optimal spatial frequency. This index has been used to classify visual cortex units as simple (MI > 1) and complex (MI < 1) in other mammals (Skottun et al., 1991). The MI is computed by dividing the cell's response at the optimal spatial frequency (AC component) by the mean response over the full range of spatial frequencies tested (DC component), when the spontaneous firing rate is subtracted. On the basis of these criteria, 37% of V1 units were complex and 63% were simple. Fig. 8B illustrates the distribution of V1 cells according to the AC/DC ratio and shows that most of the neurons have an MI > 1.

The temporal frequency preferences of 18 cells in V1 of normal hamsters were studied. These units had 'low-pass' characteristics in that there was no attenuation of neuronal responses at progressively lower temporal frequencies (Fig. 9).

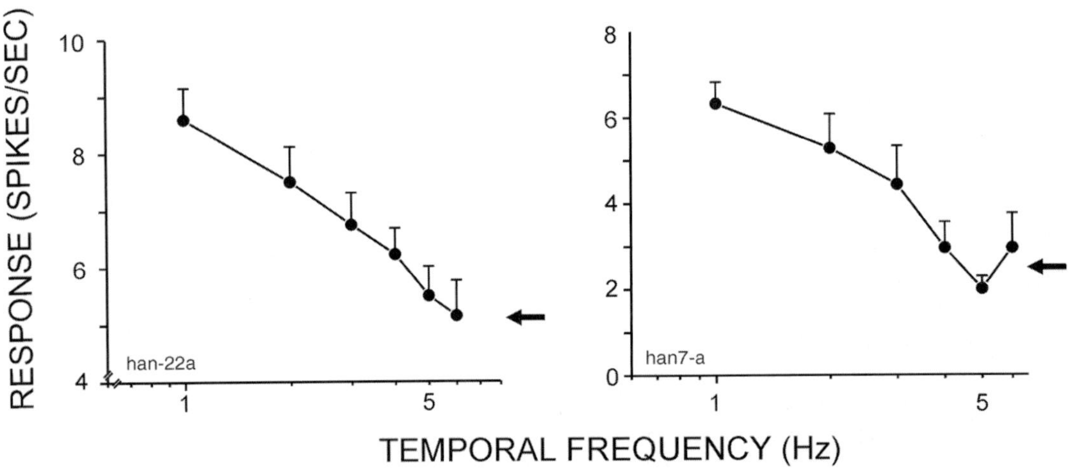

Fig. 9. Examples of temporal frequency tuning curves for two units recorded in V1 of normal hamsters. Arrows indicate spontaneous activity levels and errors bars represent SEM.

Discussion

These experiments demonstrate that distinct, surgically created neural circuits can mediate some of the functions of an ablated neural pathway. At the behavioral level, we found that rewired hamsters can use surgically induced retino-thalamo-cortical pathways to learn visual pattern discriminations that are normally mediated by the pathway from the retina (via the thalamus) to the primary visual cortex. Our physiological data show that neurons in the auditory cortex of rewired hamsters acquire visual properties that are comparable in many respects to those of neurons in V1 of normal hamsters. In A1 of 'rewired' hamsters, a subset of neurons has well-defined visual RFs and are selective for stimulus orientation or direction of movement. These data extend previous neurophysiological findings. Neurons in the primary (S1) and secondary (S2) somatosensory cortices of neonatally operated hamsters with retinal projections to VB, but of not normal hamsters, respond to visual stimulation (Frost and Métin, 1985). The visual response properties of the S1 and S2 neurons are qualitatively and quantitatively similar to those of neurons in V1 of normal hamsters (Métin and Frost, 1989). Neurons in the auditory cortex of neonatally operated ferrets with retino-MG projections are also visually responsive (Sur et al., 1988; Pallas, 1990).

The data of the present experiments suggest two hypotheses originally proposed on the basis of our neurophysiological data obtained in S1 and S2 of hamsters with retino-VB projections (Frost and Métin, 1985; Métin and Frost, 1989): The 'systems theoretic' hypothesis states that the visual response properties of neurons in V1 of normal hamsters and neurons in non-visual sensory cortices of 'rewired' hamsters are similar because the different primary sensory thalamic nuclei and cortices, respectively work similar transformations on their inputs. Thus, they are not intrinsically specialized to process information of one sensory modality and their specificity is attributable to the modality of their inputs. This hypothesis is supported by the numerous similarities in the functional organization of the sensory cortices and thalamic nuclei (Métin and Frost, 1989). The 'developmental' hypothesis states that at the developmental stage when the rewiring surgery is performed, the primary visual, auditory and somatosensory thalamic nuclei and cortices are equipotential and that they later differentiate as a function of the modality of their inputs. These hypotheses are mutually compatible: some features of the different sensory systems may be shared whereas others may differentiate in a modality-specific fashion driven by spatial and temporal patterning of electrical activity. Thus, by anatomical, neurophysiological and behavioral measures, surgically induced retino-thalamo-cortical pathways reproduce many of the essential features of the normal retino-geniculo-striate pathway.

Our data are consistent with several other findings: (1) Lesions sustained during development can cause changes in neural connectivity or synaptic efficacy that produce striking neurophysiological alterations (see Rauschecker, 1975; Frost, 1994). (2) In patients who become blind early in life, the visual cortex appears to contribute to Braille reading (Cohen et al., 1997). (3) In deaf and hearing subjects who learn American sign language early, watching signing activates cortical regions that process language, whereas this does not occur in non-signing, hearing subjects (Neville et al., 1998). One cannot say from our data whether 'rewired' hamsters perceive a visual stimulus as auditory or visual when it activates the AC. Early blind patients appear to perceive Braille characters as somatosensory stimuli despite the contribution of their visual cortex to Braille reading (Cohen et al., 1997; Sadato et al., 1998). Ferrets that have a surgically induced retino-MG-AC pathway but no visual cortex, distinguish visual from auditory stimuli (Von Melchner et al., 2000). Thus, 'rewired' hamsters with retino-MG projections may perceive light stimuli as visual, even in the absence of the visual cortex.

Our results raise the possibility that surgically created neural circuits may one day be used therapeutically. However, it should be emphasized that the visual capacities of our 'rewired' hamsters are not normal. For example, visual acuity in these animals is reduced. The extent to which surgically created neural circuits can sustain vision must be elucidated in other species that have more highly differentiated visual systems and more elaborate visual behaviors than rodents. Furthermore, it remains to be demonstrated whether neurophysiological and behavioral results similar to those we have obtained in neonatally operated animals, can be reproduced in subjects that receive lesions and reparative surgery as adults.

Acknowledgements

This research was supported by Grants MT-13359 from the Medical Research Council of Canada (M.P.), and RO1-MH49568 from the NIMH (D.O.F.), R01-EY11434 (D.O.F.).

References

Blochert, P.K., Ferrier, R.J. and Cooper, R.M. (1976) Effects of pretectal lesions on rats wearing light-diffusing occluders. *Brain Res.*, 104: 121–128.

Campbell, G. and Frost, D.O. (1987) Target-controlled differentiation of axon terminals and synaptic organization. *Proc. Natl. Acad. Sci. USA*, 84: 6929–6933.

Campbell, G. and Frost, D.O. (1988) Synaptic organization of anomalous retinal projections to the somatosensory and auditory thalamus: target-controlled morphogenesis of axon terminals and synaptic glomeruli. *J. Comp. Neurol.*, 272: 383–408.

Caviness Jr., V.S. (1975) Architectonic map of neocortex of the normal mouse. *J. Comp. Neurol.*, 164: 247–264.

Caviness Jr., V.S. and Frost, D.O. (1980) Tangential organization of thalamic projections to the neocortex in the mouse. *J. Comp. Neurol.*, 194: 335–367.

Cohen, L.G., Celnik, P., Pascual-Leone, A., Corwell, B., Falz, L., Dambrosia, J., Honda, M., Sadato, N., Gerloff, C., Catala, M.D. and Hallett, M. (1997) Functional relevance of cross-modal plasticity in blind humans. *Nature*, 389: 180–183.

Crain, B.J. and Hall, W.C. (1980a) The organization of the lateral posterior nucleus of the golden hamster after neonatal superior colliculus lesions. *J. Comp. Neurol.*, 193: 383–401.

Crain, B.J. and Hall, W.C. (1980b) The organization of afferents to the lateral posterior nucleus in the golden hamster after different combinations of neonatal lesions. *J. Comp. Neurol.*, 193: 403–412.

Frost, D.O. (1981) Orderly anomalous retinal projections to the medial geniculate, ventrobasal and lateral posterior nuclei of the hamster. *J. Comp. Neurol.*, 203: 227–256.

Frost, D.O. (1994) In: V.A. Casagrande and P. Shinkman (Eds.), *Advances in Neural and Behavioral Development*. Ablex, Norwood, NJ, pp. 123–147.

Frost, D.O. and Métin, C. (1985) Induction of functional retinal projections to the somatosensory system. *Nature*, 317: 162–164.

Frost, D.O., Boire, D., Gingras, G. and Ptito, M. (2000) Surgically created neural pathways mediate visual pattern discrimination. *Proc. Natl. Acad. Sci. USA*, 97: 11068–11073.

Kalil, R.E. and Schneider, G.E. (1975) Abnormal synaptic connections of the optic tract in the thalamus after midbrain lesions in newborn hamsters. *Brain Res.*, 100: 690–698.

Métin, C. and Frost, D.O. (1989) Visual responses of neurons in somatosensory cortex of hamsters with experimentally induced retinal projections to somatosensory thalamus. *Proc. Natl. Acad. Sci. USA*, 86: 357–361.

Neville, H.J., Bavelier, D., Corina, D., Rauschecker, J., Karni, A., Lalwani, A., Braun, A., Clark, V., Jezzard, P. and Turner, R. (1998) Cerebral organization for language in deaf and hearing subjects: biological constraints and effects of experience. *Proc. Natl. Acad. Sci. USA*, 95: 922–929.

Pallas, S.L. (1990). Cross-modal plasticity in sensory cortex. Visual responses in primary auditory cortex in ferrets with induced retinal projections to the medial geniculate nucleus.

In: B.L. Finlay (Ed.), *The Neocortex*. Plenum Press, New York, pp. 205–215.

Rauschecker, J.P. (1975) Compensatory plasticity and sensory substitution in the cerebral cortex. *Trends Neurosci.*, 18: 36–43.

Roe, A.W., Pallas, S.L., Kwon, Y.H. and Sur, M. (1992) Visual projections routed to the auditory pathway in ferrets: receptive fields of visual neurons in primary auditory cortex. *J. Neurosci.*, 12: 3651–3664.

Rothblat, L.A. and Schwartz, M.L. (1978) Complex pattern discrimination in the albino rat: role of striate cortex and ipsilateral retino-cortical-pathway. *Soc. Neurosci. Abstr.*, 4: 643.

Sadato, N., Pascual-Leone, A., Grafman, J., Deiber, M.-P., Ibanez, V. and Hallett, M. (1998) Neural networks for Braille reading by the blind. *Brain*, 121: 1213–1229.

Schneider, G.E. (1969) Two visual systems. *Science*, 163: 895–902.

Schneider, G.E. (1973) Early lesions of the superior colliculus: factors affecting the formation of abnormal retinal projections. *Brain Behav. Evol.*, 8: 73–109.

Schneider, G.E. (1975) Two visuomotor systems in the Syrian hamster. *Neurosci. Res. Program Bull.*, 13: 255–257.

Skottun, B.C., De Valois, R.L., Grosd, D.H., Movshon, J.A., Albrecht, D.G. and Bonels, A.B. (1991) Classifying simple and complex cells on the basis of response modulation. *Vision Res.*, 31: 1079–1086.

Sur, M., Garraghty, P.E. and Roe, A.W. (1988) Experimentally induced visual projections into auditory thalamus and cortex. *Science*, 242: 1437–1441.

Tiao, Y.C. and Blakemore, C. (1976) Functional organization in the visual cortex of the golden hamster. *J. Comp. Neurol.*, 168: 459–483.

Von Melchner, L., Pallas, S.L. and Sur, M. (2000) Visual behaviour mediated by retinal projections directed to the auditory pathway. *Nature*, 404: 871–876.

C. Casanova and M. Ptito (Eds.)
Progress in Brain Research, Vol. 134

CHAPTER 29

Attentional selection and the processing of task-irrelevant information: insights from fMRI examinations of the Stroop task

Marie T. Banich [1,*], Michael P. Milham [2], Benjamin L. Jacobson [1], Andrew Webb [2], Tracey Wszalek [2], Neal J. Cohen [2] and Arthur F. Kramer [2]

[1] *Department of Psychology, University of Colorado at Boulder, E213-E Muenzinger Hall, 345 UCB, Boulder, CO 80309, USA*
[2] *The Beckman Institute, University of Illinois at Urbana-Champaign, Urbana, IL 61801, USA*

Abstract: In this chapter, we discuss our research that reveals how attentional mechanisms can modulate activity of posterior brain regions responsible for processing the *unattended* attribute of a stimulus. To do so, we utilized fMRI to reveal patterns of regional brain activity for variants of the Stroop task that differ in the nature of the task-irrelevant stimulus attribute. In all variants, individuals had to identify the ink color in which an item was presented. To vary attentional demands, we manipulated whether or not the task-irrelevant information contained conflicting color information. The variants differed in whether the conflicting color information was contained in a word naming a color (e.g. the word 'red' in blue ink), a word naming an object highly associated with a specific color (e.g. the word 'frog' in red ink), or a line drawing of an object highly associated with a specific color (e.g. a drawing of a frog in red ink). When the unattended stimulus attribute contained color information that conflicted with an item's ink color, increased activity was observed in the posterior brain region that processes the aspect of the task-irrelevant attribute related to color. Increased activity was observed in the left precuneus and left superior parietal cortex when the conflicting information arose from a color word; in the middle temporal gyrus and insular cortex when the word named an object highly associated with a specific color, and included extensive regions of early portions of the ventral visual processing stream when a line drawing was highly associated with a specific color. These areas have been implicated in word processing, semantic processing, and visual processing, respectively. Our results suggest that attentional selection can occur by: (1) increasing the gain on all posterior regions responsible for processing information related to the task demands, regardless of whether that information is contained in the task-relevant or task-irrelevant dimension; (2) limiting the processing of task-irrelevant information in order to reduce interference; and (3) modulating the processing of representations varying from those of a low-level perceptual nature up through those of a higher-order semantic nature.

Introduction

Neural mechanisms of visual selective attention for task-relevant information

This chapter discusses cognitive and neurobiological mechanisms responsible for the attentional selection of task-relevant visual attributes. We have obtained insights into this issue through a series of fMRI studies examining attentional control in different

* Corresponding author: M.T. Banich, Department of Psychology, University of Colorado at Boulder, E213-E Muenzinger Hall, 345 UCB, Boulder, CO 80309, USA. Tel.: +1-303-492-6655; Fax: +1-303-492-2967; E-mail: mbanich@psych.colorado.edu

variants of the Stroop task. One of the most ubiquitous findings from both neurophysiological and neuroimaging work is that attentional selection enhances activity within brain regions most highly specialized for processing the stimulus towards which attention is directed. A classic example comes from the work of Moran and Desimone (1985). They demonstrated that selective attention modulates neuronal firing in the extrastriate cortex of rhesus monkeys. In their paradigm, two stimuli that differed in visual attributes (e.g. color, orientation, and size) were presented on each trial. One stimulus was an effective stimulus, in that it was very capable of making the cell fire, whereas the other stimulus was relatively ineffective in driving the cell's response. Neurons were isolated in area V4 that had a receptive field that included both stimuli. When the monkey's attention was directed to the location of the effective stimulus, the firing rate of the cell was greatly enhanced as compared to when attention was directed to the location of the ineffective stimulus. It is important to note that the perceptual displays are identical in both cases — both contain an effective and ineffective stimulus. The difference in firing rates between the two conditions depends on where the monkey's attention is directed. When attention is directed to the location of the effective stimulus, the firing rate increases. These results indicate that directing attention to a stimulus effective for stimulating a given brain region can cause an increase in the neuronal responsiveness of that brain region.

Neuroimaging work with humans has yielded similar findings, and also shown that these selective mechanisms can work on much more complex visual forms than those composed of simple visual attributes. One example is imaging work that examined visual selection for faces (Wojciulik et al., 1998). In this study, the region of the brain that responds differentially to faces as compared to other objects (i.e. the fusiform face area) was identified in each participant on an individual basis. Having identified this region, the researchers then examined the degree to which activity in this region could be modulated by covert attention. Individuals were shown displays that contained five items: a fixation cross, two faces, and two houses. To keep the location of spatial attention constant, individuals were told to fixate on the cross, and displays were brief enough to preclude saccadic eye movements. On half the trials, participants decided whether the faces matched, and on the other half decided whether the houses matched. Greater activation was found in the fusiform face area when faces as compared to houses were attended (i.e. the decision was about faces), even though both faces and houses were always within the same display. When covert attention is directed towards the face stimuli, attentional mechanisms increase activation of areas specialized for processing faces. These results indicate that directing attention to location, as in the case of the Moran and Desimone study, is not the only means by which attentional regulation can affect processing in posterior sensory areas. Covert attention to a specific stimulus can also increase activation of the posterior region specialized for processing that visual stimulus.

In all the studies discussed so far, the selection process has been one in which a particular visual item or class of items (e.g. faces) is selected over other items in the display. Yet selection may also require that a particular attribute of a single visual stimulus (e.g. its form) be attended to over another visual attribute (e.g. its color). The neural mechanisms that allow for such selection appear to be similar to those discussed above — an enhancement of the neuronal response in the posterior processing region most specialized for processing that visual attribute. A classic example of this phenomenon is demonstrated by the work of Corbetta et al. (1991). They utilized positron emission tomography (PET) to examine the effect of selective attention for three basic visual attributes: shape, color, and motion. In their task, individuals viewed two consecutively presented displays that contained a set of shapes (e.g. rectangles) displayed in a particular color (e.g. red) moving at a particular rate across the screen (e.g. slowly). For a given set of trials, individuals were instructed to decide whether the displays were the same based on one visual attribute (e.g. color) and not the others (e.g. form and motion). Activity was modulated in different regions of posterior cortex depending on the visual attribute to which participants attended. For example, when individuals were instructed to make decisions based on color as compared to when passively viewing the same display, activation was increased in the collateral sulcus between lingual and fusiform gyri. This area has been implicated in color perception (Zeki and Marini, 1998) and damage to it produces achromatopsia, a selective deficit in color vision (Damasio et al., 1980). In contrast, when the decision had to be based on form as compared to passively viewing the displays, increased activations were noted in different regions of extrastriate cortex — bilaterally in the fusiform and parahippocampal gyri. These results indicate that not only do attentional mechanisms increase activity in regions of extrastriate cortex, but that attentional selection for a specific attribute of a presented stimulus increases activation in areas responsible for processing that attribute.

These studies are all characterized by situations in which the relationship between the attributes of an item (e.g. shape, form, motion) or items within a display are relatively random (i.e. there is no particular reason why squares would be displayed in red as compared to blue). Hence, in all these tasks, there are no additional sources of information that conflict with, or are relevant to selection of a particular visual attribute. In contrast, in the paradigms we have used, a relationship exists between the task-relevant visual attribute and task-irrelevant information. Such a situation creates very different demands on attentional selection. In the series of studies described below, we have systematically varied the way in which task-irrelevant information is able to interfere with selection of the task-relevant visual attribute. By doing so we can further explore the mechanisms of attentional selection in visual processing areas.

Selective attention for the task-relevant attribute in the Stroop paradigm

In the Stroop task, individuals view colored words. Their task is to identify a basic visual attribute of the item, its color, while ignoring the identity of the word. Because this task requires the selection of visual information about color, it can inform us with regard to mechanisms of attentional selection for simple visual attributes. Attending to the item's color under such conditions is attentionally demanding, as word reading occurs more automatically than does color identification. Hence, attentional control is required to selectively attend to the color of the word as compared to its identity. Moreover, the word's identity can have a very large effect on how easily attention can be directed to its color. It takes longer to identify the ink color when the word is incongruent and names a different color (e.g. the word 'red' in blue ink) as compared to when the word is neutral and is unrelated to color (e.g. the word 'lot' in blue ink). Attentional demands are greater on the incongruent trials than neutral trials because the word's identity contains a task-irrelevant source of information about color.

Examining patterns of brain activation for different types of Stroop trials can provide insights into mechanisms of selective attention for the basic visual attribute of color. It has been found that a comparison of incongruent as compared to neutral Stroop stimuli generally does not reveal an increase in activation of color perception regions (i.e. V4) (e.g. Pardo et al., 1990; Bench et al., 1993; George et al., 1994; Carter et al., 1995; Taylor et al., 1997). In many ways, this finding might be considered surprising because it takes more attentional resources to direct attention to the ink color when the word contains competing color information (i.e. on incongruent trials) as compared to when it does not (i.e. on neutral trials). Likewise, increased activation in the color area is not observed for the comparison of either incongruent or neutral Stroop stimuli as compared to a line of XXXXs (Bench et al., 1993). Once again, the greater difficulty of selecting color information from words as compared to a line of XXXXs does not appear to cause increased activation of the color processing region. This lack of increased activation in the color processing area suggests that activation of this region is not influenced by the difficulty of selecting the task-relevant color information *relative* to the task-irrelevant information. Rather, as suggested by the Corbetta et al. (1991) study, activation may increase in color processing areas whenever color is the attended attribute. Because the need to extract color information is similar across incongruent words, neutral words, and a line of XXXXs, no difference in activation in V4 is observed across these conditions.

These findings are important as they suggest that there must exist other means of attentional regulation besides boosting activation of the region responsible for processing the attended attribute. The question then arises as to what other mechanisms aid in attentional control, and are sensitive to the *relative* demands placed on extracting task-relevant information in comparison to task-irrelevant information.

A neural model of attentional control in the Stroop paradigm

To answer this issue, we have performed a series of fMRI studies with variants of the Stroop task. Although there are a large number of studies that have examined patterns of brain activation during the Stroop task (Pardo et al., 1990; Bench et al., 1993; Carter et al., 1995, 1997; Bush et al., 1998; Brown et al., 1999; Petersen et al., 1999), our use of variants of the Stroop task were specifically designed to delineate the role that each of these brain regions plays in attentional control (Banich et al., 2000a,b). Before discussing the evidence in detail, we provide a brief overview of our findings.

Our results suggest that dorsolateral prefrontal regions are critically important for creating an 'attentional set' that modulates activity within posterior processing systems and facilitates selection of task-relevant representations within working memory. Furthermore, the involvement of dorsolateral prefrontal regions in task performance is more prominent when effortful control is required to select the task-relevant over the task-irrelevant dimension. In contrast, when the task-relevant dimension is processed more automatically than the task-irrelevant dimension, no such increase in dorsolateral prefrontal activation is observed (Banich et al., 2000b). The role of dorsolateral prefrontal cortex is distinct from that of medial frontal regions, such as the anterior cingulate, which appear to be involved in response selection (Milham et al., 2001a). Furthermore, the dorsolateral region identified in these studies seems to co-activate with a region of parietal cortex (precuneus). We posit that this dorsolateral/parietal circuitry is the source of attentional control, responsible for selecting and maintaining an attentional set that specifies the nature of task-relevant information.

Although this system may provide for top-down control of attention by maintaining an attentional set, there must be sites at which processing of information is modulated by this attentional set (see Posner and Petersen, 1990 for a distinction between the *site* of selective effects and the *source* of the signals producing those effects). As reviewed above, in the Stroop task this modulation *does not* occur in V4. Rather, our studies have suggested that some aspects of attentional control may occur through modulation of processing of the *task-irrelevant* attribute, rather than the task-relevant one (e.g. color). The studies that have led to these conclusions are described in detail below.

Attentional selection and task-irrelevant attributes

Initial findings

To determine how attentional control occurs in the Stroop task, we examined differences in the neural network responsible for attentional control in the face of incongruent information for pairs of variants of the Stroop task (Banich et al., 2000a). In one experiment, we examined activation that accompanied increased attentional demands for a color–word task and a color–object task (Banich et al., 2000a, Expt. 2). Our nomenclature for these tasks is to hyphenate the name, with the first word referring to the task-relevant dimension (e.g. color) and the second word referring to the task-irrelevant dimension (e.g. object). As discussed above, in the color–word task, an individual must identify the color of a word, while ignoring the word's identity. In the color–object task, an individual must identify the color of an object, while ignoring its identity. To vary attentional demands, we contrasted performance on incongruent trials to neutral trials. For the color–word task, an incongruent trial is one in which the word names a color other than the word's ink color (e.g. the word 'red' in blue ink). A neutral trial is one in which the word is unrelated to color (e.g. the word 'lot' in blue ink). For the color–object task, an incongruent trial is one in which an object is depicted in a color distinct from that with which it is highly associated (e.g. a red frog). A neutral trial is one in which the object is not strongly associated with a single color, but is shown in one of many colors with which it can be associated (e.g. a red car).

Notice that the comparison between patterns of brain activation in these two tasks can be particularly informative because in both tasks an individual must attend to the same attribute — color. Hence, those brain regions that are specifically responsible for attending to the task-relevant attribute should show similar activation across both tasks. In contrast, the source of task-irrelevant information differs across the two tasks. Therefore, the brain regions that exhibit different patterns of activation for the two tasks are those that are sensitive to the to-be-ignored information.

The behavioral results for both tasks did indeed indicate that we were successful in manipulating attentional demands. A significant Stroop effect was observed for both the color–word and color–object task as responses to incongruent trials were elongated compared to neutral trials. With regards to brain activation, we indeed found evidence that the dorsolateral prefrontal region is important for imposing an 'attentional set'. Dorsolateral prefrontal cortex was significantly more active on incongruent than neutral trials for both the color–word and color–object task. Furthermore, the region that was activated in both tasks significantly overlapped. Such a finding was expected, as in both cases the task-relevant attribute is color.

The role of the dorsolateral prefrontal region in imposing an attentional set was confirmed in another experiment in which we compared activation for a color–word Stroop task with a spatial–word Stroop task (Banich et al., 2000a, Experiment 1). In the spatial–word Stroop, individuals must decide if a word is located above, below, or inside a box. On incongruent trials, the word names a position incongruent with its location (e.g. the word 'below' positioned above the box). On neutral trials, the word has no spatial information (e.g. the word 'house' positioned above the box). For both tasks, we obtained dorsolateral prefrontal activation. In this case, however, the region of activation was overlapping, but partially distinct — more dorsal regions were only activated by the spatial–word task, and more ventral regions only by the color–word task. We interpreted these findings as indicating that dorsolateral prefrontal regions are important for imposing an attentional set, but with some degree of specialization depending on whether the task-relevant attribute is processed by the dorsal visual processing stream (i.e. space) as compared to the ventral visual processing stream (e.g. color).

These two experiments also shed light on the posterior sites at which dorsolateral prefrontal regions exert their attentional control. Most informative was the difference in the pattern of activation between the color–word and color–object task because this difference reveals which brain regions are sensitive to the task-irrelevant information (e.g. the word vs. the object). Although both tasks produced activity in the parietal lobes (BA 7 and BA 40), the color–word task produced unique activation in three regions of the parietal lobe. These were: (1) the precuneus; (2) a superior region of the left superior parietal region; and (3) a lateral region of the left inferior parietal region. In contrast, although both tasks produced activation in the left fusiform gyrus (BA 19), there was significantly more activation for the color–object than color–word task extending throughout the ventral visual processing stream, including the inferior occipital, middle occipital, fusiform, lingual, and middle temporal gyri.

This pattern of results suggests that attentional selection in the Stroop task may work by modulating processing of task-irrelevant information. All of the parietal regions specifically activated by the color–word task appear to be involved in word-related processing. The left precuneus region has been reported to become active when processing words compared to letter strings (Jessen et al., 1999). The lateral left inferior region is likely to reflect the translation of orthography to phonology (e.g. Price, 1998), as this area has been reported to be more active when viewing or naming words as compared to pictures. Finally, the left superior region becomes activated when words must be encoded into memory (Kelley et al., 1998). The extensive patterns of activation noted within ventral visual processing stream specific to the color–object task is strikingly similar to those areas activated when objects are encoded into memory (Kelley et al., 1998). The one notable difference is that our activations did not extend as far anteriorly, terminating before the parahippocampal gyrus.

Interpretation

We interpret these findings as suggesting that a series of distinct mechanisms in posterior cortex serve to regulate attentional selection. First, we interpret the parietal lobe activation that is common across the tasks (i.e. regions of BA 7 and BA 40) as reflecting activation imposed by an increased need for attentional control in the incongruent as compared to neutral condition. These brain regions have been found to be activated across a variety of attentionally demanding tasks, and have been described as being part of a general attentional activation system that allocates resources regardless of the stimulus dimension (e.g. Coull and Nobre, 1998). Such increased activation appears to be the neural correlate of the elongation of reaction time for incongruent as compared to neutral trials that is observed in the behavioral data.

In contrast, the areas uniquely activated for each task (as compared to those activated in common) in the incongruent as compared to neutral condition, represent the modulation of activity in regions responsible for processing task-irrelevant information when that information is related to color. The mechanism behind this modulation of activity is not entirely clear. One possibility is that the attentional set imposed by dorsolateral prefrontal regions may result in increased activation of any posterior brain region that is responsible for processing information related to task demands. Therefore, when the task demands require attention to color, upregulation of activity may occur in any region that is processing color-related information, regardless of its source — whether it be contained in the task-relevant or task-irrelevant dimension. This idea is consistent with the results of Moran and Desimone (1985), Wojciulik et al. (1998), Corbetta et al. (1991), and others, indicating an increase in activity of brain regions that process information about the to-be-attended attribute. Our findings, however, suggest a more broad tuning of activity of regions in posterior cortex than has been suggested previously, one that encompasses modulation of activity of all regions involved in processing any information that is color-related. Furthermore, the activation in these posterior regions does not appear to be driven by conflict between the task-relevant and task-irrelevant dimensions, but rather that information contained in the task-irrelevant dimension is *related* to the task-relevant information. Support for such a notion comes from the finding that the same ventral regions show increased activity for objects highly associated with colors, regardless of whether they are presented in congruent or incongruent colors (Banich et al., 1999).

Whenever dorsolateral regions impose an attentional set for color, *all* posterior regions are put on 'alert' for color information. The outcome of this 'alerting' function differs for neutral and incongruent trials. On neutral trials, the task-irrelevant dimension contains no color information. Even if areas sensitive to task-irrelevant information are on 'alert', no color-related information is detected, and hence activation is not increased. In contrast on incongruent trials, the task-irrelevant dimension contains color information, which leads to greater activation of those regions processing task-irrelevant information that is color related. We speculate that the increased activation might reflect a mechanism whereby prefrontal regions 're-interrogate' posterior regions after detecting that these regions are processing information related to that which is task-relevant.

In studies using paradigms in which there is no relationship between the information contained in the attended and unattended attribute such an alerting function would go undetected. For example, in any task in which one is to attend to an item's color and ignore its form, the form-processing area might become more sensitive to color information. However, if the relationship between form and color is arbitrary (as in the study by Corbetta et al., 1991 and others like it), no increased activation in the form-related area would occur since the information processed by that area is not systematically related to the task-relevant dimension.

Our findings also indicate that the processing of the task-irrelevant information is not completely suppressed, as it must be processed to some degree for its relationship to the task-relevant dimension, color, to be detected. It appears that the imposition of an attentional set by prefrontal areas is not so precise as to completely limit processing of color information only to that contained in a particular information channel (i.e. color information contained in the ink color but not in word). If suppression were total, we would not expect variations in the pattern of uniquely activated regions depending on the nature of the task-irrelevant attribute.

Other evidence from our data, however, indicates that the pattern of increased activation in these posterior regions may, at the same time, represent the end product of an attentional mechanism that serves to limit the processing of task-irrelevant information.

Supporting this suggestion, the ventral stream activations observed in our study were less extensive than those noted by Kelley et al. (1998). The activation for incongruent as compared to neutral trials in the color–object task did not extend to anterior regions of the ventral visual processing stream where there is a linkage between object form and identity. Likewise, for the color–word task, increased activation on incongruent as compared to neutral trials was observed in parietal regions associated with the mapping of orthography to phonology. This activation did not extend anterior into temporal regions that are associated with the full semantic processing of words.

Additional support for this interpretation comes from the pattern of activation observed for the color–word task in older individuals (60–75 years of age) (Milham et al., 2001b). One striking effect was that relative to younger adults, the elderly adults exhibited much more extensive activation of the ventral visual processing pathway, which was accompanied by a marginally significant increase in Stroop interference (i.e. the difference in reaction time between incongruent and neutral trials). For young adults, the color–word task only produced activation in the left fusiform gyrus. In contrast, the activation in the elderly extended further along the ventral processing stream, distributed through areas BA 18, 19 and 37. We conjecture that this more extensive activation indicates that processing of the task-irrelevant word information is not as limited in the elderly as in young adults.

Modulation of processing by task-irrelevant information can occur regardless of whether the information that elicits a competing representation of color is actually present in the stimulus or not. In the case of the color–word task, the competing color information is specified by information contained in the stimulus, as the incongruent word names a specific color that is distinct from the ink color. In contrast, in the color–object task, the incongruent stimulus does not directly specify a competing color. Rather, interference must occur via the linkage in memory of the object's form (e.g. a frog) with its prototypical color (e.g. green). It is this prototypical color that interferes with correctly identifying the actual color in which the object is depicted.

The increased activation on incongruent trials relative to neutral trials in the word processing regions in the color–word task and the ventral visual processing region in the object–word task stands in marked contrast to a lack of modulation in activity for areas associated with the processing of color information. For neither task did we observe increased activation in the region previously identified as being the area associated with color perception (e.g. $x = -12$, $y = -74$, $z = 0$) (Zeki and Marini, 1998), nor in areas of the inferior temporal lobe (BA 20) that are associated with retrieving color knowledge (Chao and Martin, 1999). Our results, therefore, are consistent with other Stroop studies that do not indicate increased activation in the color processing area.

Further examination of attentional control by modulation of task-irrelevant information

The results from these studies suggest that attentional selection can influence the processing of the task-irrelevant information, and that the site of this effect will vary depending on the nature of that task-irrelevant attribute (e.g. a word versus an object). Here we wished to further examine this issue. On the basis of our prior results, we have argued that the pattern of regional activation across Stroop tasks that differed with regards to the task-irrelevant attribute (i.e. color–word vs. color–object) could inform us as to the nature of the interfering representation. In the color–object task, we argued that the source of the interfering information about color was one that is retrieved when processing the form of the object, activating ventral object processing regions. In contrast, in the color–word task, we argued that the source of the interfering information about color was one that was intimately linked to the word's identity, activating word processing areas.

To further explore the idea that attentional selection can be linked to task-irrelevant information, we examined performance on a color–object word task. In this task, incongruent trials consist of words that name objects highly associated with a specific color (e.g. 'frog'). In the less attentionally demanding neutral trials, the words name objects that are associated with multiple colors (e.g. a car can be green, red, blue, gray, white, tan, black, etc.). In contrast to the color–object task, in which the *visual form of the object* elicits information about color, we propose that interfering color information in the color–

object word task is retrieved without the aid of object recognition areas. We also propose that the interfering color information in the color–object word task differs from that in the standard color–word task. In the case of the standard color–word Stroop task, the linkage of the word with color is direct ('blue' has a color meaning). In contrast, in the case of the color–object word task, the linkage of the word with color is indirect ('frog' has a meaning of an animal that typically is green). Therefore, we expect to see increased activation on incongruent as compared to neutral trials in different posterior areas in the color object–word task than previously observed in either the standard color–word task or the object–word task. We propose that the modulation of activation in the color–object word task will likely occur in amodal semantic areas, as semantics provides a means to link the object word with associated color information. To test this hypothesis, we conducted an experiment that allowed us to compare patterns of brain activation on the standard color–word Stroop task with that of a color–object word task. We then compared the pattern for both these tasks that we had obtained previously for the color–object task (Banich et al., 2000a, Expt. 2).

Methods

Participants

Participants were 14 right-handed native English speakers with normal or corrected to normal vision (age range: 21–35 years). All participants were screened to ensure that they did not have a history of neurological damage or color-blindness and gave informed consent prior to participation.

Stimuli and design

The stimuli were programmed using Mel V2.0 and presented using an IBM-PC compatible computer. Our task made use of three ink colors: red, orange, and green. Three trial types were included in our experiment: (1) *incongruent standard color–word trials* in which the word named a color incongruent with the ink color in which it was printed (e.g. the word 'GREEN' in red ink); (2) *incongruent color–object word trials* in which the ink color of a word was incongruent with the color highly associated with the object named by that word (e.g. the word 'FROG' printed in red ink); and (3) *neutral trials* in which the word was unrelated to color (e.g. the word 'LOT' in red ink). Half of the neutral words were matched with the color words for word frequency and length, and the other half matched the object words, in that they also described objects, except in this case the objects are not highly associated with any particular color (e.g. the word 'CAR' in red ink).

We made use of a blocked fMRI design, in which neutral blocks were alternated with incongruent standard color word and incongruent color–object word blocks (i.e. neutral; incongruent standard color–words; neutral; incongruent color–object words) such that participants were presented a total of four incongruent standard color–word and four incongruent color–object word blocks. Neutral trials were intermixed in incongruent blocks (50 : 50 mix) to prevent the development of strategies regarding the degree to which the words are read. Each block consisted of 18 trials, presented at a rate of one trial every 2 s. Each trial consisted of a 300-ms fixation cross followed by a 1200-ms presentation of the stimulus (colored word) and 500-ms pause.

Procedure

Participants were placed in a 1.5 Tesla GE Signa scanner equipped for echo-planar imaging (EPI). Head position was stabilized using a bite-bar attached to the head coil to minimize motion during the session. A total of 248 gradient T1 weighted EPI images acquired for each participant (TR = 2400 ms, TE = 40 ms, flip angle = 90°), each consisting of 15 contiguous slices (3.75 × 3.75 × 7.0 mm) parallel to the AC–PC line. A high-resolution 3D anatomical set (T1-weighted 3-dimensional spoiled gradient echo images) was collected for each participant, as well as T1-weighted images of our functional acquisition slices. Stimuli were presented on a goggle system by Magnetic Resonance Technologies, and responses were acquired on a three-button response pad.

Image processing

The first six volumes of each run were discarded to allow the MR signal to reach steady state. Functional data for each participant was then convolved using a 3D Gaussian kernel (FWHM = 8 × 8 × 8 mm, kernel width = 7 × 7 mm), temporally denoised using an ID-wavelet transform (visu-shrink, number of levels = 4), intensity normalized, and linearly detrended. MedX3.2 was used for image processing and statistical analysis.

Image analyses

For each participant, we calculated a mean image for each of the three conditions: (1) neutral; (2) incongruent standard color words; and (3) incongruent color–object words. Mean image maps were warped into a common stereotaxic space (Tailarach and Tournoux, 1988). Pair-wise comparisons of the three conditions were then carried out using a paired t-test ($n = 14$) (the paired t-test was employed due to its ability to remove the impact of between subject variability). Voxels with a z-score exceeding 3.1 ($P < 0.001$) were considered active. The peak detection algorithm described by Mintun et al. (1989) was employed for localizing activations.

Results

Behavioral results

RT to incongruent color words (750 ms) were significantly elongated compared to neutral words (625 ms) ($P < 0.001$), whereas RT to incongruent object words (666 ms) were only marginally significantly elongated compared to neutral words ($P < 0.10$).

Imaging results

Standard incongruent color–word vs. neutral word

The standard color–word task activated a set of brain structures that we have observed in our prior studies. These regions include dorsolateral prefrontal cortex ($x = -42$, $y = 10$, $z = 34$), inferior prefrontal cortex ($x = -34$, $y = 22$, $z = -2$), anterior cingulate cortex ($x = 2$, $y = 16$, $z = 42$), precuneus ($x = -6$, $y = -74$, $z = 50$), extrastriate cortex ($x = 16$, $y = -74$, $z = 14$, BA 19; $x = 2$, $y = -74$, $z = -8$, $x = 12$, $y = -86$, $y = -6$; BA 18), superior parietal ($x = -24$, $y = -74$, $z = 42$, BA 19/7), and inferior parietal ($x = -42$, $y = -44$, $z = 42$, BA 40) cortex.

Incongruent color–object word vs. neutral word

The color–object word task activated regions different from those seen active in the standard color–word task. These regions include the middle temporal gyrus ($x = -56$, $y = -10$, $z = -2$), and the insula ($x = -40$, $y = -14$, $z = 10$). Although both the color–object word task and standard color–word task activated inferior prefrontal regions bilaterally, the center of these activations in the color–object word task differed from those found in the standard color–word task. Activation in the left inferior frontal cortex during the color–object word task was more anterior, superior, and lateral ($x = -58$, $y = 26$, $x = 12$, BA 45) than the activation found in left inferior frontal regions during the standard color–word task ($x = -34$, $y = 22$, $z = -2$, BA 47).

Results from the color–word task and color–object word task compared with previous results from the color–object task

We were also interested in comparing activations in the standard color–word and the color–object word task with those obtained previously with the color–object task. In the color–object task participants viewed a line drawing of the objects depicted by the words in the color–object word task (i.e. viewed a red frog as compared to seeing the word ‘frog’ in red). We generated a mask that assigned a value of zero to brain regions activated by either the standard or color–object word task, and a value of one to the remaining voxels. This mask was then applied to previously reported results obtained during a color–object task (Banich et al., 2000a, Expt. 2). This manipulation revealed regions active in the color–object task that were not active in either the color–word or color–object word tasks. The activations found comprised an extensive band of cortex in visual processing areas extending posterior to $y = -96$, anterior to $y = -54$, superior to $z = 60$, and inferior to $z = -16$. Peaks of activation were located both dorsally ($x = -38$, $y = -48$, $z = 48$) and ventrally ($x = -38$, $y = -54$, $z = -10$), with more extensive and greater activation in the left hemisphere. Hence, this analysis indicated that the areas of the ventral visual processing stream activated by the color–object task were activated neither by the standard color–word task nor the color–object word task.

Discussion

The results of the current study accord well with our prior ones in indicating that attentional effects can be linked to the modulation of processing of task-irrelevant information. There were unique patterns of activation under conditions of increased attentional demand for regions in the posterior cortex in the standard color–word task that differed from those of the color–object word task, which in turn differed from the previous results obtained in the color–object task. The increased activation of distinct regions of posterior cortex depending on the task irrelevant-dimension may reflect part of a mechanism by which attention ultimately modulates or gates task-irrelevant information in order to reduce interference and increase task performance. We hypothesize that processing of task-irrelevant information is modulated in these tasks because the task-irrelevant information is related to that which is task-relevant (i.e. is related to color).

The regions uniquely activated across our different Stroop tasks varied, which we believe reveals the level of representation at which information from the unattended attribute influences performance. In the case of the standard color–word task, comparison of brain activity during incongruent and neutral trials yielded unique areas of activation in regions previously reported to be engaged by word processing. The region of the left precuneus that exhibited increased activation in our study has been reported to become active when processing orthography to phonology (Jessen et al., 1999). Furthermore, the left superior parietal region has been shown to become active when words must be encoded into memory (Kelley et al., 1998). Hence, in this task, the representation of color information from the task-irrelevant dimension that is influencing performance appears to be one linked to an orthographic or phonological representation.

For the color–object word task, a different set of posterior regions was uniquely activated. Increased activation on incongruent as compared to neutral trials was observed in regions of the middle temporal gyrus (BA 20/21) that have been found to become active during retrieval of previously acquired color information and during color naming of objects (Chao and Martin, 1999). Hence, the representation of color information from the task-irrelevant dimension that is influencing performance in this case appears to be one linked to form, that is the association between an object's form and its prototypical color. Finally, in the case of the color–object word task, increased activation under conditions of higher attentional demand were noted in the middle temporal and insular regions, as well as an inferior frontal region (BA 45) that was not activated by the standard color–word task. These findings suggest that the representation of color information from the task-irrelevant dimension that is influencing performance is one that is amodal and semantic. In this case, a word such as 'frog' evokes a representation of a color (i.e. green) through the semantic association of frogs with that color.

The difference in the site of activation in the left inferior prefrontal region between the standard color–word task and the color–object word task also suggests a difference between the two tasks in the nature of the representation of color information from the task-irrelevant dimension that is influencing performance. Left inferior frontal regions have been reported to become active during retrieval, selection, maintenance, or evaluation of semantic knowledge (Wagner, 1999). This region (BA 45 and BA 47) appears to be selective to semantic processing (Thompson-Schill et al., 1997) and its activation is uninfluenced by task difficulty (Demb et al., 1995). BA 47 became active during the color–word task while an area slightly more anterior, superior, and lateral (BA 45) was active during the color–word object task. We speculate that activation in these distinct regions of the inferior frontal cortex may reflect specialization for extracting meaning from color words as compared to color–object words. Alternatively, this differential activation might arise from a more general difference in retrieval mechanisms between the two tasks. Interference in the standard color–word task arises out of a one-step process in which color meaning is directly extracted from the word, whereas the interference in the color–object word task arises from a two-step process in which the object word must be processed for meaning, from which, in turn, arises the interfering color information.

The results of our research clearly suggest that attentional modulation can vary depending on the nature of the task-irrelevant attribute and the nature of the representation from which interference arises (visual, orthographic, phonological, semantic). Modulation of activation occurs in those brain regions that process the specific representation that allows information in the task-irrelevant dimension to be linked to that which is task-relevant (e.g. color). In summary, our results suggest that attentional selection can occur by: (1) increasing the gain on all posterior regions responsible for processing information related to the task demands, regardless of whether that information is contained in the task-relevant or task-irrelevant dimension; (2) limiting the processing of task-irrelevant information in order to reduce interference; and (3) modulating the processing of representations varying from those that are of low-level perceptual nature up through those of a higher-order semantic nature.

Acknowledgements

The research described in this chapter was supported by the Human Brain Mapping Project at the Beckman Institute, University of Illinois at Urbana-Champaign in conjunction with Carle Clinic, Urbana, IL.

References

Banich, M.T., Milham, M., Webb, A., Wszalek, T., Brown, C., Gullet, D., Shah, C., Barad, V., Cohen, N., Kramer, A. and Liang, Z.-P. (1999) Components of the neural network underlying the Stroop task as assessed by fMRI. *Soc. Neurosci. Abstr.*, 25: 865.3.

Banich, M.T., Milham, M.P., Atchley, R.A., Cohen, N.J., Webb, A., Wszalek, T., Kramer, A.F., Liang, Z.-P., Wright, A., Shenker, J., Magin, R., Barad, V., Gullett, D., Shah, C. and Brown, C. (2000a) fMRI studies of Stroop tasks reveal unique roles of anterior and posterior brain systems in attentional selection. *J. Cogn. Neurosci.*, 12: 988–1000.

Banich, M.T., Milham, M.P., Atchley, R.A., Cohen, N.J., Webb, A., Wszalek, T., Kramer, A.F., Liang, Z.-P., Barad, V., Gullett, D., Shah, C. and Brown, C. (2000b) Prefrontal regions play a predominant role in imposing an attentional 'set': evidence from fMRI. *Cogn. Brain Res.*, 10: 1–9.

Bench, C.J., Frith, C.D., Grasby, P.M., Friston, K.J., Paulesu, E., Frackowiak, R.S.J. and Dolan, R.J. (1993) Investigations of the functional anatomy of attention using the Stroop test. *Neuropsychologia*, 31: 907–922.

Brown, G.G., Kinderman, S.S., Siegle, G.J., Granholm, E., Wong, E.C. and Buxton, R.B. (1999) Brain activation and pupil response during covert performance of the Stroop Color Word task. *J. Int. Neuropsychol. Soc.*, 5: 308–319.

Bush, G., Whalen, P.J., Rosen, B.R., Jenike, M.A., McInerney, S.C. and Rauch, S.L. (1998) The counting Stroop: an interference task specialized for functional neuroimaging — validation study with functional MRI. *Hum. Brain Mapp.*, 6: 270–282.

Carter, C., Mintun, M. and Cohen, J.D. (1995) Interference and facilitation effects during selective attention: an H_2 ^{15}O PET study of Stroop task performance. *Neuroimage*, 2: 264–272.

Carter, C.S., Mintun, M., Nichols, T. and Cohen, J.D. (1997) Anterior cingulate gyrus dysfunction and selection attention deficits in schizophrenia: [^{15}O] H_2O PET study during single-trail Stroop task performance. *Am. J. Psychiatry*, 154: 1670–1675.

Chao, L.L. and Martin, A. (1999) Cortical regions associated with perceiving, naming, and knowing about colors. *J. Cogn. Neurosci.*, 11: 25–35.

Corbetta, M., Miezin, F.M., Dobmeyer, S., Shulman, G.L. and Petersen, S.E. (1991) Selective and divided attention during visual discriminations of shape, color, and speed: Functional anatomy by positron emission tomography. *J. Neurol.*, 11: 2383–2402.

Coull, J.T. and Nobre, A.C. (1998) Where and when to pay attention: the neural systems for directing attention to spatial locations and to time intervals as revealed by both PET and fMRI. *J. Neurol.*, 18: 7426–7435.

Damasio, A., Yamada, T., Damasio, H., Corbett, J. and McKee, J. (1980) Central achromatopsia: behavioral, anatomic, and physiologic aspects. *Neurology*, 30(10): 1065–1071.

Demb, J.B., Desmond, J.E., Wagner, A.D., Vaidya, C.J., Glover, G.H. and Gabrieli, J.D.E. (1995) Semantic encoding and retrieval in the left inferior prefrontal cortex: a functional MRI study of task difficulty and process specificity. *J. Neurol.*, 15(9): 5870–5878.

George, M., Ketter, T., Parekh, R., Ring, H., Casey, B., Trimble, M., Horwitz, B., Herscovitch, P. and Post, R. (1994) Regional brain activity when selecting a response despite interference: an H_2O PET study of the Stroop and an emotional Stroop. *Hum. Brain Mapp.*, 1: 195–209.

Jessen, F., Erb, M., Klose, U., Lotze, M., Grodd, W. and Heun, R. (1999) Activation of human language processing brain regions after the presentation of random letter strings demonstrated within event-related functional magnetic resonance imaging. *Neurosci. Lett.*, 270: 13–16.

Kelley, W.M., Miezen, F.M., McDermott, K.B., Buckner, R.L., Raichle, M.E., Cohen, N.J., Ollinger, J.M., Akbudak, E., Conturo, T.E., Synder, A.Z. and Petersen, S.E. (1998) Hemispheric specialization in human dorsal cortex and medial temporal lobe for verbal and nonverbal memory encoding. *Neuron*, 20: 927–936.

Milham, M.P., Banich, M.T., Webb, A., Barad, V., Cohen, N.J., Wszalek, T. and Kramer, A.F. (2001a) The relative involve-

ment of anterior cingulate and prefrontal cortex in attentional control depends on the nature of conflict. *Cogn. Brain Res.*, in press.
Milham, M.P., Erickson, K.I., Banich, M.T., Kramer, A.F., Webb, A., Wszalek, T. and Cohen, N.J. (2001b) Attentional control in the aging brain: Insights from an fMRI study of the Stroop task. *Brain Cogn.*, in press.
Mintun, M., Fox, P. and Raichle, M. (1989) Highly accurate method of localizating regions of neuronal activation in the human brain with positron emission tomography. *J. Cereb. Blood Flow Metab.*, 1: 96–103.
Moran, J. and Desimone, R. (1985) Selective attention gates visual processing in the extrastriate cortex. *Science*, 299: 782–784.
Pardo, J.V., Pardo, P.J., Janer, K.W. and Raichle, M.E. (1990) The anterior cingulate cortex mediates processing selection in the Stroop attentional conflict paradigm. *Proc. Natl. Acad. Sci. USA*, 87: 256–259.
Petersen, B.S., Skudlarski, P., Gatenby, J.C., Zhang, H., Anderson, A.W. and Gore, J.C. (1999) An fMRI study of Stroop word-color interference: evidence for cingulate subregions subserving multiple distributed attentional systems. *Biol. Psychiatry*, 45: 1237–1258.
Posner, M.I. and Petersen, S.E. (1990) The attention system of the human brain. *Annu. Rev. Neurosci.*, 13: 25–42.
Price, C.J. (1998) The functional anatomy of word comprehension and production. *Trends Cogn. Sci.*, 2: 281–288.
Tailarach, J. and Tournoux, P. (1988) *Co-planar Stereotactic Atlas of the Human Brain,* 2nd edn. Thieme, Stuttgart, Germany.
Taylor, S.F., Kornblum, S., Lauber, E.J., Minoshima, S. and Koeppe, R.A. (1997) Isolation of specific interference processing in the Stroop task: PET activation studies. *Neuroimage*, 6: 81–92.
Thompson-Schill, S.L., D'Esposito, M., Aguirre, G.K. and Farah, M. (1997) Role of left inferior prefrontal cortex in retrieval of semantic knowledge: a reevaluation. *Proc. Natl. Acad. Sci. USA*, 94: 14792–14797.
Wagner, A. (1999) Working memory contributions to human learning and remembering. *Neuron*, 22: 19–22.
Wojciulik, E., Kanwisher, N. and Driver, J. (1998) Covert visual attention modulates face-specific activity in the human fusiform gyrus: fMRI study. *J. Neurophysiol.*, 79: 1574–1578.
Zeki, S. and Marini, L. (1998) Three cortical stages of colour processing in the human brain. *Brain*, 121: 1669–1685.

C. Casanova and M. Ptito (Eds.)
Progress in Brain Research, Vol. 134

CHAPTER 30

Object-based attention and object working memory: overlapping processes revealed by selective interference effects in humans

Lisa L. Barnes, James K. Nelson and Patricia A. Reuter-Lorenz *

Department of Psychology, University of Michigan, Ann Arbor, MI 48109-1109, USA

Abstract: Human observers can discriminate two attributes from the same object more efficiently than attributes from two different objects even if the retinal locations of the attributes are the same in the single and dual object cases. The single object advantage challenges the spatial spotlight view of attention and suggests that attentional selection can be object based. We report that the single object advantage is reliably reduced when an object working memory task is performed concurrently, whereas concurrent verbal and spatial working memory tasks have no effect. This selective interference effect provides support for the existence of object-based attentional processes that also contribute to the short-term retention of objects in working memory. These results are consistent with the hypothesis that both attentional and memory subsystems are organized along domain-specific lines, and suggest the importance of attention in rehearsal operations. The contributions of inferior temporal and parietal mechanisms that have been implicated in attending to and remembering objects are considered.

Introduction

The rich repertoire of human behavior necessitates flexible perceptual mechanisms. Within any particular context, different properties of the environment may be more or less relevant depending upon our behavioral goals. It is now well established that the primate visual system represents sensory input within several different frames of reference that can guide spatially-directed behavior (Snyder et al., 1998; Colby and Goldberg, 1999). Distinct regions of parietal cortex have been linked to different egocentric reference frames (e.g. Colby and Goldberg, 1999). According to some models, attention serves as the mechanism that selects representations within particular reference frames in accordance with current behavioral demands and cognitive goals. Indeed, for several decades, empirical and theoretical work in humans and other primates had been dominated by the view that attention is a spatially selective mechanism that facilitates or inhibits stimulus processing according to spatial location (e.g. Posner et al., 1980; Wurtz et al., 1982; Eriksen and St. James, 1986; Colby and Goldberg, 1999). Nevertheless, there is now a good deal of evidence to indicate that a purely space-based conception of attention is inadequate and that attentional selection can also be object based (Olson and Gettner, 1996; Roelfsma et al., 1998; Behrmann and Haimson, 1999; Behrmann and Tipper, 1999). Following an overview of this evidence, we describe behavioral studies from our laboratory that support the idea that object-based selection processes are functionally related to the mechanisms underlying working memory for objects. Our work suggests that attention can indeed operate on representations of objects per se and that such operations are also part of a system that mediates object working memory. We offer several

* Corresponding author: P.A. Reuter-Lorenz, Department of Psychology, University of Michigan, Ann Arbor, MI 48109-1109, USA. E-mail: parl@umich.edu

hypotheses about the neural substrates of these object-based processing mechanisms.

Object-based visual selective attention

Generally, three lines of evidence from human studies support the existence of object-based selective attention. One line demonstrates that it is relatively difficult to ignore distracting or irrelevant information that belongs to the same object or perceptual group as task relevant information (e.g. Driver and Baylis, 1989; Kramer and Jacobson, 1991; Yantis, 1992; Baylis and Driver, 1992; O'Craven et al., 1999). The second line demonstrates that it is easier to detect or report different attributes belonging to the same object compared to different attributes belonging to different objects even when retinal distance is equated in the two conditions (e.g. Duncan, 1984; Baylis and Driver, 1993; Kramer and Watson, 1996; however see Davis et al., 2000). Both lines of research indicate that nonspatial factors constrain our ability to deal with several simultaneous sources of visual information (e.g. Driver and Baylis, 1989). Finally, neuropsychological evidence indicates that neural mechanisms underlying object-based attention may be separable from those mediating location-based or spatial attention. Parietal patients with hemispatial neglect show reduced attentional deficits when stimuli are grouped into a single object (e.g. Behrmann et al., 1990; Farah et al., 1993; Ward et al., 1994; Driver et al., 1997; Mattingley et al., 1997; see Driver and Baylis, 1998, for review). At least one neuroimaging study has found that a subset of the brain regions activated when subjects are attending to objects dissociate from the areas activated during a space-based selection task (Fink et al., 1997; see Weber et al., 1997 and Valdes-Sosa et al., 1998, for related ERP evidence). The present work aims to further our understanding of object-based attention by examining its relationship to other object processing operations.

A closer look at Duncan's seminal study (1984) offers an instructive introduction to the current research. In his study, subjects viewed stimuli that consisted of two superimposed objects: an outline box and a line struck through it. The box was either short or tall and had either a left or right-sided gap. The line was tilted clockwise or counter-clockwise and was either dotted or dashed. The subjects' task was to report either a single attribute or two attributes on every trial. When reporting two attributes, they either reported them from the same object or from different objects. Subjects were more accurate at reporting two attributes from the same object than they were at reporting two attributes from two different objects, even though the two objects were superimposed. This pattern is not readily explained by the idea that attention is allocated to spatial locations. As an alternative, Duncan proposed that attention can operate on representations of objects, one at a time. Moreover, when an object is attended, all of its attributes are selected and are therefore more accessible than attributes from unattended objects.

Although Duncan's study has been criticized on a number of grounds (e.g. Watt, 1988; Kramer and Jacobson, 1991), the basic results have been replicated in a variety of studies from different laboratories. Since that time, the evidence that selection can operate on representations of objects has come largely from studies demonstrating performance advantages for single objects compared to multiple objects that cannot be accounted for by any existing model of space-based attentional allocation (e.g. Baylis and Driver, 1993; Vecera and Farah, 1994). The prevailing logic, in other words, has been as follows: when an appeal to the spatial properties of a visual display cannot explain experimental results, object-based mechanisms are inferred. We sought to obtain positive evidence that putative object-based effects arise from mechanisms responsible for processing objects per se. Our strategy was to demonstrate that the mechanisms underlying object-based attentional selection are also necessary for other tasks that explicitly involve objects, such as retaining objects in working memory. If attending to objects and remembering objects require some of the same operations and/or representations, then the two types of tasks should interfere with one another when they are performed concurrently. On the other hand, memory tasks that do not involve objects should not interfere with object-based visual selection. Evidence for *selective* interference would suggest that components of the attentional system are domain-specific and that object-based attentional effects arise from mechanisms that also contribute to the retention of objects in working memory.

Overlap of object attention and object working memory

There is a history in the cognitive neuroscience literature of using patterns of selective interference in dual-task paradigms to probe the neurocognitive architecture. This method was used extensively by Kinsbourne and his associates (e.g. Kinsbourne and Hicks, 1978; see also Wickens, 1980) to map the hemispheric organization of mental processes. The logic of the selective interference approach is that the greater the interference produced when two tasks are performed concurrently, the greater the functional and structural overlap of their underlying mechanisms. A recent neuroimaging study supports this logic. Using PET, Klingberg and Roland (1997) showed that interference between various working memory and go/no-go tasks is related to the degree of overlap of cortical areas activated by the tasks.

The selective interference method has also played a central role in identifying the verbal and spatial subcomponents of the working memory system (Brooks, 1967; Logie et al., 1990). Numerous studies have shown, for example, that performing a linguistic task during the retention interval of a working memory task produces a greater performance decrement when the to-be-remembered items are verbal (i.e. words or letters) than when the to-be-remembered items are spatial (i.e. locations in a matrix). Likewise, performing a visual–spatial task (i.e. judging the similarity of dot patterns) selectively interferes with location memory while leaving verbal working memory relatively unaffected. These behavioral results have been interpreted to indicate that separable mechanisms mediate verbal and spatial working memory (e.g. Baddeley, 1992; Jonides et al., 1996). Along with neuropsychological evidence from studies of brain-damaged patients, functional imaging evidence has provided converging support for this conclusion. Verbal working memory is associated with a predominantly left hemisphere circuit that includes parietal loci (Brodmann's areas 40 and 7), and frontal sites in SMA, Broca's area and dorsolateral prefrontal cortex; spatial working memory activates many of these same sites, but with a right hemisphere predominance (Smith and Jonides, 1997, 1999; Reuter-Lorenz et al., 2000, for a review see Cabeza and Nyberg, 2000).

Further neuroimaging work has indicated that object working memory may be at least partially dissociable from both verbal and spatial working memory. Like verbal working memory, object working memory has been found to activate left hemisphere parietal loci more than a comparable spatial working memory task (Smith et al., 1995). However, in addition to several sites in lateral prefrontal cortex that may be unique to object working memory (see Haxby et al., 2000, for evidence from facial stimuli and Wilson et al., 1993, for evidence from monkeys) activation of temporal area 37 has been found consistently (Smith et al., 1995; Elliot and Dolan, 1998; see Cabeza and Nyberg, 2000 for a review). In many cases, this activation is bilateral although left-sided predominance has also been reported (Smith et al., 1995).

There are indications from primate and human studies that object-based selection may utilize some of the same brain mechanisms implicated in object working memory. For example, single-unit recordings from area IT in monkeys has revealed that neurons tuned to particular objects show memory-related activity and participate in the attentional selection of task-relevant target objects (Chelazzi et al., 1993, 1998). Chelazzi and colleagues suggest that visual descriptions or representations held in working memory aid selection by biasing incoming visual signals. Whereas the neural evidence from human studies is less precise, structural overlap of object working memory areas and object-based attentional processes can be identified through neuroimaging and lesion studies. Inferior temporal regions in Brodmann's area 37 along with portions of occipital area 19 are consistently implicated when human subjects perform tasks requiring discriminations based on shape and form (see Cabeza and Nyberg, 2000 for a review). In many cases, these activations are bilateral. However, in contrast to faces which yield more right hemisphere activation, visual objects are associated with a predominance of left temporo-occipital activation at least in some perceptual tasks (Haxby et al., 1991; Sergent et al., 1992; Schacter et al., 1995) as well as when attention to objects is explicitly required (Fink et al., 1997). Moreover, damage to the inferotemporal cortices can lead to deficits in visual form and object recognition (i.e. visual agnosia, see Farah, 1990). Apperceptive agnosia, a form of visual agnosia associated with diffuse ventral stream damage, can impair the single object advantage thought to be indicative of object-based attentional selection (Vecera and Behrmann, 1997).

In addition to requiring common regions within the ventral stream, left parietal loci are also implicated in object-based attention and memory. As noted above, activation of parietal areas is commonly found in object working memory tasks with some indications of a left-sided predominance (Haxby et al., 1995; Elliot and Dolan, 1998). Greater left than right parietal activation has also been found for object-based attention using PET (Fink et al., 1997). Neuropsychological evidence from patients with lateralized parietal damage indicates that the single-object attentional advantage is disrupted more by left than by right sided lesions (Egly et al., 1994a). A special role for the left hemisphere is also implicated by the results from an investigation of a split-brain patient who showed object-based selection in the right but not in the left visual field (Egly et al., 1994b). Together these findings suggest that object-based attention and object working memory share a circuitry that includes parietal and temporal loci with a possible left hemisphere predominance.

From a cognitive perspective, one motivation for suspecting overlap between object-based attention and working memory for objects is that such overlap is evident in the spatial domain. There is mounting evidence to indicate that spatial attention is the mechanism that maintains or rehearses location information in spatial working memory (Jones and Macken, 1993; Awh and Jonides, 1998; Awh et al., 1998). In fact, recent evidence suggests that when subjects hold a spatial location in memory, they are better able to perceive stimuli at that location, as if the attentional spotlight is focused there during the retention interval (Awh et al., 1998). It seems reasonable to hypothesize that attending and remembering objects may also rely on shared mechanisms. Given that object working memory is at least partially dissociable from spatial working memory, it is feasible that their rehearsal mechanisms may be domain specific. Object working memory may recruit attentional processes that are specialized for objects. The data we report support this idea.

New evidence for shared mechanisms

Here we report what we believe to be the first evidence for functional overlap between object working memory and object-based attention in humans. Using a dual-task approach, we aimed to disrupt object-based selection by having subjects simultaneously perform another task that might rely on some of the same cognitive operations. Recall that the single-object advantage is the benefit accrued when discriminating two attributes on the same object compared to when those same attributes reside on different objects. We find that this advantage is selectively diminished when subjects perform a concurrent object working memory task. In contrast, concurrent verbal or spatial working memory tasks have no effect on the single object advantage. These results indicate that the cognitive mechanisms that select perceptual objects are also involved with maintaining object representations in memory.

The experiment had three conditions. All conditions included a task intended to measure object-based attention effects. In this 'vertex task' (adapted from Baylis and Driver, 1993), subjects judge the relative height of two vertices that reside on the same object or on two different objects. The spatial distance between the vertices is equivalent in these two conditions. The subjects' task was to report whether the left or right vertex is lower. The stimuli are pictured in Fig. 1A and B. The two vertices reside on separate objects in Fig. 1A and on a single object in Fig. 1B even though these attributes are equidistant and have identical positions in space in both cases. The single object condition typically yields a reaction time advantage of approximately 30 ms relative to the dual-object condition (Baylis and Driver, 1993; Gibson, 1994). Baylis and Driver conducted further studies that ruled out such factors as spatial frequency, contour differences, and convexity as explanations for the single object advantage (Baylis and Driver, 1993; Baylis, 1994).

In all conditions subjects also performed a working memory task, but the contents of working memory changed across conditions; subjects retained either verbal items (letters), spatial locations (indicated by dots), or objects (shapes drawn from Attneave and Arnoult, 1956). See Fig. 1C–E for details on the working memory tasks.

Different groups of subjects participated in each of the three working memory conditions. For each condition, the vertex task and the working memory task were performed in two different modes. In the *pure-task* mode, subjects performed alternating blocks of the vertex task and the designated memory task. In the *dual-task* mode, the vertex task was performed during the delay period of the working memory task. Thus in the pure-task mode, subjects alternated between the vertex and the memory tasks, but always completed one task before starting the other. In the dual-task mode, subjects performed the vertex task while they held items in working memory. By comparing performance in the pure- and dual-task modes we can determine whether the two tasks interfere with each other and whether the pattern of interference depends on the type of working memory that is engaged. See Fig. 2 for details on the task conditions.

If the single object advantage requires selection mechanisms that are particular to objects, then it should be possible to reduce this advantage in a dual-task paradigm when the secondary working memory task also involves objects. Interference that is specific to object working memory would implicate shared object processing mechanisms. At the other extreme, if all three types of working memory reduce the single object advantage a more general mechanism would be implicated and no inference could be drawn about object-specific processes.

Response times and errors for each condition are presented in Table 1. The crucial results, however, are summarized in Fig. 3. This figure plots the difference between response latencies for the single-object and the two-objects displays (i.e. the single object advantage) for the pure and dual-task modes for each of the working memory conditions. In all conditions, subjects are faster when responding to a single object than to two objects, replicating the primary result of Baylis and Driver (1993). Importantly, however, this single object advantage is reduced in the dual-task condition when subjects are performing the vertex task while simultaneously holding abstract shapes in memory. There is no significant reduction, however, for either the verbal or the spatial working memory conditions. There were no significant differences in working memory performance between pure and

TABLE 1

Summary of reaction time data for vertex task

Working memory condition	Task condition	Vertex condition	Mean RT	SD	SEM
Object	Pure	1-object	276.6	43.5	10.0
		2-object	327.7	43.0	9.9
	Dual	1-object	311.0	59.8	13.7
		2-object	343.0	51.4	11.8
Verbal	Pure	1-object	274.6	51.0	11.4
		2-object	322.7	52.0	11.6
	Dual	1-object	300.3	75.2	16.8
		2-object	349.1	77.1	17.2
Spatial	Pure	1-object	297.5	73.3	18.3
		2-object	339.4	80.0	20.0
	Dual	1-object	306.7	75.7	18.9
		2-object	345.4	74.8	18.7

All errors were excluded from the analysis of the latency data. Reaction times less than 100 ms and more than two standard deviations from the mean for each subject were excluded resulting in the elimination of 2.8% of the data, 2.2% of data, and 1.7% of data for the object, verbal and spatial working memory conditions, respectively. Performance on the working memory task did not vary by task condition for object working memory (84%, SD = 9.6 in the pure-task condition and 81%, SD = 6.4 in the dual-task condition), verbal working memory (80%, SD = 9.7 pure-task condition, 81%, SD = 7.7 dual-task condition), or spatial working memory (76%, SD = 7.5 pure-task condition and 74%, SD = 7.2 dual-task condition).

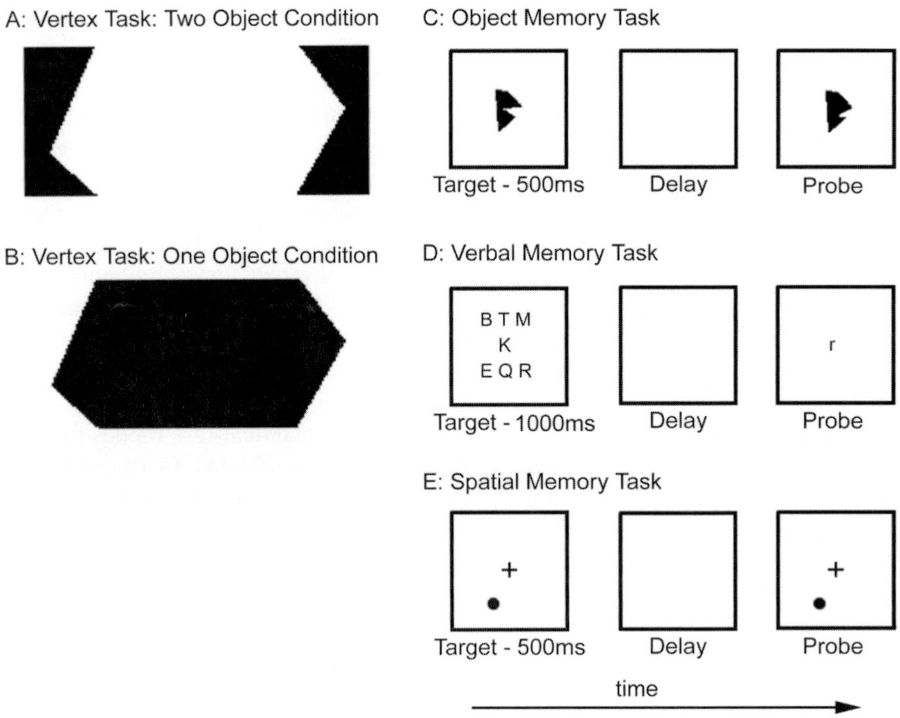

Fig. 1. Illustrations of the component tasks. (A,B) The stimuli for the vertex task, after Baylis and Driver (1993). All subjects performed this task. It began with a fixation cross for 500 ms, followed by the stimulus display for 150 ms. The stimulus display was either a hexagon (one-object) or two pentagons (two-objects). Subjects judged which vertex was lower on the screen, indicating 'left' or 'right' by a button response; a 700-ms inter-trial interval followed the response. Speed and accuracy were equally stressed. The hexagon subtended a maximum of 4.4° horizontally and 2.6° in height. The pentagons, which were formed around the outer contours of imaginary hexagons, subtended 6.0° horizontally and 2.6° vertically. The vertical offset of the vertices was always 0.8°. The fixation point could appear centered at any point within a 0.5 × 0.5° area in the center of the screen. The vertical position of the center point of the stimulus displays varied by 0.8° around the center of the screen, independent of fixation. Finally, the vertical position of the two vertices in each display varied by as much as 1.6° above and below the center of the screen independent of the variations in object location and the fixation point. Feedback was given for incorrect responses only, in the form of a loud beep. The presentation of the two types of vertex stimulus displays and their positions on the screen were randomized. (C) An example trial of the object memory task. Nineteen subjects received this task as the working memory component task. The target stimuli were 6-sided shapes from Attneave and Arnoult (1956), and were presented for 500 ms. The probe memory item was the same shape as the target item 50% of the time and a similar foil the rest of the time. The Attneave figures were presented from a preconstructed list in which no 'target' figure appeared more than once per block of trials. The experimenter recorded the subjects' verbal responses ("yes" if target and probe matched, "no" otherwise) for the memory items. (D) An example trial of the verbal memory task. Twenty subjects received this task as the working memory component task. On each trial, seven uppercase letters were presented for 1000 ms. They were arranged within an imaginary box (5.7 × 5.7°) with three letters arrayed across the top edge of the box, three across the bottom, and one letter in the center (never forming a pronounceable word). The letters (consisting of vowels and consonants) were presented in a 48-point, New York style font. A single lower-case probe letter was presented at the center of the imaginary box. The letters were selected from a set of 15 letters in which the lower case letter looked physically different from the uppercase letter (e.g., Aa; Bb; Dd, etc.). On half of the trials, the probe item had been included in the set of seven letters, and the rest of the time it had not. (E) An example trial of the spatial memory task. Sixteen subjects received this task as the working memory component task. The stimulus consisted of a single black dot with a diameter of 0.5 cm. The dot was presented on the circumference of an imaginary elliptical shape (diameter 8.8° horizontally and 5° vertically) along with a fixation cross at the center of the screen for 500 ms. After the memory delay, another black dot appeared on the circumference of the imaginary ellipse along with the central fixation cross, and subjects reported verbally whether the probe location matched the one held in memory. Half of the locations matched and the remaining half were either 1° or 2° from the memorized location. The two types of mismatches were randomized, but occurred equally often within a block of trials.

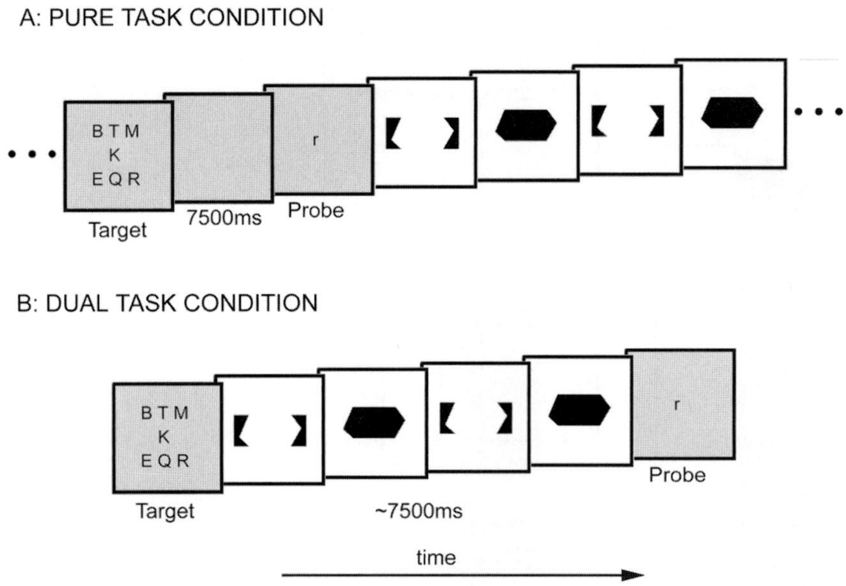

Fig. 2. Task conditions. (A) In the pure task condition, subjects alternated between the vertex task and working memory task (i.e. performed them sequentially), performing three trials of the working memory task followed by 12 consecutive trials of the vertex task (only one working memory trial and four vertex task trials are represented in the figure). During the retention interval of the memory task, the screen was blank for 7.5 s. (B) In the dual-task condition, the vertex task is performed while subjects are holding information in working memory. Subjects viewed the memory target stimulus, then performed four consecutive trials of the vertex task, which lasted approximately 7.5 s. Subjects were then presented with the memory probe stimulus. Subjects were told to treat each task with equal importance. Each subject performed the eight blocks of trials (4 dual, 4 pure) in a counterbalanced ABBA order. Half the subjects began with the dual-task and half began with the pure block. The dual-task condition consisted of 17 trials per block which provided 68 observations for the vertex task (34 observations each for the one- and two-objects displays) and 17 observations for the memory task. In the pure condition, there were four trials per block (i.e. 12 consecutive trials of the vertex task followed by three memory trials) which allowed for 48 observations for the vertex task (24 observations each for the one- and two-objects displays) and 12 observations for the memory task. Each experimental condition was practiced prior to data collection. The experiment lasted approximately 1 h.

dual task modes for any of the working memory conditions [1].

Interference with the single object advantage could conceivably result from competition for general attentional resources produced by the dual task demands. However, this possibility is unlikely be-

[1] Pilot testing revealed that subjects were significantly more accurate on the spatial memory task in the pure condition compared to the dual-task condition. One reason for this difference may have been the requirement to reorient to the center of the screen to perform the vertex task after encoding the peripheral memory location. This reorienting may have disrupted the ability to retain the location in working memory, leading to decreased accuracy. Awh et al. (1998) demonstrated that accuracy on a spatial working memory task was impaired when subjects performed a secondary task during the retention interval that required shifts of attention to non-memorized locations. In contrast, performance was not affected when the intervening task completely enclosed the memorized locations, thereby minimizing the need to shift attention. They concluded from these results that spatial attention serves a rehearsal function that maintains locations in spatial working memory. In an effort to equate memory performance in the pure and dual-task conditions of the present study our instructions emphasized accuracy on the memory task in the dual-task condition. We also enlarged the stimuli for the vertex task so that they completely overlapped the memory locations. This change reduced the need to reorient attention to the center of the screen to perform the vertex task. The vertex stimuli were enlarged such that the hexagon subtended a maximum of 8.85° horizontally and 5.26° vertically. The pentagons subtended 11.08° horizontally and 5.26° vertically.

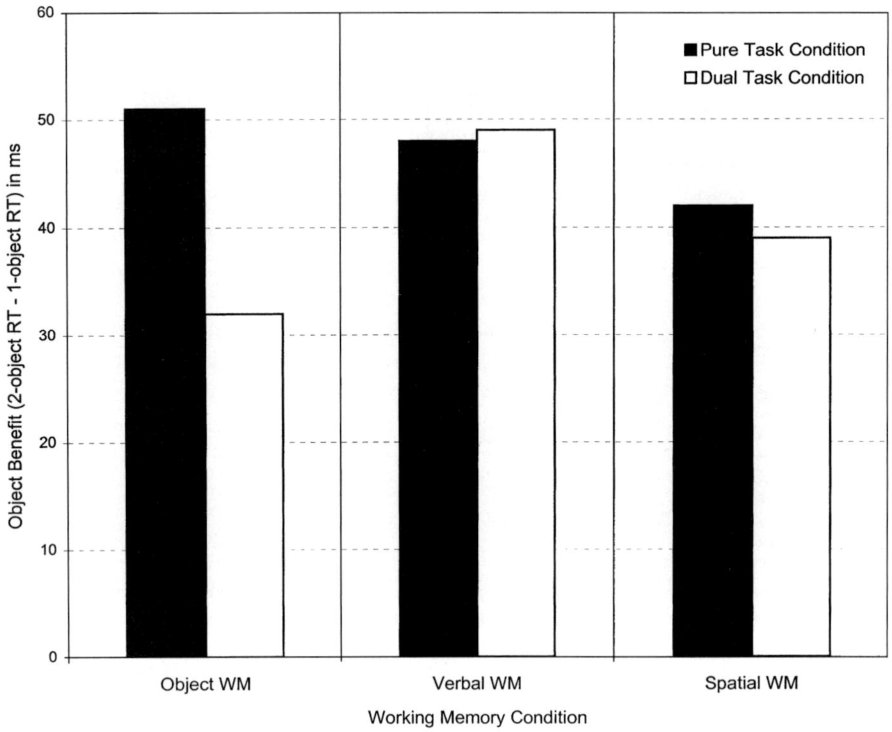

Fig. 3. The single object advantage expressed as the difference between response times for the two object and the single object condition. This advantage is selectively reduced by a concurrent object working memory task ($F(1, 18) = 16.46$, $P < 0.001$), but not by a concurrent verbal or spatial working memory task.

cause neither verbal nor spatial working memory reduced the single object advantage. The selective interference with the single object advantage that is evident in the object working memory condition is consistent with the proposal that object-based selection requires some of the same operations needed to retain objects in working memory.

It is also possible that the single object advantage relies not on *object* specific processes, but rather on more general *visuospatial* processes. The spatial memory condition addresses this possibility; again, no reduction of the object benefit was found. Based on this result, we conclude that the disruption of the single object advantage in the dual-task object-memory condition indicates their mutual engagement of domain-specific (object) processes. More specifically we suggest that attentional mechanisms that are engaged when selecting perceptual objects from the visual array are the same as those required to hold objects on line in working memory.

Before discussing what those mechanisms might be, let us consider how the attention tasks are performed with and without an object working memory load. Baylis and Driver (1993) propose that in their task, the single object discriminations are based on object-centered representations. The two-object vertex judgments are determined indirectly in that they require that the parts of objects be represented in scene-based coordinates. This indirect determination takes longer and is more prone to errors, thus leading to the single object advantage. We interpret the diminution of the single-object advantage in the dual-task/object working memory condition to mean that holding objects in working memory disrupts the ability to use perceptual objects as the basis for visual selection. Consequently, the vertex discriminations in the single and dual object displays are likely to rely on the same indirect representational processes. The present experiments do not indicate what these alternative representational processes might be, although it seems reasonable to assume that spatial representations are critical. The work of Humphreys (e.g. Humphreys, 1998) suggests that the single-object task relies on object representations mediated by the ventral stream whereas the two-object task requires between-object codes that relies to a greater extent on dorsal stream (parietal) representations. More research is needed to clarify the role of spatial attention in selecting locations within and between objects.

Activation versus representation

What mechanisms are the source of interference between object-based selection and object working memory? Two possibilities suggest themselves. One is an 'activational' process that serves to maintain representations in an activated state during the retention interval of a working memory task. This activational or rehearsal-like process, according to some models of working memory (e.g. Smyth and Scholey, 1994; Awh and Jonides, 1998) is selective attention. In a perceptual task that does not have a memory component, this same activational process selects representations in accord with the task demands. This selective process could plausibly be mediated by left parietal regions which are recruited during object working memory tasks (Smith et al., 1995) and implicated in object-based attention as well (e.g. Egly et al., 1994a; Fink et al., 1997).

The second mechanism that could be shared by object-based attention and object working memory is one that mediates the object representations themselves. Such representational processes are likely to involve regions of the inferior temporal lobe, including area 37. It is conceivable that retaining an object in working memory recruits activational processes mediated by parietal areas which interact with task-relevant object representations in the ventral visual stream. Likewise, object-based attentional selection may require similar parietal mechanisms to activate (e.g. competitively bias) object representations in the ventral pathway. While the present data do not permit us to identify the specific source of interference between object-based attention and object working memory, it is likely that both representational and activational processes may play a role.

Conclusion

Our results support the existence of object-based attention processes that are separable from space-based attention and demonstrate a functional link between attending to perceptual objects and holding objects in working memory. As such, they provide converging evidence for interactions between mechanisms for remembering objects (e.g. Chelazzi et al., 1998) and attending to objects, and extend the growing literature indicating that selective attention is closely linked to rehearsal in working memory (e.g. Awh and Jonides, 1998). We demonstrate that the rehearsal mechanisms required by object working memory differ from those engaged by verbal or spatial working memory because only the former interfered with object-based selection. Our data therefore provide evidence for domain specificity within the high level visual processes of attending to and remembering objects.

References

Attneave, R. and Arnoult, M.D. (1956) Methodological considerations in the quantitative study of shape and pattern in perception. *Psychol. Bull.*, 53: 452–471.

Awh, E. and Jonides, J. (1998) Spatial selective attention and spatial working memory. In: R. Parasuraman (Ed.), *The Attentive Brain*. MIT Press, Cambridge, MA, pp. 353–380.

Awh, E., Jonides, J. and Reuter-Lorenz, P.A. (1998) Rehearsal in spatial working memory. *J. Exp. Psychol. Hum. Percept. Perform.*, 24: 780–790.

Baddeley, A.D. (1992) Working memory: the interface between memory and cognition. *J. Cogn. Neurosci.*, 4: 281–288.

Baylis, G.C. (1994) Visual attention and objects: two-object cost with equal convexity. *J. Exp. Psychol. Hum. Percept. Perform.*, 20: 208–212.

Baylis, G.C. and Driver, J. (1992) Visual parsing and response competition: the effect of grouping factors. *Percept. Psychophys.*, 51: 145–162.

Baylis, G.C. and Driver, J. (1993) Visual attention and objects: evidence for hierarchical coding of location. *J. Exp. Psychol. Hum. Percept. Perform.*, 19: 451–470.

Behrmann, M. and Haimson, C. (1999) The cognitive neuroscience of visual attention. *Curr. Opin. Neurobiol.*, 9: 158–163.

Behrmann, M. and Tipper, S.P. (1999) Attention accesses multiple reference frames: evidence from visual neglect. *J. Exp. Psychol. Hum. Percept. Perform.*, 25: 83–101.

Behrmann, M., Moscovitch, M., Black, S.E. and Mozer, M. (1990) Perceptual and conceptual mechanisms in neglect. *Brain*, 113: 1163–1183.

Brooks, L.R. (1967) Visual and verbal components of thought. *Psychon. Bull.*, 1: 20–21.

Cabeza, R. and Nyberg, L. (2000) Imaging cognition II: an empirical review of 275 PET and fMRI studies. *J. Cogn. Neurosci.*, 12: 1–47.

Chelazzi, L., Miller, E.K., Duncan, J. and Desimone, R. (1993) A neural basis for visual search in inferior temporal cortex. *Nature*, 363: 345–347.

Chelazzi, L., Duncan, J., Miller, E.K. and Desimone, R. (1998) Responses of neurons in inferior temporal cortex during memory-guided visual search. *J. Neurophysiol.*, 80: 2918–2940.

Colby, C.L. and Goldberg, M.E. (1999) Space and attention in parietal cortex. *Annu. Rev. Neurosci.*, 22: 319-349.

Davis, G., Driver, J., Pavani, F. and Shepherd, A. (2000) Reappraising the apparent costs of attending to two separate visual objects. *Vision Res.*, 40: 1323–1332.

Driver, J. and Baylis, G.C. (1989) Movement and visual attention: the spotlight metaphor breaks down. *J. Exp. Psychol. Hum. Percept. Perform.*, 15: 448–456.

Driver, J. and Baylis, G.C. (1998) Attention and visual object segmentation. In: R. Parasuraman (Ed.), *The Attentive Brain*. MIT Press, Cambridge, MA, pp. 299–325.

Driver, J., Mattingley, J.B., Rorden, C. and Davis, G. (1997) Extinction as a paradigm measure of attentional bias and restricted capacity following brain injury. In: R. Thier and H.-O. Karanth (Eds.), *Parietal Lobe Contributions to Orientation in 3D Space*. Springer-Verlag, Berlin, pp. 401–429.

Duncan, J. (1984) Selective attention and the organization of visual information. *J. Exp. Psychol. Gen.*, 113: 501–517.

Egly, R., Driver, J. and Rafal, R.D. (1994a) Shifting visual attention between objects and locations: evidence from normal and parietal lesion subjects. *J. Exp. Psychol. Gen.*, 123: 161–177.

Egly, R., Rafal, R., Driver, J. and Starrveveld, Y. (1994b) Covert orienting in the split brain reveals hemispheric specialization for object-based attention. *Psychol. Sci.*, 5: 380–383.

Elliot, R. and Dolan, R.J. (1998) The neural response in short-term visual recognition memory for perceptual conjunctions. *NeuroImage*, 7: 14–22.

Eriksen, C.W. and St James, J.D. (1986) Visual attention within and around the field of focal attention: a zoom lens model. *Percept. Psychophys.*, 40: 225–240.

Farah, M. (1990) *Visual Agnosia: Disorders of Object Recognition and What They Tell Us about Normal Vision*. MIT Press, Cambridge, MA.

Farah, M., Wallace, M. and Vecera, S. (1993) 'What' and 'where' in visual attention. In: I.H. Robertson and J.C. Marshall (Eds.), *Unilateral Neglect*. Erlbaum, Hillsdale, NJ, pp. 123–137.

Fink, G.R., Dolan, R.J., Halligan, P.W., Marshall, J.C. and Frith, C.D. (1997) Space-based and object-based visual attention: shared and specific neural domains. *Brain*, 120: 2013–2028.

Gibson, B.S. (1994) Visual attention and objects: one versus two or convex versus concave? *J. Exp. Psychol. Hum. Percept. Perform.*, 20: 203–207.

Haxby, J.V., Grady, C.L., Horowitz, B., Ungerleider, L.G., Mishkin, M., Carson, R.E., Herscovitch, P., Shapiro, M.B. and Rapoport, S.I. (1991) Dissociation of object and spatial visual processing pathways in human extrastriate cortex. *Proc. Natl. Acad. Sci. USA*, 88: 1621–1625.

Haxby, J.V., Ungerleider, L.G., Horwitz, B., Rapoport, S.I. and Grady, C.L. (1995) Hemispheric differences in neural systems for face working memory: A PET-rCBF study. *Hum. Brain Mapp.*, 3: 68–82.

Haxby, J., Petit, L., Ungerleider, L.G. and Courtney, S. (2000) Distinguishing the functional roles of multiple regions in distributed neural systems for visual working memory. *NeuroImage*, 11: 380–391.

Humphreys, G.W. (1998) Neural representation of objects in space: a dual-coding account. *Philos. Trans. R. Soc.*, 353: 1341–1351.

Jones, D.M. and Macken, W.J. (1993) Irrelevant tones produce an irrelevant speech effect: implications for phonological coding in working memory. *J. Exp. Psychol. Learn. Mem. Cogn.*, 19: 369–381.

Jonides, J., Reuter-Lorenz, P.A., Smith, E., Awh, E., Barnes, L.L., Drain, M., Glass, J., Lauber, E.J., Patalano, A.L. and Schumacher, E.H. (1996) Verbal and spatial working memory in humans. *Psychol. Learn. Motiv.*, 35: 43–88.

Kinsbourne, M. and Hicks, R.E. (1978) Functional cerebral space: a model for overflow, transfer and interface effects in human performance: a tutorial review. In: J. Requin (Ed.), *Attention and Performance VII*. Erlbaum, Hillsdale, NJ, pp. 345–362.

Klingberg, T. and Roland, P.E. (1997) Interference between two concurrent tasks is associated with activation of overlapping fields in the cortex. *Cogn. Brain Res.*, 6: 1–8.

Kramer, A.F. and Jacobson, A. (1991) Perceptual organization and focused attention: the role of objects and proximity in visual processing. *Percept. Psychophys.*, 50: 267–284.

Kramer, A. and Watson, S.E. (1996) Object-based visual selection and the principle of uniform connectedness. In: A.F. Kramer, M.G.H. Coles and G.D. Logan (Eds.), *Converging Operations in the Study of Visual Selective Attention*. American Psychological Association, Washington, DC, pp. 395–414.

Logie, R.H., Zuco, G.M. and Baddeley, A.D. (1990) Interference with visual short-term memory. *Acta Psychol.*, 75: 55–74.

Mattingley, J.B., Davis, G. and Driver, J. (1997) Preattentive filling-in of visual surfaces in parietal extinction. *Science*, 229: 782–784.

O'Craven, K.M., Downing, P.E. and Kanwisher, N. (1999) fMRI evidence for objects as the units of attentional selection. *Nature*, 401: 584–587.

Olson, C.R. and Gettner, S.N. (1996) Representation of object-centered space in the primate frontal lobe. *Cogn. Brain Res.*, 5: 147–156.

Posner, M.I., Snyder, C.R. and Davidson, B.J. (1980) Attention and the detection of signals. *J. Exp. Psychol. Gen.*, 109: 160–174.

Reuter-Lorenz, P.A., Jonides, J., Smith, E.E., Hartley, A., Miller, A., Marshuetz, C. and Koeppe, R.A. (2000) Age differences in the frontal lateralization of verbal and spatial working memory revealed by PET. *J. Cogn. Neurosci.*, 12: 174–187.

Roelfsma, P.R., Lamme, V.A.F. and Spekreijse, H. (1998) Object-based attention in the primary visual cortex of the macaque monkey. *Nature*, 395: 376–381.

Schacter, D.L., Reiman, E., Uecker, A., Polster, M.R., Yun, L.S. and Cooper, L.A. (1995) Brain regions associated with retrieval of structurally coherent visual information. *Nature*, 376: 587–590.

Sergent, J., Ohta, S. and MacDonald, B. (1992) Functional neuroanatomy of face and object processing: a positron emission tomography study. *Brain*, 115: 15–36.

Smith, E.E. and Jonides, J. (1997) Working memory: a view from neuroimaging. *Cogn. Psychol.*, 33: 5–42.

Smith, E.E. and Jonides, J. (1999) Storage and executive processes in the frontal lobes. *Science*, 283: 1657–1660.

Smith, E.E., Jonides, J., Koeppe, R.A., Awh, E., Schumacher, E.H. and Minoshima, S. (1995) Spatial versus object working memory: PET investigations. *J. Cogn. Neurosci.*, 7: 337–356.

Smyth, M.M. and Scholey, K.A. (1994) Interference in immediate spatial memory. *Mem. Cogn.*, 22: 1–13.

Snyder, L.H., Grieve, K.L., Brotchie, P. and Andersen, R.A. (1998) Separate body- and world-referenced representations of visual space in parietal cortex. *Nature*, 394: 887–891.

Valdes-Sosa, M., Bobes, M.A., Rodriquez, V. and Pinilla, T. (1998) Switching attention without shifting the spotlight: Object-based attentional modulation of brain potentials. *J. Cogn. Neurosci.*, 10: 137–151.

Vecera, S.P. and Behrmann, M. (1997) Spatial attention does not require preattentive grouping. *Neuropsychology*, 11: 30–43.

Vecera, S.P. and Farah, M.J. (1994) Does visual attention select objects or locations? *J. Exp. Psychol. Gen.*, 123: 146–160.

Ward, R., Goodrich, S. and Driver, J. (1994) Grouping reduces visual extinction. *Vis. Cogn.*, 1: 101–129.

Watt, R.J. (1988) *Visual Processing: Computational, Psychophysical and Cognitive Research*. Erlbaum, Hillsdale, NJ.

Weber, T.A., Kramer, A.F. and Miller, G.A. (1997) Selective processing of superimposed objects: an electrophysiological analysis of object-based attentional selection. *Biol. Psychol.*, 45: 159–182.

Wickens, C.D. (1980) The structure of attentional resources. In: R. Nickerson (Ed.), *Attention and Performance VIII*. Erlbaum, Hillsdale, NJ.

Wilson, F.A.W., O'Scalaidhe, S.P. and Goldman-Rakic, P.S. (1993) Dissociation of object and spatial processing domains in primate prefrontal cortex. *Science*, 260: 1955–1957.

Wurtz, R.H., Goldberg, M.E. and Robinson, D.L. (1982) Brain mechanisms of visual attention. *Sci. Am.*, 246(June): 124–135.

Yantis, S. (1992) Multielement visual tracking: attention and perceptual organization. *Cogn. Psychol.*, 24: 295–340.

Subject Index